Occupational Therapy and Physical Dysfunction

Dedication

This edition is dedicated to our families and friends, and to all 76 of our contributors, past and present, who have been brave enough to put pen to paper.

Annie, Marg and Sybil would particularly like to thank Mary Law, our editor, who has stood by us and encouraged us throughout our ups and downs of the last 24 years.

For Churchill Livingstone

Editorial Director: Mary Law
Project Manager: Jane Dingwall
Design Direction: George Ajayi/Judith Wright

Occupational Therapy and Physical Dysfunction

Principles, Skills and Practice

Edited by

Annie Turner TDipCOT SROT MA FCOT
Head of Division of Occupational Therapy, Centre for Health Care Education, University College Northampton

Marg Foster TDipCOT SROT CertEd MMedSci
Senior Lecturer, School of Health and Community Studies, University of Derby

Sybil E Johnson DipCOT SROT DMS
Team Manager, Disability Services, Dorset Social Services, Ferndown Local Office, Dorset

Foreword by

Sheelagh E Richards DipCOT SROT FCOT
Secretary and Chief Executive, The British Association & College of Occupational Therapists, London

FIFTH EDITION

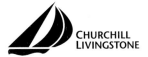
CHURCHILL
LIVINGSTONE

EDINBURGH LONDON NEW YORK OXFORD PHILADELPHIA ST LOUIS SYDNEY TORONTO 2002

CHURCHILL LIVINGSTONE
An imprint of Elsevier Limited

First edition 1981
Second edition 1987
Third edition 1992
Fourth edition 1996
Fifth edition 2002
Reprinted 2003 (twice)

ISBN 0 443 06224 2

British Library Cataloguing in Publication Data
A catalogue record for this book is available from the British Library

Library of Congress Cataloging in Publication Data
A catalog record for this book is available from the Library of Congress

Note
Medical knowledge is constantly changing. As new information
becomes available, changes in treatment, procedures, equipment and
the use of drugs become necessary. The editions, contributors and the
publishers have, as far as it is possible, taken care to ensure that the
information given in this text is accurate and up to date. However,
readers are strongly advised to confirm that the information,
especially with regard to drug usage, complies with the latest
legislation and standards of practice.

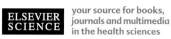

ELSEVIER SCIENCE your source for books, journals and multimedia in the health sciences

www.elsevierhealth.com

The
publisher's
policy is to use
paper manufactured
from sustainable forests

Printed in China
P/03

Contents

Contributors

Theresa Baxter DipCOT SROT IHSM MEd
Senior Lecturer, School of Health and
Community Studies, University of Derby

Qualified from Derby in 1980. Following practice
in a number of areas of physical dysfunction in
London, and a period as deputy occupational
therapy manager at Queens Medical Centre
Nottingham, Theresa moved into education.
Particular areas of interest include work rehabilitation, hand therapy and orthotics, the therapeutic value of activity, fieldwork education and
management.

Chapter 17 Upper limb trauma

Alison Beattie DipCOT SROT
Consultant Occupational Therapist, Glasgow

Alison Beattie has had wide-ranging experience,
mainly in hospitals in the Glasgow area, where
she has held posts up to Head of Department
level. She has worked for the Glasgow branch of
the Parkinson's Disease Society since 1978 and
has undertaken several research projects including one on Parkinson's Disease. She advises the
national office of the Parkinson's Disease Society
and chaired their occupational therapy working
party.

Chapter 26 Parkinson's disease

Gillian Brown DipCOT SROT MSc
Head Occupational Therapist (Paediatrics),
Barking, Havering and Redbridge
NHS Trust

Having qualified in 1977 from the London School
of Occupational Therapy Gillian Brown has
worked in paediatrics since 1978 in the hospital
setting, within the voluntary sector and also within
community paediatrics. In 1996 she completed an
MSc in Paediatric Occupational Therapy and now
combines the clinical lead role within Redbridge
with a module leader role at the University of East
London. Gillian is currently a National Executive
Committee Member for the National Association
of Paediatric Occupational Therapists.

Chapter 11 Cerebral palsy
Chapter 12 Muscular dystrophy

Carol Collins DipCOT SROT DCR
Independent occupational therapist and brain
injury case manager
Based in Bury, Lancashire

Carol Collins has a background in radiography,
creative arts and therapeutic horse riding and on
qualifying as an occupational therapist in 1992
began work with people with acquired brain
injury as a member of Highbank Health Care Ltd.
She designed rehabilitation programmes for
clients both within the unit and in the community.
In 1993 she began to provide Brain Injury Case
Management Services and is an associate member
of the British Association of Brain Injury Case

Managers. She was also involved in the setting up and commissioning of new services, including a Transitional Care Unit and a Transitional Living Unit for people with acquired brain injury. She is listed on the UK Register of Expert Witnesses and began operating as an independent occupational therapist and brain injury case manager in 1997.

Chapter 15 Acquired brain injury

Jill Cooper DipCOT SROT DMS
Head Occupational Therapist, Royal Marsden Hospital, London

Chapter 24 Oncology

Sue Cox Martin DipCOT SROT
Senior Occupational Therapist,
The Duke of Cornwall Spinal Treatment Centre, Salisbury District Hospital, Wiltshire

Sue trained at Newcastle upon Tyne and qualified as an O.T. in 1980. She joined Pinderfields Hospital in Wakefield as a Basic grade for two years, where she developed an interest in spinal cord injury. To build on this she joined the team at Hexham Spinal Unit and soon after the opportunity arose to contribute to the development of a newly built spinal unit at Salisbury. There Sue has remained for the last eighteen years during which time she has married Bill and they have two children: Jessie and Charlie.

Chapter 16 Spinal cord lesions

Michael Curtin MPhil BOCCThy SROT
Lecturer in Occupational Therapy, School of Health Professions and Rehabilitation Sciences, University of Southampton

Trained in Australia. Worked in a variety of physical rehabilitation fields, in both children and adults, in Australia, Botswana and England. Previously employed as a research occupational therapist at the National Spinal Injuries Centre, Stoke Mandeville Hospital. Currently working as a lecturer in occupational therapy.

Chapter 16 Spinal cord lesions

Jackie Dean DipCOT SROT
Independent occupational therapist and brain injury case manager.
Based in Wirral, Merseyside

Jackie Dean qualified as an occupational therapist in 1978. She developed an interest in acquired brain injury during her first job at Frenchay Hospital in Bristol. Subsequently she has worked in acute, statutory, voluntary and private positions with this client group. She has worked as a visiting lecturer on several occupational therapy courses and has designed and run workshops in the treatment of various neurological disorders. She became an independent occupational therapist in 1985. In 1992 she became involved in medico-legal assessment work and she assisted in the development of the Transitional Rehabilitation Unit (TRU Ltd). She left the unit in 1997 to expand her role as a brain injury case manager. She is a full member of the British Association of Brain Injury Case Managers.

Chapter 15 Acquired brain injury

Cath Doman DipCOT SROT
Principal Occupational Therapist, Doncaster Metropolitan Borough Council Social Services Directorate, Doncaster

Graduated from St Loyes School of Occupational Therapy in 1991. First post was in Bournemouth Social Services followed by a Senior Practitioner post in Dorset Social Services. She is currently Principal Occupational Therapist for Doncaster Social Services. Lives in Harrogate with husband Mark.

Chapter 7 Tools for living
Chapter 20 Motor neurone disease

Alison Laver Fawcett DipCOT SROT OT(C) PhD
Mental Health Project Worker, Harrogate Healthcare NHS Trust and North Yorkshire Social Services, Ripon, North Yorkshire

Qualified as an occupational therapist from Dorset House, Oxford in 1986. She obtained a PhD in Psychology (Neuropsychology and psychometrics) from the University of Surrey in 1995. The focus of her doctoral work was the development of the Structured Observational Test of Function (SOTOF). She worked as a clinician at several hospitals in London and then as a researcher and educator at Canterbury Christ Church College, Washington University School of Medicine, USA, McMaster University Faculty of Health Sciences, Canada and the University of Teesside. She currently works part-time as Mental Health Project Worker in a joint funded post evaluating statutory and non-statutory services for older people with mental health problems residing in and around Ripon, North Yorkshire.

Chapter 5 Assessment

Marg Foster TDipCOT SROT CertEd MMedSci
Programme Leader, School of Health and Community Studies, University of Derby

Qualified in 1966. Worked in areas of physical disability and paediatric practice. Researched personal care equipment with Department of Consumer Ergonomics at Loughborough University before moving into occupational therapy education. Currently programme leader for undergraduate full-time, part-time and accelerated pathways for BSc(Hons) Occupational Therapy and Education Representative on Council of College of Occupational Therapists.

Chapter 3 Theoretical frameworks
Chapter 4 Skills for practice
Chapter 6 Activity analysis
Chapter 10 Life skills

Stephanie Gething DipCOT SROT
Senior Occupational Therapist Cardiac Rehabilitation, Nevill Hall Hospital, Abergavenny

Qualified from St Loyes School of Occupational Therapy in 1982. Worked in Nevill Hall Hospital throughout career, covered all areas of hospital-based care. In 1992 helped to set up Multi-disciplinary Cardiac Rehabilitation Programme at Nevill Hall Hospital. Also involved in training and development of staff and students.

Chapter 19 Cerebrovascular accident

Rosemary Gollop DipCOT SROT MPH
Formerly Senior Occupational Therapist, Occupational Therapy Department, City Hospital, Nottingham

Has worked as a senior occupational therapist in the field of burns for 16 years. A long-standing interest in involving users and carers in health planning has led to a recent move from secondary care into the field of public health. She is currently completing a Masters degree in Public Health and is working on patient and public involvement at Nottingham Health Authority.

Chapter 13 Burns

Sue Griffiths BA DipCOT SROT PGDip MSc
Senior Lecturer, Division of Occupational Therapy, Centre for Healthcare Education, University College Northampton

Sue Griffiths qualified in 1981 from Derby School of Occupational Therapy. She worked in a range of clinical settings in both physical and mental health, before working as a contract manager for a district-wide OT service. She is currently a senior lecturer at University College Northampton and has recently completed an MSc in Evidence Based Healthcare at Oxford University. Her special interests are management, research and creative activity.

Chapter 8 Professional context

Alison Hammond DipCOT SROT BSc(Hons) MSc PhD
Senior Research Therapist, Rheumatology, Derbyshire Royal Infirmary, Derby

Has been evaluating the effectiveness of OT and patient education in rheumatology for over 10 years.

Chapter 23 Rheumatoid arthritis

Jan Harrison DipCOT SROT FETC MSc
Consultant Occupational Therapist,
Research House, Perivale, Middlesex

Trained in London and worked for many years at
the National Hospital for Neurology and Neurosurgery, Queen Square, latterly as Lead
Professional Advisor. She has a Master's degree in
Rehabilitation and now runs her own consultancy
with associates. She has served as a nationally
elected member of Council. She founded and was
twice chair of NANOT (the National Association
of Neurological Occupational Therapists).

Chapter 26 Parkinson's disease

Camilla Hawkins DipCOT(LHMC) BA(Hons)
Senior Occupational Therapist
Mildmay Hospital, London

Camilla Hawkins qualified in 1992 from the postgraduate accelerated Diploma course at The
London Hospital Medical College. She has developed her long-standing interest in palliative care
and the care of individuals with a life-limiting
illness through community-based work, as well
as within a hospital-based oncology service.

For the past five years Camilla has worked
within a service specifically for the care of individuals with an HIV or AIDS diagnosis. This has
enabled her to develop her interests in psychological care as well as developing links with clinical
education. Camilla is the HIV and AIDS representative on the specialist section of HOPE
(HIV/AIDS, Oncology, Palliative Care Education)
and is currently completing an MSc in Occupational Therapy at the University of East London.

Chapter 18 HIV/AIDS

Vivienne Ibbotson DipCOT SROT
Senior Occupational Therapist,
Mobility and Specialised Rehabilitation Centre,
Northern General Hospital, Sheffield

Qualified 1970 from Derby School of Occupational
Therapy. Worked in Hillingdon Hospital, followed by Berne, Switzerland before returning to
community in Sheffield. For past 14 years worked
with upper limb amputees and limb-deficient chil-

dren. Also involved in writing articles and papers
on this speciality as well as attending and presenting papers at national and international conferences. Co-organised four upper limb symposia
(5th currently in planning), which is now recognised internationally as the only dedicated upper
limb symposium of its kind.

*Chapter 14 Upper limb amputees and limb-deficient
children*

Paula Jeffreson DipCOT SROT
Head Occupational Therapist, Robert Jones and
Agnes Hunt Orthopaedic and District Hospital
NHS Trust, Oswestry, Shropshire

Chapter 23 Rheumatoid arthritis
Chapter 27 Osteoarthritis

Hilary Johnson DipCOT SROT BA Cert Ed(PCE)
Senior Lecturer, Division of Occupational
Therapy, Centre for Healthcare Education,
University College, Northampton

Hilary Johnson qualified as an occupational
therapist in 1968 at the York School. She has had
a long and varied career in clinical occupational
therapy, having worked in general medicine,
brain injury, hand injury rehabilitation, learning
disabilities and community mental health. As a
clinician she regularly supervised students on
placement. In 1993 she took her up her current
post in higher education at University College
Northampton, where she lectures in clinical reasoning and psychological theory applied to
occupational therapy practice.

*Chapter 9 Psychosocial perspectives in person-
centred practice*

Sybil E Johnson DipCOT SROT DMS
Team Manager, Disability Services, Dorset Social
Services, Ferndown Local Office, Dorset

Sarah Jane Kelly DipCOT SROT
Senior Occupational Therapist, Back Pain Unit,
Kings Mill Centre, Sutton in Ashfield

Chapter 22 Spinal disorder (back pain)

Helen McKenna DipCOT SROT
Senior Hand Therapist, Pulvertaft Hand Unit,
Derbyshire Royal Infirmary, Derby

Qualified from Derby in 1983. Worked in a
variety of areas of practice in the Midlands.
Recent experience in trauma and orthopaedics at
Queens Medical Centre, Nottingham. Designed a
number of commercially produced hand splints
and received Prince of Wales Award to investigate hand therapy systems in the USA. Currently
working in the Pulvertaft Hand Unit, Derbyshire
Royal Infirmary.

Chapter 17 Upper limb trauma

Linda Morgans DipCOT SROT
Senior Occupational Therapist
Neurology/Rehabilitation, Nevill Hall Hospital,
Abergavenny

Qualified from St Loyes School of Occupational
Therapy in 1974. Has worked from South
Wales since, working in Nevill Hall Hospital for
most of her career covering all areas of hospital-
based care; particularly interested in Care of the
Elderly, Stroke and Neurological Rehabilitation.

Chapter 19 Cerebrovascular accident

Kim Oliver BSc(Hons) SROT
Senior Occupational Therapist, Cardiac and
Respiratory Medicine, Glenfield Hospital,
Leicester

Qualified from Derby in 1997. Variety of experience in different areas of physical dysfunction
and rehabilitation. Currently senior 1 in cardiac
and respiratory medicine involved with the management of chronic disease, cardiac rehabilitation, lung cancer and palliative care.

Chapter 25 Cardiac and respiratory disease

Joanne Pratt DipCOT SROT GCE BA MSc
Lecturer and Programme Organiser
BSc/BscHonsOT, Division of Occupational
Therapy, School of Social Sciences, Glasgow
Caledonian University, Glasgow

Qualified from Derby in 1997. Has had experience across a diverse range of practice including
acute care and rehabilitation. Current professional interests and energies lie in raising the
profile of occupational therapy in industrial settings, especially with regard to disability and
ageing management, job retention and work
rehabilitation.

Chapter 6 Activity analysis

Pauline Rowe DipCOT SROT CertEd MEd
Senior Lecturer in Occupational Therapy,
School of Health and Community Studies,
University of Derby

Worked in a range of clinical settings in both
physical and mental health. Since taking up
current post as senior lecturer subject areas
involved in include anatomy and physiology,
clinical sciences, orthotics, interpersonal communication, group dynamics, the use of the arts as
therapeutic media and qualitative research.

Chapter 7 Tools for living

Donna Schell DipCOT SROT CMS
Occupational Therapy Service Manager,
St Andrews Group of Hospitals, Northampton

Chapter 8 Professional context

Louise Sewell BSc SROT
Research Occupational Therapist,
Pulmonary Rehabilitation, Department of
Respiratory Medicine, Glenfield Hospital,
Leicester

Louise Sewell qualified as an occupational
therapist from Liverpool University in 1993 and
has worked in a variety of clinical specialties
including stroke rehabilitation, pain management and cardiac rehabilitation. She is now
employed as a research occupational therapist
in pulmonary and cardiac rehabilitation at
Glenfield Hospital in Leicester.

Chapter 25 Cardiac and respiratory disease

Liz Tipping DipCOT SROT LPC(Back Care Management)
Lecturer in Occupational Therapy,
St Loyes School of Health Studies, Exeter

Graduated from Exeter. Majority of clinical experience in social sevices plus several years in a GP practice. Now at St Loyes teaching across the curriculum and responsible for training undergraduates in manual handling. Currently undertaking an MSc in Health Ergonomics at Surrey University.

Chapter 7 Tools for living
Chapter 21 Multiple sclerosis

Annie Turner TDipCOT SROT MA FCOT
Head of Division of Occupational Therapy,
Centre for Health Care Education,
University College Northampton

Chapter 1 History and philosophy of occupational therapy
Chapter 2 Occupation for therapy

Elizabeth White DipCOT SROT DKC PhD
Lecturer in Occupational Therapy, School of
Occupational Therapy, Barts and the London,
Queen Mary's School of Medicine and Dentistry,
University of London

Chapter 7 Tools for living

Sandie Woods DipCOT SROT BSc(Hons) BA
Head Occupational Therapist, Mildmay
Hospital, London

Sandie Woods qualified in 1977 from the London School of Occupational Therapy. She worked for five years, in two posts, at Enfield General Hospital, gaining experience in a number of different fields. Sandie then moved to the London Borough of Hackney, where she had three posts over fourteen years, the last five years as team manager, specialising in care in the community. For the past four and a half years Sandie has been Head of Occupational Therapy at Mildmay Hospital, specialising in the care of individuals with HIV and AIDS. Sandie is a great believer in continuing professional development. Following her training Sandie went on to complete two degrees with the Open University. Following this Sandie completed a postgraduate diploma in Health Psychology at City University and Certificates in Counselling Skills and Theory from the Central School of Counselling and Therapy. Sandie is currently completing her dissertation as the final part of an MSc in Occupational Therapy at the University of East London.

Chapter 18 HIV/AIDS

Foreword

By anyone's definition, setting out to write an authoritative textbook is challenging. Bringing a team from diverse specialties together to assemble the best of contemporary practice in a coherent volume must be doubly foreboding. That success will inevitably be followed by demand for a follow-up edition would make most of us recoil from the venture in the first place. But 'Turner, Foster and Johnson' has become a seminal text in the education of undergraduate occupational therapists in the UK and its success has sustained this team's commitment since the first edition was published in 1981. They deserve our warmest congratulations and admiration for this fifth edition 20 years later.

Their team includes six experienced contributors from the last edition and twenty-four new contributors; some are well-established authors and others perhaps less well known outside their specialist arena. However well-seasoned or novice the writers, the reader of any authoritative text will have high expectations and in this fifth edition all achieve a consistently high quality, which attests to the status of the 'advanced practitioner' now being valued and recognised across the healthcare professions. They too deserve our thanks and appreciation for their willingness not only to share their knowledge and expertise, but to subject their theories and practice to the profession's judgement.

Over the last decade, in particular, the organisational and policy context for health and social care has been under constant change and reform. Yet within this environment, frequently constrained by tight resources, there is an outstanding wealth of innovation and creativity. The pursuit of knowledge and the constant determination to find new approaches to managing disease and working with individuals and their carers to solve their problems continues to excite hard-pressed professionals; pushing forward the frontiers is immensely rewarding. In the past that was left to the few – to the academic, the specialist or the researcher. Now critical appraisal, reflective practice, systematic audit, peer review, best value review, service evaluation, clinical governance and a host of other methodologies are accepted parts of the professional's landscape. The need to deliver evidence-based practice is well understood and all professionals have to play their part in the 'total quality management' of service delivery. This agenda is challenging but none would resist its morality or appeal, only question how long it has been in arriving and appreciate how time-consuming and difficult it is to achieve.

Against that background, this volume makes excellent use of a developing evidence base for the value of occupational therapy interventions. In their preface, the editors focus on the novice practitioner but the text would prove an invaluable refresher to all those practising in the broad field of physical illness and disability, or in any of the specialisms it features. Inevitably, different audiences will seek out different qualities. This is primarily a text for the undergraduate and so our educators will want to know that it reflects the best of contemporary practice. I believe it does.

This edition embodies the theoretical underpinnings of interventions throughout the text, in an accessible manner and in a way which roundly demonstrates the importance of models and frames of reference as the clear foundations or 'building blocks' to practice. Annie Turner's revision of the history and philosophy of occupational therapy provides new insights but also illustrates that the basic, even simple, foundations of the profession – that occupation matters to humans and that the individual should 'share the effort of rehabilitation' (see p. 4) – remain valid as the very bedrocks of modern occupational therapy. The new chapter on 'Occupation for therapy' then provides a sound and questioning critique on the role of occupation, drawing on the most recent writings of international experts such as Finlay, Whiteford, Wilcock, Zemke and Clark. This chapter provides an excellent platform for the better appreciation of Marg Foster's overview of theoretical frameworks. Similarly, the new structure of Section 2 is a welcome development from the fourth edition as it brings a new coherence to, and appreciation of, the range of skills which are essential to the provision of effective therapy. The 'novice' is led smoothly into the consideration of principles for practice, followed by expert contributions on key areas of practice.

From a national policy perspective, I was also keen to find a text bedded in the reality of modern health and social care delivery. New practitioners need a firm theoretical and practical foundation but they also need to enter employment with a keen sense of the organisational drivers and the policy pressures that will influence their everyday practice. Turner quickly challenges the institutional pressure for 'safe discharge' and rapid hospital throughput with its consequent neglect of the individual's wider occupational needs. However, throughout the text, 'client-centred' practice is a constant theme. This is not simply expounded as a fashionable theme – how convenient that would be when in UK we have a new NHS plan that extols its vision as 'a health service designed around the patient'. Instead it is reinforced as the very embodiment of the way good occupational therapy is practised: that ill or disabled people, and their carers, are partners in the process. Hilary Johnson provides an excellent overview of psychosocial frameworks in Chapter 9 and gives due prominence to the influence of the Independent Living Movement, citing some of its chief proponents, including Oliver, Finkelstein and Morris. If new occupational therapists emerge with the art of client-centred practice instilled in their very being, they will be better able to challenge the institutional pressures that prevent the full use of their skills in helping individuals to achieve the personal goals and lifestyle priorities that matter to them.

Johnson's concluding thoughts on the therapist relinquishing some of her power and sharing her professional knowledge in a spirit of genuine partnership with the service user (see p. 272) have an added resonance with the pressure for improved team-working described by Griffiths and Schell in Chapter 8. Again, this is a central tenet of the NHS plan. Similarly, a sound connection is made with the Lawrence Enquiry (see p. 262) in challenging any professional cosiness about the extent to which our services are appropriate and sensitive to the needs of those from different religious or cultural backgrounds. Laver emphasises the importance of standardised assessments (see p. 135) and firmly challenges the rationale for continued retreat into home-made variations. As the Government sets out to achieve a single assessment process across health and social care, it behoves occupational therapists to contribute expert assessments which stand up to scrutiny, form a sound foundation for their intervention and link with valid outcome measures that clearly demonstrate the value of their contribution to efficient and effective service provision.

In this fifth edition, the authors should be proud of the new theoretical depth they have brought to undergraduate education. But readers will be equally grateful to find the little 'gems' that restore their heart; mine arrived quickly on page 9 – Stanton Wood's 1940 quote that 'occupation is essential to the maintenance of health' and that the concept had the 'simplicity of genius'. Sixty-one years later, as the debate about occupational science is lively and the evidence base still needs improving, that simple belief is worth hanging on to. I hope it serves as an inspiration to all those students who will embark upon this text. I wish them happy studies and a bright future in a most worthwhile profession.

Thanks to Annie, Marg, Sybil and colleagues for another winner.

London 2001   Sheelagh E Richards

Preface

The many changes in thinking, knowledge, legislation and practice which have occurred in recent years have shaped this 'new look' fifth edition. The authors have reflected the enormous change in culture which has surrounded both the practice and theory of occupational therapy in the UK and have endeavoured to capture this and use it as the basis for this edition.

This changing culture has seen a growth in the need for occupational therapists to demonstrate that their interventions are based on sound clinical reasoning, with a specific brief to provide evidence for the efficacy of their practice. The introduction of clinical governance, evidence-based practice and quality audit has shaped the remit of therapists in health, social care and private practice.

The practice chapters within the text reflect this growth by basing their guidance for interventions on existing evidence. For a number of practice fields, however, this has not been an easy task. Several practitioners have, despite extensive searching, found little or no concrete evidence of the effectiveness of practice in their particular field. The profession is clearly at the dawn of a new era where, having reflected on its raison d'être and reaffirmed its roots, it is only too aware of the need to produce an evidence base for its practice. Whilst, for many years, occupational therapy has been thought to be 'a good idea' the evidence to back this thinking has been sadly lacking. Today, however, all practitioners are equipped with the skills to produce this evidence and, facilitated by the culture in which they work, are discovering, through scientific means, that the 'good idea' which has been around for so long in theory can be proven to work in practice.

Whilst the evidence for the effectiveness of occupational therapy is mounting there is also an accompanying growth in the theoretical foundations which underpin and shape its practice. A veritable explosion of literature in recent years has enabled practitioners to internalise and articulate occupational therapy's identity, theories and boundaries. The profession is developing a more universally acknowledged language to describe its theories and practices and to proclaim its own knowledge base and relationship to the biopsychosocial sciences.

To this end this fifth edition, for the first time, has been able to place occupation at the centre of all its writing. Practice chapters debate the principles of assessment and intervention around the occupational needs of the individual. The individual's occupational performance needs, in their unique environment, provide the driving force which shape intervention. These chapters give little medical information, as this can easily be obtained elsewhere; however, they are focused around areas of clinical expertise to enable the novice practitioner to link occupational theory more readily to the practice context.

The fifth edition enables the novice therapist to gain a firm understanding of the identity and theories which underpin the profession and to link these theories directly into practice. It is not a text which provides all the answers, nor would it try to do so. It should be seen as a 'starter for ten', a text which will spark understanding and enquiry and will lead the novice to explore further the concepts and principles which are introduced.

The book is divided into four sections, the first of which presents the roundations for practice. This expanded section explores the roots and philosophy of the profession and debates the concept of the use of occupation as therapy and the theoretical frameworks which spring from this. Whilst many foundation chapters have a universal application to practice, the book emphasises concepts which focus on those whose occupational needs arise primarily from physical dysfunction. The second and third sections explore the universal principles and skills required by the therapist working with people who have physical dysfunction. Section four addresses intervention strategies which may be considered in a number of clinical specialties. These specialties are presented in a way that reflects the lifespan theme, commencing with those chapters which address the needs of children and moving on to those which address the needs of younger, and then older adults. The chapters have moved away from the technical and somewhat prescriptive descriptions of earlier editions to a style which explores principles and their links to practice. The book continues to retain its currency by using senior practitioners and academics to share their particular areas of expertise in both theory and practice.

The three editors have continued to enjoy working together. Without doubt this edition has faced more practical setbacks than any other. Many personal challenges have been met and we have remained a tight and supportive trio of friends who have now worked together on this project for more that twenty years. Without doubt we must include in our cohort the continued support from Churchill Livingstone in particular from Jane Dingwall, for her patience and perseverance and from Mary Law, who has remained our advocate throughout all five editions. We have also seen, during this edition, the mounting pressures on authors from all fields of work. Lack of time and pressures of work for all contributors have tested our cajoling skills to the limit and we hope that these universal pressures will not stifle the desire held by many therapists to explore, research and communicate their profession.

We hope that the text will continue to provide a current and challenging foundation text which will serve the novice practitioner through the early years of the twenty-first century.

2001

Annie Turner
Marg Foster
Sybil Johnson

Foundations for practice

1

History and philosophy of occupational therapy

Annie Turner

INTRODUCTION

In the year 2000, the College of Occupational Therapists (2000a) contended that:

Occupational therapists treat people of all ages with mental and physical problems through meaningful occupation to improve everyday function and prevent disability.

The concepts within this statement thus reflect the current thinking and practice of occupational therapy within the United Kingdom today.

In 1962, Mary Reilly, an American professor of occupational therapy, wrote that: 'Man, through the use of his hands, as they are energised by his mind and will, can influence the state of his own health'. In this much-quoted statement, Reilly encapsulated the concepts that had underpinned occupational therapy since its inception at the beginning of the 20th century. As a profession, occupational therapy was established and grew throughout the 20th century. The term 'occupational therapy' was first coined by George Barton, a disabled American architect, at the start of the 20th century. Barton established Consolation House, an institution in Clifton Springs, New York in which, by means of occupation, people were retrained and helped to readjust to gainful living (Licht 1948). His use of the term 'occupational therapy' helped focus the work and writings of the time and reflected the growing realisation that occupation could be used as a health-promoting agent. However, although the profession itself is relatively young, the idea of using occupation as a means of helping the sick is by no means a new one. This chapter traces some of the concepts and events that led to the way in which occupational therapy is practised and thought about today and proposes a philosophy that can be used to underpin and evaluate our current and future practice.

A HISTORY OF OCCUPATIONAL THERAPY

ROOTS FROM ANCIENT TIMES

Although there is no historical reference to occupational therapy, as such, until the beginning of the 20th century, Egyptian writings dating from as long ago as 2000 BC tell of temples where melancholics congregated in large numbers to seek relief. Games and recreations were instituted and everyone's time was taken up 'by some pleasurable occupation' (Pinel 1803, cited in Howarth & MacDonald 1946). The classical Greek god of healing, Asclepius, was reported to have quietened delirium with songs, farces and music (Le Clerc 1699, cited in MacDonald et al 1970). In AD 430 the Roman writer Martianus Capella quoted the Greek physician Asclepiades' belief in the curative use of music and song for the treatment of disturbances of the mind and disease of the body (cited in Licht 1948). Around 30 BC, Seneca, the Roman writer and orator, recommended employment for any kind of mental agitation (Howarth & MacDonald 1940) whilst the Greek physician Soranus (AD 98–138) believed in pleasant surroundings and activities for his patients. In the first century AD, Aulus Cornelius Celsus, a Roman encyclopaedist whose writings included an account of surgical practice, also recommended music, conversation, reading, exercise to the point of fatigue, travel and a change of scenery in order to ease troubled minds. The celebrated Greek physician, Galen (AD c. 130–200), advocated treatment by occupation, suggesting digging, fishing, housebuilding and shipbuilding. Galen is also famously quoted as saying that: 'Employment is nature's best

physician and is essential to human happiness' (cited in Howarth & MacDonald 1940). Interestingly, Licht (1948 p81) disputes this statement, feeling that Galen was quoted out of context. He argues that:

Galen did say that 'Exercise is nature's physician' but the exercise to which he referred was entirely unrelated to the objectives of occupational therapy ... he clearly indicates that he prefers exercise to medication or diet for its effect on the digestive tract.

Licht felt that the origin of this statement, so widely quoted and advocated by occupational therapists, is, in fact, a misinterpreted quotation from a poor translation.

Despite this, many other examples of the therapeutic use of occupation have been cited through the ages. Rhazes (AD 852–932), an Arabian physician, advocated chess-playing and emphasised that the patient should share the effort of rehabilitation. A few centuries later, Bartholemew, a 13th-century clergyman writing in his encyclopaedia, felt that insane people should be 'gladded with instruments and some deal be occupied' (Licht 1948 p5).

THE 18TH AND 19TH CENTURIES

Our modern understanding of the nature and treatment of disease in the United Kingdom has its roots in the 18th century. Prior to this time it was felt that the key to the treatment of 'lunatics' lay in fear, and that the best means of producing this was through punishment. Deriving from practices of the Dark Ages, many forms of cruel and torturous 'treatments' were devised. 'Lunatics' were not seen as having rights or needs, but as deserving ridicule, confinement and punishment. The French physician, Philippe Pinel (1745–1826), took a more enlightened view and instituted reforms in the treatment of the mentally ill, the most renowned of which was to release the shackles of asylum inmates. He prescribed physical exercises and manual occupations, believing that 'Rigorously executed manual labour is the best method of securing good morale and discipline' (Pinel 1806, reprinted in Licht 1948 p19). Pinel wrote of a

Spanish hospital, which received patients from all ranks of society, pointing out that the recovery rate was higher among the lower classes, who were employed in the work of the hospital, than amongst the 'idle grandees'. However, the idea of patients undertaking work met with resistance in the private hospitals, where it was thought that those who paid for treatment should not be put to work.

In the same period, William Tuke established The Retreat at York, a hospital for those with mental illness based on the humane thinking that reflected the beliefs of The Society of Friends (the Quakers) who ran it. Many physicians followed his ideas and the 19th century saw more widespread acceptance of occupation for treatment, particularly of the mentally ill. At around this time, in 1798, Dr Benjamin Rush from Philadelphia prescribed spinning, sewing and churning for women and grinding corn, gardening and reaping for men, whilst Percy Anecdotes, writing in a 'Madhouse in Aversa' (Italy) in 1821 found that moderate work, combined with amusement, provided the best means of cure and advocated printing, translating, music and manufacturing woollen cloth (Howarth & MacDonald 1940). In October 1897, G Blumer, an American physician, wrote in the Journal of Insanity, how he considered that: 'Compared with drug treatment, so far as the great mass of asylum population is concerned, occupation, properly systemized and diversified, is of immeasurably greater consequence' (cited in Licht 1948 p14) whilst Dunton (Dunton & Licht 1950 p4) remarked that older practitioners of that time recorded: 'Instances … of women patients who ravelled out their stockings in order to obtain thread with which to knit, using straight hair pins of an old fashioned type for needles'.

Until the turn of the 20th century, therefore, there were growing, although isolated, incidents of practice and writing that produced anecdotal evidence of the natural drive for occupation and its effectiveness in the treatment of people with mental health difficulties. Haas (1925), the director of Men's Therapeutic Activities in Bloomingdale Hospital, White Plain, New York, felt that prior to this time all that was written was 'a large number of brief statements that the employment of patients was believed to be beneficial' (Haas 1925 p9), although Dunton (Dunton & Licht, 1950 p3) muses that 'It is probable that economic factors determined the placement of a patient in a laundry or kitchen or at farm work rather than the idea that by such work or occupation the patient might benefit'. Despite these affirmations, statements were based on observations or feelings, rather than scientific research, a situation that has dogged the profession during the rise of empirical science in the 20th century.

THE 20TH CENTURY

It seems to be generally accepted (Haas 1925, Licht 1948, Willard & Spackman 1947) that the first person to establish a course in what could be seen as occupational therapy was Susan Tracey (1878–1928), head nurse at Adams Nervine Hospital, Boston. In 1906 she ran a course called Invalid Occupation for student nurses, and published her lectures in a book of that title in 1910. Around this time, in 1908, the Chicago School of Civics and Philanthropy offered a course of training in occupations to trained nurses in institutes for the 'insane and feebleminded'. This work was continued by Eleanor Clarke Slagle, who became Director of Occupational Therapy for the New York State Mental Health Commission. Clearly, there was much activity related to the foundations of the profession at this time (Box 1.1). As stated at the beginning of the chapter, it was during this time that George Barton coined the term 'occupational therapy' and it was in 1915 that Dr William Rush Dunton first published lectures from his training course under the title 'Occupational Therapy'. Thus, by the beginning of the 20th century, the idea of using occupation in the treatment of the mentally ill had become quite widely established. Also at this time, it was becoming more socially acceptable for women to take up careers and join the professions; their traditional roles of caring for the sick could now incorporate the expanding knowledge related to that care and, along with the pioneering work taking place in nursing, these caring professions gained more respectability.

Box 1.1 An outline of some historical ideas, which led to the formation of occupational therapy, and the milestones in the development of the British profession

2600 BC	The Chinese thought that disease resulted from organic inactivity, so used physical training as therapy
2000 BC	The Egyptians dedicated temples for the treatment of melancholics. Here patients' time was spent in pleasurable activity such as games and recreation
1000 BC	The Persians used physical therapy to train their youth
600 BC	Asclepius, the Greek classical god of healing, soothed delirium with songs, farces and music
600 BC–AD 200	Pythagorus, Thales and Orpheus used music to sooth troubled minds. Hippocrates emphasised the link between mind and body and recommended wrestling, riding, labour and vigorous exercise. Cornelius Celcus, who studied anatomy and medicine, recommended sailing, hunting, handling of arms, ball games, running and walking for their therapeutic benefits
1250–1700	Leonardo da Vinci, Decartes and Francis Bacon studied anatomy, movement, rhythm, posture and energy expenditure. Ramazzini, Professor of Practical Medicine, stressed the importance of the prevention of illness–He observed his patients–workers in his workshop, and placed high value on weaving, cobbling, tailoring and pottery as exercise. This was early movement analysis
1780	Tissot used occupational exercise for the treatment of the mentally ill. He advocated sewing, playing the violin, sweeping, sawing, bell ringing, hammering, chopping wood, riding and swimming
1786	Philippe Pinel used work as therapy in Paris. His name is associated with the concept of Moral Treatment
1786	William Cowper, in a letter to Lady Hesketh, dated 16 January 1786, described the malady which had seized him and how he improved his own state of mind by the use of carpentry, gardening, writing and poetry. This may be the first recorded account of a patient's own experience in English literature
1792	The Quaker William Tuke opened The Retreat in York. Tuke's name is very much associated with Moral Treatment
1850	The Crimean War enabled many women to take up careers. The nursing profession began to develop under Florence Nightingale
1914–1918	The First World War – physiotherapy began to develop

The development of occupational therapy as a profession

End of 19th century	An increasing awareness of the value of occupation as a treatment. The term 'occupational therapy' began to evolve. The emphasis was still very much on the use of occupation within the psychiatric field
1924	Dr Elizabeth Casson introduced occupational therapy into her nursing home in Clifton, Bristol, after attending a conference by Professor Sir David Henderson and visiting a newly established occupational therapy school in Philadelphia, USA
1925	Margaret Fulton, the first qualified occupational therapist to work in the UK (after training in Philadelphia) established an occupational therapy department at the Royal Comhill Hospital, Aberdeen. Dr Elizabeth Casson sent Constance Tebbit to train in the USA. She returned to work in the Dorset House Psychiatric Nursing Home in Bristol
1930	Dr Casson established the first British occupational training school at Dorset House, with Constance Tebbit as principal
1932	In Scotland the first professional association was formed. It had 30 members
1936	The Astley Ainslie school was established in Edinburgh. The Association of Occupational Therapists (AOT) was formed in England
1938	The first public examinations were held
1939–1945	The AOT set up short courses for occupational therapy auxiliaries. This could be upgraded to full professional status with further study
	The War Emergency Diploma allowed professionals with previous qualifications, e.g. teachers and nurses, to qualify as occupational therapists
1941	St Andrews School of Occupational Therapy in Northampton was established as the second English school
1943	AOT included England, Wales and Northern Ireland
1947	The National Health Service Act. Occupational therapy schools were privately funded at this time
1950s	A Joint Council was formed to look at matters common to the AOT and Scottish AOT
1951	First International Congress run by the AOT
1952	World Federation of Occupational Therapists was inaugurated, with Margaret Fulton as president and Constance Glyn-Owens (née Tebbit) as secretary
1954	First World Congress, held in Edinburgh

continued

Box 1.1   (*continued*)

1960/1	The establishment of the Council for the Professions Supplementary to Medicine leads to State Registration
1974	The British Association of Occupational Therapists was formed from a merger between AOT and SAOT
1977	First European Congress
1978	The Association divided into: The College of Occupational Therapists (which deals with professional and educational matters) and The British Association of Occupational Therapists (the trade union)
1990s	Training to first degree level is established on all pre-registration courses

---

The establishment, in the late 19th and early 20th centuries, of public health measures to control infectious diseases included the building of fever hospitals and sanatoria. A regime of prolonged bedrest, followed by a gradual increase in exercise, was established for those with tuberculosis (Paterson 1997). Dr Philip, a Scottish physician, gave an address on 'Rest and movement in tuberculosis' (Philip 1910, cited in Groundes-Peace 1957) in which he described the prescription of graded activity and showed people's progression from complete rest (indicated by the wearing of a white badge) through regulated exercise (yellow badge) and thence through various stages of regulated work to the wearing of a red badge, where activities included digging, sawing, carpentry and window cleaning. During this period, a farm colony was established near Edinburgh and a village settlement near Papworth in Cambridgeshire, both of which aimed to employ people in appropriate long-term work prior to their return to open employment.

During and after the First World War, casualties amongst young men resulted in an acute shortage of manpower in the workforce. The need to re-establish these men in open employment undoubtedly facilitated the growth of occupational therapy in the treatment of those with physical disabilities. Sir Robert Jones, Inspector of Military Orthopaedics during the First World War, persuaded the War Office to allow him to open Curative Workshops throughout military hospitals in the United Kingdom and these became the models for occupational therapy departments for the treatment of those with physical dysfunction. Influenced by workshops established in the United States, they were equipped with tools and machinery to exercise joints and muscles. Treadle exercising machines, carpentry, window cleaning and painting were used.

Influenced additionally by the work of two American engineers, Frederick W Taylor (1856–1915) and Frank Gilbreth (1868–1924), these workshops incorporated the principles of scientific management, which had its foundations in the analysis of work processes (Paterson 1997). Taylor and Gilbreth were also advocates of the need to adapt work, rearrange the environment and modify machinery in order to help 'cripples' resume 'a man's job' (Gilbreth 1917 p278, cited in Paterson 1997 p28).

Based on these workshops, the first occupational therapy department in Scotland, fully equipped with saws and lathes, was opened in 1936 at the Astley Ainslie Institution in Edinburgh, by Lieutenant Colonel John Cunningham, the medical superintendent. In the same year, the first Occupational Therapy Training Centre was also opened at the Institution (Groundes-Peace 1957).

Occupational therapy was introduced into England by Dr Elizabeth Casson who, having visited both the Bloomingdale Hospital in New York and the Boston School of Occupational Therapy in 1926, established the Dorset House School of Occupational Therapy in Bristol in 1930, which today is part of Oxford Brookes University. Dr Casson opened the Allendale Curative Workshop for people with physical disabilities in 1939 (Paterson 1997) (Fig. 1.1).

The Second World War also added impetus to the development of occupational therapy and the work undertaken played a vital role in the

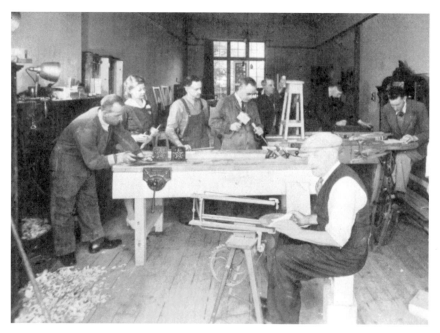

Fig. 1.1 The Allendale Curative Workshop, established in Bristol by Dr Elizabeth Casson in 1939 (reproduced from Howarth & MacDonald 1946 The Theory of Occupational Therapy, 3rd edn, by kind permission of Baillière, Tindall & Cox, London).

rehabilitation and re-establishment of wounded soldiers into the workforce. Balme (1953), cited by Paterson (1997) quotes from the Official Medical History of the Second World War that: 'Occupational therapy departments should be built and equipped as an integral part of the scheme …'. The Allendale Curative Workshop became a model for the development of similar occupational therapy departments and, in order to meet increased demands, the Dorset House School trained additional numbers of students in emergency courses (Fig. 1.2). Established and run, therefore, along military lines, and constrained to make use of 'crafts' by government limitations on materials, the ethos and work practices of early occupational therapy departments were developed from these post-war needs.

CONCEPTS AND LEGACIES FROM EARLY WRITINGS

In reviewing the increasing bank of opinion and experience that led to the creation and growth of occupational therapy, it is easy to see the emerging concepts that began to shape the profession. Once established, definitions and articles began to appear, to consolidate its foundations and explain them to others. Analysis of these early writings help to explain not only the concepts on which the profession was founded but also the legacies, both positive and negative, that have surrounded the profession throughout the greater part of the 20th century.

There appear to be three general concepts running through the early writings:

- that occupation is a natural state and is linked to health
- that people should be treated as individuals
- that occupation should be used as a therapeutic agent.

OCCUPATION IS A NATURAL STATE AND IS LINKED TO HEALTH

This fundamental concept continues to drive the profession and is strongly evident throughout the early writings. In 1922 Meyer wrote in the

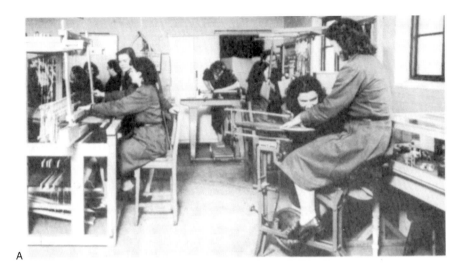

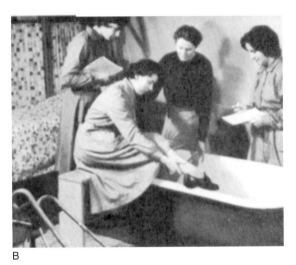

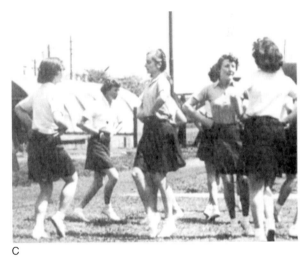

Fig. 1.2 Students training in the early days of the Dorset House School. (A) In the workshop, (B) in activities of daily living, (C) in recreational activities (reproduced by kind permission of the School of Occupational Therapy, Oxford Brookes University, Oxford).

Archives of Occupational Therapy of the link between health and occupation. He saw occupation as comprising not only doing, but also thinking and being, and its absence or interruption resulting in the breakdown of roles, habits and health (Meyer 1922). In 1948 Licht (p19) wrote of occupations: 'There is no longer any question about the desirability of such practices since continuous and unanimous experience ... has demonstrated its effectiveness in maintaining health'. He goes on to say that 'the surest and most effective method of restoration of reason is occupation' (Licht 1948 p20).

In an early text on occupational therapy, Stanton Woods, a consultant adviser in physical medicine, wrote in Howarth and MacDonald (1940) that 'occupation is essential to the maintenance of health' and that the concept had the 'simplicity of genius'. He saw occupation as having a normalising effect that helps rouse interest, develop attention and build self-esteem. He was conscious, however, that occupation alone does not cure, a sentiment echoed by Licht, who criticised George Barton's unbridled enthusiasms for occupational therapy and maintained it did much 'to retard the acceptance of occupational therapy by physicians as a result of his unbounded claims concerning the therapeutic value of work' (Licht 1948 p16).

Occupation was seen as an agent in helping people return to the world of normal activity and strongly linked with this was the concept that 'the patient corrects for himself the deficient factors' (Willard & Spackman 1947). Willard and Spackman saw the therapeutic use of occupation as an active, as opposed to a passive, process and noted that the measure of success was the change that occurred in the person rather than the product of the activity in which the person was engaged. They saw that 'the patient [was] the architect of his own reconstruction', a concept held dear today and reflected in the logo created by the British occupational therapy profession of the phoenix rising from the ashes through its own efforts (Fig. 1.3).

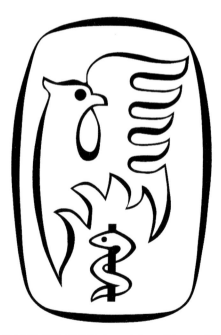

Fig. 1.3 Logo of the British Association of Occupational Therapists, which uses the image of the phoenix rising from the ashes through its own efforts (copyright held by the British Association of Occupational Therapy and reproduced by kind permission of the British Association of Occupational Therapists, London).

PEOPLE AS INDIVIDUALS

Although clearly functioning within the medical model, early writers reflected the importance of relating to people as individuals. They saw the importance of treating the whole person and of the motivation to be gained by working towards self-identified goals. In 1925, Haas recognised that 'all instruction is individual [and] will vary according to the patient's condition and needs'.

This concept was echoed by Howarth and MacDonald in 1940 who, whilst endeavouring to define and explain occupational therapy, described it as consisting of 'occupations selected and prescribed for each individual patient with his or her particular needs in view'. This concept of people as individuals was further developed within occupational therapy in 1947, when Clare Spackman postulated the need for the occupational therapists to expand their knowledge of the person beyond that available from the physician. Spackman began to refer to 'people' as opposed to 'patients', a concept the authors of this text have felt vital for many years. Spackman stated (Willard & Spackman 1947 p181): 'It is important that the person be considered as a whole, a human being with problems and interests, not as a case. In some instances information is available before the first interview but, more often than not, this is purely medical in nature'. She saw a knowledge of human nature to be of advantage and emphasised that 'each patient must be considered as an individual'. Today, the concept of the individual is central to our practice and our increased knowledge of psychology and sociology, which greatly expanded during the 1950s and 1960s, together with our more recent knowledge of person-centred approaches and occupational science, have enabled us to learn much about this concept and to keep it as a central theme within the practice of occupational therapy.

THE USE OF OCCUPATION AS A THERAPEUTIC AGENT

Very early writings showed a wide variety of occupations in use as therapeutic agents, although it was not until the early 20th century that the fundamental link between health and occupation in daily life was articulated. Indeed, not until the creation of occupational science in the late 20th century was the occupational nature of humans explored scientifically. Earlier parts of this chapter make reference to the use of music, farming, walking, reading, debating and playing chess, amongst others, as occupations used until the beginning of the 20th century. These writings often referred to work or labour as the therapeutic tool. However, in the early 20th century, the Arts and Crafts movement held sway and, in reflecting this, writers of the time extolled the virtue of more creative activities at the expense of those previously used. In 1925, Haas, writing in his text 'Occupational Therapy for the Mentally and Nervously Ill', saw that the introduction or revival of fine handicrafts had been most influential in the advancement of occupational therapy.

Whilst occupations (or, at least, labours) of a domestic and rural nature clearly continued for the first half of the century, Haas wrote at great length of the value of crafts, including jewellery making, enamelling, weaving, woodturning, rush seating and printing. His great love, however, was basketry, about which he spoke highly, and at length, going so far as to say that 'Basketry can be used to meet all needs in a way that no other craft can' (Haas 1925 p26). However, he acknowledged that many might question this, and went on to say that its popularity arose because 'it was the only suitable craft with which those interested in the use of occupation for its therapeutic use were familiar' (Haas 1925 p26).

The legacy of Haas's writings, and that of others at the time, could be said to have plagued occupational therapy for many years (Fig. 1.4). Some may argue that the idea of 'basket ladies' still lurks not far under the surface of some people's concept of occupational therapy. Any therapists trained as late as the 1970s will recognise many of those crafts mentioned above as central to their syllabus. Those of us who spent many (although often happily indulgent) hours lost in the intricacies of basketry, weaving, spinning, woodturning, jewellery making and print-

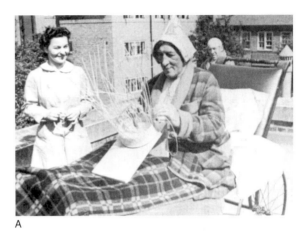

A

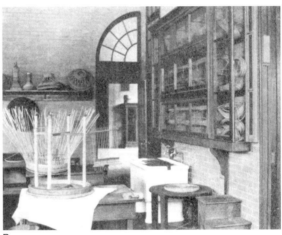

B

Fig. 1.4 (A) Basketry (and sun hat!) for the long-term bed-bound patient, St John's and St Elizabeth's Hospital, London, c. 1940 (reproduced by kind permission of the School of Occupational Therapy, Oxford Brookes University, Oxford), (B) the basket room at the Occupational Building of Bloomingdale Hospital, White Plains, New York in 1925 (as illustrated in Haas 1925 Occupational Therapy for the Mentally and Nervously Ill, the Bruce Publishing Company, Wisconsin).

ing will be more than aware of the legacy left from this time.

As the concept developed, advice began to be given on which activities would be most suitable for which conditions and how their therapeutic characteristics could be gauged. Haas (1925) explained that simply being busy was not necessarily therapeutic in itself, a thought echoed by Willard and Spackman (1947), who warned that 'an activity entered into without a purpose is not occupational therapy'! They felt that the ability to relate an activity to the individual need of the person is what distinguishes the occupational therapist from the craft instructor and that 'therapy came about as a result of prescribed activities intelligently planned'. They emphasised that an activity must be analysed to ensure it met the exact exercise required and, where necessary, adapted to meet special needs. However, Haas (1925 p149) approached the idea of patient choice with caution saying 'It is not considered any more essentially therapeutic that the patient … be always allowed to select what he wishes to do than it is for [him] to decide which medicine he likes'. In this, and similar statements, one can begin to see how a person-centred philosophy can easily be subsumed within the prescription of occupation.

Much was written on the standard of work to be achieved. It was generally felt that the work produced should be of a high standard, that the materials used should be of good quality and that design was important. Haas felt that where work contained mistakes these should be rectified by the individual. However, he remained focused on the idea that it was the process, rather than the product, that was the essence of therapy, stating that 'No thought should be given to the importance of the product as this must surely be considered secondary to the therapeutic needs' (Haas 1925). Howarth and MacDonald (1946) also told therapists that they should not be satisfied with poor standards of work, whilst Edgerton (1947, cited in Willard & Spackman 1947 p43), clearly felt strongly about standards, stating: 'There is little excuse for the tinselled, garish gadget for which the most that can be said is that it will catch the dust that might otherwise fall upon something of greater value'. Her message, I think, conveys the sentiment without confusion!

LINKS WITH MEDICINE

Early writings show that the use of occupation to help treat the sick had its roots in the medical profession, who treated the sick in hospitals,

rather than in non-medical establishments, such as the church or other welfare institutions, who cared for the sick. As occupational therapy was forming into a profession it was established as a treatment to be prescribed by a doctor, much as a medicine would be. Early occupational therapists were pleased, and indeed proud, that their profession was given credibility through the part it played in the rehabilitation of wounded soldiers, and were at pains to emphasise the importance of adhering to the doctor's wishes. Haas (1925) directed that 'the work must necessarily be carried out under medical direction'. Howarth and MacDonald (1946) concurred, stating 'every patient accepted for treatment should have a prescription card signed by the medical officer in charge of his case'. They saw that occupational therapy should be 'definitely prescribed and guided' by the doctor, while Willard and Spackman (1947 p183) felt that 'the fact that the physician has prescribed the occupational therapy programme helps the patient to realise it is a type of medical treatment'. They wrote that the person who comes for occupational therapy is carrying out the doctor's orders and warned that no change should be made to the prescribed treatment without the approval of the physician who is the recognised authority. Even in the 1960s Mary Jones (1964) wrote 'It is stressed that the work is planned to fulfil the doctor's aims of treatment'.

Such adhesion to the medical model must seem strange to today's new practitioner, brought up within a professional Code of Ethics and Professional Conduct that states 'Occupational therapists shall accept referrals which they deem to be appropriate and for which they have the resources'. Confirming that 'it is the duty of occupational therapists to obtain sufficient information to enable them to determine the appropriateness of the referral' (College of Occupational Therapists 2000 p5) occupational therapists are required to 'decline to accept a referral' if they cannot meet the basic standards of treatment. Whilst acknowledging a limited pot of resources, therefore, the College of Occupational Therapists expects occupational therapists to be responsible for the decisions they make about those they accept onto their case load

(College of Occupational Therapists 2000b p5). However, it must be remembered that early practitioners during the formation of the profession were also playing an integral role in the effort to re-establish a workforce depleted by war, and that this post-war work was driven by medical and military doctrine.

Despite this early type of relationship with medicine, occupational therapy gained considerable credibility through its medical links, gaining the right to control its own register through the establishment of the Council for the Professions Supplementary to Medicine Act in 1960. The revision of this, by the Health Act in 1999 (Department of Health 1999), gave wider and stronger powers to the health professions.

Although the establishment of occupational therapy under the wing of medicine gave it many advantages, it is also clear that there were many disadvantages. The close links with, and dominance by, the medical model led to a shift from early, person-centred practice to a medically modelled one. Despite early writings to the contrary, people were classed as cases, or patients, whose input from the occupational therapist was led primarily by their diagnosis rather than their self-identified occupational needs. Writings in the middle of the 20th century gave detailed and complex descriptions of how a particular diagnosis should be treated with designated crafts (Table 1.1, Box 1.2). Haas (1925) stated, for example, that 'Network [net making] serves well with confused and depressed cases'. Dunton and Licht (1950) advocated brushwork, bookbinding, chaircaning, leatherwork, printing and metalwork for increasing flexion of the elbow, while basketry, braided rugs, knotting, weaving and woodwork were recommended for elbow extension.

Table 1.1 Crafts recommended for the treatment of 'cases following fractures and injury' (reproduced from Howarth and MacDonald 1946 The Theory of Occupational Therapy, 3rd edn. by kind permission of Baillière, Tindall & Cox, London)

Joint	Movements involved	Suggested occupations
Fingers	Flexion, extension, abduction, adduction	Canework Cord-knotting Leather punching and thonging Modelling (wedging clay) Netting Rug-making Rug-plaiting Weaving-tapestry, weaving, shuttle throwing by finger movements, etc. Willow-work Woodwork – gripping tools Games: Bagatelle – with fingers, chess, draughts, peg solitaire, marbles, puff billiards
Wrist	Flexion, extension, abduction, adduction	Block-printing Canework Drilling Plaiting rushes and twisting Painting Rug-weaving Sandpapering and painting large surfaces upright Sawing and planing wood Weaving on special loom Work with hammer or screwdriver
Forearm	Supination, pronation	Cord-knotting Embroidery on a horizontal frame Netting Plaiting Screwdriving Weaving on special loom

continued

Table 1.1 (*continued*)

Joint	Movements involved	Suggested occupations
Elbow	Flexion, extension	Big loom weaving Cord-knotting Digging Sandpapering and painting large upright surfaces Sawing and planing wood Stool-seating

Shoulder	Flexion, extension, abduction,
	    adduction, circumduction,
	    rotation in and out
		Canework
		Cord-knotting
		Cross-cut wood sawing
		Hedge-clipping
		Sandpapering and painting at a height
		Sewing (long threads)
		Warping on board or mill
		Weaving (long threads) on upright loom
		Woodwork
		Games: Darts, billiards, bowls, skittles
		Bicycle saw

Hip	Flexion, extension, abduction, adduction, rotation	Cycling Foot bellows Lathe Loom with foot heddle change on spring Bicycle saw
Knee	Flexion, extension, rotation of tibia in and out	Foot bellows Digging Lathe Pottery wheel Weaving on loom Bicycle saw adjusted
Ankle and foot	Flexion, extension, inversion, eversion	Sewing machine Treadle saw Weaving

Many experienced therapists practising today will remember undertaking their education when this thinking predominated. Many hours were spent rote learning the origins and insertions of muscles, the names of bony structures and in completing 'muscle analysis' of craft activities. In line with this thinking was the birth of specialist adapted equipment for undertaking craft work, aimed at ensuring precision in the treatment of orthopaedic and some neurological conditions. Bicycle fretsaws; specialist woodturning lathes; ankle rotators and quadriceps switches and flexion, extension, pronation and supination (FEPS) apparatus for attaching to printing presses or weaving looms via rope circuits, were widely used. Their basic concept was to ensure that the crafts used could be precisely adapted to move or strengthen particular joints and muscle groups (Fig. 1.5).

However, it must be remembered that, in the post-war period, an individual's rehabilitation needs stretched over several months. Medical and surgical techniques were not as sophisticated as procedures used today and this machinery, used with appropriate crafts by people who were often skilled at making things by hand, were appropriate for their time. This equipment had its heyday in the 1960s and 1970s and was still in active use in the 1980s and beyond. The original concept of the development of this equipment worked well with the medical and rehabilitation needs of the times. The use of specific crafts, combined with the application of biomechanics, served well in helping fundamentally fit young people return to work and daily life.

Box 1.2   An analysis of wood working for the treatment of limitation of motion in the elbow and shoulder (reproduced from Willard and Spackman 1947 Principles of Occupational Therapy, by kind permission of JB Lippincott, Philadelphia)

Elbow

FLEXION AND EXTENSION

Use of a coping saw: The arm is held at the side. The range of motion is limited to about 40°. The resistance is dependent upon whether the saw is placed with the teeth up or down. With the teeth of the saw up, resistance is given in flexion; with them down, in extension.

Ripsawing: In the natural position the greatest resistance is offered in extension.

Flat sanding: The wood should be placed slightly below shoulder height and should extend in front of the patient. The use of both hands on the sander will help prevent compensatory motion of the back when one end of the wood is placed near the patient's chest. A motor sander that moves away from the patient gives passive stretching of the flexor muscles of the arm and active contraction of them in pulling the machine back toward the body.

Hammering (arm at side): This may be made a resistive exercise with stretching by placing the nail just out of the patient's reach. Resistance will be greater in extension. The weight of the tool gives resistance to flexion.

Planing: General elbow and shoulder exercise is obtained to a greater or less degree depending upon the length of the stroke. The greater resistance is in extension of the elbow and flexion of the shoulder.

Shoulder

FLEXION AND EXTENSION

Sanding: The wood should be placed vertically and raised to increase the range of motion. Wood finishing provides the same motions.

Ripsawing: If the wood is in a normal position, the greatest resistance is in elbow extension, but the return stroke of the saw gives good hyperextension of the shoulder. To increase range of motion in flexion the wood should be placed vertically. When raised above shoulder level the greatest resistance is in flexion.

Use of coping saw: This is a very light exercise for early use in treatment and provides only a limited range of motion.

ABDUCTION AND ADDUCTION, LATERAL PLANE

Sanding: Wood should be placed vertically at the patient's side and raised to give greater range of motion. The greater resistance is in abduction.

Ripsawing: The wood should be placed vertically at the patient's side and raised to give greater range of motion. The greater resistance is in abduction.

ABDUCTION AND ADDUCTION, HORIZONTAL PLANE

Sanding: The wood is placed in a horizontal position slightly below shoulder height and in front of the patient.

INTERNAL AND EXTERNAL ROTATION

Screwing: The elbow is held in complete extension to reduce forearm pronation and supination. Resistance is greater for the right arm in external rotation, for the left arm in internal rotation. Use of left-handed screws reverses resistance.

Unfortunately, occupational therapists appear not to have kept abreast of change and, by allowing the use of the equipment to outweigh the use of occupation as therapy, were instrumental in the profession losing its way, particularly with regard to the treatment of physical dysfunction. In many instances, the equipment was used but the craft discarded. Fretsaws were ridden, lathes were pedalled and FEPS handles were turned, but no wood or warp were attached to them. In many instances it was impossible to distinguish occupational therapy from physiotherapy. Many therapists (myself amongst them) were embarrassed when they set up a complex rope circuit on a weaving loom to help restore the knee extension of a young sportsman, or when they tried to convince an elderly lady that making a jigsaw whilst pedalling gingerly on a bicycle fretsaw was essential to the functioning of her newly replaced hip joint.

The realisation of the universal loss of identity within occupational therapy prompted occupational therapists to question its true values and examine what had gone wrong. Shannon (1977) felt that occupational therapy had become 'derailed' and quoted Truman (1965, cited in Shannon 1977) warning that 'A science that hesitates to forget its founders is lost', reflecting that a discipline that does indeed forget its founders may also be lost. Shannon advocated a return to the philosophy postulated by Meyer and Slagle as the profession's best hope for arresting this derailment. Such writings drove occupational therapists to investigate the roots of their practice. The original concepts of the use of occupation were revisited and our relationship with medicine explored.

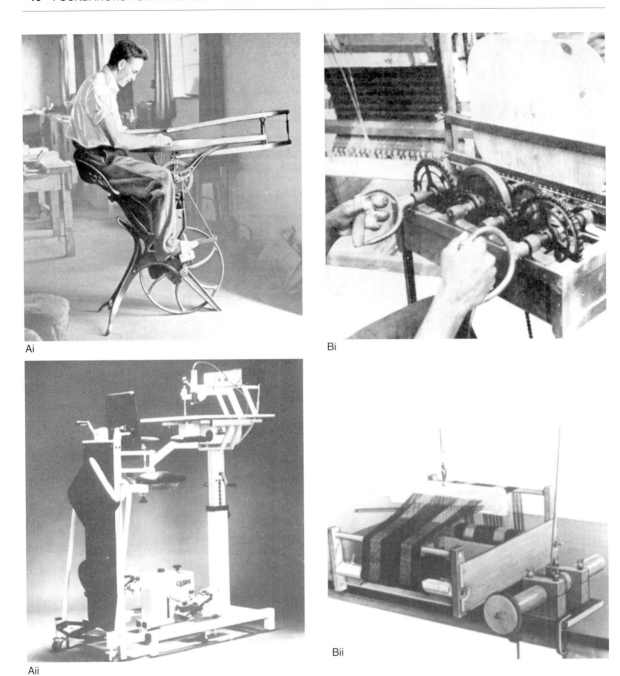

Ai

Bi

Aii

Bii

Fig. 1.5 Equipment to be used in conjunction with crafts were initially adapted, and later specially manufactured, to address limitations of strength and range of movement. (Ai) An early bicycle fretsaw (from Howarth and MacDonald 1946 The Theory of Occupational Therapy, 3rd edn, reproduced by kind permission of Ballière, Tindall & Cox, London), (Aii) the electronic cycle (from Turner 1987 The Practice of Occupational Therapy, 2nd edn, reproduced with kind permission of Churchill Livingstone, Edinburgh), (B) equipment designed to assist pronation and supination of the forearm has stood the test of time: (i) pronation and supination drilling machine (from Jones 1964 An Approach to Occupational Therapy, reproduced with kind permission of Butterworths, London), (ii) FEPS (flexion, extension, pronation and supination) apparatus attached to a rigid heddle loom (from Turner 1987 The Practice of Occupational Therapy, 2nd edn, reproduced with kind permission of Churchill Livingstone, Edinburgh), (iii) MULE (micro-processor controlled upper limb exerciser) exerciser used with a word processor.

Fig. 1.5(Biii) see opposite (top)

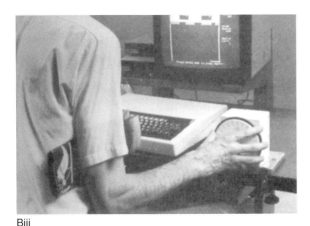

Biii

Fig. 1.5 (*continued*)

Increased knowledge and understanding of our values and beliefs led to the development of profession-specific thinking tools and language and the instigation of occupational science as a tool through which to investigate and establish the efficacy of the profession's practice.

A PHILOSOPHY FOR OCCUPATIONAL THERAPY

A philosophy can be described as a set of beliefs, values and principles that underpins actions. For a profession, a philosophy acts as a creed that shapes the thinking and actions of its members. Without a firm philosophical base against which occupational therapists can evaluate and judge their practice, research and theory, they are vulnerable to pressures, fashions, domination and erroneous developments, as we have seen (Fig. 1.6). Creek and Ormston (1996) see a philosophical base as vital to ensure that practice remains person-centred and does not become focused on techniques or theories; it provides a base against which to test and modify theories and prevents occupational therapy being subsumed in the theories of other groups.

The original concepts of early writers, recently revisited and enhanced by an expanding knowledge base in both foundation sciences and practice skills, provide a sound springboard for the philosophy of our profession. Many authors, in an attempt to identify the uniqueness of our profession, have explored and proposed a philosophy on which it may be based. Shannon (1977) quoted Meyer (1922) and Eleanor Clarke Slagle (1928, cited in Shannon 1977), who both emphasised the importance for humans of rhythm and balance between work, play, rest and sleep as requirements for healthy living. He vehemently denies any benefit occupational therapy may have gained from its adherence to the medical model, condemning the reductionism it introduced into the profession, and advocates a return to the basic theoretical tenets of the profession, which were focused on the balance and rhythm of occupations in healthy daily living and on temporal adaptation, which enables us to function competently whilst influencing, and being influenced, by our environment. Roles and rhythms were seen as vital considerations, as was the 'transforming of patients into agents managing their own lives insofar as is possible' (Smith 1974, cited in Shannon 1977).

A position statement issued by the College of Occupational Therapists in 1994 saw the essential elements of the profession being the promotion of health and wellbeing through the use of purposeful activity, with particular attention being paid to the person's roles, skills and priorities. In 1997 Kielhofner discussed what he saw as the emerging paradigm of occupational therapy and explored its core constructs: the occupational nature of humans, the problems of occupational dysfunction and the use of occupation as a health determinant.

These examples are but a few of the many writings about the philosophical basis of occupational therapy, which was explored and articulated at length in the last two decades of the 20th century. An analysis of these enables us to see a pattern of concepts emerge which leads this text to postulate the following as a philosophy on which to base the profession's practice, theory and research (Box 1.3).

PEOPLE ARE INDIVIDUAL AND INHERENTLY DIFFERENT FROM ONE ANOTHER

The basis for this element of the philosophy is found in the development of Moral Treatment –

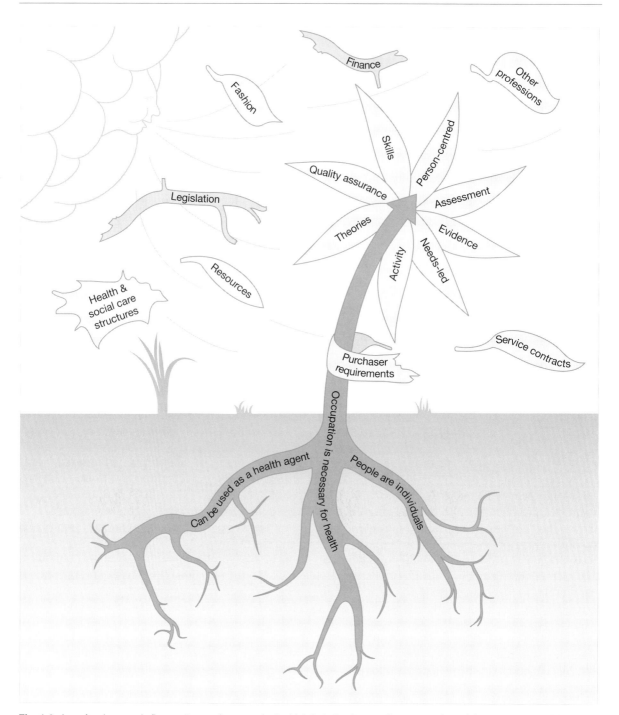

Fig. 1.6 A profession needs firm roots as a base against which to judge its practice, research and theory and to avoid being swayed by fashions and pressures.

an 18th-century movement of Anglo-French origins that was based on the fundamental belief in the essential worth of each individual and the right of each person to humane care when ill. In 1791, moved by their spiritual and humanistic beliefs, the Society of Friends, a Quaker group,

---

Box 1.3   A philosophy for occupational therapy

- People are individual and inherently different from one another
- Occupation is fundamental to health and wellbeing
- Where occupational performance has been interrupted a person can:
  - use occupation and/or activity to develop the adaptive skills required to acquire, maintain or restore occupational performance
  - modify their occupations and/or activities to facilitate occupational performance

---

felt the need to establish its own institution 'in which a milder and more appropriate system of treatment than that usually practised, might be adopted' (Tuke 1813 p23). The Society believed that existing treatment 'was too frequently calculated to depress and degrade, rather than to awaken the slumbering reason' (Tuke 1813 p23). Their institution, The Retreat, near York, was established in 1796 under the charge of a Quaker tea merchant, William Tuke.

Tuke's fundamental beliefs in people's individuality and worth were reflected in the respect and kindness with which he treated them and also by giving them responsibility for their own actions and behaviour, such that both staff and the sick person had a part to play in the individual's recovery. He reflected 'I can truly declare that by gentleness of manner, and kindness of treatment, I have seldom failed to obtain the confidence and conciliate the esteem [of people]' (Tuke 1813 p135).

Humanistic psychology

These early ideas were further developed by humanistic psychologists in the 20th century, and their belief in the concepts of personal freedom, self-determination and creativity. Two important exponents of this theory, Abraham Maslow and Carl Rogers, expanded our understanding of, and belief in, treating people as individuals.

Abraham Maslow

Maslow (1970) believed that the essence of being was that people are whole, free, healthy and purposeful. He studied healthy, well-functioning people and saw the person's motivations as being key to their wellbeing. He placed these motivations in a hierarchy (Fig. 1.7), with self-actualisation, that is the full use and exploration of talents, capacities and potentials, at the top. Maslow concluded that there is, in all individuals, a drive towards actualisation of inherent potentials, thus enhancing life, and a desire to satisfy self-identified needs, which ensures physical and psychological survival and wellbeing, thus maintaining life. Maslow postulated that a person could strive towards actualisation only once their survival needs had been satisfied. In everyday terms this would mean that a person

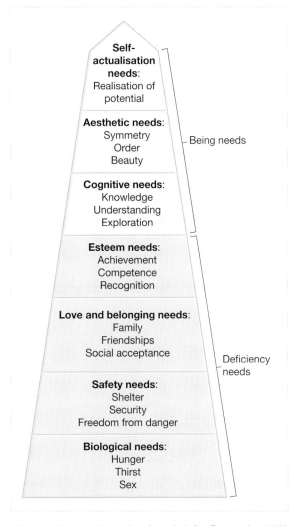

Fig. 1.7 Maslow's hierarchy of needs (after Dworetzky 1988).

could not enjoy the challenge of mastering a new computer program (esteem and self-esteem) if he had an unresolved argument with a partner (love and belonging), nor could he perform well in an examination (self-actualisation) if he was suffering from a hangover (physiological needs).

Carl Rogers

Rogers (1967) also studied individuals' abilities to maintain their health and wellbeing. He believed that people are free, are normally capable of dealing with the limitations of life and are able to be in charge of their own destiny and make choices concerning their future. He saw people as having the capacity to change and grow and, like Maslow, believed that a desire for self-actualisation underlies our actions. From these beliefs came the idea that people should exercise their capacity to develop and change in order to achieve their self-identified needs and, indeed, had a responsibility to do so.

Humanistic psychology also stressed the importance of a person's own subjective and individual view of themselves and their world. Humanists saw that subjectivity, that is, the way an individual sees a situation or event, and intuition (a person's natural instinctive feeling for something) as vital and important elements in the way people experience things. Therefore, an individual's own view of a situation is valid and important for him (see also Chapter 9).

How these beliefs influence practice

Such beliefs, as a fundamental element in the philosophy of occupational therapy, are reflected in the attitudes therapists have towards the people they work with and the ways in which they work with them.

First, occupational therapists believe that people are individuals. They do not treat them all alike, or see their opinions as being of lesser value, and should, as a result, get to know the person and facilitate him* to identify his needs in order to be

---

* Throughout the text, and purely for the sake of ease, 'he/his' is used to refer to the person receiving occupational therapy and 'she/her' is used to refer to the therapist.

able to organise appropriate intervention strategies. A belief that people are different should lead to tolerance of those who do not conform to social norms. The therapist should not be led in her decisions primarily by the person's diagnosis, nor by the needs, fashions and pressures of the service in which she works – an element that is sometimes difficult to identify and overcome. Thus, the therapist's belief in humanistic principles gives rise to a person-centred approach (see Chapter 2).

Second, occupational therapists believe that the way a person views something is important and should be treated as reality for that individual. She shows this belief through expressing an understanding of the person's feeling and accepting it as valid for him. For example, if a person has undergone trauma that has affected coordination in all four limbs, the therapist should not dismiss the fact that his primary concern is that he cannot hold a newspaper simply because she feels his overriding difficulty is that he cannot walk. Related to this is the therapist's belief in the worth of individuals. If she believes people are of worth then her action must be to respect their opinions. Where, for instance, a decision has to be made about the discharge destination for an elderly person, or where assessment is being made for a piece of equipment, the person's opinions and expectations are of equal importance and value to those of the therapist. The therapist's knowledge of motivation, coupled with her respect for people's opinions, lead her to believe that a decision made primarily by a person himself is more likely to be upheld than one that is made by others on his behalf. How many occupational therapists, with the wisdom of hindsight, can remember occasions in which they have seen equipment ordered for an individual, or have advised on different strategies, only to discover some time later that the equipment has not been used, or that the person is adhering to their old ways because they had not been sufficiently involved in the decision-making process and do not want to incorporate the change suggested by another.

Such beliefs also affect and dictate the relationship developed with an individual, which should be one based on mutual respect and cooperation. The therapist, in believing that an individual is responsible for his life and in charge of his destiny, will work with him to help facilitate his ability to make decisions regarding his treatment and to develop skills that the person sees as appropriate.

Occupational therapists also believe that a healthy person has the ability to adapt to unforeseen circumstances so that he can carry on with his life in a way that is meaningful to him. Whilst not everyone will adapt to a similar circumstance in the same way (for example, one person whose car fails to start on the way to work in the morning may ask for a lift from a neighbour, another may fetch his toolkit and tackle the job himself, a third may call a taxi whilst another may telephone a motoring organisation or perhaps phone in sick to work!) each person will be able to alter his behaviour in order to deal effectively with the unforeseen circumstance. The therapist is optimistic about the person's ability to shape his life. In believing that he has a responsibility for his own life the therapist will encourage the person to strive actively to reshape it. She will, therefore, use only those strategies that will actively involve the person in participating towards achieving his own aims and will not use media that require the person to be passive. She will, however, be sensitive to cultural differences, which may not concur with this element of our philosophy.

Last, in believing that actualisation is the prime motivator for action, the occupational therapist should work with the person to identify the areas he sees as important and in which he wishes to fulfil his potential. Intervention should be based on activities that have meaning for that person and these will then act as inherent motivators. For example, for an elderly person aiming to regain upper limb function, activities related to his grandchildren (making cakes for the school fête or a rack to hold CDs) would be meaningful, whereas for a young person with similar difficulties, activities that incorporate his interest in sport or music may help towards regaining skills.

Having a knowledge of, and a respect for, the people she is working with is of prime importance to the occupational therapist. Treating people as individuals, accepting their view of events, encouraging them to take responsibility for the way their life progresses, and believing in

their ability to do so, are the main ways in which the occupational therapist's belief in people as individuals is translated into her everyday professional practice.

OCCUPATION IS FUNDAMENTAL TO HEALTH AND WELLBEING

'To do is to be' (Mill, cited in Cracknell 1993). If we watch people going about their daily business it is easy to concur with the idea that humans are occupational by nature (Box 1.4). Occupation continues to occur spontaneously through the life of healthy individuals. As a person grows older the nature of their 'doing' will change. This change, and the content of their occupations, will be determined, in part, by their perceived roles and responsibilities and influenced by the culture and society in which they live (see also Chapter 9). Deviation from the boundaries of occupation set by the group within which the person lives is often not acceptable and can lead to negative feedback and lowered self-esteem.

Occupation is that which defines and organises a sphere of action over a period of time and is perceived by the individual as part of his identity, that is, it is something that the person 'owns'. By contrast, within the context of occupational therapy, activity is seen as the short-term tasks undertaken by individuals in relation to the development and meeting of occupational goals. Occupation, therefore, drives activity. Occupation may be related to a role title, such as farmer or dancer, or may organise a sphere of activity that reflects the person's self-identity but which brings no particular role

---

Box 1.4   Meyer's five fundamental assumptions regarding the occupational nature of humans

- A fundamental link exists between health and occupation
- Healthy occupation maintains a balance between existing, thinking and acting
- A unity exists between mind and body
- When participation in occupation is interrupted mind and body deteriorate
- As occupation maintains mind and body it is suited to the restoration of functional ability

with the title, such as the image of oneself as an independent person or one who believes in helping the welfare of others. Thus, a person's occupations are reflected in the content and manner of the activities he performs. A young adult, for example, may spend his day in personal care activities, eating, travelling to work or college, meeting and talking with friends, working, playing in a band and organising a charity event, and each of his activities will reflect the image he holds of himself as, for example, an independent person, student, musician and charity worker. As a person progresses through life his occupations, roles and beliefs, will vary as do the number and pace of activities he performs to undertake them (for further information see also Chapter 2).

It can be seen, therefore, that to maintain a state of occupational wellbeing, people require a balance of occupations and this is reflected in the habits and routines that control the rhythm of our lives. Routines and habits that are balanced between activities of productivity (which may be related to maintaining our environment and/or acquiring sustenance), self-maintenance (related to the care of the individual) and leisure activities (in which the person has the opportunity to fulfil his own creative, aesthetic, physical, social or intellectual pursuits) will maintain a state of wellbeing. Healthy individuals have flexible and adaptable routines that reflect their abilities, responsibilities and potentials.

The therapist sees her area of concern as the restoration or acquisition of occupational wellbeing in a person who is in a state of occupational dysfunction. In being aware of the need for balance in occupations the therapist will address dysfunctions in all areas of the person's life and, where necessary, encourage the restoration or acquisition of a balance of occupations related to his daily living skills, productivity and leisure. The therapist, in believing that occupation brings its own reward, will use, either as a therapeutic medium or as an aim for the restoration of occupational wellbeing, those activities that hold particular interest and meaning for the individual and will therefore act as prime motivators. In carrying forward this belief into practice, the therapist will be able to assess the person's need and use, or facilitate, meaningful activity in order to help the person acquire occupational wellbeing. This concept is discussed in greater length in Chapter 2.

THE USE OF OCCUPATION AND ACTIVITY TO RESTORE OCCUPATIONAL PERFORMANCE

Where occupational performance has been interrupted a person can:

- use occupation and/or activity to develop the adaptive skills required to acquire, maintain or restore occupational performance
- modify their occupations and/or activities in order to facilitate occupational performance.

Within the philosophy of Moral Treatment was the belief that mental illness occurred when people failed to adapt successfully to external pressures. As a result they were seen to either adopt faulty coping strategies or, indeed, to adopt no alternative strategies at all. These early assumptions have formed the basis of the belief that occupational dysfunction in any aspect of a person's life can occur as a result of the person's inability to acquire adaptive skills. This may occur for a variety of reasons.

First, a child may fail to develop adaptive skills as a result of dysfunction manifest at birth or in early childhood. A child, for example, who cannot explore the environment as a result of motor or sensory dysfunction, and possibly also because of overprotection by his parents, will be unable to develop the normal movement patterns or motor skills required to participate in everyday physical activities. His inability to move normally will not only prevent him developing adaptive motor and sensory skills (so that he can learn, for example, not to lose his balance while playing on his rocking horse or not to put his hand too near to the teapot because it is hot) but will also impede his development of social, language and other global skills because of his inability to participate in everyday experiences and relationships.

Alternatively, physical dysfunction as a result of an acquired illness, such as a traumatic, metabolic or vascular condition, may inhibit or curtail a person's ability to use existing adaptive skills. His situation can appear so overwhelming that he cannot, on his own, acquire the necessary new adaptive skills he needs for successful occupational performance. For example, an adult who has suffered a head injury will need assistance to acquire new adaptive skills, such as improving motor and cognitive function in order to regain his ability to look after his garden, drive his car or return to his job. Additionally, he will need help in modifying activities in order to restore occupational performance. He may, for example, need to learn strategies to assist with shortfall in memory, or need help to adapt his telephone to compensate for poor speech.

However, it may be considered that maladaptive performance can be the cause, as well as the outcome, of some physical dysfunctions. Circumstances in which a person fails to adapt successfully to external stresses and adopts maladaptive coping strategies have been shown to lead to physical or psychological disorders.

Developing adaptive skills

It can be seen, therefore, that when successful adaptation is impaired, for whatever reason, occupational performance will be interrupted. It is this interruption of occupational performance that is the prime concern of the occupational therapist. Thus it is the impact that a dysfunction has on a person, rather than the dysfunction itself, that is the focus of occupational therapy. For example, for an occupational therapist working with a person who has an amputation of a lower limb, the main focus of intervention of occupational therapy is not on the state of the remaining part of the limb, nor primarily on the way the person uses his prosthetic limb, but rather on the impact this change, and the related loss of adaptive skills, has on those activities the person wishes or needs to perform in his everyday life.

Because of their belief in individuals' abilities and responsibility to influence their environment and their health, occupational therapists see that a person's way forward in gaining or regaining adaptive skills is through his own efforts, that is, through active participation in their treatment. Such active participation may take many forms and occupational therapists develop and encourage this by facilitating the person to make decisions, solve problems, develop new behaviours

and habits, determine priorities and other similar strategies in order to help the person gain control over his dysfunction. When this approach to facilitating occupational performance is taken the therapist generally draws on the principles of the learning, biomechanical, developmental or adaptive frames of reference (see Chapter 3).

Modifying occupation

Where occupational performance has been limited by dysfunction and the occupational therapist considers that intervention to restore adaptive skills is not feasible, she may feel that the most appropriate method of restoring that performance is through adaptation not of the person, but of the occupation or the activity. For example, where a person has limited respiratory function because of a chronic respiratory condition, efforts to restore his abilities to their previous level would seem inappropriate. In this instance, therefore, the occupational therapist would endeavour not to change the person's capacities to fit the existing occupations or activities but to adapt them in order that they can be performed within his existing level of performance. She may, for example, modify or negate the need to climb upstairs to visit the bathroom or bedroom by discussing the installation of a banister or stairlift, the creation of a downstairs facility, or the possibility of moving to a flat or bungalow. Alternatively, for a person who has difficulty doing the laundry, she may discuss with him the possibility of using different equipment (a lightweight iron, for example, or a combined washer/dryer), of paying for a laundry service or of employing a homecarer. Where this approach to facilitating occupational performance is taken, the therapist should always work through a hierarchy of methods, starting with the least complex and invasive, in order to meet the person's needs (see Chapter 7). This approach to intervention and problem solving utilises the principles of the compensatory frame of reference (see Chapter 3).

It is interesting to note that with current demographic, medical and legislative changes, the use of this frame of reference to facilitate occupational performance in those with long-term occupational dysfunction, is forming an ever-increasing part of the occupational therapist's role.

CONCLUSION

In conclusion, it can be seen that the concepts that form the basis of occupational therapy today have their roots in ancient times, even though the profession itself was established at the beginning of the 20th century. Throughout the development of the profession, beliefs have been held about occupation as fundamental to the establishment, maintenance and restoration of health and of the need to see each person as an individual with their own identified needs. This chapter has debated how these concepts drive occupational therapy practice and how loss of identification with them can damage the profession's progress.

ACKNOWLEDGEMENT

I would like to thank Irene Paterson, MEd, FCOT, T Dip COT, SROT, for her constructive and challenging thoughts, and for her help in the production of this chapter.

REFERENCES

College of Occupational Therapists 1994 Core skills and a conceptual framework for practice – a position statement. College of Occupational Therapists, London

College of Occupational Therapists 2000a A definition of occupational therapy. College of Occupational Therapists, London

College of Occupational Therapists 2000b Code of ethics and professional conduct for occupational therapists. College of Occupational Therapists, London

Cracknell E 1993 British Journal of Occupational Therapy 56(11):39

Creek J, Ormston C 1996 The essential elements of professional motivation. British Journal of Occupational Therapy 59(1):7–10

Department of Health 1999 The Health Act. HMSO, London

Dunton WR 1950 A history of occupational therapy. In: Dunton WR, Licht S (eds) Occupational therapy, principles and practice. Charles C Thomas, Springfield, IL

Groundes-Peace ZC 1957 An outline of the development of occupational therapy in Scotland. Scottish Journal of Occupational Therapy 30(9):16–43

Haas LJ 1925 Occupational therapy for the mentally and nervously ill. Bruce Publishing Company, Wisconsin

Howarth NA, MacDonald EM 1940 Theory of occupational therapy for students and nurses. Baillière, Tindall & Cox, London

Howarth NA, MacDonald EM 1946 Theory of occupational therapy, 3rd edn. Baillière, Tindall & Cox, London

Jones MS 1964 An approach to occupational therapy, 2nd edn. Butterworths, London

Kielhofner G 1997 Conceptual foundations of occupational therapy, 2nd edn. FA Davis, Philadelphia, PA

Licht S 1948 Occupational therapy source book. Williams and Wilkins Company, Baltimore, MD

MacDonald EM, MacCaul G, Murrey L 1970 Occupational therapy in rehabilitation, 3rd edn. Baillière Tindall, London

Maslow A 1970 Motivation and personality, 2nd edn. Harper & Row, New York

Meyer A 1922 A philosophy of occupational therapy. Reprinted from The Archives of Occupational Therapy, vol 1, pp 1–10 in American Journal of Occupational Therapy 1977 31(10):639–642

Paterson CF 1997 An historical perspective of work practice services. In: Pratt Z, Jacobs K (eds) Work practice: international perspectives pages. Butterworth-Heinemann, Oxford, pp 25–28

Reilly M 1962 Occupational therapy can be one of the great ideas of twentieth century medicine. American Journal of Occupational Therapy 16(1):1–9

Rogers C 1967 On becoming a person. Constable, London

Shannon PD 1977 The derailment of occupational therapy. American Journal of Occupational Therapy 31(4):229–234

Tuke S 1813 Description of the retreat. Reprinted 1964 by Dawsons, London

Willard HS, Spackman CS 1947 Principles of occupational therapy. JB Lippincott Company, Philadelphia

FURTHER READING

Dunton WR 1945 Prescribing occupational therapy, 2nd edn. Charles C Thomas, Springfield, IL

Glover MR 1984 The Retreat, York, An early experiment in the treatment of mental illness. William Sessions, York

Licht S 1967 The founding and founders of the American Occupational Therapy Association. American Journal of Occupational Therapy xx1(5):269–277

Mayers CA 1990 A philosophy unique to occupational therapy. British Journal of Occupational Therapy 53(9):379–380

2

Occupation for therapy

Annie Turner

INTRODUCTION

The use of occupation as therapy is the central core of our profession. Chapter 1 explored how this concept forms the philosophical basis from which occupational therapists work and how it is used to judge the boundaries of our professional activities. What, however, do we really mean by the term 'occupation'?

Throughout the history of the profession there has been active debate about the meaning of the term and its relationship to other terms and phrases commonly used by occupational therapists. 'Activity', 'meaningful activity' and 'purposeful activity', for example, are often used interchangeably with 'occupation'. However, can we really say we have a true understanding of the specific meaning of each of these terms? The term 'occupation' has also been used as a basis from which profession-specific terminology has been developed. We hear about 'occupational performance', 'occupational need' and 'occupational form'. These terms have been coined relatively recently to enhance concepts within the profession and provide bases for thinking and practice.

Surely, then, it behoves us to own a clear understanding of the term from which the title and concept of our profession stems. In order to use occupation successfully and confidently as therapy it is essential for all occupational therapists to understand the concepts underlying the term 'occupation'. Equally, our own understanding will enhance, demonstrate and direct the clarity and boundaries of our professional activities. It will enable us to clearly articulate, evaluate and develop these from a sound base. We will be able to use our own understanding to explain and judge what we do and, as importantly, what we don't do, in order to contain and control our profession's growth and development.

DEFINING OCCUPATION

In recent years attempts have been made to define the term occupation within the context of occupational therapy. What emerges from these attempts is that 'occupation', as used by occupational therapists, cannot be defined in a trite phrase which will trip off the tongue with ease. Certain themes, however, emerge consistently (Box 2.1).

Occupations are the fabric of 'doings' of people's everyday lives

Golledge (1998a) describes occupations as 'part of an individual's lifestyle' performed 'in a manner that reflects an individual's personal style'. Occupation is seen as the core aspect of people's existence through which they fulfil basic needs. Wilcock (1993a) defines occupation as the 'central aspect of human experience' and a 'natural human phenomenon' whilst Darnel and Heater (1994) state that occupation refers to 'human doing'.

Box 2.1   Concepts within the ways occupational therapists use the term occupation

- Occupations are the fabric of 'doings' of people's everyday lives.
- Occupations are driven by people's aspirations, needs and environments.
- Occupations relate to the purposeful use of time as defined by the individual.
- Occupations are the means through which people control the balance of their lives.

Occupations are driven by people's aspirations, needs and environments

People 'do' according to what they wish, need or feel obliged to achieve and do so in a way that reflects their roles, culture, environment, experience and abilities. People adapt their 'doing' to control, or in response to, the environments in which they perform. The relationship between roles and occupation is indivisible, for these determine the duties, expectations, desires and rhythms of our lives. Kielhofner and Forsyth (1997) felt that roles organise our behaviour through influencing the sets of tasks we undertake, the partitioning of our daily and weekly cycles and the manner and style in which we interact with others.

Occupations relate to the purposeful use of time as defined by the individual

Occupations are unique to each individual because their content relates to the importance that person places on the outcomes they wish, need or feel obliged to achieve. Occupation is therefore individually defined, valued, given meaning and organised. A purposeful occupation is one that fulfils goals that are meaningful to the person. It is true to say, therefore, that there can be no such thing as universally meaningful or purposeful occupations.

Occupations are the means through which people control and balance their lives

People make decisions about what they will and won't, should and shouldn't, prefer and don't prefer to do and when, where, how and with whom they will do it. Leaky (1978, cited in Wilcock 1993b), contends that 'humans are different, not so much for what we do ... but the fact that we can [i.e. are able to] do more or less what we want'. Whilst this may be so, humans are both facilitated and constrained by their skills, roles, responsibilities and environment. Levels of control change during a lifetime and according to a person's circumstances. Few people, if any, are free to choose exactly what they do but, as adults, they can possess the ability to control the balance of their occupations.

In endeavouring to establish what occupation does mean in the context of occupational therapy, it is equally important to look at what it doesn't mean. Also, it is especially important to differentiate occupation from activity. Kielhofner (1993) suggested that occupation was not related to sexual, survival or social activities while Mocellin (1992) suggests that occupation 'does not relate to activities concerned with bodily function'. Other authors have endeavoured to separate and define activity from occupation. Hagedorn (1995) reviews occupation using the concepts of organisation and fulfilment of roles; she describes activity in terms of task and purpose within a finite period. Similar concepts emerge in Kielhofner and Forsyth's (1997) proposal of the difference between activity choices and occupational choices. Activity choices are seen as 'short term, deliberate decisions to enter and exit occupational activities'; occupational choices are a 'deliberate commitment to enter an occupational role, acquire a new habit or undertake a personal project'. Whilst it could be contended that perhaps not all occupational roles are entered into deliberately (inherited roles within a family, for example, such as becoming 'head' of a family or being responsible for ageing parents), the concepts within the many definitions of 'activity' appear to portray it as a specific, time-defined task. Within the context of occupational therapy therefore, activities form the short-term tasks undertaken by individuals in relation to the development and meeting of longer-term occupational needs. By contrast, 'occupation' defines and organises a sphere of action over a period of time and is part of a person's personal and social identity.

OCCUPATION, HEALTH AND WELLBEING

In defining occupation as a natural and central human phenomenon it is important to explore the fundamental reasons why people undertake occupation.

At its simplest, occupation is seen as an innate drive to fulfil the needs through which humans survive. If survival is seen first and foremost as the fulfilment of basic needs for food, water, sleep, reproduction, shelter and safety, humans undertake occupations in order to survive and remain healthy. Needs, therefore, can be viewed as 'inbuilt health agents' (Wilcock 1993b). Wilcock also proposes that needs warn and protect people by causing discomforts (such as pain, fear and hunger), which require action in order to be allayed. Needs also reward the use of capacities through providing the need for the pursuit of satisfaction, fulfilment, belonging and pleasure, and are also seen as a means of preventing disorder through drives for exploration, thought, communication and understanding. Needs are therefore seen as physiological phenomena that provide motivation and, as such, cause humans to be seen as occupational by nature. Wilcock (1993b) quotes extracts from the diaries of the explorer James Cook, written between 1768 and 1771, which record that he found people from primitive societies to be happy and healthy, whilst Virey, a French physician/philosopher, wrote in 1828 that 'people living a culturally primitive life are generally more physically perfect than those from affluent societies'. In fulfilling basic needs within a 'natural' environment humans were seen to maintain health and happiness. According to Wilcock, therefore, it would seem that the fulfilment of fundamental needs by means of occupational behaviour is the foundation of healthy living.

Linked to health is wellbeing, a state variously described as a subjective assessment of health and related to feelings such as self-esteem, happiness, possessing energy and having satisfying relationships. Health, too, is viewed as much as a self-defined mental, as a physical, state. Indeed, as far back as 1946, the World Health Organization (WHO) defined health as 'A state of physical and mental wellbeing, not merely the absence of disease or infirmity' (WHO 1946, cited in Wilcock 1998c), a definition that is still in use today.

Table 2.1 Human drives and needs – behaviour is seen as being driven by the fulfilment of physiological needs or of genetically based desires (based on Reiss 2000 and Wilcock 1993)

Wilcock (1993)	Reiss (2000)
Human needs that drive behaviour	*Genetically based desires and values that drive behaviour*
Those that warn and protect through experiences of discomfort	
Needs to avoid:	*Desires to:*
pain/tension	avoid aversive sensations
hunger	eat
anxiety/fear/anger	avoid aversive sensations
loneliness	seek social contact
Those that prevent disorder and use capacities	
Needs to:	*Desires for:*
expend energy	physical activity
explore and understand	learning
spend time with others	spending time with relatives
Those that reward the use of capacities	
Needs for:	*Desires for:*
purpose	social prestige
pleasure	public service prestige
satisfaction	
fulfilment	
	Additional desires for:
Additional needs for:	order
expression of thought	sex
utilisation of ideas	independence
	vengeance
	power

Recent research appears to confirm these findings. Warburton (1998) has shown that the pursuit of pleasure can boost the immune system and thus enhance health whilst Reiss (2000) postulates that human behaviour is driven by 16 fundamental desires and values, which, he claims, have a genetic basis. These values appear to link closely to Wilcock's groups of needs and include drives and values related to curiosity, food, social contact, exercise and assertive behaviour (Table 2.1).

OCCUPATIONAL BALANCE AND IDENTITY

The satisfaction of basic needs directed the occupational behaviour of primitive humans. As humans developed their capacities so their societies grew and satisfying survival needs occupied relatively less time, thus leaving more space for creativity and the pursuit of pleasure. As different cultures and societies emerged, occupa-tional behaviours were moulded by the environments, beliefs, characteristics and skills that the different cultures developed and valued. Today it is felt that in order to maintain health, people's occupations must comprise a balance between the ability to look after themselves (self care), their contribution to their social and economic environments (productivity) and the fulfilment and enjoyment of life (leisure).

Self care

Self care relates to the occupations a person performs in order to take care of himself and are often referred to as personal activities of daily living. These include bathing, hair care, dental care, using the WC, eating, sleeping and dressing. With the exception of eating, the majority of the components of these activities are usually performed in private and within an individual's personal style, manner and standard.

Productivity

Productivity involves occupations in which a person contributes in some way to the maintenance of his social and/or economic community. Included here are tasks related to homecare (housework, gardening, household and car maintenance); family care (food preparation, care of family members, shopping and pet care) and work (paid, unpaid or study).

Leisure

Leisure, described by Kielhofner and Forsyth (1997) as 'adult play', comprises those occupations said to be undertaken for pleasure. Their range is enormous and particularly culturally determined. My own research (Turner 1997) found the most frequently identified leisure pursuits by British adults who considered themselves to be healthy to be watching TV; reading; socialising in pubs, cafés and at home; attending clubs, events and meetings; sports; holidays and travel; listening to music and telephoning family and friends.

While it is relatively straightforward to view occupations within these three categories it must be remembered that, because occupations are self-identified in terms of their meaning, it may not be as simple as it seems to classify them. Closer examination shows, for example, that shopping and gardening have been classed as leisure by some whilst for others they are seen as productivity. Pet care is also classed in both these categories whilst keeping fit and eating are mentioned under both self care and leisure. Driving, whilst predominantly seen as productivity, is classed according to the activity to which it is linked. Driving to one's place of employment is seen as part of work, driving to the supermarket is linked to family care (both are productivity), driving to and from a pub is classified by some as leisure and driving to the gym as self care (Fig. 2.1). These classifications reinforce the notion that meaning, and therefore purpose, are in the mind of the performer and not in the eye of the beholder.

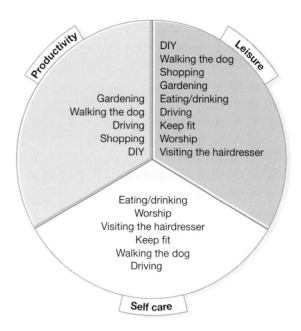

Fig. 2.1 Differences in the classifications of some occupations by healthy adults (Turner 1997).

However viewed, the balance of occupations classed under these categories is seen as essential to the maintenance of health. We appear to have an inherent knowledge that this is so and expressions such as 'All work and no play make Jack a dull boy' (an adage originating in the 17th century) are passed down through generations. Similar adages can be traced back in history. In the Bible, for instance, we are told that 'God blessed the seventh day ...: because that in it he had rested from all his work' (Genesis 1:3). Primeau (1995) cites 'If a man insists always in being serious and never allowing himself a bit of fun and relaxation, he would go mad or become unstable without knowing it' (taken from the 'Histories of Herodutus' bk 1 ch 173, cited in Bartlett 1980 p78). Also along this line, Primeau quotes Meyer, a founder of occupational therapy, who wrote in 1922 'The whole of human organisation has its shape in a kind of rhythm ... work and play, rest and sleep, which our organism must be able to balance even under difficulty. The only way to attain balance in all this is actual doing'. My research (Turner 1997) appears to confirm that adults who consider themselves to

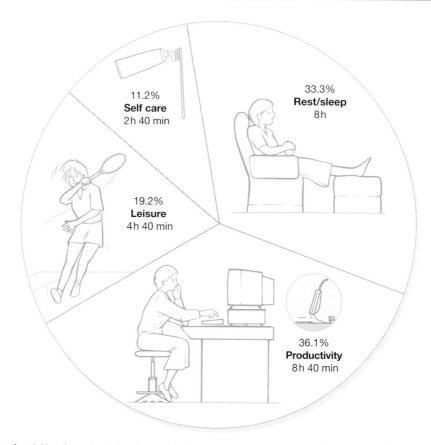

11.2%
Self care
2 h 40 min

33.3%
Rest/sleep
8 h

19.2%
Leisure
4 h 40 min

36.1%
Productivity
8 h 40 min

Fig. 2.2 Balance of activities throughout the day as identified by people who consider themselves to be healthy (Turner 1997).

be healthy demonstrate a balance between these self-identified occupational categories throughout the day (Fig. 2.2). The importance of balance, then, would seem inherent and paramount for health.

IS OCCUPATION ALWAYS HEALTH GIVING?

We have seen that the balance of occupational behaviours in primitive cultures leads to health and happiness. There is also evidence that early civilisations valued a balance of work and leisure. Aristotle, a 3rd century Greek philosopher, believed happiness depended on leisure and that people worked in order to enjoy leisure. He felt that leisure should be freely chosen.

Prior to the industrial revolution, people's lives were dictated more by the rhythms of nature than they are today. The seasons, the spring births of farm animals, harvesting and tides all controlled the rhythms of people's lives. With industrialisation, this natural rhythm was compromised, to be overprinted for many by indoor factory work, where lives were dictated not by nature but by industrialists. Hours were long, conditions poor and work and leisure were separated in time and place. New rhythms and concepts eventually arose: the weekend, holidays, retirement and prolonged childhood, and it is from these rhythms that the balance within industrialised societies must now exist. Today, modern technology has removed our appreciation of the rhythms of nature still further. We can buy strawberries in December, turn up the central heating to maintain a constant temperature at home all year round and use a machine to wash and dry the laundry. On a different scale, developments in cloning farm animals mean that farmers will not have to wait for the natural birthing season – spring.

So how possible is it to retain natural rhythms and balance in the 21st century? Many people's lives are controlled by contracts, public transport or road systems, fashions, the clock and consumerism. Increasing expectations at work, in self-presentation, in childcare and in standards of living and leisure pursuits have led to many people feeling time-pressured (Primeau 1995). The increasing use of technology, people's pursuit of ever more technology and the resultant reduction in the use of our human survival capacities has had profound changes on the way people act. Mocellin (1992) states that 'It is through personal income that an individual is normally able to satisfy the need that he or she may have for engaging in other occupations [than paid work]'. Where we once walked, we now drive; where we once did housework, we now press a button; where we once laboured in the field, we may now sit at a desk. In 1968 Maslow (cited in Wilcock 1993b, p21) observed: 'capacities clamor to be used, and cease their clamor only when they are well used. That is, capacities are also needs. Not only is it fun to use our capacities, but it is also necessary for growth. The unused skill can become a disease centre or else atrophy and disappear'.

Modern industrialised lifestyles have been linked increasingly with stress and the results of over- or underemployment and inactivity. Many circulatory, digestive and malignant diseases have been traced, in part at least, to lack of physical activity, overprocessed diets, smoking and chemicals in food and the environment. Indeed, Mocellin (1995) feels that 'it is difficult to deny that occupation, however it might be defined, is today a significant cause of unhappiness and ill health'. In substantiation he cites concepts that underpin not only wage labour but unemployment, industrial hazards and sweatshop working as examples to counter the idea that health and occupation are necessarily always interlinked. We are also aware of the problems people experience through role conflict and role overload.

In recent years, however, it appears that a rise in humane awareness and evidence of the effects of modern Western lifestyles are causing a shift in the collective consciousness. The desire to gain more contact with the natural world and to drop out of a fast track existence, the popularity of gardening and the increased uptake of sport, the use of gymnasia and attention to diet and wholefoods have resulted from an awareness of the negative, unhealthy effects of some modern occupational behaviour. They aim to redress the balance of productivity, leisure, self care and rest. Looking back to different times in history when societal pressures and changes have caused a dramatic imbalance in occupational behaviour, there has been an inherent, corresponding drive to restore the balance. As a counter to the hustle and bustle of modern life, Handsaker (1998) extolled the importance of meaningful inactivity such as reflection, quietude and contemplation.

Where, then, does this leave occupational therapists? Is our fundamental belief in the links between health and occupation under threat? I believe not. It would be foolhardy for any profession not to challenge and evaluate its basic beliefs and, indeed, professional growth is often achieved from this process. A true understanding of the debate around health and occupation, alluded to only briefly here, is essential for occupational therapists. Not only does it help us understand the polarised effects of occupation on health but it allows us to be confident, rather than defensive, when our beliefs are questioned. There are inevitably elements of truth in these challenges and a mature profession will address these and learn from them. There has been an explosion of evidence in the last few years related to the efficacy of occupational therapy based on the belief that occupation is related to health, but clearly we need to learn yet more about this link in order to evaluate the criticisms.

OCCUPATION AS A PERSON-CENTRED CONCEPT

In understanding that occupational behaviour is driven by individual needs and aspirations it has been appreciated that occupation is a personal construct. This, therefore, must lead the therapist to believe that, because occupational behaviour is individual to each person's view of their life, there can be no such thing as a generic purposeful activity. Radomski (1995) reminded us that quality of life is personally defined and emphasised the importance for occupational therapists to look at the potency, rather than just the frequency and duration of the occupations and activities a person undertakes. How, then, can we begin to define a purposeful activity for each individual?

Based on their philosophical concepts, occupational therapists have for many years endeavoured to empathise with a person's situation. They have based the direction of their intervention on helping the person re-establish those functions that are most important to him and embraced a person-centred approach within their practice. Sumsion (1999) defines person (client)-centred occupational therapy as a partnership between the therapist and the individual receiving intervention. She states (Sumsion 1999 p56) that:

The client's occupational goals are given priority and are at the centre of assessment and treatment. The therapist listens to and respects the client's standards and adapts the intervention to meet the client's needs. The client participates actively in negotiating goals for intervention and is empowered to make decisions. The therapist and the client work together to address the issues presented by a variety of environments to enable the client to fulfil his or her role expectations.

A phenomenological approach, which sits comfortably with an occupational therapist's belief in the need for person-centred practice, is one way to achieve this. This type of approach was defined by Finlay (1999) as one that seeks to understand, describe and interpret human behaviour from the perspective of the person being studied, in order to help establish the meaning and impact a person's situation has on his life. It helps the therapist enter the person's life world and see things from his point of view. To achieve this, Finlay emphasised the importance of suspending one's own presuppositions, interpretations and prior understandings in order to understand the other person's way of looking at things. Story telling, personal accounts and narratives, observation, reflective interviews, diaries and the writing of a personal mission statement are all methods that help people articulate their understanding of their situation and begin to compare the 'what was' with the 'what is'. They can then begin to discuss, make decisions about, and form expectations regarding the 'what's to come'. In this way the importance of different losses may be identified, prioritised and addressed. Mattingly (1991), cited in Wood (1995), proposed the use of applied phenomenology to help gain an understanding of a person's occupational behaviours from his own perspective. She stated that this approach enabled occupational therapists to 'walk into people's personal worlds in order to understand the meaning that patients ascribe to their illness and other life experience' (Mattingley 1991, cited in Wood 1995 p48).

MAKING ASSUMPTIONS ABOUT MEANINGFUL AND PURPOSEFUL OCCUPATIONS

To be truly person-centred, therefore, means that we should always work with the individual's specific needs and goals and endeavour to see things from his perspective. In reality, though, this can be difficult. In a busy service, do we not tend to make assumptions about what will be a meaningful occupation for the people we treat and have a repertoire of activities readily available to draw on? This is perhaps a situation that we need to consider objectively. How often have we undertaken 'dressing practice' routinely because a functional assessment shows a person cannot dress himself and we have made the assumption that independence in this area is meaningful for him? Fair and Barnitt (1999) have suggested that there is an assumption by occupational therapists that they know how certain activities, such as dressing and getting in and out of the bath, 'should' be done, even though there is little evidence to support these assumptions. Equally, do we ever assume that making a hot drink and a snack is more meaningful to the person than, for example, using the telephone? Again, Fair and Barnitt (1999) demonstrated that tea making, for example, was not always culturally relevant or held a place within a person's lifestyle. Do we concentrate our efforts so strongly on personal care activities in order to make someone 'safe' for discharge that we ignore the real fears and needs in his life? Are we too focused on serving the institution by clearing beds and enhancing throughput figures?

That being said, we undertake these activities in part because we feel that the expectations, choices and routines that govern many people contain common factors. We see it as reasonable to assume that within our culture there is a pool of core activities from which we can draw that will be meaningful to many. Could we argue that without pulling, in some way, from a repertoire of generic activities our service would become too expensive in time and resources, and thus non-viable within current restraints? Perhaps the answer lies somewhere along a continuum of total individualism on the one hand and stereotypical, routine interventions on the other.

The problem is that if we make illegitimate assumptions about the purposefulness and meaningfulness of occupations within people's lives we may well get it wrong. Knutas and Borall (1995) demonstrated this in a study looking at the outcomes, for two men, of intervention following stroke. They showed that the interventions had failed to address the fact that the most important impact of stroke for them had related to their view of it within their lives. Their subsequent outcomes and attitudes following therapy related to the retention or loss of roles within the family more than their level of functional ability. One man, who saw no advantage to being cast in the sick role, retained his roles at work and within the family, whilst accepting that these were now carried out within limitations. However, the other man, who planned to do things 'when he was better' gave his role as central man in the family to his son. The evaluation of the interventions a year later showed that the outcomes related to the men's attitudes, values and interests rather than to their initial levels of functional ability. In making assumptions about their needs based mainly on their functional level, the occupational therapist had missed the point about what was really necessary.

Radomski (1995) confirmed this, stating that factors contributing to poor quality of life (also following stroke) are linked to loss of roles and lack of self-confidence rather than to functional ability. She felt that occupational therapists overemphasise the recovery of physical skills and also that these are often defined as being purposeful by the therapist, rather than the individual.

Incorrect assumptions can be made not only from asking insufficient questions but also from not remembering to ask questions at all. Stephenson and Wiles (2000) showed that the assumption made by many occupational therapists was that home-based treatment was of greater relevance and more motivating than hospital-based treatment. Whilst this was supported by legislation it was not seen as such by users. Similarly, Nocon and Pleace (1997) showed how disabled people felt that they were not consulted or listened to by professional staff when housing decisions were made. Incorrect assumptions were made about their needs and wishes.

Offering person-centred intervention within a large institutional service is not easy. The occupational therapist needs to strike a balance between providing interventions that truly meet people's needs and running a viable service that draws from a portfolio of activities. She must ensure that she asks the right questions in order to provide for a person's needs whilst, at the same time, working within the demands of the service provider.

MAKING DECISIONS FOR ACUTELY ILL PEOPLE

The issue of making assumptions also arises when people cannot identify, or articulate, their own needs and wishes. When people are acutely ill decisions are made on their behalf. This relationship works well at this stage but, as the person recovers and is able to discuss and express his own needs, he should be encouraged to do so (Fig. 2.3). The process of making decisions that will best serve the person's needs is traced by Cracknell (1995) in an article entitled 'A small achievable task', which documents the

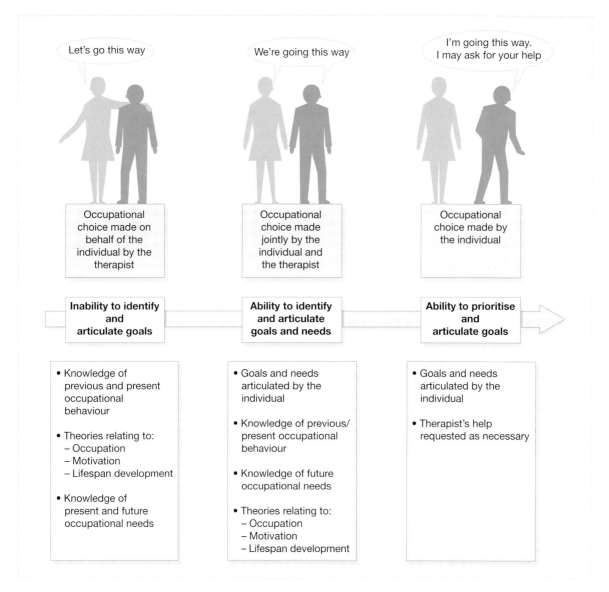

Fig. 2.3 Continuum of decision making during the occupational therapy programme.

progress of her daughter's rehabilitation from the time when she undertook activities suggested by others through to the point when she could make joint, and then independent, decisions about her own needs. In order to make decisions for others we must use our theory base to guide us, rather than make assumptions. The occupational therapist can use phenomenological concepts as a guide to discover meaningful occu-

pations for a person who cannot articulate them for himself. She can either use her knowledge of life development theory (see Chapter 3) to help identify a likely meaningful and appropriate occupation and/or she will be able to approach family and friends and ask them to describe the person's life world. In this way the therapist can make decisions based, as far as possible, on the person's individual lifestyle and motivators.

Our knowledge of psychology shows us that people perform better when they are motivated. If we can identify an individual's unique motivators, and the potency of each of these, we can truly undertake person-centred intervention. Writing in the *Sunday Times*, John Diamond (2000) showed that the levels of people's ambitions may need to change in their new situation, but need not altogether be dashed. Drawing on his own experience while undertaking treatment for cancer he writes (Diamond 2000 p81) 'While I know that I'll probably never play poker in Vegas … or write the great British novel … there are still a few minor ambitions which I have no real excuse for putting off'. To be truly person-centred, therefore, the occupational therapist must help the individual identify the potency of their everyday occupations and prioritise these so that he is motivated to recover those areas that he identifies as most important to him and not those assumed to be so by the therapist or others. Functional ability alone, in the absence of meaning, will not fulfil needs and ambitions. Lester (1999), reporting on a study day for support workers, quoted one speaker, an RAF pilot recovering from Guillain–Barré syndrome, as suggesting to the audience that the individual's dealings with the therapist should be one in which the unspoken relationship reflects 'It's my life and you may help if necessary'. A mantra, perhaps, to be used when considering the use of meaningful occupation in a person-centred profession.

THE CONSEQUENCES OF OCCUPATIONAL LOSS

Having proposed occupation as a basis for health and debated the need for balance in order for this to be maintained, it is important to look at what happens when occupational behaviour is interrupted or lost, either through disability or another disorder. A state of occupational deprivation exists when a person cannot undertake what is meaningful to him. Whiteford (2000) emphasises that the important concept within occupational deprivation is that someone or something external to the individual is doing the depriving and that this force is outside the individual's control.

Studies give evidence that loss of occupation and role have a negative effect on a person's health and wellbeing. One of the overriding themes to emerge from studies and accounts of people whose normal occupations and roles have been disrupted is the resultant negative emotions that individuals display. Boredom, frustration, monotony and restricted lifestyles are reported as the main feelings associated with loss of occupation (Box 2.2). Jacobsen (1997) reported the phenomenon of hostages held in Peru and showed how the group established routines, roles and rotas to counter these negative feelings. Rotas for cleaning and cooking were developed and a daily pattern evolved, including morning physical exercises and classes in language teaching and lectures. Following a post-lunch rest period, board games, reading, model making and puzzles were undertaken in the afternoon while in the evening there were singsongs and music making. Whether through need alone, or combined with socialisation, it is interesting to note the establishment of a routine involving leisure, self-maintenance, productivity and rest.

A phenomenological study by Lister (1999) showed feelings of uselessness and loss of choice,

---

Box 2.2 Some identified consequences of long-term occupational loss

Physical

Joint stiffness	Muscle loss and aching
Lowered bone density	Reduced circulation
Constipation and bloating	Reduced vital capacity
Skill loss	

Psychological

Boredom	Frustration
Monotony	Helplessness
Hopelessness	Anger
Loss of interest	Skill loss
Loss of control	

Social

Loss of roles and routine	Feelings of isolation
Increased dependency	Long-term plans dashed
Feeling useless	Loss of spontaneity

spontaneity and control amongst people who had lost the ability to drive following stroke. Linked to this loss was a feeling of being cut-off, of being dependent and having long-term plans obliterated. A wider look shows that it appears that humans are not the only species to react to loss of occupation in this way. Zoocheck (2000), investigating stereotypical behaviour in caged animals, concluded that this arose 'after a long period of being denied the opportunity to perform constructive behaviours designed to achieve pleasure or avoid pain'. It was felt that such behaviour indicated chronic suffering caused by frustration, boredom and inactivity and reflected feelings of hopelessness amongst the animals.

It is perhaps easier to draw on our own experience to understand the physical effects of occupational loss. We know that even a long car journey or flight, or a short period of sickness spent in bed leaves us with aching muscles and stiff joints. The human body is very much a 'use it or lose it' machine. Long-term loss or diminution of physical occupational behaviour has been shown to result in lower bone density and respiratory capacity, sluggish circulation and reduced digestive activity causing bloating and constipation. Studies of unemployed people and prisoners showing increased incidence of ill health are now widespread and we know that babies deprived of a stimulating environment fail to develop. Di Bona (2000) found that physically demanding leisure activities satisfied more needs than passive ones such as watching TV or reading and quoted Yerxa and Baum Locker's study (1990, cited in Di Bona 2000), which showed that disabled people watched significantly more TV than their able-bodied peers.

MOTIVATION

Closely linked to the loss of occupational and role loss is the idea that motivation plays a large part in people's ability to restore and reorganise their lives after loss. We saw earlier in this chapter (p33) the significant difference in outcome between two people, one of whom retained his roles after a stroke and one who

didn't. Wilcock (1998c) sites studies of the mortality rates of prisoners of war being higher in those who 'did not find a purpose'. We have seen that our occupational behaviour is best motivated by the intrinsic desire or need to perform activities that are most meaningful to us. While each person contributes their own idea of what is meaningful, we can see that certain things are more universally potent than others. In my research (Turner 1997), it was shown that a person's family, satisfying one's own desires, earning a living and creating and maintaining a comfortable personal environment were the four most potent motivators amongst a group of adults who identified themselves as being in good health (Box 2.3). Potent motivators, then, appear to be a mixture of intrinsic and extrinsic concepts.

It is also interesting to note that, during informal conversations with several groups of practitioners when discussing these findings, it was often pointed out that people with enduring mental health problems (including the homeless) lack these potent motivators and responsibilities. Equally, for many people in care homes these potent responsibilities no longer exist. What can emerge, then, may be the creation of a responsibility/motivator to take their place. Examination of the list shows that, hovering closely beneath these prime motivators of 'healthy' people are motivations from pets, faith and friendships.

In recent years we have confirmed, through research, an awareness we have always held of the role that pets can play in helping to give meaning and friendship in life. We can perhaps also think of people for whom friendships and faith play an important role in the absence of family. Perelle and Granville (1993) in their study of the effectiveness of pet therapy programmes in care homes found that pets facilitated a dramatic improvement in residents' social and self-maintenance behaviours, with an increase in smiling and independence. Citing previous work (Corson & Corson 1978, Levinson 1969) they found that pets decreased feelings of loneliness and increased interactions. 'A pet can provide, in boundless measure, love and unqualified approval. Many elderly and lonely people have

---

Box 2.3 Prime motivators and responsibilities (Turner 1997)

Motivators	Score	Responsibilities	Score

1. Family
  care for
  children
  grandchildren
  parents
  partner/spouse
	101	1. Family
		  care of
		  contact with
		  role member
			80

2. Self
  health
  happiness
  achieving ambitions
	37	2. Job, finance, earn money	60

		3. Responsibility to self
		  health
		  avoid dependency
		  pursuit of happiness
			43

3. Job/money/earn a living	36	4. House/garden
		  care of
		  repair
		  decoration
			35

4. Personal environment
  garden
  'nice things'
  'pleasant home'
  house
	27		

		5. Pets care of	16=

5. Socialising
  friends
  meeting people
	24	6. Friendship/social
		  socialising
			16=

6. Faith	15	7. Spiritual commitments
		  attend church
		  serve God
			12

7. Leisure
  interests
  creativity
	14	8. Non-employment commitments
		  community care
		  youth groups
			9

8. Non-family responsibilities including pets	13=		

9. Getting out and about
  holidays
  mobility
	13=	9. Other	5

10. 'Living'
  love of life
  love
  waking each day
	11		

Subjects were asked to rank their top three perceived motivators and responsibilities. These were then weighted (3 = top priority, 1 = lowest priority), grouped, and totalled.

---

discovered that pets satisfy vital emotional needs.' (Levinson 1969 p368, cited in Perelle & Granville 2000).

ROUTINE

When roles and occupations are lost not only are physical and psychological health affected but routines are frequently lost along with roles. Most people's daily lives are made up of the routines and habits that reflect their roles and occupational needs, motivators and responsibilities. Kielhofner and Forsyth (1997) state 'habituation thus holds together the ordinary fabric of our lives'. What happens then, when these are interrupted?

For some, where losses have perhaps been gradual, routines may remain in the absence or diminution of roles. We may know an elderly person, or couple, who stick rigidly to routines established when their lives were full of family, social and employment responsibilities, or we may know someone made redundant who continues their life around routines established when they went to work. Both these examples allow people to retain, even if temporarily, patterns that enable certain occupational behaviours to be continued in the absence of roles – the motivators have been removed and the routine has become dominant and is now itself the motivator. However, when routines are disturbed either through functional and/or role loss, difficulties can arise. Loss of potent roles that control major chunks of time can result in a lack of motivation to perform those roles that remain. Roles and routines, based upon needs and goals and served by skills, may all need intervention to restore balance and meaning to a person's life.

OCCUPATIONAL DYSFUNCTION

Occupational dysfunction can be seen as the outcome of ongoing occupational deprivation. Where dysfunction leads to loss of skills to undertake desired occupational behaviours the effects can be devastating and widespread. Activities that touch all areas of self-maintenance, leisure and productivity may be affected, with the result that roles may be lost and routines interrupted. Where occupations can no longer be undertaken, the ability to fulfil desires, needs and responsibilities can be dashed. In classifying disability in terms of activity loss, the World Health Organization recognises that the impact, and therefore the evaluation, of functional loss sits squarely on the effect it has on people's daily lives, both qualitatively (phemomenologically) and quantitatively (through empirical research) (de Kleijn-de Vrankrijker et al 1998). Whilst the focus of medicine is to alleviate impairment, the focus of occupational therapy is to reinstate occupational function.

In order, then, to re-establish occupational behaviour, readjustments to the way in which they are executed and, perhaps more importantly, examination of the potency of motivators and responsibilities, is essential. Identification and facilitation of the process of adaptation to new circumstances will enable the person to continue to fulfil these within the limits imposed by his dysfunction. He may retain roles, for example, but devolve functions to others; he may adjust the focus of his ambition and/or he may strive to reinstate function. Facilitating this adaptive process is the paramount domain of the occupational therapist. Kielhofner and Forsyth (1997) felt that 'therapy has the ominous challenge of enabling the human system to achieve a new dynamic order' and states that '... therapy becomes the means by which the life course is redirected. Even when a person's goal is to reinstate, as far as possible, a previous way of life, a change will be required to approximate life as it was before the onset of impairment.' (Keilhofner & Forsyth 1997 p110). The means through which we do this is occupation itself.

THE NEED FOR EVIDENCE

Recently, occupational therapy, as with all disciplines within healthcare, has come under increasing pressure to provide evidence for the efficacy and effectiveness of its treatment base. In 1996, Lloyd-Smith observed 'in fact, little is known about the effectiveness or otherwise of most treatments [offered to the NHS]'. Driven through legislation, notably 'The New NHS: Modern, Dependable' (Department of Health 1997), purchasers are increasingly requiring therapists to demonstrate clinical effectiveness. Clinical governance, the mechanism through which standards are set, delivered and monitored, today demands a framework through which therapists must demonstrate the quality of the treatments they use. Indeed, Ellenburg (1996) foresaw a time when purchasers will only buy procedures for which there is proven effectiveness.

Do we, however, have this evidence? Can we prove that occupational therapy is effective? We have been aware for many years that, whilst occupational therapy is a 'good idea', when it was challenged, occupational therapists had little, if any, concrete evidence that what they are doing was effective. Growing up, as we did, under the wing of medicine, the pressure to produce empirical data to support our work has long been around and equally we have been aware of our inability to produce this. As far back as 1925, Haas wrote:

Little was written [about occupational therapy] prior to 1910 other than a large number of brief statements that the employment of patients was believed to be beneficial. If the science of occupational therapy is to develop … this progress can only come through the careful recording of experience and the presentation of these data.

In extolling the virtues of basketry as a therapeutic medium he wrote 'basketry holds an important place but few have stopped to analyse the reasons for this'. Continuing this theme, Licht (1948) observed that:

Recent critics have seriously questioned its [occupational therapy's] value. To this charge the response is usually emotional. Unfortunately the charge is not without some justification because the available data are inadequate and must wait for research to factually prove the clinically obvious.

In 1981 Bing (cited in Paterson 1997), felt that 'occupational therapists believe in the efficacy of meaningful occupation but are striving for a theoretical base to support it'. It is sad then that in 1990, 65 years after Haas's observations, Yerxa et al concluded that occupational therapy was still 'an applied discipline in search of a science to apply'.

To answer these criticisms, and indeed to produce for ourselves the evidence, and thus the confidence, to articulate and support our thoughts on occupation, occupational science came into being (Box 2.4). In an article introducing this new science, Yerxa et al (1989) defined it as 'the study of the human as an occupational being including the need for, and capacity to engage in and orchestrate daily occupations in the environment over the lifespan'. They saw it as a scientific foundation for practice that will:

Box 2.4   Definition and purpose of occupational science (Based on Illott 1995 and Yerxa et al 1989.)

Definition
'The study of the human as an occupational being including the need for, and capacity to engage in and orchestrate daily occupations in the environment over a lifespan' (Yerxa et al 1989)

Its purpose is to explore:
- the human need to be occupied
- the purpose of occupation in survival and health
- the effects of occupation or occupational deprivation
- how social, cultural and political structures affect occupation
- why humans strive for occupational competence and mastery
- how occupation provides for biological and sociocultural needs
- how occupation is necessary in the development of human capacities
- understanding what prevents or enhances occupational performance

Additionally it aims to:
- Provide practitioners with the support for what they do
- Distinguish occupational therapy from other disciplines
- Provide new understanding of what it means to be disabled
- Help the profession contribute new knowledge and skills
- Provide occupational therapists with more effective ideas and approaches for practice

---

… provide practitioners with support for what they do, justify the significance of occupational therapy to health and differentiate it from other disciplines, … provide new understanding of what it means to be disabled, help the profession contribute new knowledge and skills and provide individual occupational therapists with more effective ideas and approaches for practise.

(Yerxa et al 1989 p3)

Burke (1996) reflected the need for a unique science to serve occupation. She acknowledged our lack of evidence but felt that because of our close links with medicine we had been 'citizens in a reductionist world' where status and funding were given to the production of hard, empirical, quantitative data alone, whereas our interests are equally served through the production of qualitative, phenomenological, narrative data. Thus, occupational therapists have lagged behind in the quest to research their profession. It has been argued that, in part, this has been because we were trying to prove the unprovable; that research may challenge long-held assumptions and so would be an uncomfortable process. Indeed, this may be true, given the results of research carried out at the University of Nottingham, which showed that while occupational therapy does effect an improvement in people treated following stroke, the difference does not reach statistical significance (*Therapy Weekly* 2000). However, avoiding the issue will not advance our cause. The recent interest in, and recognition of the validity of 'soft' qualitative data as a legitimate means of providing evidence has facilitated and given many therapists the confidence to investigate the efficacy of their profession. Equally, the advance of quantitative evidence is growing apace.

Some may, and indeed have, criticised what they consider to be the artificial creation of occupational science. Mocellin (1996), for example, contends that because occupational science is over-inclusive, because 'practise [is] informed by wrong theories' and because we have 'adopted scientific jargon in an attempt to solve many of the problems thought to be confronting the profession', occupational science is in danger of being patronising and inherently weak. However, Wood (1995) counterargues by showing that, throughout the history of scientific investigation 'knowing how' has always preceded 'knowing that'. She proposes that knowledge of how to do something to the point where it is seen to be obviously effective is in itself the stimulation for the formation of theory. Others have questioned whether occupational science should be developed as a pure or applied science. Yerxa et al's (1989) original description of its purpose inextricably links it to occupational therapy while Burke (1996) sees it developing in its own right. Time alone will show us the path of its development.

SO WHAT IS THE EVIDENCE?

It would seem that in recent years the need to prove the effectiveness of our intervention and the efficacy of our knowledge base has entered the collective consciousness of the profession. As the need for evidence continued to be articulated and the external pressures mounted and became

backed by legislation, as a wider range of research tools gained respectability and education for therapists moved to first-degree level, as more practitioners gained higher academic awards thus producing a wealth of therapists with research interests and abilities, the evidence began to mount.

On the down side, however, we see that, within the hierarchy of acceptable evidence, much of what we have produced sits within the lower levels (Fig. 2.4) and very little, if any at present, reaches gold standard (Class A). Clearly, the evidence we have will help our confidence and standards but, within the field of status and reflected through initiatives such as the National Institute for Clinical Effectiveness (NICE), we do not necessarily do so well. This is an area that we all need to address when undertaking professional research.

Nevertheless, the evidence that is emerging appears to confirm our assumptions. Earlier sections of this chapter began to explore several issues identified by Zemke and Clark (1996) in their text relating to the evolution of occupational

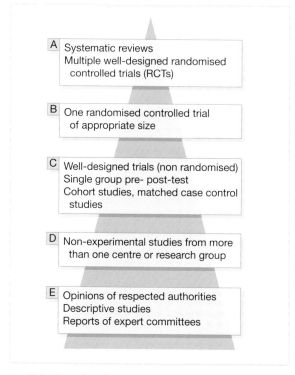

A Systematic reviews
Multiple well-designed randomised controlled trials (RCTs)

B One randomised controlled trial of appropriate size

C Well-designed trials (non randomised)
Single group pre- post-test
Cohort studies, matched case control studies

D Non-experimental studies from more than one centre or research group

E Opinions of respected authorities
Descriptive studies
Reports of expert committees

Fig. 2.4 Hierarchy of acceptable research evidence (after Muir Gray 1996).

science. Increasing evidence in these areas begins to explore and confirm the complex dimensions of occupation. However, for many practitioners the day-to-day need is for evidence of the use of occupation as an effective, measurable means of intervention. With the explosion of emerging data it would be impossible to address here in any meaningful way the concepts developing within this evidence. A dip into the sea of data shows evidence to support a huge range of practice domains. Articles, study days, conferences and texts all present and evaluate research findings. To be current and aware, the practitioner must become adept at searching and analysing data. She must become an active hunter–gatherer of evidence to confirm and advance her practice, and of course she must read the practice chapters in this text to inform herself of the current body of knowledge related to her domains of practice!

USING OCCUPATION AS THERAPY

A knowledge of a person's past, present and desired occupational behaviour informs and guides the assessment and intervention undertaken by occupational therapists. Information is gathered through the assessment process, priorities are negotiated and established using a combination of theoretical frameworks and information gained about the individual. Aims and goals are established based on these person-centred priorities, interventions executed and outcomes measured and evaluated. Throughout this process of clinical reasoning and judgement, the occupational therapist is informed by her knowledge of occupation. She will need to understand normal occupational patterns for the individual, judge the impact of loss and imbalance on his occupational performance, seek information about the person's motivations, desires and needs and then use meaningful occupations as the therapeutic medium through which to elicit adaptation to the desired new pattern of occupational performance. This she will do based, as far as possible, on the evidence and knowledge she has of the efficacy of the different skills, media and techniques she has at her disposal. Tea making, for

example, is an oft-used occupational therapy intervention. Figure 2.5 shows how specific evidence can be used to help inform tea making as part of an intervention programme.

Using occupation as therapy involves an understanding of the many elements that contribute to successful occupational performance. Figure 2.6 shows the relationship of these elements and how occupation can be seen as both the means and ends of intervention. Ensuring that occupation remains the central focus of practice is essential. Whether working on performance components that form the building blocks necessary for undertaking occupations, whether analysing occupation and/or activity to discover and remediate shortfalls in performance areas, whether working at the level of occupational performance to facilitate the desired outcomes for the individual in terms of roles and responsibilities or whether considering the individual's performance context, the occupational therapist must, at all times, ensure that the person's occupational performance needs drive and shape practice. These needs must be individually and clearly identified, articulated and evaluated as the central thread of any intervention programme.

To be purposeful and meaningful the occupations the therapist uses must be current and culturally relevant. Fashions come and go and political and financial pressures wax and wane. It is easy to decry the creative media based on the Arts and Crafts movement at the turn of the 20th century and the therapeutic machinery developed during our subservience to the medical model, but what has replaced them? Indeed, within the culture in which occupational therapists work in acute medicine today, could it be argued that to use activities specifically to reinstate function is inappropriate? Do we feel we do not have the resources to undertake them? Are pressures from employers such that they are no longer a viable tool within our repertoire? We have seen, and are hopefully emerging from, the era of occupational therapists using 'activities' such as water siphoning, polishing table tops, stretching rubber bands and endless remedial games (many of which may not be remedial or fun or, indeed, played as a game) to address performance components alone rather than occupational performance needs. We

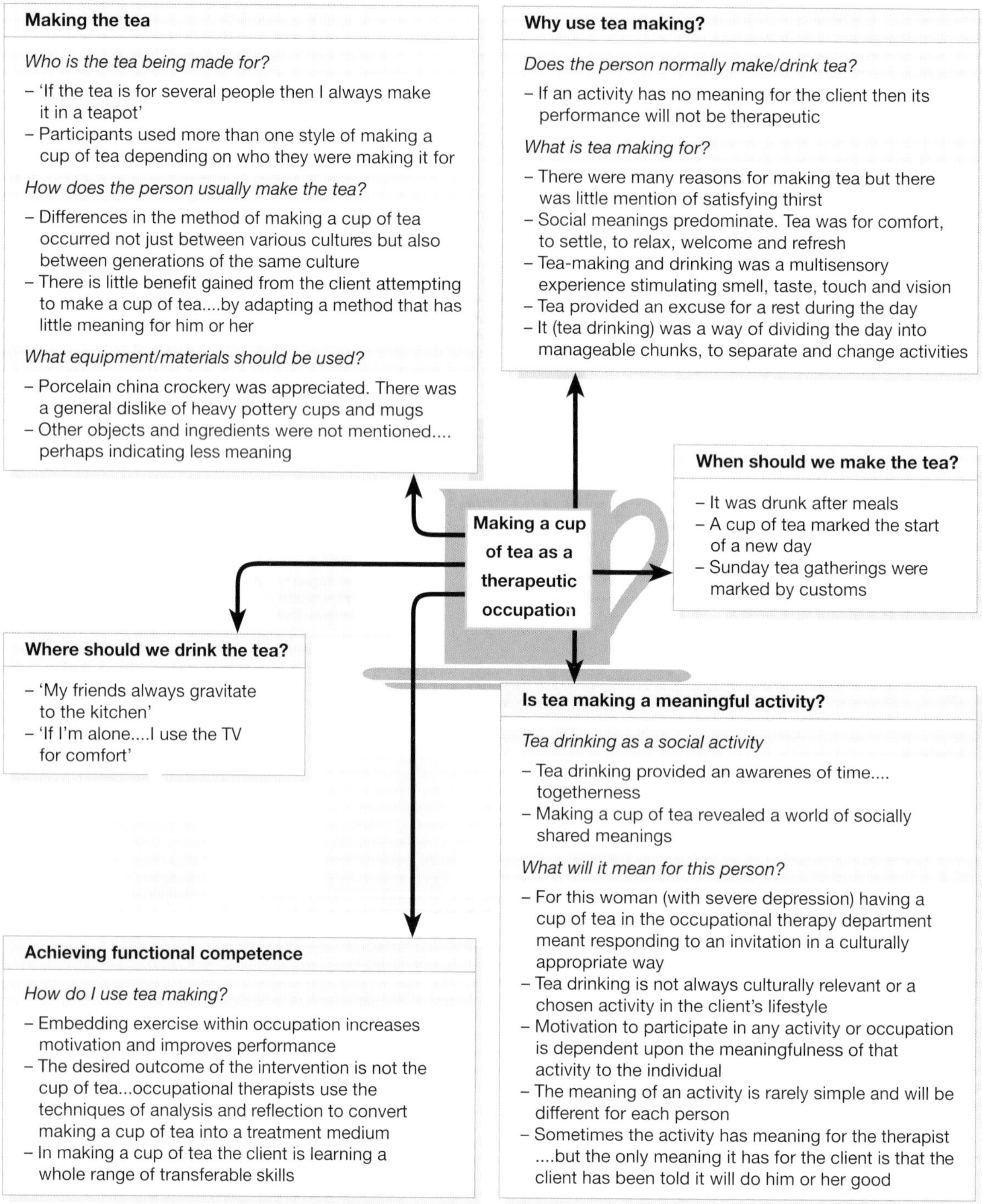

Making the tea

Who is the tea being made for?

– 'If the tea is for several people then I always make it in a teapot'
– Participants used more than one style of making a cup of tea depending on who they were making it for

How does the person usually make the tea?

– Differences in the method of making a cup of tea occurred not just between various cultures but also between generations of the same culture
– There is little benefit gained from the client attempting to make a cup of tea....by adapting a method that has little meaning for him or her

What equipment/materials should be used?

– Porcelain china crockery was appreciated. There was a general dislike of heavy pottery cups and mugs
– Other objects and ingredients were not mentioned.... perhaps indicating less meaning

Why use tea making?

Does the person normally make/drink tea?

– If an activity has no meaning for the client then its performance will not be therapeutic

What is tea making for?

– There were many reasons for making tea but there was little mention of satisfying thirst
– Social meanings predominate. Tea was for comfort, to settle, to relax, welcome and refresh
– Tea-making and drinking was a multisensory experience stimulating smell, taste, touch and vision
– Tea provided an excuse for a rest during the day
– It (tea drinking) was a way of dividing the day into manageable chunks, to separate and change activities

When should we make the tea?

– It was drunk after meals
– A cup of tea marked the start of a new day
– Sunday tea gatherings were marked by customs

Making a cup of tea as a therapeutic occupation

Where should we drink the tea?

– 'My friends always gravitate to the kitchen'
– 'If I'm alone....I use the TV for comfort'

Is tea making a meaningful activity?

Tea drinking as a social activity

– Tea drinking provided an awarenes of time.... togetherness
– Making a cup of tea revealed a world of socially shared meanings

What will it mean for this person?

– For this woman (with severe depression) having a cup of tea in the occupational therapy department meant responding to an invitation in a culturally appropriate way
– Tea drinking is not always culturally relevant or a chosen activity in the client's lifestyle
– Motivation to participate in any activity or occupation is dependent upon the meaningfulness of that activity to the individual
– The meaning of an activity is rarely simple and will be different for each person
– Sometimes the activity has meaning for the therapist ....but the only meaning it has for the client is that the client has been told it will do him or her good

Achieving functional competence

How do I use tea making?

– Embedding exercise within occupation increases motivation and improves performance
– The desired outcome of the intervention is not the cup of tea...occupational therapists use the techniques of analysis and reflection to convert making a cup of tea into a treatment medium
– In making a cup of tea the client is learning a whole range of transferable skills

Fig. 2.5 How evidence related to tea making can be used to inform its use as a therapeutic occupation. Evidence is drawn from Greek (1996), De Kuiper et al (1993), Hannam (1997) and Fair and Barnitt (1999).

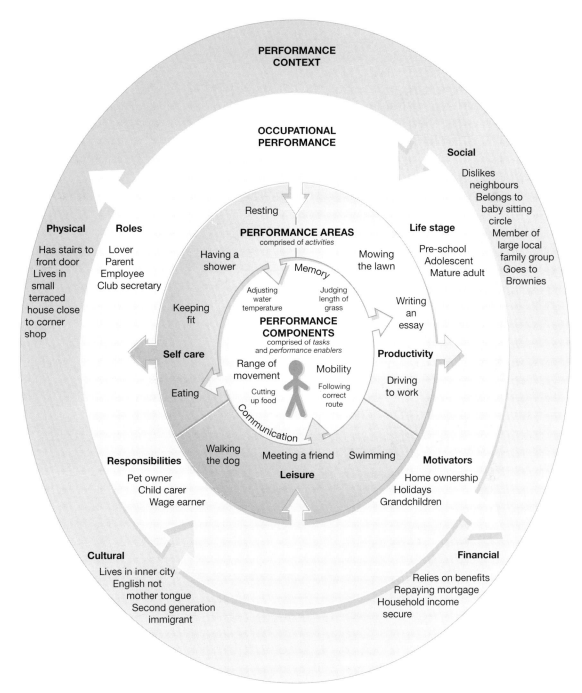

Fig. 2.6 The relationship of the elements of occupational performance that may be addressed during intervention, showing how each impacts, and is impacted on, by the others.

are also, hopefully, developing sufficient professional identity to prevent us venturing into the domains of other professions by using wax baths, massage and functional bracing. Miller (1999), reviewing over 800 interventions used by occupational therapists, found that 51% of these could be categorised as 'solving performance problems' (learning new techniques, adapting performance or providing equipment were included); 43% were categorised as the 'therapeutic use of activity' (using woodwork, cookery and singing to promote performance were cited as examples of this) while the remaining 6%, he suggested, were outside the brief of occupational therapy and included the use of techniques not taught within

the remit of occupational therapy education and not linked to the person's occupational performance. When we review our practice, can we be sure that our interventions do not fall within this last category? And if they do, why are we using them? Do we not have enough to do within the boundaries of our own profession? The government's agenda for the future development of professions licensed by the Health Professions

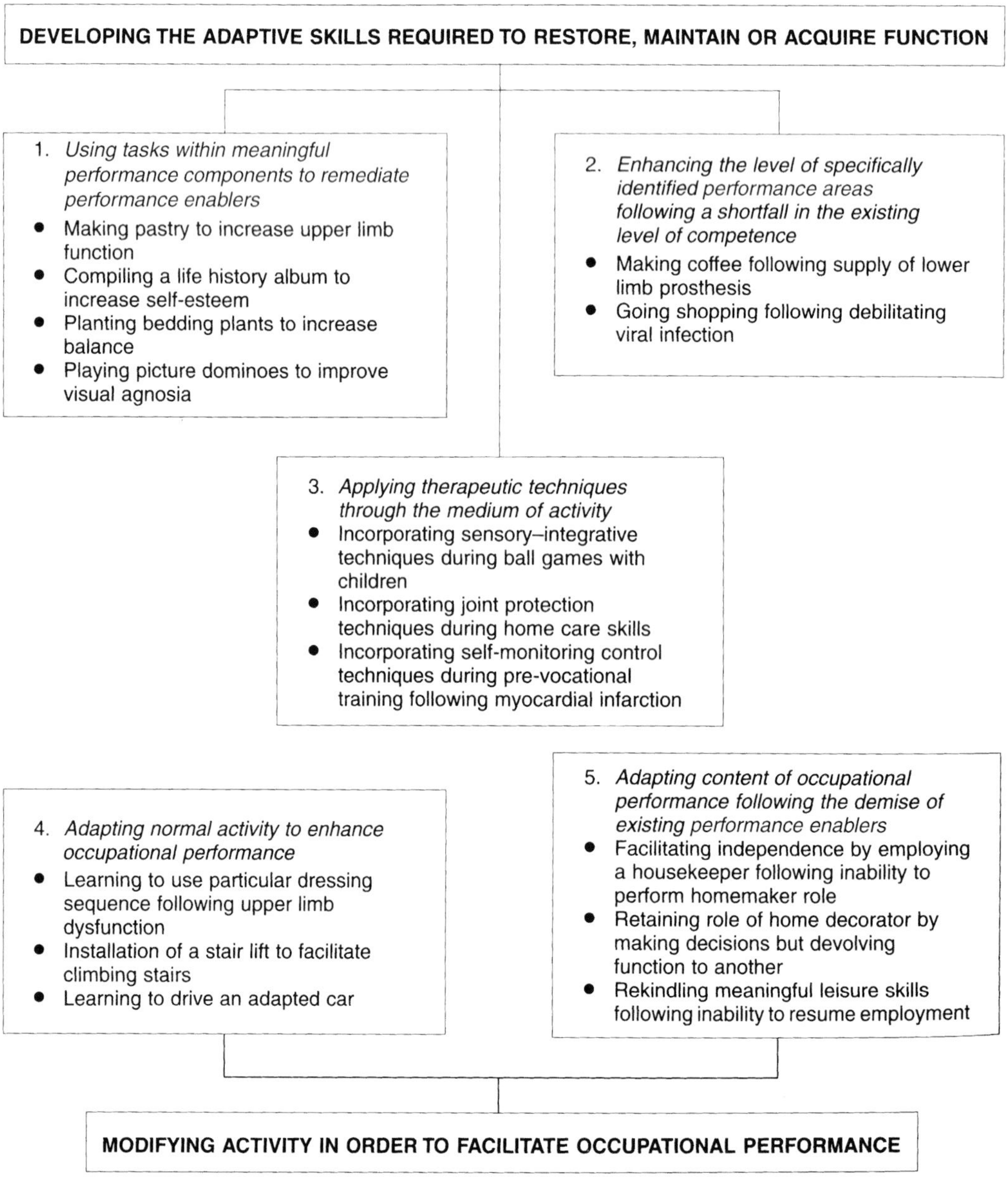

DEVELOPING THE ADAPTIVE SKILLS REQUIRED TO RESTORE, MAINTAIN OR ACQUIRE FUNCTION

1. *Using tasks within meaningful performance components to remediate performance enablers*
   - Making pastry to increase upper limb function
   - Compiling a life history album to increase self-esteem
   - Planting bedding plants to increase balance
   - Playing picture dominoes to improve visual agnosia

2. *Enhancing the level of specifically identified performance areas following a shortfall in the existing level of competence*
   - Making coffee following supply of lower limb prosthesis
   - Going shopping following debilitating viral infection

3. *Applying therapeutic techniques through the medium of activity*
   - Incorporating sensory–integrative techniques during ball games with children
   - Incorporating joint protection techniques during home care skills
   - Incorporating self-monitoring control techniques during pre-vocational training following myocardial infarction

4. *Adapting normal activity to enhance occupational performance*
   - Learning to use particular dressing sequence following upper limb dysfunction
   - Installation of a stair lift to facilitate climbing stairs
   - Learning to drive an adapted car

5. *Adapting content of occupational performance following the demise of existing performance enablers*
   - Facilitating independence by employing a housekeeper following inability to perform homemaker role
   - Retaining role of home decorator by making decisions but devolving function to another
   - Rekindling meaningful leisure skills following inability to resume employment

MODIFYING ACTIVITY IN ORDER TO FACILITATE OCCUPATIONAL PERFORMANCE

Fig. 2.7 How occupational therapists use activities for the treatment of physical dysfunction.

Council strongly supports the identification of generic core skills. If occupational therapy does not clearly define the usefulness of its practice, we may find that we are inadvertently supporting this change. Indeed, Hagedorn (1995) states 'I assert that if this element [occupation] is removed, whatever is happening may still be therapy, but it is not occupational therapy'. Without a sound framework to guide our practice, occupational therapists can easily become side-tracked down non-occupational pathways that lead to non-occupational and indefensible practice.

CONCLUSION

Without doubt, times are changing and occupational therapists must move with them or be left behind. We must evaluate our knowledge of occupation in this ever-changing culture of healthcare, but with speed. A model to guide the ways in which occupational therapists use their skills in occupation and activity to inform an intervention programme is proposed in Figure 2.7. However, the extent to which each of these skills is used will be determined by the needs of the individual and the therapeutic context in which the therapist works. Her knowledge of occupation, therefore, forms a fundamental guide throughout the intervention process. Without the application of this knowledge, intervention becomes at best repetitious, based solely on custom and practice, and at worst a technical, stereotypical programme based more on clinical diagnosis than the person's occupational needs. If our knowledge and practice are to advance, we must make sure this is not the case.

REFERENCES

Bartlett J 1980 Familiar quotation, 15th edn. Little Brown, Boston

Burke J 1996 Moving occupation into treatment: clinical interpretation of 'legitimizing occupational therapy's knowledge'. The American Journal of Occupational Therapy 50(8):635–638

Cracknell E 1995 A small, achievable task. British Journal of Occupational Therapy 58(8):343–344

Creek J 1996 Making a cup of tea as an honours degree subject. British Journal of Occupational Therapy 59(3):128–130

Darnell J, Heater S 1994 Occupational therapist or activity therapist – which do you choose to be? American Journal of Occupational Therapy 48(5):467–468

de Kleijn-de Vrankrijker M, Heerkens YF, van Ravensburg CD 1998 In: McColl MA, Bichenbach JE (eds) Introduction to disability. WB Saunders, London

De Kuiper W, Nelson D, White B 1993 Materials based occupation vs. imagery based occupation vs. rote exercise: a replication and extension. Occupational Therapy Journal of Research 13(3):183–197

Department of Health 1997 The new NHS: modern, dependable. HMSO, London

Diamond J 2000 The last word. The Times Magazine 5(3):81

Di Bona L 2000 What are the benefits of leisure? An exploration using the leisure satisfaction scale. The British Journal of Occupational Therapy 63(2):50–58

Ellenburg D 1996 Outcomes research: the history, debate and inplications for the field of occupational therapy. American Journal of Occupational Therapy 50(4):435–441

Fair A, Barnitt R 1999 Making a cup of tea as part of a culturally sensitive service. British Journal of Occupational Therapy 62(5):199–205

Finlay L 1999 Applying phenomenology in research: problems, principles and practice. British Journal of Occupational Therapy 62(7):299–306

Golledge J 1998a Distinguishing between occupation, purposeful activity and activity. Part 1: Review and explanation. The British Journal of Occupational Therapy 61(3):100–105

Golledge J 1998b Distinguishing between occupation, purposeful activity and activity. Part 2: Why is the distinction important? The British Journal of Occupational Therapy 61(4):157–160

Haas LJ 1925 Occupational therapy for the mentally and nervously ill. The Bruce Publishing Co, Wisconsin

Hagedorn R 1995 Occupational therapy, perspectives and processes. Churchill Livingstone, Edinburgh

Handsaker S 1998 Therapy from within. Therapy Weekly, 29 September, 6

Hannam D 1997 More than a cup of tea: meaning construction in an everyday occupation. Journal of Occupational Science: Australia 4(2):69–74

Illott I 1995 Occupational science: the foundation for practice. British Journal of Therapy and Rehabilitation 2(7):367–370

Jacobson P 1997 Surviving the siege. Telegraph Magazine, 14 June, 24–30

Kielhofner G 1993 In: Hopkins H, Smith H (eds) Willard and Spackman's occupational therapy, 8th edn. Lippincott, Philadelphia, PA

Kielhofner G, Forsyth K 1997 The model of human occupation: an overview of current concepts. The British Journal of Occupational Therapy 60(3):103–110

Knutas A, Borall L 1995 The meaning of stroke in everyday life – a comparative case study of two persons. Scandinavian Journal of Occupational Therapy 95(2):56–62

Lester M 1999 It's my life, you may help. Occupational Therapy News 7(5):12

Licht S 1948 Occupational therapy source book. Williams & Wilkins, Baltimore, MD

Lister R 1999 Loss of ability to drive following a stroke: the early experiences of three elderly people on discharge from hospital. British Journal of Occupational Therapy 62(11):514–520

Lloyd-Smith W 1996 Where's the evidence? British Journal of Therapy and Rehabilitation 3(12):659–662

Miller S 1999 The use of activity as therapy: a review of the arguments. Paper presented to the College of Occupational Therapists Annual Conference, Liverpool

Mocellin G 1992 An overview of occupational therapy in the context of American influence on the profession. British Journal of Occupational Therapy: Part 1 55(1):7–12

Mocellin G 1996 Occupational therapy: a critical overview. Part 1 58(12):502–506, Part 2 59(1):11–16

Muir Gray JA 1997 Evidence based healthcare. Churchill Livingstone, Edinburgh

Nocon A, Pleace N 1997 'Until disabled people get consulted …': the role of occupational therapy in meeting housing needs. The British Journal of Occupational Therapy 60(3):115–122

Paterson C 1997 Rationales for the use of occupation in 19th century asylums. British Journal of Occupational Therapy 60(4):179–183

Perelle I, Granville D 1993 Assessment of the effectiveness of a pet facilitated therapy program in a nursing home setting. Society and Animals 1(1):91–100

Primeau L 1995 Work and leisure: transending the dichotomy. American Journal of Occupational Therapy 50(7):569–576

Radomski M 1995 There is more to life than putting on your pants. The American Journal of Occupational Therapy 49(6):487–490

Reiss S 2000 Who am I: the 16 basic desires that motivate our actions and determine our personality. GP Pitman and Sous, New York

Sumsion T 1999 A study to determine a British occupational therapy definition of client centred practice. British Journal of Occupational Therapy 62(2):52–58

Stephenson S, Wiles R 2000 Advantages and disadvantages of the home setting for therapy: views of patients and therapists. The British Journal of Occupational Therapy 63(2):59–64

Therapy Weekly 2000 Stroke: new study is a total shock for OTs. Therapy Weekly, 13 April, 3

Turner A 1997 Do current activity media used within occupational therapy education reflect the changing activity patterns of living today? Paper presented to the College of Occupational Therapists Annual Conference, Southampton

Warburton DM 1996 Pleasure is good for you. Institute for Public Affairs, review 49:24–28

Whiteford G 2000 Occupational deprivation: Global challenge in the new milleneum. British Journal of Occupational Therapy 63(5):200–204

Wilcock A 1993 A theory of the human need for occupation. Occupational Science: Australia 1(1):17–24

Wilcock A 1995 The occupational brain: a theory of human nature. Journal of Occupational Science: Australia 2(1):68–73

Wilcock A, van der Arend H, Darling K et al 1998a An exploratory study of people's perceptions and experiences of wellbeing. The British Journal of Occupational Therapy 61(2):75–82

Wilcock A 1998b Occupation for health. The British Journal of Occupational Therapy 61(8):340–345

Wilcock A 1998c An occupational perspective of health. Slack, New York

Wood W 1995 Weaving the warp and weft of occupational therapy: an art and science for all times. American Journal of Occupational Therapy 49(1):44–52

Wood W 1996 Legitimizing occupational therapy's knowledge. American Journal of Occupational Therapy 50(8):626–634

Yerxa EJ, Clark F, Frank G et al 1989 An introduction to occupational science, a foundation to occupational therapy in the 21st century. Occupational Therapy in Health Care 6(4):1–17

Zemke R, Clark F 1996 Occupational science, the evolving discipline. FA Davis, Philadelphia

Zoocheck Canada Inc. 1997 Zoos in Ontario: a discussion. Available on www.Zoocheck.com/programs/zoocheck/-lindley/discussion97.shtml

---

FURTHER READING

Breines E 1995 Understanding 'occupation' as the founders did. British Journal of Occupational Therapy 58(11):458–460

Dickerson A 1995 Action indentification may explain why the doing of activities in occupational therapy effects positive changes in clients. British Journal of Occupational Therapy 58(11):461–464

Green S 1995 Elderly mentally ill people and quality of life: who wants activities? British Journal of Occupational Therapy 58(9):377–382

Law M, Steinwender S, Leclair L 1998 Occupation, health and wellbeing. Canadian Journal of Occupational Therapy, April, 81–91

Murray I 1999 Pets for patients may save the NHS £1b a year. The Times, 9 September, 5

Polatajko HJ, Mandich A, Martini R 1999 Dynamic performance analysis: a framework for understanding occupational performance. American Journal of Occupational Therapy 54(1):65–72

Sealey C 1999 Clinical governance: an information guide for occupational therapists. British Journal of Occupational Therapy 62(6):263–268

Townsend E 1997 Occupation: potential for personal and social transformation. Journal of Occupational Science: Australia 4(1):18–26

Wilcock A 1993 Keynote paper: biological and sociocultural aspects of occupation, health and health promotion. British Journal of Occupational Therapy 56(6):200–203

Wilcock A 1999 The Doris Sym lecture: developing a philosophy of occupation for health. British Journal of Occupational Therapy 62(5):192–198

3

Theoretical frameworks

Marg Foster

INTRODUCTION

Occupational therapy is a rapidly developing profession that is increasingly consolidating its theoretical basis in order to provide a solid foundation for research and evaluation and to more clearly explain its philosophy and practices to others.

For many years, occupational therapists have been using a variety of techniques in treatment and intervention, but in recent years there has been a reappraisal of the value of individual methods and practices, the basis on which these have developed, and the ways in which they interlink within the various branches of occupational therapy.

Competence in any profession depends upon an understanding of the theory that underlies it. 'Theory' in this general sense encompasses philosophical viewpoints, paradigms, frames of reference, models, approaches, and particular *theories*. The occupational therapist needs to be conversant with these elements of theory as they have developed within her own profession, so that she has a clear understanding of the principles of her discipline and a sound basis from which to plan, implement and justify her interventions.

Many texts present in-depth discussion of particular aspects of theory (see Reference section, p80), and this chapter aims to provide an overview of the main aspects of occupational therapy theory that have application to the treatment of people with physical dysfunction.

The first sections of the chapter discuss the importance of theory to the profession of occupational therapy as a whole and to the individual therapist. Various terms used in the discussion of theory, such as 'paradigm', 'frame of reference', 'approach' and 'model', are defined. The interconnections between these areas of theory are then illustrated.

The next sections of the chapter turn to the application of theory to practice. First, specific theories that have had an important influence upon occupational therapy are discussed; these are the humanistic, occupations/activities and psychosocial theories. The basic assumptions of each theory are outlined and particular refinements on these theories as they have evolved within occupational therapy are described.

The remaining sections of the chapter are devoted to particular frames of reference that have had an important influence on the treatment of physical dysfunction, namely the developmental, biomechanical, compensatory and learning frames of reference. The merits and limitations of each frame of reference are set out, and their relevance to today's changing practice is discussed.

THE IMPORTANCE OF THEORY

PROFESSIONALISM

In the present competitive health and social care market, occupational therapy must have a sound theoretical framework by which it can define itself and justify its actions in order to maintain and enhance its professional standing. The 1989 Report of the Commission of Inquiry entitled 'Occupational Therapy, an Emerging Profession in Health Care', recommended that therapists should 'seek to validate the profession's claim to professional status by devising ways of measuring and monitoring the effectiveness and efficiency of practices, procedures and organisational arrangements' (Blom Cooper 1989). Since the publication of this report, considerable research and evaluation of practice has been carried out, much of which has been devoted to investigation

and development of the theoretical base of occupational therapy. Before considering the nature and importance of this theoretical base, it is advantageous to consider the qualities essential to a profession.

What is a profession?

Professions do not come into existence by historical accident. Rather a complex interplay of forces over time ushers a profession into being. Internally there must be the vision and energy of those who found and develop the profession. Externally social movements provide ideas and support for its mission. Governmental systems legitimise and regulate the members' activities … underlying these factors is an implicit social contract … the profession meets a basic social need … Professions are able to provide their distinctive service because they have accumulated and developed a conceptual foundation that explains and directs their practical efforts.

(Kielhofner 1992)

No one definition exists that defines a profession, although various texts that outline the characteristics representative of a profession agree on a number of points. In addition to the social constructs of the profession, the following points are considered to be fundamental to any profession (Wallis 1987):

- A unique body of knowledge which is pertinent to the practices and beliefs of the profession. Some knowledge may overlap with that of other professions, but the particular integration and utilisation of knowledge is unique to each profession.
- A sound theory base on which to explain the profession's philosophies and values. Many texts state that this theory base should be proven by investigation and research.
- Educational requirements in order to become a member of the profession; continuing education within the profession to maintain standards in the light of change.
- Autonomy in determining the rules of the profession and maintaining standards.
- Ethical responsibility to regulate the modes of behaviour of those within the profession and to protect the client.

- Professional commitment within the membership to adhere to the practices and beliefs of the profession and to further its development.

The British Association of Occupational Therapists (2000) Code of Ethics and Professional Conduct defines the ways in which practitioners should meet professional obligations in relation to consumers in terms of responsibilities, relationships, professional integrity and standards of practice. Included in these are articles concerning professional demeanour, clinical competence, personal behaviour and professional development.

The College of Occupational Therapists, the Council for Professions Allied to Medicine and the Privy Council, together with the educational establishments, validate the educational programmes for entry into the profession.

Implications for occupational therapy

It is vital for occupational therapy to have a proven theory base if it is to continue to be recognised as a profession. Study of the theory base on which it is founded, and the basis on which its practices are carried out, should be an essential part of any profession's development. Skill as a 'doer' based on practice, repetition and experience reflects a technical level of competence. Professionalism, however, requires skill in thinking, in reflecting on previous experiences, and in linking these to theory and learning (Parham 1987) and to the presenting situation, in order that the choice of 'doing' is the most appropriate to the particular problem – clinical reasoning. Barnitt (1990) in a keynote paper to the World Federation of Occupational Therapists (WFOT) 10th International Congress stressed the value of thinking. She outlined the structure of the profession as the 'shared body of knowledge, the skills practised by its members and the shared values and beliefs which underpin the ethics and motivation of its members'. She stated that 'the structure is dependent on the thinking which brought it into existence, which then propels it forward through change, progress and decline' and thinking is the means by which the structure is 'held together or separated out'. A high standard of thinking and clinical reasoning

enhances not only the individual but also the recognition of the profession as a whole. This may be reflected in academic credentials (diplomas, degrees, doctorates) and through validated research, but should also be evident in the ways in which members of the profession are conversant with current theory and reflect these theories and beliefs positively in their practice.

A therapist's confidence in addressing issues, making considered decisions and defending outcomes is supported by a sound understanding of the theoretical principles of the profession. The ability to justify actions is a vital component of today's health and social care provision, where there is an increased demand for evidence-based practice. Clinical audit and demands for efficiency and cost effectiveness require professionals to be able to explain or defend their practices to managers, purchasers and consumers. The Health Councils Act (1999) has formalised the requirement for therapists to continue their own personal development and learning to ensure their professional practices remain current, competent and ethical.

CLARITY OF PURPOSE

Theory is the lens through which we see reality more clearly.

(Kielhofner 1985)

The history of occupational therapy demonstrates the consequences of basing a profession on a weak theory base. Lacking a solid theoretical framework, the profession was, particularly in the 1960s, diverted from its original purpose and allied itself more closely to theories from other professions, which appeared to have a sounder proven knowledge base or which were particularly valued or fashionable at the time (see Chapter 1).

Since then, occupational therapists have begun both to question and to value their own basic philosophy. Through the development of conceptual models, the analysis of approaches and the evaluation of practices, they have been able to justify the basis on which therapy intervention is founded and more clearly explain the aims and goals of practice to themselves and to others.

Without a theoretical framework a profession is like a ship afloat without a compass in a sea of change. It is at the mercy of the waves and tides of fashion, regularly changing course according to their ebb and flow, without ever reaching its proper destination. It is at risk of washing up on an unknown shore, where its crew will be likely to modify their behaviour to match the customs or culture of the natives and thereby gain acceptance.

Theory is the compass that guides the profession's progress, keeping its direction true whatever storms or changes in tides it encounters. Theory sets the course (the therapy process) and guides the passage (the intervention) to ensure that the ship reaches its chosen shore.

Theory provides a means by which our professional practice can be explained and clarified – for our own benefit and in response to others. It is a framework in which we can explain the philosophy of our practice, justify the value of interventions, and measure the efficacy of treatment.

The move to increase community-based services places more occupational therapists in multidisciplinary situations where they work with colleagues from disciplines other than their own. Sound professional knowledge and expertise is therefore essential to retain identity, educate others, and integrate occupational therapy practices into the multidisciplinary framework. The practitioner needs to be self-reliant within her discipline and demonstrate skills of independent thinking and clinical reasoning to meet people's needs and justify actions to others. To do this efficiently, she needs a sound theoretical base to guide her judgements and develop practice expertise.

Theory is an integral part of competent professional practice (Fig. 3.1). Mont and Ross (cited in Black & Champion 1976) remind us that 'there is nothing impractical about good theory ... Action divorced from theory is the random scurrying of a rat in a new maze. Good theory is the power to find the way to the goal with a minimum of lost motion and electric shock'.

COMMON UNDERSTANDING

In a profession that has such a broad spectrum of practice, it is essential to have a common under-

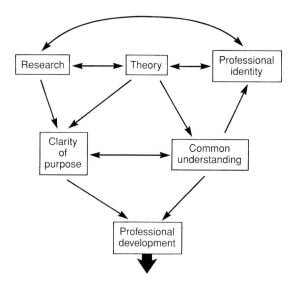

Fig. 3.1 The importance of theory to practice.

standing to retain professional identity within the membership, and in the perceptions of the purchasers and consumers.

Clark et al (1991), in an article concerning occupational science, indicated the need for the profession to have 'a unified vision of what is at the heart of our practice'. In the 1960s, the alliance of some areas of occupational therapy to the medical model led to a divergence in practice, with the development of specialist techniques based on medical factors rather than on individuals' occupational needs. Such divergencies did nothing to enhance the understanding of the profession by clients, other professionals and employers. When individuals received different treatments and advice from different therapists there was understandably some confusion, often followed by a loss of respect for the methods used or the information given.

How can such a situation be explained? Much was due to the emphasis on competence in 'doing' rather than on the value of knowing the *why* behind the 'doing', or on clarity regarding the philosophy and process of intervention. The development of theory based on holism and humanism and the organisation of problem-based intervention strategies has enabled therapists to understand and explain more clearly the projected aims and goals of their practices and thereby justify the variations in the methods used to achieve specific outcomes to meet individual requirements.

The occupational therapist has been recognised for the unique breadth of her practice, but only at the risk of being considered a 'Jack of all trades and master of none'. Mastery in combination with breadth is increasingly important in the present climate of healthcare, in which there is more diversity in services and service delivery, and intervention is 'needs led'.

The clientele of occupational therapy has changed in recent years, and will change further in the future, to include more people with multiple and complex problems. This is occurring for various reasons, including:

- demographic changes, including an increase in the number of elderly people
- advances in surgical and survival techniques, which enable people to survive longer following severe trauma and to live much longer with chronic medical conditions such as multiple sclerosis and cancer
- improved antenatal and neonatal care and diagnostic techniques, which have enabled children with multiple handicaps to survive
- manpower demands, which have led to simple orthopaedic conditions not being seen by occupational therapists in many areas because of the more pressing needs of those with chronic or more complex problems.

As a result of this shift in clientele, the narrow focus of earlier treatment techniques will be insufficient to meet people's needs. An increasing emphasis on a broad based understanding of the individual will be a spur to research into the merits of particular frames of reference and to investigation of how the many theories can be cohesively integrated to meet the complex needs of a changing clientele.

A BASIS FOR RESEARCH AND DEVELOPMENT

The interrelationship between theory and research in all areas of knowledge and development is well known. Theory forms the basis on which research is carried out, and research leads to the proving or disproving of theory.

The Concise Oxford Dictionary defines research as 'careful search or enquiry into a subject to discover facts by study or critical investigation'. Research is a question in search of an answer. In the present climate of therapy, as the professions re-examine their practices in order to justify them to employers, managers and other professions, and with a view to meeting changing patterns of need, research and investigation are vital. Occupational therapists need to investigate the premises on which their interventions are founded, prove the efficacy of those interventions to others and justify the evidence base of their practices.

While many therapists, and others, intuitively recognise the benefits of various occupational therapy practices, there is currently a dearth of research by which the effectiveness of these has been measured or proven. Reliance on intuition and face validity does not provide a sound basis on which to assess the value of a given practice or to build further developments.

Many people view research as something done by others from which they are able to gain information. This is quite true as far as it goes. However, this view is often linked to a hesitancy to personally embark on research because it is perceived to be specialist, complex, highly intellectual, remote or even 'detached from the real world'.

In the past, occupational therapists have gained recognition as 'doers'. They have been active in devising and utilising methods to facilitate patients' and clients' abilities as doers, and have been under pressure themselves to be doers as the number of people requiring their assistance has increased and the profession has expanded. This has inevitably been at the expense of time for research to qualify and quantify the results of the 'doing', or to promote new thinking.

Occupational therapists should all be involved in research in some aspect of their work, even if only to prove their own worth. This may be through the simplest form of evaluation of a particular practice or intervention, or through a more complex investigation of needs or modes of provision for future planning strategies. Research is also needed to develop more valid and reliable assessment instruments on which clinicians can confidently base their intervention strategies (Ellis 1981).

Investigation by Taylor and Mitchell (1990) revealed that many clinicians were not personally carrying out research because of the constraints of time, finance, skills and caseload needs, but were in favour of clinical research and keen to collaborate with experienced researchers. Since this time, many more practitioners have become actively involved with research, through work-based projects to investigate particular facets of their service or practice, through further academic studies in conjunction with educational establishments, or through temporary or permanent research appointments.

No profession can afford to stand still if it is to retain its credibility, but change should not occur for the sake of change. While occupational therapy needs to keep pace with changing conditions, it should not lose sight of its original purpose.

Lyons (1985) stated that therapists had 'acquired a modest but respectable body of knowledge', which should be 'defined, researched and systematised, so that it becomes evident, definable, defensible and saleable'. In today's health and social care climate, these factors are increasingly important to maintain and enhance the profession's standing in service provision.

Theory guides the attitudes and values of a profession. It forms the basis for clinical reasoning (the questioning, analysis and determining of actions) and of the reflection on outcomes and appropriateness of present practices. Theory based on sound reflection and proven findings makes a major contribution to the development of proactive thinking for future needs (Parnham 1987). The history of the profession's divergence from its originating philosophy in the 1960s and 1970s, when developments occurred without the support of a strong, defined and proven theory base, provides further argument for research and planned development based on sound theory.

DEFINING TERMS

There are frequently slight differences among healthcare professionals in their understanding of theoretical terms. This may occur because some words are used differently between one profession and another. Additionally, the analysis of occupational therapy is a worldwide process and there are differences in the use and understanding of terms between nations and, depending on which source of information has been used, between individuals within one country. Therefore, definitions of terms as they are used in this text are given below.

PHILOSOPHY

A common use of the word 'philosophy' refers to a set of ultimate values, i.e. a view of the meaning of life and of the significance of the world we live in. Moral philosophy is the branch of knowledge that deals with the principles of human behaviour and ethics.

The philosophy of occupational therapy is based on the profession's view of what constitutes an acceptable or desirable quality of life. It determines the values, beliefs and practices of the profession, which are founded in what therapists consider is inherently good and provide a basis from which to approach theory and practice (Yerxa 1979).

One of the earliest philosophies for the profession, put forward by Adolph Meyer in 1922, identified occupational therapy as 'an awakening to the fullest meaning of time as the biggest wonder and asset of our lives and the valuation of opportunity and performance as the greatest measure of time'. The philosophy of occupational therapy is discussed in greater depth in Chapter 1.

PARADIGMS

The use of the word 'paradigm' became popular following the writings of the philosopher Thomas Kuhn in the 1960s (Kuhn 1970). Kielhofner (1992) uses the word 'paradigm' to refer to 'an agreed body of theory explaining and rationalising professional unity and practice, that incorporates all the profession's concerns, concepts and expertise, and guides values and commitments'.

A paradigm imposes a shape upon a science. It derives from the values, principles and knowledge shared by members of a professional community, and determines the scope and boundaries of the profession, thus guiding practice, research and future development.

Paradigms are built by members of a profession. They are formulated to guide the development of theory and practice, and are eventually discarded as new findings and beliefs emerge to form a new paradigm. This is a natural process of development, which occurs in all areas of science. To take an historical example, after the explorations of Christopher Columbus and others, the paradigm of a flat world was replaced by the paradigm of a round world. This shift in understanding further changed thinking and beliefs, and stimulated and guided new thinking and promoted other discoveries.

Paradigm developments have occurred in occupational therapy. The profession's initial paradigm was based on a view of man's need to be 'occupied'. This was replaced by a reductionist paradigm, which emphasised body and mind mechanisms as discrete parts of a whole. The present paradigm combines elements from the previous two into a new whole reflecting occupational behaviour and performance. This paradigm has led to the development of new models, for example the Human Occupation Model (Reed & Sanderson 1983), the Model of Human Occupation (Kielhofner 1985), the Activities Health Model (Cynkin & Robinson 1990) and the Canadian Model of Occupational Performance (Townsend et al 1997).

THEORIES

The new Shorter Oxford English Dictionary (1993) defines 'theory' as:

- a mental scheme of something to be done
- a way of doing something, a systematic statement of rules or principles to be followed

- the principles or methods of an art or science, especially as distinguished from the practice of it
- a system of ideas or statements explaining something.

In the present text, 'theory' might be used in any of these ways. Thus a theory is a mental scheme of something to be done and should portray the the rules and principles for the task in hand. In the introductory section of this chapter, 'theory' was used in the general sense to refer to the discussion of the 'principles' of the profession as opposed to its 'practice'. It should be borne in mind, however, that just as our practice should be firmly grounded in theory, our theory should never be far removed from practice. A theory that is not readily applicable to and verified by practice may have to be revised or discarded. Practice research to gather evidence regularly brings theory into question. Where inconsistences are found, revisions of thinking or modification of ideas result in an ever-developing process.

A slight shift in meaning occurs when the text moves from the discussion of 'theory' in its widest sense (i.e. a type of discourse as in: 'the subject of this chapter is occupational therapy theory') to the discussion of a particular 'theory' or 'theories' (e.g. Piaget's theory of intellectual development). Thus, within the philosophy and paradigm of occupational therapy 'theory', various particular 'theories' come into play, some of which are unique to the profession and some of which have been borrowed from and adapted from other disciplines.

FRAMES OF REFERENCE

A frame of reference is an organised body of knowledge, principles and research findings that forms the conceptual basis of a particular aspect of practice. Mosey (1981) defined a frame of reference as a 'set of inter-related internally consistant concepts, definitions and postulates that provide a systematic description of, and prescription for, a practitioner's interaction with a particular aspect of a profession's domain of concern'.

Unlike a paradigm, which provides a general structure for thought, a frame of reference rationalises and explains a particular facet of practice. It consists of a 'group of compatible theories that can be applied within a particular field of practice' (Creek & Feaver 1993). Young and Quinn (1992) defined frames of reference as 'those aspects which influence our perceptions, decisions and practice'. They form a basis for clinical reasoning (Rogers 1983).

Occupational therapy models have evolved partly through experienced individuals using frames of reference to develop structures for practice. They have built on their own theories, values, knowledge, practice and research findings to develop patterns and processes that may be used by many members of the profession.

Frames of reference are therefore important to the professional development of the individual therapist and of the discipline as a whole. They lead to the use of 'a standard set of facts to judge, control or direct some action or expression' (Reed & Sanderson 1983) and to clarity in the explanation, evaluation and evolution of professional theory.

As Mosey (1981) writes:

A frame of reference delineates a particular aspect of a profession and provides a central theme to which to refer for decisions regarding the appropriateness of the programme design and content ... It influences the practitioner's choices and approach to treatment and thus gives unity, balance and direction to the treatment programme.

However, confusion occurs because of the different labels given to frames of reference by different practitioners, according to their thinking and interlinking of ideas (Table 3.1). Variations occur between American theorists. Mosey (1981) named three frames of reference – 'analytical, acquisitional and developmental' – while Hopkins and Smith (1988) outline nine – 'behavioural, biomechanical, cognitive, developmental, neurodevelopmental, sensorimotor, occupational behaviour, rehabilitation and psychoanalytic'. These different labels indicate differences in thinking in what actually constitutes a 'frame of reference'. Mosey uses broader terms to reflect modes of progress than do Hopkins and Smith,

Table 3.1 Different authors' representations and terminology for occupational therapy frames of reference

Authors	Frames of reference
Mosey (1981)	Analytical, acquisitional, developmental
Hopkins & Smith (1988)	Behavioural, biomechanical, cognitive, developmental, neurodevelopmental, sensorimotor, occupational behaviour, rehabilitation, psychoanalytical
Young & Quinn (1992)	Adaptive performance, developmental, sensorimotor, cognitive, role performance, rehabilitation
Creek (1997)	Rehabilitative, psychodynamic, behavioural, human developmental, occupational behaviour, cognitive behavioural, cognitive
Hagedorn (1997)	Biomechanical, neurodevelopmental, sensory integration, behavioural, cognitive, psychodynamic, humanistic
Turner et al (1996)	Phenomenological, developmental, biomechanical, learning, compensatory

whose titles are more allied to particular intervention strategies.

Variations also occur in British texts. Young and Quinn (1992) identified six frames of reference 'adaptive performance, developmental, sensorimotor, cognitive, role performance and rehabilitation'. In 1997, Hagedorn divided frames of reference between those that are primary and those that are applied. The physiological primary frame of reference underpins the biomechanical, neurodevelopmental and sensory integration applied frames of reference. Similarly, the psychological primary frame of reference supports cognitive and behavioural applied frames of reference; psychiatry and psychotherapy link with the psychodynamic frame of reference and humanism supports the humanistic applied frame of reference. Creek (1997) identified seven frames of reference: rehabilitative, psychodynamic, behavioural, human developmental, occupational behaviour, cognitive behavioural and cognitive. Application of these to the field of mental health through different models and approaches is described in some detail in the text (Creek 1997).

Kielhofner (1992) challenges the title 'frames of reference', stating that he prefers to label them as conceptual models for practice. Other authors argue that a model is a diagrammatic representation, whereas a frame of reference is an interlinking of compatible ideas and themes to explain particular similarities in practices and occurrences.

The authors of this text agree with the term 'frame of reference' as an interlinking of compatible ideas and themes that may be used to direct the thinking for methods of intervention, once goals and priorities have been established.

The confusion and conflict have been addressed by identifying five fundamental frames of reference that guide occupational therapy for physical dysfunction, based on discussion with practitioners and the writings of others. These are the phenomenological frame of reference (founded in humanistic thinking), together with the developmental, biomechanical, learning and compensatory frames of reference (to reflect theories that influence therapeutic intervention). In some instances, one primary frame of reference may be used to address a number of problems. In other cases, a number of different frames of reference may be used to treat different problem areas. Similarly, a number of frames of reference may be used to address one area at different stages of intervention; for example, it may be advisable to use a biomechanical or developmental frame of reference to guide intervention in the recovery stages, but this may have less value in addressing problems resulting from residual impairment once improvement has reached a plateau, when a compensatory frame of reference may be more appropriate.

APPROACHES

Approaches are the ways and means of 'doing', that is, of implementing frames of reference. An approach consists of the rationale behind a specific technique and the way in which it is used in practice. An approach may be used singly, or in combination with others, to achieve an aim or goal. For example, the adaptive approach, which is based on the compensatory frame of reference – the belief that a problem can best be overcome by compensating for it, rather than through biomechanical or developmental means to improve anatomical or physiological functioning – may be used exclusively to treat a permanent impairment. However, where the impairment is likely to be temporary, the adaptive approach may only be used for a short time, to be phased out in favour of another approach as recovery commences.

An approach determines how an activity may be used. Within the adaptive approach, the therapist will assist a keen gardener to devise different techniques to continue his hobby, for example placing seed trays on the bench to prick out seedlings to avoid stooping and bending. Within the neurodevelopmental approach, gardening activities involving stooping and bending may be encouraged to promote balance and weight transfer. A heavy gardening activity, such as digging, may be used in the biomechanical approach to improve muscle strength and activity tolerance in the lower limbs.

MODELS

According to the Shorter Oxford English Dictionary, a model is 'a simplified description of a system or process put forward as a basis for theoretical or empirical understanding; a conceptual or mental representation of something showing the arrangement of its component parts'.

A conceptual practice model has been described as 'an abstract representation of practice' (Hopkins & Smith 1988 p383). It presents theories or ideas in schematic form, for example, through charts, plans, pictures or flow diagrams, often showing the interrelationship between the parts in the whole.

A conceptual model for professional practice represents the basic concepts or theories behind intervention in diagram or chart form, delineating a framework for professional action and thinking. This is based on professional values and beliefs, and displays the links between theory and practice. Such a model may be used to promote clearer understanding of professional actions, to clarify the boundaries and roles of intervention, to determine tasks within the intervention process, and to deduce anticipated outcomes.

A professional practice model may apply to various aspects of the profession, providing a framework for a number of areas of intervention in a variety of realms of practice. It may be used as a diagrammatic tool to explain the application of complex theories.

Models occur at different levels, depending on what they depict. Some models show the inter-linking of frames of reference with theory – for example, the Model of Human Occupation portraying Kielhofner's interpretation of occupational behaviour theory. Reed and Sanderson (1983) refer to this type of model as a 'generic' model, because it can be applied across a number of areas of practice with a number of approaches. Other models are designed at a more specific level to delineate the process of application of a

particular approach. Reed and Sanderson (1983) call these 'descriptive' models. Examples of these are the neurodevelopmental and sensorimotor models, which reflect the sequence of stages of particular aspects of development within the developmental frame of reference. Generic models may be used to determine the overall picture of a particular situation, whereas descriptive models may guide the application of particular frames of reference in intervention (Fig. 3.2).

Confusion occurs between authors on the use of the term 'model'. Kielhofner (1992) prefers to use the term 'model' to describe what others refer to as a frame of reference. The definition of a conceptual practice model used within this text is based on those used by Creek (1997), Turner (1996) and Hagedorn (1997), as a 'simplified

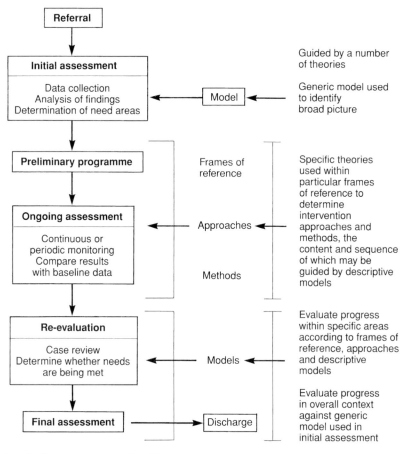

Fig. 3.2 Theoretical applications in the occupational therapy process.

representation of the structure and content of a phenomenon or system, that describes or explains the complex relationships between concepts within the system and integrates elements of theory and practice'.

LINKING TERMS

There is frequently difficulty in linking the terms defined above, particularly when there is no consistent interpretation of the terms between texts.

In the context of the present volume, the *paradigm* of occupational therapy will be considered as the basis of the fundamental principles of the profession. It comprises the concepts that therapists hold in common concerning the ways in which people use and benefit from occupation, that is, from involvement, interaction and activity in life. These concepts derive from and are supported by the profession's *philosophy* regarding the essential humanity of man and his participation with and in his environment.

Theories have developed from this paradigm (as well as from other areas of knowledge and learning) to reflect therapists' values and beliefs about the nature of occupation, the criteria for defining and achieving competence and the essence of humanism. These theories have further led to the development of a number of *frames of reference* with regard to how humans learn, develop and perform within their environment. *Approaches* have been devised in order to apply the philosophies and theories within these frames of reference in clinical practice.

Within this hierarchy of professional thinking, *models* exist at two levels. Some models have been devised and drawn up to explain particular approaches in relation to frames of reference. Other models show the integration of frames of reference with theories. Thus, some models, such as the behavioural model, may be confined to a particular aspect or area of practice, while others, such as the Model of Human Occupation, may be more broadly based, explaining the interrelation of a number of frames of reference in a theoretical whole.

THEORY IN PRACTICE

The practice of occupational therapy is eclectic in that it draws selectively upon various schools of thought in addressing a wide variety of needs. This eclecticism has permitted the use of a number of frames of reference, each of which may be used to determine particular techniques and approaches in practice. Inevitably, these frames of reference overlap and to some degree may be integrated with one another, but each is significantly different in its underlying theories and beliefs. Humanistic occupations/activities and psychosocial theories support individual aspects of practice but also underpin wider frames of reference and are used concurrently to form the basis of many approaches to practice. In this way, theories and frames of reference complement one another. Within the occupational therapy process therapists focus on different aspects of theory at particular stages to guide their thinking and actions (see Fig. 3.2). During the initial assessments, the therapist may use a broad theoretical base, to remain 'open minded' and unbiased towards the particular area of deficit. Frequently, the individual may be referred for a particular item but this may be only part of the problem. The therapist may therefore use one or more broad-based 'generic' models to identify the overall situation and gain a fuller picture of the problem in the context of the individual's unique circumstances. Following this, the therapist may use one or more specific frames of reference to guide her thinking towards, and assessment of, individual aspects of deficit or need.

When making decisions regarding intervention, the overall 'generic' picture remains in focus but particular frames of reference and individual theories guide the chosen specific approaches to meet the person's biomechanical, developmental or learning needs, or to compensate for dysfunction that cannot be overcome by other methods. The structure and sequences of these approaches and methods are more likely to be directed according to a 'descriptive' model, which defines the processes and procedures of the particular approach.

The progress made in a specific area will be analysed and assessed according to the descriptive model. However, it will also be viewed in the overall context of the person's situation and needs, as identified in the generic model during the initial assessment.

THE USE OF THEORIES

The humanistic theory

This theory is based in phenomenology and existential psychology. Phenomenology focuses on subjective experiences – individuals' personal views of events in their own current environment – and believes that people are not acted on by external forces but are themselves 'actors capable of controlling their own destiny' (Atkinson et al 1985). Existentialists believe that knowledge differs for each individual and is constantly changing as the result of personal experiences and the subsequent interpretations of these experiences. The person is seen as a whole being – a Gestalt – rather than a collection of parts.

Humanism perceives the person optimistically, believing that human nature is essentially 'good'. Such positive beliefs are reflected in the view that human beings have an innate drive to be creative, to love, to grow and to be productive. These views are demonstrated in the belief in 'the self' (as described by Rogers 1984a) in the client-centred approach, which views the individual as a free and responsible agent capable of determining his own development. Maslow (1968) also reflected this positive view that humans are motivated by a drive to satisfy needs. He described these needs in a hierarchy, the lower levels of this being devoted to satisfying needs for personal existence. When these needs have been largely met, the person is able to move on to strive to achieve higher needs for growth, self-esteem and aesthetic pleasure, and finally try to reach his full potential – self-actualisation.

Humanistic theory in practice

In practice, occupational therapists' use of phenomenological beliefs are widely applied through the humanistic ways by which the therapist respects people's autonomy and individuality throughout intervention. The therapist recognises the person's capacity for self-awareness and his right and freedom to choose his own actions. This is the opposite of didactic authoritarianism, which dominated the earlier practices of many professions – the 'professional knows best' syndrome – and is in line with current ideologies of patient autonomy, empowerment and patient-focused healthcare. When applying humanistic theory, the therapist respects the individual as a partner in therapy. Partnership in assessment of needs and priorities and in the negotiation of realistic, purposeful opportunities, is the basis on which the therapeutic relationship grows. The therapist's essential belief in individual self-determination is reflected in the ways in which she helps the individual to make informed choices from a range of suitable options without exerting control over his decisions.

Basic assumptions

- The person has the potential for awareness of personal needs, drives and goals and has the ability to change through opportunities and experiences.
- The quality of intrapersonal and interpersonal relationships and rapport are important in the development of self-esteem.
- The individual has the right to make choices and prioritise according to his personal perceptions of strengths and needs and the right to preserve or develop an internal locus of control.
- The positive strengths and abilities of the individual to overcome difficulties, rather than his weaknesses, should be emphasised.
- Merely 'being able to do' is not sufficient. Feelings of purposefulness, skill and achievement are vital components in self-actualisation and self-esteem.

Practices that reflect humanism

- Self-rating assessments.
- Recognition of values, roles and beliefs.

- Non-directive counselling.
- Providing opportunities for expressive interactions.
- Providing opportunities for informed prioritising.
- Acceptance of opinions and choices.

The occupations/activities theory

This, the earliest theoretical base for occupational therapy, was founded on the belief that occupation and activity are instrumental in achieving and maintaining health. Theories regarding the value of occupation and activities developed from studies by Meyer (1922), Reilly (1962) and many others, but have their beginnings in the view of the relationship between activity and health as understood by the Romans and ancient Greeks.

The basis of the use of this theory in occupational therapy was summed up in Mary Reilly's (1962) well-known statement: 'Man through the use of his own hands, as they are energised by mind and will, can influence the state of his own health'.

In recent years, many therapists have striven to explain the differences in meaning between 'occupation' and 'activity', in order to clarify the profession's philosophy. Occupation has been defined as:

- 'Volitional goal directed behaviour aimed at the development of play, work and life skills for optimal time management' (Rogers 1984b).
- 'The dominant activity of human beings that includes serious productive pursuits, and playful, creative and festive behaviours' (Kielhofner 1983).
- 'Man's goal directed use of time, energy, interests and attention' (American Occupational Therapy Association 1976).
- 'Those activities and tasks which engage a person's time, energy and resources and are composed of skills and values' (Reed & Sanderson 1983).
- 'An active doing process of a person engaged in goal directed, intrinsically gratifying and culturally appropriate activity' (Evans 1987).

The majority of these definitions are American. The Concise Oxford Dictionary defines 'activity' as a 'task or action' or 'being active', and 'occupation' as 'profession or employment' and 'occupying or being occupied'. In order to clarify the meaning of terms, Hagedorn, Creek, Turner and others met in 1993 to discuss definitions. The definitions suggested by this group are that 'activity is an action performed by an individual for a specific purpose on a particular occasion', whereas 'occupation defines and organises a sphere of action over a period of time and is perceived by the individual as part of his/her personal and social identity'.

In summary, activity is *doing*, whereas occupation is a state of *being*, most frequently achieved through active participation in activity. Occupational therapy is based on the belief that, to be therapeutic, activity should be purposeful. Within the realm of occupational therapy, activity is said to be purposeful when the value of its use is to 'facilitate the integration of an individual into or maintenance in his or her community' (Golledge 1998) or provides a medium by which specific skills may be developed through an activity in which the client is interested.

While there was some deviation from the occupations/activities theory in the 1960s and 1970s, the belief in the value of occupation has remained central to the profession. This may be seen through the use of purposeful activities in therapy, or through the problem-solving strategies to enhance an individual's ability in daily living tasks, thus achieving 'occupational' goals, and successful 'occupational performance'.

Analysis of occupations/activities theory (Cynkin & Robinson 1990, Kielhofner 1983, Townsend et al 1997) has led to considerable debate on the different terms, a fuller appreciation of 'occupation' and a greater recognition of the value of purposeful activity in healthy living. This has been reflected in the modern 'generic' occupational therapy models, which have frequently been organised to show factors and stages in the development of successful occupational performance. They have been able to integrate professional values concerning the belief of an individual, theories of achievement and motivation, and the implications of the individual's interrelationship with the material and social environment, to explain ways by which a broad range of activities may be used purposefully to achieve goals and a balance in health.

Basic assumptions

- Occupations and activities are vital components of balanced healthy living.
- Occupations and activities can be used in a variety of ways to overcome dysfunction, and promote health in body and mind.
- The most positive outcomes are achieved through activities that are purposeful and goal directed, offering realistic challenges and achievable outcomes.
- The greatest personal commitment is obtained when the activities chosen are relevant to the individual's lifestyle, roles, aspirations and needs within his environment, and relate realistically to his present level of function.

Generic models

Several conceptual occupational performance models have been based on the occupations/activities theory. Recent examples include:

- Cynkin and Robinson (1990) – Activities Health Model
- Kielhofner et al (1985, 1997) – Model of Human Occupation
- Reed and Sanderson (1992) – Personal Adaptation through Occupation Model
- Townsend et al (1997) – Canadian Model of Occupational Performance.

Psychosocial theory

This theory concentrates on the attainment of interpersonal and intrapersonal skills in the environment. Initially, it was considered particularly important for people with mental health problems but many of its principles are equally important in areas of physical or cognitive dysfunction to achieve social integration and role performance. Psychosocial theory may have

application for those who have to make adjustments to living as the result of trauma that affects cognitive function (for example, following head injury) or for those who have disease or injury resulting in physical or perceptual dysfunction, or gross disfigurement. Additionally, the initial acquisition of competent psychosocial performance may be limited or constrained through lack of opportunity or ability for those who suffer congenital impairment.

Many practitioners, recognising the psychological and social implications of impairment, have incorporated aspects of psychosocial theory into their frames of reference. These have been considered as factors to be included in planning holistic, humanistic intervention programmes, but have been combined with other aspects within the frame of reference rather than being considered as a theory per se.

Mosey's psychosocial theory

Use of psychosocial theory in occupational therapy was expounded by Mosey in the 1970s and 1980s. Mosey based her views on psychoanalytical and developmental theories, together with earlier learning theories used in occupational therapy. These included limitations identified in early habit training as used by Slagle (1988), Fidler and Fidler's (1978) communication processes, and Ayres' (1973) neurobehavioural orientation theory, together with her own previous theories of adaptive skill responses, described in her article entitled 'Recapitulation of Ontogenesis' (1966), a reflective summary of the stages of development of the individual.

Mosey's theory is based on the belief that individuals have an inherent need to explore the environment, which leads to a desire to be competent within that environment. The requirements to achieve competence are dependent on the nature of the society in which the individual wishes to function and on the social roles expected of and anticipated by him. The nature of the environment also has a significant effect on the process of learning.

According to Mosey (1986), the performance components which underpin psychosocial achievement are sensory integration, cognitive and psychological functioning, and social interactions.

Mosey (1986) defined sensory integration as 'processing of sensory information in such a way that the individual can act on the environment … the central nervous system translates sensory impulses into meaningful information and organises that information so as to initiate an appropriate response'. This involves a process of filtering the many stimuli that are received from the different senses – sight, hearing, smell, and vestibular, proprioceptive and tactile sensations – and, by using cognitive functioning, perceiving and organising them to make the desired response.

Mosey identified these cognitive functions as attention, concentration, memory, orientation to the environment and thought processes that 'combine, re-combine and manipulate' associations of ideas through conceptualisation, intellect, known facts and problem-solving sequences, to plan and organise the most appropriate action.

Actions also depend on psychological functioning – individuals' own perception of 'being'. This involves the person's values, needs, emotions, interests and motivation, his conscious and unconscious thought processes, and the psychodynamics of his behaviours, as well as his understanding or insight into his own and others' mental processes and actions. Psychological functioning also includes the self-concept – identity, sexual identity and body image, self-esteem and the awareness of one's own assets and limitations. Actions are also affected by object relations – 'the ways in which objects satisfy needs or interfere with satisfaction' – and the ways in which the individual 'seeks need-satisfying objects and attempts to eliminate objects that interfere with satisfaction'. This includes people's deliberate drives and courses of action, self-discipline, self-control and personal responsibilities, and the ways in which individuals deal with stress, failure and frustration. Besides their own perceptions of themselves, psychological functioning also includes individuals' concepts of others – how they view other people and how they come to these views.

Mosey (1981) identified the final element – social interaction – as the interpretation of people's perceptions and understanding of situations, their social skills in 'initiating, responding to, and sustaining interactions'. This includes communication, 'the ability to engage in meaningful interaction with another person – dyadic interaction' and group interaction skills in both structured and unstructured situations.

Basic assumptions

- The process of social integration occurs through psychosocial learning regarding roles and role needs.
- The individual may lose skills during illness but these can be relearned and regained.
- Development of skills may be delayed by congenital impairment but skills may be learned later through supported opportunities.
- Adaptation in each skill area occurs developmentally and is dependent on, and related to, adaptation in other skill areas.
- Change (adaptation) occurs as a continuum from conscious learning and doing, through non-conscious action to the adoption of unconscious habit as mastery develops.
- Most adaptation occurs through practical interaction in a 'growth facilitating' environment that is realistic with regard to the area of need and provides opportunity to explore the skill area and receive feedback from it.

Psychosocial theories have been important in models and frames of reference used by occupational therapists to underpin intervention to promote integration of the individual within the environment.

GENERIC MODELS

Generic models aim to provide a structure or format by which practitioners can integrate thinking to guide their intervention. Generic models can be applied across a number of areas of practice. While these models may draw predominantly on one theory, most draw on a number of different theories, which reflects the eclectic nature of occupational therapy practice. They interlink a number of frames of reference with these theories to enable therapists to consider various different options for intervention according to the needs and situation of the individual and particular demands or preferences.

The Model of Human Occupation

This was first devised by Kielhofner, Burke and Igi in the late 1970s and early 1980s (Kielhofner et al 1980) and was revised and refined in the early 1990s (The Model of Human Occupation: Theory and Application, Kielhofner 1995).

The model was originally based on an open systems theory but later thinking related it more to chaos theory and dynamic systems theory. These emphasise the 'dynamic nature of occupational performance and the role of occupational performance in maintaining a system's organisation and achieving change' (Kielhofner & Forsyth 1997). Kielhofner believes that the human system, the environment and the task all contribute to occupational performance (Fig. 3.3). This means that the therapist must consider the

context and meaning in which the person is performing an activity, as well as the actual performance, in order to understand and influence the performance. Kielhofner also believes that action is 'a central force in health, wellbeing, development and change' (Kielhofner & Forsyth 1997), which is the central belief of occupational therapists. Through experiences in occupational behaviours, the organisation of bodies and minds are maintained or improved. Individuals create their social identities, self-concepts and motor skills through occupational behaviour.

The Model of Human Occupation describes the structure of occupational behaviour in three subsystems that determine the motives for choosing activity (volition), the patterns and routines used to carry out the activity (habituations) and the capacity for production of the activity (performance):

- Volition is the self-awareness and drive that enables people to choose activity. It is divided into three aspects: personal causation (self-knowledge of capability and efficacy), values (significance and standards) and interests (positive desires for participation).
- Habituation is composed of roles (role scripts) and habits (habit maps), which structure occupational routines and behaviours. Roles determine the routines and range of activities that are carried out in a particular way (role scripts) as part of an internally and socially perceived role. Habits determine the style of behaviour and the ways by which particular activities are performed regularly and are internalised in habit maps.
- Performance includes the skills through which an individual carries out activity. This is a combination of musculoskeletal, neurological, cardiopulmonary, perceptual and cognitive components, which act together to provide mind–brain–body performance. Symbolic images guide the body in planning, interpreting and producing actions and behaviours and provide a way of 'knowing how to do something' in a given situation.

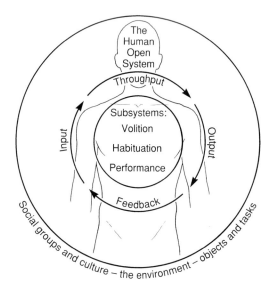

Fig. 3.3 Kielhofner's Model of Human Occupation (adapted from Kielhofner 1985 and reproduced with kind permission of Williams & Wilkins, Baltimore).

All behaviours are influenced by the environment in which the action takes place. Kielhofner considers environmental influences to be those that 'afford' opportunities and those that are 'presses' – the pressures and constraints in the environment in terms of expectations and demands. These may be considered in terms of the physical environment (the inhabited space and the objects used within it) and the social environment (people, social groups and cultures). In many instances, the environment both affords opportunities and provides pressures, and these must be understood by the therapist if she is to evaluate each individual's occupational performance in context.

Many assessment tools have been developed to support the use of the Model of Human Occupation in practice. These include interview schedules (for example, the Functional Screening Tool and the Occupational Performance History), self-administered checklists and tests (such as the Belief in Skills Test, the Interest Checklist and the Occupational Questionnaire), as well as a number of assessments for observation of function (for example, AMPS – the Assessment of Motor and Process Skills).

The Model of Human Occupation has the potential to encompass the physical, psychological and social aspects of performance and to recognise the effects of the environment upon the individual. It can therefore be used in conjunction with a number of frames of reference to organise and structure investigation, support analysis and clinical reasoning, and prioritise intervention. It can include a variety of therapeutic approaches to meet the particular volitional, habituational and performance requirements of the individual.

Canadian Model of Occupational Performance (CMOP)

This model, previously known as the Canadian Guidelines for Client Centred Practice, was originally devised in 1982 by a task force supported by the Canadian Association of Occupational Therapists and the Department of National Health and Welfare and, following revision in 1983 and later in 1997, was renamed the Canadian Model of Occupational Performance. The model is essentially based on a client-centred philosophy, viewing the client's values and beliefs as the core, giving meaning to activity, recognising the human skills that contribute to performance and the range of performance areas, all of which are surrounded and influenced by the impact of the environment.

Occupational performance is 'the result of a dynamic relationship between persons, environment and occupation over a person's lifespan' (Townsend et al 1997). The model is displayed in a circular form, superimposed by a triangle (Fig. 3.4), which represents the interacting elements of occupational performance. This inner triangle displays the four basic components of performance (affective, spirituality, cognitive and physical) with spirituality at the core. Beneath this triangle is the inner circle of the components of occupation (self care, productivity and leisure) and surrounding this circle is the outer circle representing the environments (physical, institutional, cultural and social).

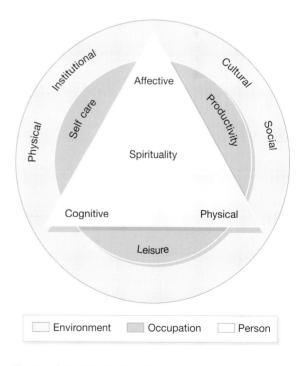

Fig. 3.4 Canadian Model of Occupational Performance.

The decision to site spirituality at the core of the performance triangle is based on the premise that this is central to all activity and gives meaning to occupation and daily living. It is linked to cultural beliefs but also embodies personal values, meaning and worth – the inner self – which is the basis for action and drive. The performance is carried out through the three following components:

- doing – physical components which comprise motor, sensory and sensorimotor skills
- thinking – cognitive components of intellect, perception, comprehension, concentration, judgement and reasoning
- feeling – affective components related to emotional and social areas in personal and interpersonal relationships.

The inner circle displays occupation under three familiar areas – self care, productivity and leisure – but with the review of the model these were redefined from those in the original model. The Canadian Association of Occupational Therapists (CAOT) (Townsend et al 1997) defined self care as 'occupations for looking after self', which includes all the activities necessary for self care and self-management. Similarly, for the purpose of the model, productivity was redefined as 'occupations that make a social or economic contribution or that provide for economic sustenance' (Townsend et al 1997). This includes those activities that enable individuals to consider themselves productive, whether or not there is any end product or financial reward involved. Leisure broadly encompasses all those occupations that are carried out for enjoyment.

Surrounding the inner triangle and circle is the outer circle, which represents the environment. Four different areas of environmental influence are considered, namely the:

- physical environment composed of the range of natural surroundings – buildings, equipment, roads, trees, nature, climate and weather, technology
- social environment, including social priorities within the community, social groups, common interests, attitudes, beliefs and relationships

- cultural environment, which includes ethnicity and race, routines and practice based on cultural beliefs
- institutional environment, which determines policies, procedures and practices and includes such areas as legal, political and economic elements.

All occupations are to some degree influenced by the environment and it is considered an important part of the occupational therapist's role to understand this interrelationship between the individual and the environment. Sumsion (1999) gives detailed coverage of the impact of environmental influences.

The application of the model in practice is based on a client-centred approach. When using this approach, therapists demonstrate 'respect for clients, involve clients in the decision making, advocate with and for clients in meeting clients' needs, and otherwise recognise clients' experience and knowledge' (Townsend et al 1997). Research with British occupational therapists (Sumsion 1997) resulted in the following draft definition of client-centred occupational therapy:

A partnership between client and therapist. The client's occupational goals are given priority and are the centre of assessment and treatment. The therapist listens to and respects the client's standards and adapts the intervention to meet the client's needs. The client actively participates in negotiating goals for intervention and is empowered to make decisions through training and education. The therapist and client work together to address the issues presented by a variety of environments to enable the client to fulfil his/her role expectations.

(Sumsion 1999)

The Canadian Association of Occupational Therapists advocate a seven-stage process for the application of the model in practice. This comprises:

- Stage 1 – name, validate and prioritise occupational performance issues with the client in areas of self care, productivity and leisure.
- Stage 2 – select theoretical approach or approaches with the client to address the issues identified.

- Stage 3 – identify occupational performance components and environmental conditions that are contributing to the performance issue.
- Stage 4 – identify the client's personal strengths and environmental resources (structural, social, familial and community) and the therapist's experience, expertise and resources.
- Stage 5 – negotiate targeted outcomes and develop an action plan. This specifies what the client and occupational therapist will do to 'resolve or minimise limitations to occupational performance in order to achieve the targeted outcomes' (Townsend et al 1997).
- Stage 6 – implement plans through occupation.
- Stage 7 – evaluate occupational performance outcomes. This may result in completion of the intervention if the targets are achieved, review of the activities or the targets if targets have not been achieved, or continuation if this is still beneficial to the client.

This model may be used with a number of different approaches, assessments and interventions, and the Canadian Association of Occupational Therapists developed the Canadian Occupational Performance Measure as an outcome measure to evaluate the effectiveness of this client-centred approach. The measure is used as an initial assessment to enable the client to identify and prioritise areas of concern, and is used again in the latter stages of treatment to evaluate outcomes in terms of the client's perceptions of changes in performance and satisfaction levels.

Activities Health Model

This model (Cynkin & Robinson 1990; Fig. 3.5) is also based on Reilly's thinking regarding occupational behaviour that 'for attainment of optimal function (or health) it is imperative that every human being be involved consciously in problem solving and creative activity' (Cynkin & Robinson 1990).

The model defines activities health as 'a state of well being in which the individual is able to carry out the activities of everyday living with satisfac-

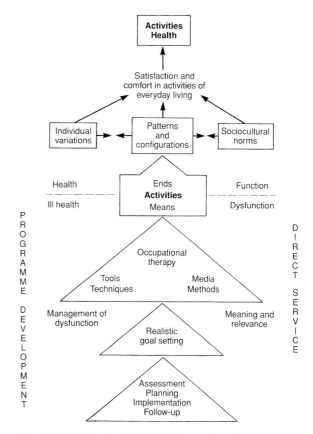

Fig. 3.5 Activities Health Model (adapted from Cynkin & Robinson 1990).

tion and comfort, in patterns and configurations that reflect sociocultural norms and idiosyncratic variation in number, variety, balance, and context of activities'.

The authors identify particular indicators of this state within the individual as the:

- number and variety of activities of everyday living that are appropriate in terms of sociocultural relevance (role, age, gender and culture)
- number and variety of activities of everyday living that are balanced in terms of personal preferences and choice, and the allocation of time to these
- overall feeling of comfort – being able to cope, feelings of accomplishment
- overall feeling of satisfaction – general feeling of wellbeing, contentment and happiness.

The Activities Health Model provides a number of assessments that may be used to determine individuals' 'daily use of time, feelings, learned history, preferences, sense of autonomy, and the social and spatial environment in which the activities take place' – 'the idiosyncratic activities configuration' – and an activities health assessment to determine the person's 'quality of life related to activities of everyday living'.

The application of the model to occupational therapy is clearly explained. Activity analysis is central to the model, demonstrating the need for the activity to be considered from two perspectives:

- the activity-centred elements – the 'essential properties and characteristics that are intrinsic to the activity, always present, in spite of individual differences in the way the activity is performed' and the acquired characteristics which 'come from variations among individuals and groups in the ways they perceive, associate to, and carry out the activity'
- the actor-centred perspective – the 'degree to which the patient/client's activities performance adheres to sociocultural standards and norms, and individual's idiosyncratic approach to the activity, and the specific performance components that a particular actor uses to carry out the activity'.

The model identifies how activities may be used as a means to achieving activities health through learning of activities (client centred and developmentally) and through the various psychosocial, behavioural and developmental approaches.

The model also shows how an activities health approach can be used in the process of practice for clinical problem-solving through the stages of assessment, planning, implementation and evaluation.

Personal Adaptation Through Occupation Model

This generic model outlined by Reed and Sanderson (1992; Fig. 3.6) is also based on the assumption that 'a person adapts or adjusts through the use of various occupations'. It is based on a number of assumptions:

- By participating in occupations a person may adapt to the environment, and occupations may be a means of adapting the environment to the person.
- The degree of adaptation is determined by 'the occupations a person learns and is able to perform'.
- All occupations require knowledge, skills and attitudes in variable amounts.
- 'All occupations are determined by the environment.' They occur because of the need to maintain the physical environment for physical existence, because of sociocultural expectations, or because of the desire for particular pleasurable occupations.
- 'Change in occupation is affected by environmental change.' Change may occur at an individual level in terms of opportunities for skill acquisition and adaptation, or change may occur in the broader environment (medical, structural or geographical), which will impact on a number of people or whole populations. This may be positive change, which enhances individuals' situations and opportunities, or negative change, which restricts occupation. Occupational therapists can assist in the development of positive change in the environment and in restricting the impact of negative change on the individual.
- Occupational therapists can have a positive effect on the extent and speed of an individual's abilities to adjust occupations through providing opportunities to relearn skills, to develop alternative skills and to adapt the environment to facilitate occupation. 'Occupational therapy media and methods are designed to assist the individual toward maximum functional independence or adaptation to the least resistive environment that will meet the individual's needs' (Reed & Sanderson 1992).
- 'Functional independence and satisfaction can be achieved by promoting a balance of occupational performance in the areas of self-

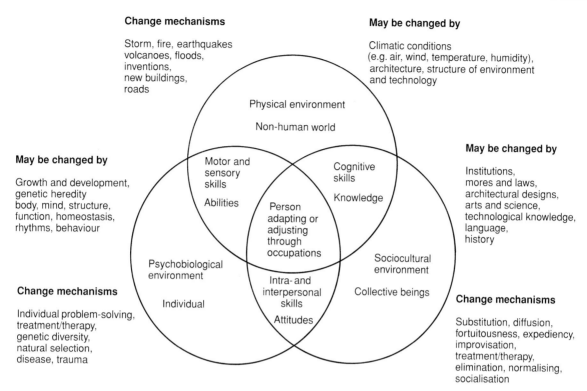

Change mechanisms

Storm, fire, earthquakes
volcanoes, floods,
inventions,
new buildings,
roads

May be changed by

Climatic conditions
(e.g. air, wind, temperature, humidity),
architecture, structure of environment
and technology

Physical environment

Non-human world

May be changed by

Growth and development,
genetic heredity
body, mind, structure,
function, homeostasis,
rhythms, behaviour

Motor and
sensory
skills

Abilities

Cognitive
skills

Knowledge

May be changed by

Institutions,
mores and laws,
architectural designs,
arts and science,
technological knowledge,
language,
history

Person
adapting or
adjusting
through
occupations

Sociocultural
environment

Psychobiological
environment

Intra- and
interpersonal
skills

Collective beings

Change mechanisms

Individual problem-solving,
treatment/therapy,
genetic diversity,
natural selection,
disease, trauma

Individual

Attitudes

Change mechanisms

Substitution, diffusion,
fortuitousness, expediency,
improvisation,
treatment/therapy,
elimination, normalising,
socialisation

Fig. 3.6 Reed and Sanderson's conceptual model – Personal Adaptation Through Occupation (from Reed & Sanderson 1992, reproduced with kind permission of Williams & Wilkins, Baltimore).

maintenance, productivity and leisure' (Reed & Sanderson 1992).

- Occupational therapy aims to develop people's knowledge, skills and attitudes consistent with individual needs, to 'promote the maximum occupational performance to which the individual is capable'.
- Maintenance and development of skills is dependent on the occupations in which they are used, being 'relevant and useful to the individual in relation to the environment'.

The model is represented as three overlapping circles, at the centre of which is the person adapting or adjusting through occupation (see Fig. 3.5). Fanning out from the person are three skill areas, which are used for adjustment and adaptation, namely motor and sensory skills (abilities), cognitive skills (knowledge) and intrapersonal and interpersonal skills (attitudes). The outer portion of each circle represents an area of the environ-

ment and is surrounded by the elements that may cause change, and by the change mechanisms that may alter the performance of skills or occupations. The physical environment or non-human world may be changed by gravity, temperature, altitude, humidity, soil, water, chemicals, air/wind, architecture and technology, and the change mechanisms that bring about these changes are cited as storms, fire, earthquakes, volcanoes, floods, inventions, new buildings and roads. The sociocultural environment made up of collective beings may be changed by institutions, mores and laws, architectural design, arts and science, technological knowledge, language and history. In this environment, the change mechanisms are substitution, diffusion, fortuitousness, expediency, improvisation, therapy/treatment, elimination, normalisation and socialisation. The third aspect of the environment portrayed in the model is the 'psychobiological' environment – the organic features of the individual. These may be changed by growth and development, genetic heredity, mind, body, structure, function, homeostasis, rhythms and behaviour, through change mechanisms such as natural selection, disease, trauma, genetic diversity, individual problem-solving, and therapy or treatment.

Reed and Sanderson (1992) outline a number of concepts that are inherent in the model and the assumptions they make. These include detailed analysis of the different environments, exploration of change mechanisms, outlines of skill acquisition, maintenance and loss, and the definition and meaning of occupation. They also explore the ideas of need and satisfaction, the nature of adaptation and adaptive potential, and the meaning of functional independence. The authors do not give details of the sequence or process of specific application of the model but offer it as a means of guiding thinking towards the attainment of functional independence. They conclude with nine proposed principles, which should be further explored and researched to establish their validity. These principles are that occupational therapists can:

- analyse with the client those occupations that will be most useful to him
- analyse the skills needed to perform specific occupations
- assess problems in skill development and acquisition by evaluating the functional components of sensorimotor, cognitive and psychosocial performance
- predict problems in occupational performance based on the analysis of problems in skill development and acquisition
- enable an individual to learn or relearn skills that are required to perform the occupations needed by the individual
- assist the individual to integrate the skills needed to perform occupations
- enable an individual to adapt to the environment through use of selected occupations
- assist the sociocultural environment to adapt to an individual through the use of selected occupations

- produce change in occupational performance and skill development and acquisition faster than a person could obtain the results using individual resources alone.

Psychosocial model

Mosey (1986) developed a psychosocial model based on three main areas: analysis, development and acquisition. Within these areas she defined three frames of reference – the reconciliation of universal issues in the analytical area, the attainment of adaptive skills in the developmental area and the adoption of roles in the acquisitional area.

Reconciliation of universal issues

This is 'concerned with the modification of intrapsychic content in such a manner that the individual is able to reconcile universal issues in a more adaptive manner' (Mosey 1986). Mosey identified eight 'universal issues': reality, trust, intimacy, adequacy, dependence/independence, sexuality, aggression and loss. She described change as occurring in four phases – communication, insight, assessment and working through. The individual is encouraged to become aware of his unconscious or unshared feelings, thoughts or beliefs about an aspect of one of the universal issues and to share or communicate them. These feelings are then explored and examined in order to promote insight. Following this, assessment occurs with a view to deciding whether to maintain the same beliefs or behaviours or to make changes in accordance with new insights. When the decision is to make a change, the individual will need support and help to work through any resulting anxieties or conflicts. Much of the process is facilitated through activities that promote transference, association and interpretation.

Attainment of adaptive skills

These form a 'developmental frame of reference addressed to those aspects of development considered to be crucial for adequate and satisfactory participation in a variety of social roles' (Mosey 1986). Adaptation occurs in seven main areas:

- perceptual/motor skill: the ability to recognise and make appropriate responses to sensory stimuli
- cognitive skill: the ability to process information and solve problems
- drive/object skill: the ability to manage and control personal drives in relation to current existing human and non-human objects
- dyadic interaction skill: the ability to engage and perform in a variety of one-to-one relationships
- group interaction skill: the ability to participate in a variety of group situations
- self-identity skill: the ability to recognise the self as an autonomous, competent, valued and developing being
- sexual identity skill: the ability to perceive one's sexual nature as 'good' and participate in long-term sexual relationships which are mutually pleasurable for those involved.

Mosey related these skills to stages of human development and identified ways through which an individual may be assisted to achieve such skills through learning in the environment.

Role acquisition

This is 'an acquisitional frame of reference addressed to those behaviours considered important for adequate participation in the major social roles' (Mosey 1986; Fig. 3.7).

Acquisition of social roles is facilitated through group explorations, which develop awareness and skills for successful interactions and performance within particular roles. The most basic skills for role acquisition are individual awareness of the needs of the role, competence in necessary personal tasks and interpersonal communicative skills. These are initially explored within the context of personal and family roles.

Social roles outside the family are developed through experiential group activities in which the task skills and interpersonal skills related to roles in school, at work and in social and leisure

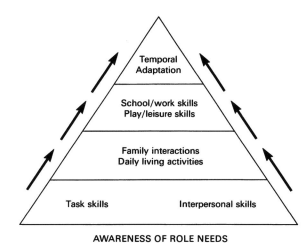

Fig. 3.7 Mosey's psychosocial theory: role acquisition (Mosey 1986).

pursuits are explored. The culmination of role acquisition is 'temporal adaptation' – the ability of the person to recognise the appropriateness of each action or activity within a role and to prioritise a number of tasks and needs realistically, so that the requirements of different roles are adequately met.

Mosey's psychosocial model may be used in a number of ways in interventions for people with physical dysfunction. It may be used to address a particular aspect of intrapersonal or interpersonal dysfunction, or it may form a more general basis for determining approaches within a developmental or occupations/activities approach.

FRAMES OF REFERENCE

Within the context of this text, a frame of reference is considered as a system of theories, serving to orient or give particular meaning to a set of circumstances, which provides a coherent conceptual basis for therapeutic intervention.

Frames of reference relating to physical dysfunction

The frames of reference most frequently used in the United Kingdom since the late 1970s to overcome or compensate for physical dysfunction are based on biomechanical, developmental and compensatory thinking. New ideas gained increasing favour as more research became available to validate their use; for example, the use of sensorimotor and sensory integration techniques with children affected by cerebral palsy.

Alongside these frames of reference occupational therapists employed humanism, to a greater or lesser extent, to address individuals' unique situations and problems. Client-centred beliefs were fundamental to identifying particular problems and the most appropriate solution *with* rather than *for* the individual.

Changes in the nature of healthcare, with greater diversity of provision and increasing numbers of people with chronic, complex conditions, has led to increased emphasis on the individual's development of coping strategies for managing their own situations. Use of cognitive problem-solving techniques, and transference and adaptation of skills, is crucial to successful functioning, particularly when impairments are likely to be permanent. Additionally, added recognition of the value of preventive as well as restorative care has increased the use of educative techniques to develop people's knowledge base, learning and understanding in order that they may make informed judgements regarding their own health.

The frames of reference that will be described in this text as they may be applied to physical dysfunction are based on thinking regarding development, biomechanics, learning and compensation. Within the scope of the text, it is not possible to address all the approaches that may be used within each frame, so the following will be given as illustrative examples of the application of the frame of reference:

- developmental frame of reference:
  - neurodevelopmental approach: Bobath techniques
  - sensory integration approach: Ayres
- biomechanical frame of reference:
  - biomechanical approach
- learning frame of reference:
  - educative approach
  - behavioural approach
  - cognitive approach

- compensatory frame of reference:
  - adaptive skills approach
  - compensatory approach.

Developmental

This frame of reference has had a significant influence upon occupational therapy practice since the 1940s; many approaches have been based on the theories of physical development and human development described by Piaget (1950), Erikson (1950), Freud (1965) and others.

Development occurs because of continuous interactions between nature (heredity, genetic factors and maturation) and nurture (the effects of experiences and the environment upon the individual). The development process affects the sensorimotor, cognitive, perceptual, personal and social domains of life. It can be attributed to: natural maturation; conscious interactions with the environment and external stimuli; the processes of learning; analysis, evaluation and making choices; and uncontrolled occurrences that influence the individual.

Most frames of reference take into account some element of growth, progression and evolution but an understanding of human development is at the core of this frame of reference, dictating and guiding the stages of the approaches that derive from it.

Basic assumptions

- Dysfunction is due to incomplete, maladaptive or retarded behaviour. This may be the result of incomplete maturation, the inability to utilise input effectively or the paucity of stimuli and opportunity.
- The person has the potential for development.
- Development occurs sequentially, each stage building on the previous one. Approaches relate closely to the stages of normal chronological human development.
- Development occurs in sequential stages from the person's present level of capability. Missing or jumping stages is usually counterproductive.

- Active cooperation rather than passive participation on behalf of the person involved facilitates greater development in most cases.

Examples

Some examples of developmental frames of reference that have influenced approaches to physical dysfunction are:

- Ayres' (1973) sensory integration model
- Rood's (1954) sensorimotor approach
- Llorens' (1970) developmental model
- Bobath and Bobath's (1975) neurodevelopmental approach
- Brunnstrom's (1970) movement therapy
- Voss et al's (1985) proprioceptive neuromuscular facilitation approach
- Gilfoyle and Grady's (1990) spatiotemporal adaptation
- Mosey's (1986) sociodevelopmental approach.

Merits

- The developmental frame of reference uses developmental theory to good effect by incorporating the normal processes of physiological and psychological progression and maturation into intervention strategies.
- The belief is one of optimism for each stage's completion, and there is a defined progression.
- The commencement point for intervention is flexible, reflecting the person's present state, and there is no defined rate of progress. The programme is therefore adaptable to a variety of levels of need and rates of development.

Limitations

- Progress to functional performance may appear slower than in some approaches, as each stage should be successfully achieved before moving on to the next.
- In the majority of situations the developmental frame of reference has limited application for people suffering with deteriorating conditions.

- Most individual approaches within this frame of reference require high levels of expertise and tend to be labour intensive.
- In order to attain maximum progress a coordinated, consistent approach is required from all members of the intervention team.

Approaches within the developmental frame of reference

The neurodevelopmental approach. A widely used approach that is developmentally based is the neurodevelopmental approach as proposed by Karel and Bertha Bobath in the 1940s and 1950s in the treatment of children with cerebral palsy. In recent years this has been extended and modified for the treatment of some adult neurological disorders, particularly hemiplegia as the result of cerebrovascular accident (CVA) or head injury.

This approach makes use of positions that inhibit abnormal postures and patterns of movement but facilitate normal equilibrium, balance and righting reactions and encourage normal movement patterns. Its basic principles are derived from the neurological learning theory and from theories of normal human development. The approach attempts to apply these principles to all aspects of activity throughout the day. It considers that the immature or damaged brain, because of the lack of opportunity to develop sophisticated balance control or because of interruption or blocking of such patterns by trauma to pathways within the brain, gives rise to primitive or abnormal muscle tone and movement patterns. By inhibiting or suppressing these abnormal patterns, and then stimulating normal sensory, postural and motor patterns, the brain may be stimulated to develop normal patterns through alternative pathways. The neurodevelopmental approach is most successful if begun in very early life for the child with cerebral palsy, or as early as is practicable after a CVA or head injury.

The sequence of treatment follows the normal sequence of development of movement in children. Humans are essentially symmetrical, and positioning and movement patterns aim to simulate and encourage bilaterality and symmetry while developing normal movement sequences. Alongside the development of motor patterns, stimulation of sensation and body awareness through touch and positioning is encouraged in order to assist the re-education of sensory pathways and to enhance the ability of the brain to interpret perceptual stimuli.

Integration of these principles within a programme of purposeful activities facilitates the development of sensorimotor control, which will then enable successful occupational performance.

Concern has been expressed by some occupational therapists that the exclusive use of neurodevelopmental approaches in occupational therapy neglects such aspects as volition, motivation or occupational needs. For use in the occupational therapy framework 'it is necessary to expand knowledge of the logical continuity beyond inhibition–facilitation techniques to activity, and to ways in which sensori-motor treatment principles can be applied during the performance of purposeful activity' (Pedretti 1985 p5).

Examples of the use of neurodevelopmental techniques with hemiplegia are:

- games such as a posting box or bead-threading to promote bilaterality with the cerebral palsied child; these involve holding the container or thread with one hand while posting shaped objects or threading beads with the other
- positioning components (for example tools, ingredients or plants) on a table or bench in cooking or greenhouse gardening, which will necessitate the individual maintaining his sitting or standing balance and crossing the midline when making the cake or potting seedlings.

The sensory integration approach. This well-researched approach is based on the theories of neurosciences as expounded by Jean Ayres. Sensory integration is the process of organising sensory information in the brain to make an adaptive response (Ayres 1973). The approach focuses on information received by the brain from the auditory, visual, vestibular, propriocep-

tive and tactile systems, particular emphasis being placed on the latter three systems.

Basic assumptions of the approach, which aim to explain the organisation of sensory stimuli in the central nervous system, are:

- the plasticity of the central nervous system
- that normal human development occurs sequentially
- that the brain is innately organised to programme a person to seek out stimulation that is organising and beneficial in itself
- that input from one system has an effect on other systems and the whole organism
- that the central nervous system is organised hierarchically – processing that occurs in the cortex depends on adequate organisation of stimuli received in the lower brain centres
- that stimuli must be registered meaningfully before the central nervous system is able to make a response and permit higher level functioning to occur (Hinojosa & Kramer 1993).

Therapy aims to improve the ability to integrate sensory information by changing the organisation of the brain. Change occurs as the result of accumulated stimuli and brain maturation, which open up new neural pathways to allow sensory information to flow through appropriate channels and integrate with other sensory information. The approach stresses the importance of the control of sensory arousal and the use of functional support systems to stimulate and develop adaptive responses according to the person's developmental stage.

A number of assessments may be used to determine:

- tactile and vestibular proprioceptive sensory processing
- form and space perception and visual–motor coordination
- bilateral integration and sequencing
- coordination, dexterity and motor skills
- practice abilities and behaviours.

Activities are designed to include a variety of sensory stimuli, with the aim of facilitating appropriate physical and emotional responses, which can be transferred according to need to other situations. Through variation and variety in activities the person is able to build up a repertoire of responses to multiple stimuli. This usually commences with basic primitive responses and gradually builds up to more complex adaptive responses to multisensory stimuli according to the person's developmental level. These adaptive responses, or 'end-product abilities', aim to facilitate adaptation within the environment through independent emotional and motor control. The approach is particularly useful with children who are brain damaged or developmentally delayed, for whom play activities may be used as the therapeutic medium, but it may also be used with adults who have suffered brain damage or have learning disabilities.

Activities such as press-button games or obstacle courses may be used to integrate actions with verbal or visual stimuli. Similarly activities involving hammocks or swings enable the individual to experience changes of positioning and to make choices regarding whether to increase or diminish these by swinging with or counteracting the pendulum movement.

Biomechanical

This frame of reference was the basis of many medical interventions throughout the 20th century. It views the body as a functioning machine, made up of specific parts that may be damaged by disease or injury. This frame of reference is based in the desire to explain function anatomically and physiologically. Many of its basic premises formed the foundations on which exercise physiology, kinetics and dynamic orthoses developed within the medical model.

The body is seen as a combination of parts that work together to form a whole; however, the Gestalt (the sum of the whole being more than a combination of the parts) is not acknowledged. Treatment to overcome damage to a particular part results in return of function. Therapeutic exercise or activity improves functional performance; this in turn leads to a sense of wellbeing, which promotes recovery. There is the risk, however, that the exercise or movement becomes the main focus, at the expense of the activity medium.

Basic assumptions

- Successful human motor activity is based on physical mobility and strength.
- Participation in activity involving repeated specific graded movements maintains and improves function.
- Activity can be graded progressively to meet particular demands within an intervention programme.

Merits

- The biomechanical frame of reference makes good use of media and equipment to promote physical function.
- It can be applied to a variety of creative and constructive activities.
- It uses knowledge of activity analysis to good effect.
- It utilises the increased knowledge of anatomical, physiological and kinaesthetic processes in humans.
- It has led to the development of specific techniques for measuring movements, strength and endurance.

Limitations

- The biomechanical frame of reference focuses on physical performance in the absence of volition, role duties or environmental influences. It is specifically based in physical activity, with no reference to motivation or the psychological, emotional or social aspects of rehabilitation.
- It does not address the need for balance in activity in daily life. It emphasises lower levels for survival – mobility and physical function – but does not follow through to the higher levels of self-esteem and self-actualisation.
- It is not applicable to people whose central nervous system is impaired. The emphasis is on the promotion of physical mobility, therefore this frame of reference has limited

application to people with chronic or deteriorating conditions which affect mobility.

- There is the risk of didactic reductionism – the therapist controlling the programme and the person being the passive participant in an exercise regimen that does not necessarily reflect personal interests or promote internal locus of control. The exercise may become the focus at the expense of the activity.

Current use of the biomechanical approach

Three slightly different biomechanical approaches have been developed:

- Baldwin's reconstruction approach (presented in 1918, and one of the earliest documented 'physical' approaches) (Baldwin 1919)
- Taylor's (1934) orthopaedic approach
- Licht's (1957) kinetic approach.

While each of these approaches has a slightly different emphasis, all are based on the biomechanical frame of reference. They are used in physical rehabilitation in physiotherapy and occupational therapy to promote mobility, strength and activity tolerance (stamina). Their early popularity reflected the essentially scientific nature of medical development in the physical field in the 1960s but they are less popular today, forming only a small part of the occupational therapist's treatment methods. The need to improve range of movement, muscle strength and endurance has also been reduced by modern medical and surgical techniques, which no longer require long-term immobilisation.

The mechanistic compartmentalisation of functional performance into physical actions contradicts the holism and humanism of occupational therapy's philosophy. Overcoming specific biomechanical dysfunction is only part of the management of the individual's total needs, mobility being only one part of function. However, as mobility is an important aspect of life, the principles of the biomechanical approach may form a part, if not the whole, of the therapeutic programme.

The changing nature of occupational therapy practice (which can be seen in the shift from hospital- to community-based work and in the increase in the proportion of people with complex, chronic disabilities and neurological conditions) further limits the use of this approach. Increased awareness of the merits of broadly based intervention as opposed to specialisation may further reduce the importance of this frame of reference in the total intervention programme.

Many occupational therapists have already abandoned the exclusive use of many biomechanical practices, although certain measurement techniques and activity analyses are useful in particular aspects of treatment. Some features of the biomechanical frame of reference combined with other, less reductionist, approaches retain importance in specific areas of practice, particularly orthopaedics, sports medicine and the treatment of physical damage resulting from trauma. Other professions, including physical medicine, nursing and physiotherapy, are adopting more humanistic, holistic philosophies, which may further contribute to the decline in popularity of the biomechanical frame of reference.

Learning

This frame of reference is based on the work of educational and developmental psychologists, behaviourists and teachers. It is founded on the assumption that adaptation and change are based on the ability to learn. Learning may be cognitive, gained by insight from personal interpretations of subjective responses to sensory stimuli and cues based on studies by Beck (1976) and Piaget (1950). Learning may also occur through behavioural change based on predetermined objectives and reinforcement of good behaviours, as described by Thorndike (1932) and Bandura (1971). Formal teaching – the provision of information and guidance – also promotes learning for informed action and decision-making.

Therapists employ teaching skills in many aspects of intervention, but not all aim to promote learning. Similarly, there may be an element of learning as a secondary gain with some interventions in other frames of reference, but theories of learning are central to the beliefs and aims in this frame of reference.

Basic assumptions

- The person has the capacity to learn through education and experiences.
- The acquisition of knowledge, and insight into behaviour, will promote learning.
- Learning occurs through different educational modes, which may be cognitive, conditioned or educative.
- Behaviours are learned. Poor or non-advantageous habits can be unlearned and replaced by lasting, helpful, 'good' habits through positive experiences and practice.

This frame of reference is used to support some of the approaches within other frames of reference. It is a major influence in particular aspects of practice, for example:

- social skills training
- assertiveness training
- anxiety/stress management
- joint protection and time management education
- behaviour modification.

These techniques may be used in a number of ways in the management of physical dysfunction, not only with children to advance the stages of developmental learning but also in facilitating the relearning processes following head injury, CVA or other changed circumstances resulting from trauma and physical dysfunction.

Approaches within the learning frame of reference

The educative approach. Occupational therapists aim to work in partnership with individuals and their family/carers, identifying a range of options for problem solving and working with them to make the most appropriate choices of interventions.

If individuals and carers are to make informed choices, it is essential that they have information concerning the importance of the issue at hand, the range of options available and the implications of choice of particular decisions. An educative approach aims to provide the knowledge on which such choices may be made.

Education may be provided through verbal discussion, but this depends on the recipient's memory and interpretation of what is heard. Many therapists now use visual educational means to support verbal guidance, in the form of booklets or leaflets, which the individual may take away and study at leisure or discuss further with other people. These leaflets may provide information concerning the medical condition, the importance of particular aspects of health, and ways in which the individual may take some responsibility for his future personal healthcare. Such leaflets may be used to inform people regarding the methods of joint protection in rheumatic disease; the importance of correct posture, exercise and suitable seating in the management of back pain; the care of the residual limb following amputation; and many other areas of self care. In some instances this written information may also be supported by audio-visual means, such as tapes or instruction videos. Many such educative materials are provided in a number of languages and reflect the needs of people from a variety of cultural groups.

The therapist should discuss the information with the individual and be available to answer any queries concerning the content. The information may form the basis of decisions regarding intervention and the individual's future self-management. In many instances, the provision of written or audiovisual information will be supported by other therapeutic approaches, usually involving practical and/or experiential techniques, to further the person's learning regarding a particular technique or issue.

The behavioural approach. This is based on the findings of behaviourists who believed that behaviours are learned in response to stimuli. Undesirable behaviours can be unlearned or modified through negative reinforcement of inappropriate behaviours and positive reinforcement of advantageous behaviours. A number of techniques may be used to change behaviour. Modelling may be used and the individual encouraged to model their behaviour on good behaviour observed in others. Desensitisation, a gradual, controlled build-up of exposure to a sensitive situation, may be used to change behaviour in relation to particular circumstances. Behaviour modification may be used to change inappropriate behaviours. This usually involves writing a contract with clearly defined predetermined objectives that the individual needs to achieve. Positive reinforcement or reward is given when such objectives are achieved and this is gradually diminished as the new behaviours become established. However, at this stage care must be taken to ensure that the newly learned skills do not 'fade'.

Other modes of behavioural learning involve chaining – the gradual build-up of actions towards completion of the task – and backward chaining. In backward chaining the individual is first responsible for completing the final stage of the task, and then gradually learns to do more towards the task in reverse sequence. Biofeedback is a behavioural technique that may be used in conjunction with other techniques, for example, relaxation techniques, to develop individuals' abilities to learn how to cope with particular situations.

Behavioural techniques are rarely used in isolation by occupational therapists because of their reductionist nature. They are time-consuming to implement and monitor and demand consistency of approach by all those involved with the individual if they are to succeed. However, they are useful in situations in which particular disadvantageous behaviours need to be unlearned, for example, in cases of phobia following a particular incident, to develop appropriate social behaviours following head injury or to change unsuitable practices in daily living or work settings.

The cognitive approach. This is based on the thought processes by which individuals link memories, perceptions, ideas and experiences within the context of their own environment and use these to plan actions and problem-solve. Cognition is based on past experiences and on past and present images and perceptions of oneself. If these are faulty or negative they will affect individuals' abilities rationally to address issues, process information and take a positive role in problem solving. Analysis of the individual's reasoning processes forms the basis for the cognitive approach, which aims to re-focus thought processes to develop a more positive 'train of thought'.

A cognitive approach may be used to help individuals make informed adjustments to temporary or permanent changes in their circumstances. They aim to facilitate insight into the person's thought processes, to correct misinterpretations or distortions of ideas, and to promote a positive approach to future activities. By providing opportunities through information sharing, role play, reminiscence, reality orientation or exploration of stress management techniques, individuals are able to gain insight into their own and others' interpretations of the situation and to explore coping strategies for management of the situation in the future. Examples of how such techniques may be used with physical dysfunction may be seen in ways by which imagery or re-labelling may be used in the management of pain, or the development of assertiveness and stress management techniques to build self-confidence following disfigurement. Similarly, perceptual or memory training may be used to develop cognitive skills and awareness following CVA or head injury, or with people suffering memory problems.

The prime focus in the learning frame of reference is for the person to learn coping skills. While the three approaches have been outlined separately, they are frequently used in conjunction with each other and with other approaches, to facilitate a broad-based approach to problem-solving, which employs theoretical, experiential and practical learning.

Compensatory

This frame of reference is based on the belief that humans are functional animals and that their ability to function – by whatever means – is essential to their wellbeing. It stresses the secondary benefit to be gained by improving performance in activity or occupation despite ongoing physical, cognitive, psychological or social dysfunction. A number of different compensatory methods may be used to perform an activity. The successful completion of the activity, rather than a specific change in anatomical, physiological or psychological attributes, is the primary goal, as this will enable the individual to survive in society.

Compensation may be used to facilitate performance in a variety of activities in daily life, through the use and adaptation of remaining abilities and strengths, by adapting the activities or by the provision of external compensatory means. These methods do not directly contribute to changing the person's biological, physiological or psychological deficits.

This is one of the oldest frames of reference for rehabilitation. It is not unique to occupational therapy and is also used by physiotherapists (for example, in the provision of walking frames to compensate for lower limb weakness), by orthotists and prosthetists, and to some degree by speech and language therapists when alternative communication equipment or techniques are recommended.

Basic assumptions

- Completion of daily role activities is a basic human need; the disabled individual can benefit by learning alternative methods for carrying out these activities.
- People suffer short- and long-term dysfunction that cannot be immediately or significantly improved by other therapeutic methods, so there is a need for compensation for lost or limited abilities.
- Residual capabilities can be supplemented by external aids to promote problem solving.
- The individual's involvement in choosing appropriate methods can be advantageous in promoting some general aspects of 'wellbeing'.

Merits

- The compensatory frame of reference is a widely documented and widely used basis for therapy practice. Many therapists are familiar with it.
- It is easy to explain and understand.
- It makes good use of a problem-solving approach.
- It can be used to meet immediate short-term needs or to compensate for long-term loss. It

is therefore appropriate for acute needs, for example, immediately following surgery or for people with chronic or deteriorating disorders who are not likely to recover or improve.
- A range of options is available, with considerable choice within them to meet a wide variety of needs.
- There is no rigidly structured sequence of progression, so there can be flexibility to meet the particular needs of the individual.
- It is concrete and often visual. It is easy to understand and frequently brings speedy results.

Limitations

- Historically, this frame of reference has had a long association with the medical model and so may be prone to reductionist or recipe-like thinking. The therapist may be tempted to 'prescribe' the 'best' method of compensating for a particular problem, rather than evaluate the range of options with the person concerned. A tendency, deriving from the medical model, to compartmentalise problems may fragment this potentially holistic approach into arbitrary divisions.
- The recognition of permanence of loss of function as the basis for instigating this frame of reference may have negative connotations for the individual, who will then require considerable support.
- In choosing solutions, the therapist may be at risk of succumbing to external pressures concerning the quickest or cheapest way of compensating, thereby denying personal choice. Compensation per se may be seen as a solution in cases where the use of other approaches and frames of reference may in fact promote or facilitate physical or psychological recovery or improvement.

Approaches within the compensatory frame of reference

The adaptive skills approach. An effective method of compensation for dysfunction is for the individual to adapt his existing skills to master problems and cope independently in particular situations. This method uses existing strengths to compensate for deficits. Techniques are based on:

● detailed knowledge of the present level of skill attributes
● clear identification of any previous techniques used for performing the activity
● exploration and identification of alternative techniques to perform activity using existing skills.

Solutions may involve:

● modification of the techniques required to perform the activity
● development of new skills through exploration and practice
● transfer of existing skills to different activities
● the use of 'trick' movements to compensate for particular movement deficits
● adapting role or function to eliminate the need to perform the activity.

Techniques will obviously differ according to individual attributes and limitations. New techniques may be learned through exploration and development of skills and practising using these skills in the task or situation. Techniques such as cognitive prompts may be used to aid memory, and individual movement skills may be transferred to perform activities in a particular manner, for example, using manipulative hand skills in the non-affected hand to tie shoe-laces and dress one-handed or using upper limb strength for non-standing transfers. Equally, the addition or omission of a particular stage to a sequence of activity may facilitate independent performance. Regular practice develops familiarity and expertise in the adapted skills until they become automatic, and can be used with confidence.

The advantage of these methods of compensation over the provision of external support are:

● the enhancement of self-confidence and self-esteem through independent personal achievement – the methods are personalised and reflect individuals' skills and attributes

● that they are flexible, adaptable and transportable – they may be used in a number of situations to a greater or lesser extent, depending on need, and are constantly available to the individual wherever he may be
● that, despite the time needed for the exploration of techniques, tuition and practice, they are usually cost-effective and their effect is long term
● that they reflect the basic philosophy of the profession regarding personal potential.

The compensatory approach. This approach is widely used to compensate for dysfunction in mobility, self-maintenance and domestic activities and is also used to enable individuals to pursue work and leisure pursuits. It applies the basic beliefs of the compensatory frame of reference. Occupational therapists using this approach must recognise that the individual and carers need to be consulted and involved in the choice of the most appropriate form of compensation; this involvement will help to motivate users to accept and persevere with the chosen solution.

Methods of compensation may include:

● supply of adapted tools or equipment
● provision of prostheses or support orthoses
● modification of the environment
● provision of financial help
● organisation of manual/social assistance.

The therapist using this approach must acknowledge the need for flexibility and adaptability in responding to a person's individual circumstances. Support orthoses have the potential to solve a variety of problems in different locations, providing they are worn consistently and correctly. Adapted tools and equipment may have a wide application in some instances but some equipment or tools may be specific to one particular task and may not be easily transferable or transportable.

Environmental adaptations are often considered a more drastic measure, as they are more likely to overtly stigmatise the person with the problem and affect other members of the family;

they are also more costly. An adaptation can usually be made to particular environments pertinent to the individual, e.g. home, work, school or vehicle, but their rehabilitative value is limited to these locations. The implications of restricted freedom in the wider environment will still have to be addressed.

Financial benefits may be used to purchase equipment or services to compensate for deficit; for example, a person who is unable to perform the full range of food preparation might buy an electric food mixer or microwave oven, or make arrangements for prepared food delivery. Such financial benefits may enable the person to pursue personal preferences, depending upon the range of options available and the funding provided; for example, the Disability Living Allowance.

Arranging for helpers to assist with certain tasks will require the person to recognise his limitations and to decide that the tasks in question are essential to him, despite the loss of independence they entail. Increased dependence upon others may be viewed positively, by virtue of the social contact it brings. It also enables the person to conserve his energy for other personal priorities. Employing others to assist with particular activities also enables the individual to remain 'in charge', rather than being a grateful recipient of help.

Obviously, as there is such a wide variety of options available in the compensatory approach, detailed assessment of functional capabilities and lifestyle needs is essential. From these findings, the priorities and options for problem solving should be discussed so that optimum solutions are found. These will depend on personal preferences and volition, the level, nature and probable duration of the dysfunction, and on the social environment. Additionally, the person's potential to learn new skills and use equipment or other resources should be considered.

It may sometimes be necessary to explore a number of different options before the optimal solution is found. For the person with a progressive condition it will be necessary to re-evaluate the choice of options as the condition progresses, but this should be minimised by forward thinking and proactive planning.

CONCLUSION

Without a theory base a profession has no foundation and no planned direction. Without a theory base a professional will be ill-equipped to assess the situations she is faced with and to respond to them in a realistic and organised manner.

Understanding the theory base of occupational therapy is a complex task, given the eclectic nature of today's practice, the diversity of individuals' needs and the current emphasis upon humanistic principles in therapy. Appreciation of the individual needs and drives of her clientele and an understanding of theory will assist the therapist in her professional reasoning and reflection.

The therapist herself is an individual, with personal values and beliefs that influence her choice of frames of reference. Recognition of these within the context of other frames of reference and the broader pattern of theory will enable her to more fully understand her own professional approach and that of others.

No profession stands alone; a sound theory base is necessary to identify the strengths and boundaries of a profession in the context of multiprofessional healthcare provision.

No society stands still; theory is essential in guiding research and development in the profession to meet the changing needs of individuals and ensure that the profession of occupational therapy remains up-to-date in its practices.

REFERENCES

American Occupational Therapy Association 1976 Occupational therapy: its definition and functions. American Journal of Occupational Therapy 20:204

Atkinson RL, Atkinson C, Smith ET, Benn DJ, Hilgard ER 1985 Introduction to psychology, 10th edn. Harcourt Brace Jovanovich, San Diego, CA

Ayres AJ 1973 Sensory integration and learning disorders. Western Psychological Service, Los Angeles, CA

Baldwin BT 1919 Occupational therapy. American Journal for Care of Cripples 8:447–451

Bandura AL 1971 Social learning theory. General Learning Press, New York

Barnitt R 1990 Knowledge, skills and attitudes: what happened to thinking? British Journal of Occupational Therapy 53(11):450–456

Beck AT 1976 Cognitive therapy and emotional disorders. International University Press, New York

Black JA, Champion DJ 1976 Methods and issues in social research. John Wiley, New York

Blom Cooper L 1989 Occupational therapy, an emerging profession in healthcare. Report of a Commission of Inquiry. British Association of Occupational Therapists, London

Bobath B, Bobath K 1975 Motor development in the different types of cerebral palsy. Heinemann Medical, London

British Association of Occupational Therapists 2000 Code of Ethics and Professional Conduct. British Association of Occupational Therapists, London

Brunnstrom S 1970 Movement therapy in hemiplegia. Harper & Row, New York

Clark FA, Parham D, Carlson ME et al 1991 Occupational science – academic innovation in the service of occupational therapy's future. American Journal of Occupational Therapy 45(4):300–310

Creek J 1997 Occupational therapy and mental health. Churchill Livingstone, Edinburgh

Creek J, Feaver S 1993 Models for practice in occupational therapy. Part 1. Defining terms. British Journal of Occupational Therapy 56(1):4–6

Cynkin S, Robinson AM 1990 Occupational therapy and activities health: toward health through activities. Little, Brown, Boston, MA

Department of Health 1999 The Health Act. HMSO, London

Ellis M 1981 Why bother with research? British Journal of Occupational Therapy 44(4):115–116

Erikson E 1950 Childhood and society. WW Norton, New York

Evans KA 1987 Definition of occupation as the core concept of occupational therapy. American Journal of Occupational Therapy 41(10):627–628

Fidler G, Fidler J 1978 Doing and becoming: purposeful action and self actualisation. American Journal of Occupational Therapy 32(5):305–310

Freud A 1965 Normality and pathology in childhood. Assessment and development. International Universities Press, New York

Gilfoyle EM, Grady AP 1990 Children adapt, 2nd edn. Slack, New Jersey

Golledge J 1998 Distinguishing between occupation, purposeful activity and activity. Part 1. Review and explanation British Journal of Occupational Therapy 61(3):100–105

Hagedorn R 1997 Occupational therapy. Foundations for practice. Churchill Livingstone, Edinburgh

Hinojosa J, Kramer P 1993 Frames of reference for paediatric occupational therapy. Williams & Wilkins, Baltimore, MD

Hopkins HL, Smith HD (eds) 1988 Willard and Spackman's occupational therapy. JB Lippincott, Philadelphia, PA

Kielhofner G 1983 Health through occupation. Theory and practice in occupational therapy. FA Davis, Philadelphia, PA

Kielhofner G 1985 The model of human occupation. Theory and application. Williams & Wilkins, Baltimore, MD

Kielhofner G 1992 Conceptual foundations of occupational therapy. FA Davis, Philadelphia, MD

Kielhofner G, Burke JP, Igi CH 1980 The model of human occupation, parts 1–4. American Journal of Occupational Therapy 34(9–12):572–581, 663–675, 731–737, 777–788

Kielhofner G, Forsyth K 1997 The model of human occupation: an overview of the concept. British Journal of Occupational Therapy 60(3):103–110

Kuhn T 1970 The structure of scientific revolutions, 2nd edn. University of Chicago Press, Chicago, IL

Licht S 1957 Kinetic occupational therapy. In: Dunton WR, Licht S (eds) Occupational therapy principles and practice. Thomas, Springfield, IL

Llorens LA 1970 Facilitating growth and development. The promise of occupational therapy. American Journal of Occupational Therapy 24(1):93–101

Lyons M 1985 Paradise lost! Paradise regained? Putting the promise of occupational therapy into practice. Australian Journal of Occupational Therapy 32(2):45–53

Maslow A 1968 Toward a psychology of being. Van Nostrand, New York

Mattingley C, Fleming MH 1994 Clinical reasoning: forms of inquiry in practice. FA Davis, Philadelphia, PA

Meyer A 1922 The philosophy of occupational therapy. Archives of Occupational Therapy 1:1–10

Mosey AC 1966 Recapitulation of ontogenesis: a theory for practice of occupational therapy. American Journal of Occupational Therapy 22:426–432

Mosey AC 1981 Configuration of a profession. Raven Press, New York

Mosey AC 1986 Psychosocial components of occupational therapy. Raven Press, New York

Parham D 1987 Toward professionalism: the reflective practitioner. American Journal of Occupational Therapy. 41(9):555–560

Pedretti LW 1985 Occupational therapy: practice skills for physical dysfunction, 2nd edn. C V Mosby, St Louis, MO

Piaget J 1950 Psychology of intelligence. Routledge & Kegan Paul, London

Reed K, Sanderson S 1983 Concepts of occupational therapy. Williams & Wilkins, Baltimore, MD

Reed K, Sanderson S 1992 Concepts of occupational therapy, 3rd edn. Williams & Wilkins, Baltimore, MD

Reilly M 1962 Occupational therapy can be one of the great ideas of 20th century medicine. American Journal of Occupational Therapy 16:1

Rogers C 1984a Client centred therapy: its current practice, implications and theory. Houghton Mifflin, Boston, MA

Rogers JC 1983 Eleanor Clark Slagle Lecture. Clinical reasoning: the ethics, science and art. American Journal of Occupational Therapy 37(9):601–616

Rogers JC 1984b The foundation: why study human occupation? American Journal of Occupational Therapy 38:47–49

Rood MS 1954 Neurophysiology reactions as a basis for physical therapy. Physical Therapy Review 34:444–449

Slagle EC 1988 Historical perspectives of occupational therapy. In: Hopkins HL, Smith HD (eds) Willard and Spackman's occupational therapy. JB Lippincott, Philadelphia, PA, pp 20–21

Sumsion T 1997 Environmental challenges and opportunities of client-centred practice. British Journal of Occupational therapy 60(2):53–56

Sumsion T 1999 Client centred practice in occupational therapy. Churchill Livingstone, Edinburgh

Taylor E, Mitchell M 1990 Research attitudes and activities of occupational therapy clinicians. American Journal of Occupational Therapy 44(4):350–355

Taylor M 1934 The treatment of orthopaedic conditions. Canadian Journal of Occupational Therapy 2:1–8

Thorndike EL 1932 The fundamentals of learning. Teachers College, Columbia University, New York

Townsend E (ed) et al 1997 Enabling occupation. An occupational therapy perspective. Canadian Association of Occupational Therapists, Ottawa

Turner A, Foster M, Johnson S 1996 Occupational therapy and physical dysfunction, 4th edn. Churchill Livingstone, Edinburgh

Voss DE, Ionta MK, Myers BJ 1985 Proprioceptive neuromuscular facilitation: patterns and techniques, 3rd edn. Harper & Row, New York

Wallis MA 1987 'Profession' and 'professionalism' and the emerging profession of occupational therapy, part 1. British Journal of Occupational Therapy 50(8):264–265

Yerxa EJ 1979 The philosophical base of occupational therapy in 2001AD. American Occupational Therapy Association, Rockville, MD

Young M, Quinn E 1992 Theories and practice of occupational therapy. Churchill Livingstone, Edinburgh

Skills

SECTION CONTENTS

4

Skills for practice

Marg Foster

INTRODUCTION

During the course of her duties, an occupational therapist must, of necessity, use a very wide range of skills (Box 4.1). The exact skills used will depend on the needs of the individual and relevant others, the situation in which she is practising and the intervention chosen. Commonly, she will use skills of assessment, information-giving and receiving, reasoning, planning, communication, education and negotiation with individuals, carers and relevant others. However, during specific interventions involving individuals or groups, she may use more diverse skills to assist people to overcome or come to terms with their difficulties. Much will depend on the nature of the problems, whether the dysfunction is likely to be short term, long term or permanent, whether the individual has no other previous life experience (as in the case of congenital impairment), or whether the person's functional ability is likely to deteriorate or become life threatening. Skills in advocacy, negotiation, reflection, mentoring and caring may all be used to a greater or lesser degree, depending on the individual's needs and the prevailing situation.

An occupational therapist's key tool is her 'self', along with core skills, knowledge, attitudes and other attributes. It is often the approach – the roles adopted by the therapist and her clinical reasoning skills – that is the most significant factor for progress within the intervention regimen. A therapist continuously evaluates and modifies her roles, and the skills within them,

---

Box 4.1 Occupational therapist's skills

Advising	Imparting information, knowledge and skills to others
Advocating	Understanding individuals' needs and requirements and acting on their behalf
Assessing	Identifying assests and problems as a basis for decision making in intervention
Caring	Showing concern for an individual within a therapeutic professional relationship, providing appropriate intervention to meet his needs
Communicating	Giving and receiving information – verbal, non-verbal, written and technological
Decision making	Selecting from a range of options and encouraging the individual to make their own decisions
Educating	Transferring skills, knowledge and abilities to others
Facilitating	Providing opportunities for action/development, promoting enablement
Goal setting	Establishing aims and planning strategies for achieving them
Interviewing	Gathering information through verbal communication
Listening	Giving attention to what is being said, hearing with purpose/interest
Mentoring	Guiding others through advice and trusting support
Negotiating	Facilitating mutual decision making through exploration of a range of options
Planning	Exploring options in relation to needs and resources (Requires objectivity and realism)
Problem solving	Exploring a range of solutions and identifying the most suitable options to meet specific needs
Reasoning	Using logical thought processes, lateral thinking and/or intuition to guide decision making and actions
Reflecting	Reviewing and analysing real or created situations to question issues and develop fuller understanding
Role modelling	Demonstrating a desired set of behaviours or skills

---

and adjusts her expectations of the recipient accordingly. By gradually increasing the degree of independence and autonomy offered, and by gradually reducing her support, she can pass responsibility to the individual (Box 4.1).

This chapter considers the skills necessary for carrying out the intervention process. Many different approaches and techniques are used by an occupational therapist but the process of her interventions will usually be consistent, even when intervention is relatively short. Four basic stages are necessary to address the needs of the individual (Fig. 4.1):

- Stage 1: gathering and analysing information
- Stage 2: planning and preparing for intervention
- Stage 3: implementing intervention
- Stage 4: evaluating outcomes.

The success of each stage depends on the thoroughness and accuracy of the previous stage. There should be a logical progression from one stage to the next and the needs of the individual

and of the carers or significant others should determine the intervention strategies and activities. The needs of individuals and the approaches and skills used by the therapist will vary greatly according to the situation of each individual – whether he is experiencing short-term dysfunction from which recovery is likely or whether problems relate to long-term or permanent impairment, life-threatening situations or terminal illness, or are the result of congenital dysfunction. The therapist will also utilise different skills according to the location of her practice, whether it be hospital-based, where the emphasis may be towards return to the community, or in community or primary care, where maintaining independent or interdependent living is the focus of intervention.

The first section of this chapter describes the process by which the therapist identifies the individual's problems and negotiates priorities in the context of needs, aspirations, occupational performance and the environment. Assessments are carried out by the therapist in cooperation with

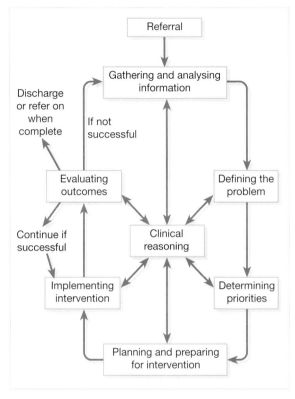

Fig. 4.1 The intervention process.

based care has resulted in a broader mixture of provision to meet the different requirements of individuals in their own homes, or in short-stay residential settings. Good liaison with other members of the wider multidisciplinary team is essential to ensure that all available resources are being used with maximum efficiency and effectiveness.

The intervention process is cyclical, particularly where the impairment has progressive or long-term implications. When evaluating the outcome of the intervention, the therapist may need to reconsider the early stages of assessment and gathering of information if the process has not provided the success anticipated. The therapist should discuss the possible reasons for limitation of this success with the individual and the multidisciplinary team and consider whether the intervention should be continued, changed or concluded. This may mean referral to another agency, or the individual and carers may, in some instances, be satisfied with what has been achieved and accept the reality of the situation, having had the opportunity to explore a number of options, and feel ready to discontinue the intervention. As always, the therapist's ability to make a sound judgement will depend upon her clinical expertise, her past experience and use of resources and, above all, her realistic, reasoned approach to meeting the individual's needs.

individuals and carers. The choice of methods should be guided by the therapist's skills in clinical reasoning, based on her scientific knowledge and research evidence, her understanding of the situation, of the individual and carers and of their needs and wishes. The therapist uses her analytical and communication skills to investigate and process the findings.

Planning and preparation requires the negotiation of aims and goals with the individual concerned. Skills in determining clear aims and breaking these down into realistic achievable goals require the therapist to understand the individual's priorities, the nature of the problem being addressed, the theoretical basis and potential outcomes of different intervention approaches and the range of resources available to her.

In the implementation stage, the therapist must consider practical constraints upon time and resources. The reduction in hospital-based services and the move to much more community-

REASONING AND REFLECTION IN CLINICAL ANALYSIS AND APPLICATION

Therapists use reasoning skills throughout all stages of the intervention process. These are the connected thought processes that are used to interpret information and reach a conclusion. Reasoning may be used deductively to identify the logical sequence of what is likely to follow a particular situation or action: 'if this is done then that will result'. Similarly, reasoning may be used inductively to analyse and weigh-up the consequences from a number of possible sequences of actions: the 'what if' scenarios.

Reasoning is based on a range of skills and experiences and is therefore likely to differ between individuals. The basis for making judgements depends upon the person's thought process development – whether this is based on logical sequencing, lateral thinking or intuitive factors – and on past experiences and reflective analysis, together with their own personal beliefs and biases. Awareness of these individual factors is an important element in the application of reasoning to clinical analysis.

Mattingley (1994) stated 'there is no one-sentence definition that captures the subtlety of how therapists think in the midst of practice … Clinical reasoning in occupational therapy is directed not only to a biological world of disease but to a human world of motives and values and beliefs – a world of human meaning … a form of phenomenological thinking'. Clinical reasoning is the term given to the thinking that guides the therapist's analysis and helps her to work with the individual to come to a clinical judgement – an opinion or decision based on the pertinent facts. Rogers (1983) maintains that clinical reasoning demands three basic attributes – science, ethics and artistry – and that 'without science clinical inquiry is not systematic; without ethics, it is not responsible; and without art, it is not convincing'.

The scientific component includes the therapist's knowledge base from clinical learning and experience, together with the systematic and formulated scientific skills in information analysis.

The ethical component is based in the therapist's philosophy and beliefs with regard to the importance of occupational performance and her respect for human values and dignity. It is founded in the therapist's recognition and respect for the person's own values and is underpinned by the Code of Ethics and Professional Conduct for Occupational Therapists (COT 2000). The ethical element is reflected in the cooperative manner in which priorities are determined and decisions are made for the benefit of the individual. It underlies the beliefs of what *ought* to be done.

The artistry component lies in the way in which the therapist uses her own personal skills to perfect her information gathering and analysis

and in her ability to interpret findings, impart values and guide decisions without imposing her own opinions. Rogers (1983 p601) states that 'the artistry of clinical reasoning is exhibited in the craftsmanship with which the therapist executes the series of steps that culminates in a clinical decision'. This is the most difficult element to define, as a wide range of skills and personal attributes determine this element.

Some believe that reasoning may be developed through 'convergent modes' – bringing factors together through scientific logical processing – whilst others may use more 'divergent modes', which 'employ lateral thinking, intuitive or creative processing and a generally phemonenological approach' (Hagedorn 1995). These different modes are explained in detail in a number of texts and articles (Hagedorn 1995, Mattingley 1994, Trombly 1995) and there is considerable research into the understanding and development of these skills (Crabtree & Lyons 1997, Flemming 1991, Mattingley 1994, Roberts 1996, Slater & Cohn 1991).

Reflection is another factor that makes a significant contribution to many of the aspects of the intervention process and clinical reasoning. Johns (2000) summed up reflection as 'a window through which the practitioner can view and focus self within the context of her own lived experience in ways that enable her to confront, understand and work towards resolving the contradictions within her practice between what is desirable and actual practice'. Schon (1987) related reflection to 'constructing knowing' and stated that 'Our knowing is ordinarily tacit, implicit in our patterns of action and in our feel for the stuff with which we are dealing. It seems right to say that our knowing is in our doing'.

Gibbs (1988) identified a reflective cycle, based in reflection *on* action, which outlined how therapists can explore their own thinking and feelings about a practice experience, evaluate what is good and bad about that experience and analyse the reasons for the occurrence. Through this analysis, therapists can develop a greater understanding of the situation and explore 'what else could have been done', in order to establish how the situation may be managed differently if it arose again.

Therapists also use reflection *in* action, to guide their thinking processes and decision making within the intervention process when unexpected events occur which have not been anticipated. Schon (1987) states that reflection in action 'has a critical function, questioning the assumptional structure of knowing-in-action'. It involves reflecting on the rationale for the action: 'why did this occur?', the questioning of the method: 'is this the most suitable way to do this?' and the anticipation of the outcomes 'what will be the benefits and constraints of changing the method?'. As a result of thinking and questioning, the therapist may change the intervention to overcome or accommodate the unanticipated event.

There are a number ways to develop reflective skills – through group work, individual diaries and narratives, and guided formal processes. Reflection forms part of a developmental cycle, enabling the individual to integrate new knowledge with previous learning to change practice. Used effectively, it has the potential to contribute to the overall advancement of the practitioner's 'intuitive knowing' in the developmental continuum from novice to expert.

GATHERING AND ANALYSING INFORMATION

Procedures for gathering information are more fully explored in Chapter 5 on assessment but this aspect is usually the first element of any intervention process and, as such, is the foundation on which later decisions are made. In many instances it is also an essential element of the management process, providing basic data for outcome measurement, clinical audit and quality assurance.

Information gathering aims to provide a basis on which to identify problems and establish an individual's priorities and needs. It is a two-stage process that consists of gathering the information followed by its interpretation, which together require specific communication, technical and analytical skills. Information gathered should be appropriate, valid and reliable and should be recorded accurately and concisely. Leonardelli-

Haertlein (1992) suggests that user competence for carrying out this stage ethically demands 'adequate and appropriate training, interpretation of results and theoretical orientation'. She states that the basic competencies for this include the ability to:

- recognise the value of standardised tests
- distinguish standardised from non-standardised tests
- distinguish objective from subjective data
- know that using standardised assessments in an unstandardised adapted manner invalidates these assessments
- recognise one's own abilities and limitations in using evaluations.

The sequence and methods by which the information is gathered will be determined by the nature of the dysfunction, the theoretical basis of practice, the therapist's expertise and the area of living under investigation. The knowledge base, experience and skill of the assessor, together with the opinions of the individual and his carers, will determine the importance of particular information for intervention planning. The neglect of a vital area of need or an unrealistic programme of intervention could result from omission or misinterpretation of information.

When considering therapists' skills, Maurer et al (1984) stated that 'occupational therapy personnel are professionally and ethically obliged to use only those evaluations for which their education and experience are sufficient and to obtain specialised training to use instruments and techniques critical to their practice area'. More recently, when addressing managerial issues, de Clive-Lowe (1996) stated that 'training in the technical rationale and procedures is essential for any clinician to have received if he or she is to use the tests responsibly and to obtain maximum benefit from them for his or her clients. Training courses must also include the most important part of assessment, the interpretation of results'.

DEFINING THE PROBLEM

Problems are the difficulties that occur for a particular individual or group of individuals in relation to a number of factors. These may be associated with specific impairments or beliefs, or occur through the constraints imposed by the structure of the environment or societal attitudes. Problems may vary greatly from person to person, depending upon personality, life aspirations, needs and social setting.

Individual perceptions and definitions of the problem will influence its severity and, at times, the person and/or the carers may have different opinions and perceptions. In this situation, the therapist's negotiation skills may be significant in achieving mutual understanding between the person and his carers. Additionally, one person may perceive the inability to perform a particular task as a major problem, whilst another may dismiss it as a minor inconvenience that can easily be overcome.

Other, less obvious, agendas may also mask the outward presentation of the true problem, such as the individual's confidence when performing the assessment, the efficiency of the assessment process and the quality of the information obtained, nature of the dysfunction and perceived locus of control, the individual's personal strengths and the degree of success of other interventions (Fig. 4.2). Identification of the true extent of the problems requires the therapist to use listening and observation skills; exploration and reflection on the information obtained will be valuable in analysis and evaluation of the total situation.

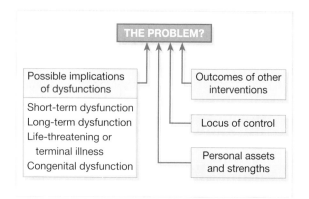

Fig. 4.2 Defining the problem.

POSSIBLE IMPLICATIONS OF THE DYSFUNCTION

Short-term dysfunction

Following a traumatic incident or acute medical condition, there is frequently an anticipation of improvement or recovery. If the condition has occurred suddenly there may be a period of shock and adjustment prior to recovery commencing, which could affect the identification of the true problem. Other interventions – surgical, medical or therapeutic – together with the person's own motivation and support systems may significantly affect the severity of the problem. The therapist's skills in recognising the impact of shock and adjustment, and of understanding the recovery process, will be basic factors when considering the possible prognosis. Good communication to develop a rapport with the individual may give insight into personal and social factors affecting that person's behaviour and motivation. Where recovery is not progressing at an anticipated rate, these latter factors may be crucial in addressing the true nature of the problem.

Long-term or permanent dysfunction

For some people, the permanence of the situation is evident at the outset, such as early amputation following trauma, whilst for others the recognition that recovery will be limited is a gradual process following a short or long period of treatment. Much will depend upon the person's residual psychological, physical and/or social skills to compensate for the limitations or losses. In many instances, these personal assets are the major determinants of the individual's management of quality of life. Additionally, the availability of resources to address the difficulties presented will play an important part in enabling the individual to continue previous activities or make any necessary changes. The therapist's skills in recognising the extent of the potential support systems and supporting the individual and those close to him through the acceptance and adjustment process play an important part in facing and addressing the problems. Problem-solving skills and knowledge of resources enable individuals to make choices according to their own needs, and regain some control over their lives.

Life-threatening or terminal illness

Many people have attempted to define the emotional stages of the grief reaction through which people pass when they are faced with a life-threatening or terminal illness. The most widely accepted processes are those described by Kubler-Ross (1970), who defined them as denial and isolation, anger, bargaining, depression and acceptance. However, everyone is an individual and reactions will vary according to one's own personality and external circumstances. Many people will not experience these stages in a given order and may pass between different stages at given times. Feelings of helplessness and hopelessness in the face of the clinical condition are not unusual but recognition of individuality helps to maintain some dignity and sense of personal value. Dame Cecily Saunders' statement (cited in Spilling 1986) 'You matter because you are you. You matter to the last moment of your life and we will do what we can, not only to help you to die peacefully, but to live until you die', underpins the philosophy of the hospice movement.

Much will depend upon when the therapist makes the initial contact with the individual and/or their carers as to their feelings at the particular time. Good, sensitive communication and attentive listening skills, together with the ability to interpret non-verbal signals, may enable the therapist to gain some insight into both the individual's and carers feelings and perceptions. Liaison with other members of the multidisciplinary team to identify clinical and/or social factors will assist the therapist in gaining a broader appreciation of the person's circumstances. Preservation of dignity and self-esteem through respect for the person's opinions and sensitive understanding of his priorities and needs enable the therapist to develop a supportive rapport for intervention planning. In some instances, the primary aim of therapeutic intervention is to maintain a quality of life when the person is experiencing a sense of hopelessness.

Opportunities to successfully participate in a chosen meaningful activity, however small, can add to the quality of the day and may help to maintain a sense of purposefulness, self-esteem and motivation to continue similar or different tasks. Recognition of the need for support for family and carers in practical and emotional terms can also help to maintain a positive relationship between the individual and those near and dear to him.

Congenital dysfunction

A diverse range of conditions may be categorised under this label, some of which, such as congenital limb absence, may change little clinically throughout life, whilst others, such as cerebral palsy, may have changing patterns of functional capability and occupational performance dependent on developmental progress. Occupational therapists are frequently involved with children with congenital impairments from a very early age, and at this stage many parents are in the process of trying to cope with the loss of the 'perfect child'. If they are to become partners in the therapeutic process, they may need considerable assistance to accept the child's problems and support the therapeutic intervention process. The therapist's knowledge of practical and emotional parenting skills, as well as her skills in assessing and recognising the child's physical and intellectual developmental stages, will be necessary in order to identify the extent of the problems for both parents and child. If the parents are to become the 'expert therapists', the practitioner's expertise in evaluating their relationship with the child and imparting skills for teaching and learning will be necessary to build parental therapeutic competence and confidence.

AWARENESS OF LOCUS OF CONTROL AND DEVELOPMENT OF AUTONOMY

Studies of locus of control may also assist the occupational therapist by providing another insight into understanding a person's problems (Lau 1982, Rotter 1966, 1975). People differ in their beliefs regarding how much control and autonomy they have in their lives. A person who believes that control is located outside the self may feel that outcomes are dependent on fate, or alternatively he may feel he is actively controlled by others. Such a person may be resistant to taking responsibility for his own decision making and may show ready compliance with any suggestions made by the therapist because he perceives her as representing 'powerful others'; he may not even attempt to strive for success, believing his fate to be 'already sealed'.

Encouraging such an individual to exercise some control over his own situation through education and an understanding approach will take time but, if successful, may contribute significantly to the short- and long-term outcomes. The therapist should endeavour to educate him about his situation and involve him in making choices and initiating ideas at all stages of the intervention. People who perceive control as lying within their own realm of responsibility are more likely to contribute their own ideas and be more evaluative of others' suggestions. They are usually more motivated to overcome difficulties, provided that the goals are realistic in view of the person's perceived needs and wishes and that emphasis is given to choice and personal responsibility in a client-centred approach.

THE IMPORTANCE OF PERSONAL ASSETS AND STRENGTHS

The basis of problem solving is the ability to identify the true problems. The therapist who focuses on the dysfunction does so at the expense of consideration of positive assets, strengths and skills. It is equally important to identify and focus on these assets and strengths, as they will be the foundations on which the individual will build his future and form the basis for intervention. Almost everyone, with the exception of very young children, will have personal life experiences, some of which may be used beneficially to address the existing problems. Particularly in the early intervention, when successful outcomes are important in maintaining a person's motivation to continue, the identification and use of these

assets and skills to achieve success, however small, will boost morale. Personal strengths may be the means by which a problem is overcome or minimised in the long term. Such an example is regularly seen through individuals who, despite substantial limitations in their physical levels of occupational performance, are able to use their strength of character and engaging personality, in maintaining a willing support team to assist with demanding daily care activities.

The therapist's skills in identifying such attributes and utilising them in the intervention programme not only encourages a more successful outcome but also maintains the individual's dignity, autonomy and personal responsibility.

EVALUATION OF THE QUALITY OF INFORMATION

Therapists frequently receive referrals for a specific issue, which is only part of the total picture. By addressing the situation from a wide perspective, using a client-centred approach, the therapist is more likely to identify associated issues and areas of difficulty that are contributing to the total problem. Despite a wealth of information gained from case notes, interviews, observations and specific assessments, the true extent of the person's problems may not be clearly defined. The individual, and his carers, may not, for whatever reason, wish to reveal their real concerns. Language difficulties, limited understanding by either the individual or the therapist, or other communication problems may restrict the exchange and evaluation of information.

The therapist needs to appraise the quality of the information gathered. In some instances, her experience and skills in utilising her knowledge and understanding of the physical, psychological, social and clinical factors of the person's dysfunction and the possible environmental influences, may enable her to identify potential areas of difficulty that have not been recognised by the individual or the carers. A person who has difficulty rising from a chair is also likely to have problems getting up from the toilet, bath, bed or car seat. The therapist's understanding of movement from her learning in biological sciences, together with her awareness of occupational performance needs in daily living activities and knowledge of environmental design, will enable her to identify those tasks that are likely to cause problems. Her clinical science base, skills in activity analysis and research evidence, together with her clinical reasoning skills, will assist her in planning the most appropriate approach to the occupational dysfunction.

Additionally, understanding of interpersonal dynamics and behavioural processes, together with astute observation, can help the therapist to identify whether the individual is able to perform a given activity, or whether he is prevented from attempting to do so by, for example, an over-anxious or overprotective carer. Equally, the individual may not be motivated to perform independently because of secondary gains from the attention provided by the carer, which may compensate for loneliness or because the activity is not perceived as personally valuable or important.

IMPACT OF OUTCOMES OF OTHER INTERVENTIONS

Other interventions or treatments the person is currently receiving, or has received in the past, should also be considered when attempting to identify the true extent of the problems. The interrelationship of other interventions with occupational therapy in both the clinical and community setting can be a significant factor in success. Progress in other areas may favourably influence the progress of occupational therapy intervention. A lack of progress may indicate the depth and extent of the individual's problems or may be the result of conflicting interventions or guidance. Similarly, a previous negative experience may affect current motivation and progress. The activities of the multidisciplinary team, both formal and informal, should be focused towards a cohesive partnership approach to the different facets of the situation.

DETERMINING PRIORITIES

Once the individual and the therapist have jointly identified the problems that must be addressed, the next task is to establish their relative importance and urgency. As it is unlikely that all the problems can be addressed simultaneously, it is important to prioritise them before planning the intervention programme. Factors contributing to priority include the:

- urgency of need
- wishes of the individual and carers and their perspectives of the most vital needs
- nature of the dysfunction and the complexity of the tasks to be performed
- culture of the individual and the social climate in which he lives.

Urgency of need

Factors contributing to urgency may be related to health and safety legislation, the professional duty of care and the Code of Ethics and Professional Conduct (College of Occupational Therapists 2000, item 3.3), as well as to local employment regulations with regard to the identification of problems and management of people's safety. The setting in which the therapist is working, together with specific factors regarding the individual and his occupational performance levels all contribute to the perceived urgency of need when planning and prioritising interventions. In acute or long-term clinical settings, the priorities for people leaving these settings may relate to their limitations in occupational performance and the proposals and arrangements for the impending discharge. An assessment of risk and provision of relevant preventive measures, interventions and support should aim to ensure safe return to the community. Similar issues concerning the possible risks within the environment and occupational performance levels also occur in community settings.

The nature of the risk should be identified and recorded through the assessment process, including the probability of the risk occurring and estimation of the consequences. If these are considered significant, their urgency may determine the priority needs for intervention in terms of 'what action would be reasonable to prevent such risks occurring' (Dimond 1997). Once identified, if attempts are not made to record and address such issues, the intervention may be considered negligent.

Where there is a rapid change in the individual's and/or carer's performance level, it may be necessary to prioritise interventions to meet the new situation. Examples of this may be seen where there is an urgent need for a piece of equipment following a rapid deterioration in a progressive disorder. Similarly, the development of a particular skill may be a necessity for transferring to a new environment; for example, a new school or work setting. Urgent support services may be required when a carer becomes unavailable due to illness or other cause.

Respecting the wishes of the individual

Individual personal drives, often referred to in American texts as 'personal causation' and 'volition', are the underlying factors that affect wishes and aspirations. Some of the factors that contribute to a person's drives are:

- spirituality, meaning and personal values
- past individual lifestyle experiences
- current lifestyle needs and social pressures.

The occupational therapist's belief in autonomy, dignity and the personal potential of the individual should lead her to take time to identify each individual's desires and drives. If intervention is to be client centred and needs led, she should *not* be tempted to interpret the range of a person's problems in terms of her own priorities and values. Similarly, care must be taken in the application of theoretical models to individual cases. Maslow's hierarchy of needs (1968), for example, identifies a structure of needs that applies to many people, basic personal needs requiring satisfaction before higher intellectual ones. This may help the therapist to understand human nature and most people's personal preferences but, like all models, it may not be directly applicable when considering *every* individual's intervention priorities.

Each individual who is faced with a problem will bring to the situation his own personality and drives, his past experiences and his particular personal values. Personal values and meaning are often particularly evident when working with people who are facing lifestyle change as the result of a permanent dysfunction or a life-threatening or terminal illness. Therapists regularly see individuals who have overcome tremendous difficulties in order to succeed, but may also be faced with those who do not wish to attempt the first hurdle in the recovery process. These spiritual and personal attributes often contribute to the priority factors in the choice of activity and the determination to succeed (Christiansen 1997). The Canadian Association of Occupational Therapists (1997) has stated that the role of the occupational therapist is to 'enable individuals, groups and communities to develop the means and opportunities to identify, engage in, and achieve desired potentials in the occupations of life'. Egan and DeLaat (1994) consider that in order to do this 'consideration of spirituality is essential in assisting the client to engage or re-engage in occupation. The therapist helps the client identify occupations which have, or could have, positive meaning'. When discussing spirituality as a part of total care, Hume (1999) considers that as therapists 'we need to regain our sense of this aspect of life and to take a global approach to treatment planning. This is not easy within the constraints of clinical audit and financial stringency, or where the focus is often on brief intervention rather than long term care. However, if we are to give the holistic care we claim to provide, we need to take hold of our roots more firmly. Patients are often aware of a spiritual dimension, even if they cannot articulate it as such, and it our responsibility to meet their needs'.

Identifying personal meaning and wishes may be relatively easy with some people. An individual with arthritis may be able to express a particular need in a daily living activity. However, when cognitive or communication skills are impaired, for example, following stroke or head injury, or where the person has no previous life experience on which to base a judgement (as in the case of cerebral palsy in childhood) identification of personal meaning and drives may be more difficult. Observation of the person's non-verbal responses to suggestions, or levels of enthusiasm when participating in particular activities, may give an indication of personal inclinations.

Many expressed priorities are based on previous life experience and life roles – parent, partner, breadwinner, independent being. Additionally, lifestyle needs and social pressures will almost certainly contribute to most people's priorities. A person who lives alone may perceive mobility and safety in self-care activities as his most vital need. The breadwinner may rate gaining competence in work-related tasks in order to retain employment as more important than achieving independence in all aspects of personal and domestic care.

Nature of the dysfunction and complexity of the tasks to be performed

It is usual to prioritise intervention according to the expected sequence of recovery, which in most cases results in addressing more simple tasks earlier in the programme and progressing at a later stage to those activities which are more complex and make greater demands on the individual's functional performance. However, people with progressive deteriorating conditions may need to downgrade activities from more complex tasks to those which require a lesser level of skill, in accordance with their remaining attributes. Additionally, in some instances, as a result of a person's specific individual lifestyle needs, it may be necessary to address a complex task early in the intervention, because of the necessity for early success, or because of the anticipated time necessary to achieve a suitable outcome.

Culture of the individual and social climate in which he lives

Culture affects many aspects of occupational performance and lifestyle activities, and determines those tasks which are valued above others, and the ways in which particular activities are performed. Within some cultures the work ethic takes preference, whilst in others the ability to perform daily self care or social activities to an acceptable standard is paramount. Different role, gender and generational demands occur in different cultures, which may affect individual priorities according to the person's perceived role expectations, and those of his cultural group.

The social climate in which an individual lives also has an impact on personal priorities. A person living alone, with no additional assistance and support, may prioritise activities differently to someone who resides in a family which provides loving care and assistance. The nature of the priorities for the person living alone may not relate to personal survival needs, but may be chosen with regard to quality of life and social outlets. Issues regarding a person's role or social standing may also affect choice of priority activities, for example a person with a responsible job who is the breadwinner may choose activities related to returning to employment in preference to independence in activities of daily living, if assistance with these personal care activities is readily provided by a family member or carer. The therapist's interview and assessment skills, as well as her knowledge of different cultures and social climates, should enable her to identify and negotiate individual preferences in order to provide client-centred intervention.

PLANNING AND PROBLEM SOLVING

Once a person's problems have been identified and prioritised, the next stage is to determine the aims and goals to be achieved. When these have been decided upon, it will be necessary to consider the range of ways of attaining them, the approaches and media to be used and the specific responsibilities for individual aspects of the intervention (Fig. 4.3).

SETTING AIMS AND GOALS

A clear understanding of the difference between aims and goals, as well as their relative value in the intervention process, is necessary for the

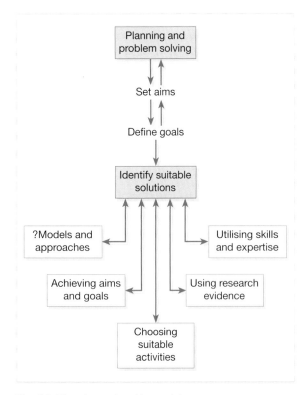

Fig. 4.3 Planning and problem solving.

individual, the therapist and anyone else who is closely involved in achieving the appropriate outcome.

An aim is a general statement of the situation one hopes to achieve, usually in the long term. Goals, sometimes called short-term or specific objectives, are much more concise descriptions of specific outcomes, usually stated in positive terms on the part of the participant. Goals state the activity the person will perform, under specified conditions and to a particular degree of success. The activity is expressed in assessable, achievable terms. The conditions are the particular circumstances in which the person will perform the activity. The degree of success is the acceptable level of performance. It is usual for a progressive sequence of goals to contribute to the attainment of an aim.

An example of an aim may be: Mrs Smith will achieve maximum independence in mobility for safe discharge. A specific goal towards this aim may be: Mrs Smith will be able to transfer safely from bed to bedside chair using her zimmer frame, without manual assistance or verbal prompts, by the end of the week. Once this has been achieved, goals for other transfer skills may be negotiated.

When negotiating goals with the person and/or their carer, the therapist should ensure they are appropriate and specific to the individual and they must be measurable and attainable. Incorporating aims and goals into the planning process:

• makes completion of total tasks less onerous by tackling the problems in small achievable steps
• encourages accurate assessment and clear identification of strengths and weaknesses in order to write specific goals
• facilitates flexibility within the programme by focusing on specific needs at a given time within the total process
• provides a consistent method for planning in a variety of situations which can be applied to many areas of activity and practice
• encourages consistency in care and facilitates understanding of the reasons for particular practices by presenting a systematic, ordered approach that can be used by staff from a variety of disciplines as well as by the individual and his carers
• assists in identifying each intervention activity, the learning methods and anticipated outcome
• provides opportunities to measure achievement to enable the success of the activity to be clearly evaluated.

It is usual to plan a small number of aims, some of which may be addressed simultaneously. Similarly, the achievement of one specific goal may involve the acquisition of a particular skill that contributes to more than one aim. The example of the goal concerning transfer skills may contribute to long-term aims in areas of self care, work activities and leisure pursuits.

The value of the therapist's analytical skills in determining particular strengths and needs and developing these into specific aims and goals in partnership with the person concerned, and with relevant others, cannot be underestimated. Negotiated aims and goals provide a foundation for clear, concise, accurate, individual intervention, in which the person concerned is an active participant. They provide a system that may be understood by all concerned, thereby promoting liaison and cooperation between the individual and all members of the team, and forming a basis for outcome measurement.

IDENTIFYING SUITABLE SOLUTIONS

ACHIEVING AIMS AND GOALS

Having negotiated the overall aims, the range of solutions to achieve any particular aim will vary greatly depending upon the level of occupational performance, the tasks to be achieved, the person's culture, the environment of intervention and the urgency of need. When exploring the range of possibilities, the therapist needs to consider the merits and constraints of specific options to achieve individual goals. This may be illustrated by the different ways by which independence in toileting may be attained, that is, through the use of specific activities to improve strength and mobility in order to perform transfer techniques independently; by adapting clothing, either in choice of design or modification of fastenings; through the use of assistive equipment such as seat raises, rails, frames or commodes; or through alterations to the environment to provide an accessible toilet. Through exploration of the merits and constraints of each option, the individual, the carers and the therapist can decide upon the most suitable solution for all concerned and design specific goals accordingly.

CHOOSING A MODEL OF PRACTICE AND THE INTERVENTION APPROACH(ES)

The philosophy and design of theoretical models and intervention approaches is discussed in detail in Chapter 3. When working in certain locations, the model of practice may be determined by the practice setting. This could be a profession-specific model, which is followed only by occupational therapy staff, or there may be multidisciplinary models, which are used by a number of different personnel. Consideration and review of the appropriateness of the chosen model/s to meet the needs of the service users should be carried out regularly to ensure they meet people's needs and provide a quality service. Through formal research and informal monitoring, new models develop and modifications to existing models occur to meet changing requirements of clients and services.

The approach is related to the chosen model, but is also determined by the person's clinical condition and occupational performance needs. Where dysfunction is likely to be permanent or continue for some time, a compensatory approach may be necessary to address deficits in the short or long term. However, if positive change or improvement is anticipated, other approaches relevant to the problems and desired outcomes will be more appropriate. The therapist may use a number of approaches within the intervention, some sequentially as improvement occurs and others concurrently dependent upon the area addressed. It is vital that the therapist is conversant with and skilled in the application and interpretation of individual models and approaches if she is to use them proficiently. Where a number of approaches are being used, she needs to understand the merits and limitation of each approach to ensure they are complementary to each other and not contradictory to her own or others' interventions.

IDENTIFYING SUITABLE ACTIVITIES

One of the earliest British professional texts, 'Occupational Therapy in Rehabilitation' (Macdonald 1960), stated 'almost *any* activity can be used. What matters is the *aim* of its use, and whether it achieves, or is suitable to achieve, the purpose for which it is employed'. This statement is still true today, despite major changes in the range of activities available to the therapist, the developments in healthcare and the changing needs of disabled persons and their carers. Choice of activities must be realistic in terms of the lifestyle and needs of the individual, taking account of his personal circumstances, domestic, work and leisure experiences and his socio-cultural environment. Activity should be chosen in light of previous physical, cognitive and social competence, and should be graded according to his present strengths and deficits. The therapist's understanding of activity analysis, application and grading, in conjunction with a thorough baseline assessment and good negotiation skills, are essential to determining the choice of an appropriate activity to facilitate needs-led provision.

Activities should be appropriate to the person's age, gender and culture but care must be taken to ascertain suitability in each case, and not to adhere to sexist, generational or cultural stereotypes. Activities employing the use of modern technology may be particularly appropriate for the person wishing to return to paid employment, whilst cookery or creative leisure activities may have more appeal to the elderly housewife. However, such assumptions must not be made without due consultation with the person concerned, as the elderly housewife may be an enthusiastic computer user. Such enthusiasm may motivate her to pursue computing and thereby gain cognitive skills, fine motor control or social attributes in excess of those acquired through cookery or leisure pursuits.

The needs of the carer frequently require equal consideration in the choice of activity. If the carer is willing to continue assistance with dressing activities but risks personal injury through helping with moving and handling techniques, specific activities to improve the person's strength, their motor performance and balance for independent transfers or education in the use of mechanical lifting equipment, may be more appropriate than daily dressing practice. A carer's continued assistance with dressing activities, if given out of a genuine desire to help, may be the basis of trust and secure friendship, while the risk of personal injury through helping with transfers may cause the carer anxiety and make him or her reluctant to continue in the caring role. Mechanical hoists may overcome risks to the carer, but such equipment offers less flexibility than acquisition of skills in independent transfers and is often more costly to provide. Personal interests provide a strong emotive element in choice of activity. An activity chosen predominantly for pleasure may be the driving force in motivating the person to pursue other therapeutic activities, despite some discomfort and considerable effort in their execution. However, choosing an activity in which the person has had a previously good level of skill should be considered with care, as the negative effects of reduced capabilities because of the present level of impairment may serve only to reinforce the sense of loss.

THE THERAPIST'S ROLES AND SKILLS

Occupational therapists are recognised for their flexible approach to problem solving. However, the therapist herself is an individual with particular skills that extend or limit her own capabilities and expertise. Many therapists maintain a broad spectrum of experience and have well developed transferable skills that can be applied to different situations. Some therapists prefer to specialise in particular roles or intervention approaches and may develop in-depth knowledge and skills in these areas, often at the expense of other facets of practice. The recognition of both types of expertise through changes in service provision and development of clinical specialisms is an essential part of the development of the profession. However, all therapists must 'only provide services and use techniques for which they are qualified by education, training and/or experience, and are within their professional competence' (College of Occupational Therapists 2000).

Occupational therapists rarely work in isolation. Recognition of the roles and expertise of others within and outside the multidisciplinary team is an essential part of the therapist's role in today's complex mixed service provision. Skill in communication and liaison with relevant other individuals or organisations facilitates multi-agency service delivery. Whilst providing only a small part of the total intervention, it may still be necessary for the therapist to maintain a key worker or care manager role in certain instances, while the direct provision of specific aspects of intervention is the responsibility of others. The therapist's role may then become one of co-ordination, monitoring and review, to ensure the provision is comprehensive and cohesive and continues to meet the needs of the individual. This is particularly important when working with people with long-term, complex or deteriorating conditions, where the duration of need, the multiplicity of the problems or the changing levels of individuals' skills require regular appraisal and review to ensure the individual and the carers are receiving the most efficient and effective services.

The primary aim of therapeutic intervention for children with congenital dysfunction is to promote maximum competence in occupational performance for lifelong activity, frequently based on an absence of any previous experience. The therapist will therefore have to use a range of creative skills to provide opportunities to explore unknown activities with the child and initiate enthusiasm for participation in same. An educative approach, with both the child and parents/carers, employing a range of strategies for teaching and learning will be used. This involves exploration of abilities and identification of opportunities to perform tasks according to the child's developmental progress, individual interests and personal needs. Good communication skills appropriate to each child's functional capabilities and individual personality may be required to motivate both the child and the parents/carers. The child, whilst being the primary focus, is not alone, and obtaining the support of parents or carers should be included throughout the intervention, as success may be dependent on them continuing such activities throughout the child's early life. This requires sensitivity on the part of the therapist to identify the parent's/carer's attitudes and approaches to the child, and their reasons for these. Support for parents is an equal part of the therapeutic process, to enable them to further the child's progress throughout the early years of learning.

Where dysfunction is likely to be short term, the individual's motivation to participate actively in the rehabilitation process may be crucial to the extent and speed of recovery. Pain and discomfort frequently predominate in the acute phase and the therapist's acknowledgement of these helps to develop an understanding relationship. It is important for the therapist to appreciate that, whilst for some people the short-term dysfunction may be perceived as less of a problem than long-term or permanent dysfunction, nevertheless, for the individual concerned at the time, it is likely to be a major issue. An understanding of the anticipated recovery process, supported by a clear explanation of the therapeutic application of chosen techniques, enables individuals to appreciate the specific value of these techniques in the total intervention programme. Using meaningful occupations and setting small achievable targets and goals maintains interest and enthusiasm for the rehabilitation programme.

USING RESEARCH EVIDENCE TO DETERMINE INTERVENTION

'Research will be done by some, facilitated by others and implemented by all' (College of Occupational Therapists 2000).

In today's climate of health and social care, where emphasis is on efficient and effective use of resources and evidence-based provision, it is essential that therapists are informed regarding the value and limitations of current interventions. Continuing professional development to remain conversant with the latest research evidence, together with practical evaluation and reflection on one's own practices, facilitates quality service delivery and development. Whilst such analysis and reflection will contribute some evidence to the development of practice within one's own specific professional context, the sharing of information between professionals and with other professions, through study groups, papers, journals or conferences, enables the individual therapist to choose best practice for her own interventions. Recognition of the value of research and the ability to analyse the quality of investigation and findings, and, where appropriate, apply it in one's own area, supports professional accountability and evidence-based client care.

SKILLS IN IMPLEMENTING INTERVENTION

An intervention plan should set out how to meet short-term goals in the most appropriate way for the individual in a particular setting. It is not always possible to choose where the activity will take place, as the urgency of need and the location of the original contact may determine this. Within the community, intervention may take place in the person's home, a day centre, school, GP surgery, health clinic or other suitable location. In the clinical setting it may be in the ward, the therapy unit, the outpatient or casualty department or the specialist clinic. Therapists' awareness of the resources available at each of these locations will to some degree affect the range of options available, and impact of the location on the individual and urgency of need may determine priorities and the intervention strategy.

Factors to consider

Time

This is an important element to address in all situations but it should not be the prime factor in determining the quality of intervention. The therapist's time management skills to manage not only the caseload interventions but also the recording, reporting, liaison and development requirements are an essential part of practice in all settings. Whilst the intervention process of information collection, analysis, intervention and evaluation will be similar in each location, the amount of time devoted to each aspect will differ significantly dependent upon the urgency and extent of need, the priorities, the service location and type of provision, and the resources available. When addressing intervention, time may be considered in terms of overall duration or in terms of the most appropriate time within the daily or weekly routine.

When considering the duration of intervention, some therapists have a major role in discharge facilitation or admission prevention and this frequently results in pressure of time to assess risk and implement appropriate management strategies for safe return to the community. The therapist's skills in assessment, problem identification and prioritisation, communication and education of others, as well as her awareness of resources and liaison with others, are essential to the quality and efficiency of the management of the situation and health and safety requirements.

Home assessment with people in hospital is a time-consuming activity and is not necessary in many cases but, where it is considered essential, the pressures of time should not overrule it and the therapist should adhere to professional standards when carrying out such a visit (College of Occupational Therapists 2000).

In other situations, external pressures on time may be less important to the intervention and the therapist may be able to plan an intervention programme and timetable according to the individual's needs. This should take account of the optimum length of time for each therapy session and how frequently these should occur. It may be based on the nature of the dysfunction, its cause, course and prognosis, the advantages gained by regular intervention, as well as the requirements of the referring agent.

Assessment for, and management of, major adaptations may require intermittent but long-term contact during the planning and construction of the adaptation whereas a person with an acute short-term dysfunction may benefit from intensive regular treatment to facilitate speedy recovery. Children with congenital problems may require regular treatment at some stages of their development but at other times may require only intermittent contact to monitor progress or address a particular problem.

When considering the particular time of day for intervention, there may be particular times when therapy is likely to be more advantageous. Activities to improve physical performance for a person with an arthritic disorder characterised by morning stiffness may be more successful in the afternoon. Similarly, in a situation where the person has an increasing level of fatigue through the day, activities in the morning may be especially successful. However, it will be necessary for the therapist to observe some self-maintenance activities when the person is at the worst stage of the day, so that she can consider methods by which he can cope successfully throughout his daily routine.

When a person has cognitive problems, particularly those affecting orientation in time or place, the timing and the location of activities should equate, as far as possible, to his 'normal' daily routine.

Choosing the format of intervention

The therapist should consider the most appropriate format for the intervention process. In some instances a one-to-one approach will be essential whilst for others a group activity may provide an opportunity for shared experiences. In many instances, the therapy location and setting (such as the hospital bed or home environment) or the person's circumstances may determine the format and the nature of the individual needs may demand a one-to-one approach. However, some goals, especially those related to the development of social and communication skills, may be more readily achieved by participation in group activities.

The format of the intervention may also be affected by the choice of activity medium and the amount of direction or guidance required by the person to safely succeed in achieving the desired goal.

The therapist's knowledge of the individual's needs and wishes, the resources available and the different ways by which certain goals may be achieved will affect the choice of format.

Resource management

Resources are infinite in the ideal world but in the real world there are many constraints that have to be managed to the best advantage to the particular situation. Efficient and effective management of resources is an essential skill in today's health and social care provision. This includes the best use of each individual's expertise in evidence-based practice and the efficient and effective use of material and non-material resources for service delivery and client care. Having planned a possible theoretical programme of intervention, the therapist should analyse and evaluate its feasibility in terms of whether it is realistic and achievable in practice. Limitations in the therapist's knowledge and skills should be acknowledged, together with constraints on practical resources such as staff, a suitable location, transport, tools and materials, equipment and finance, all of which may affect the intervention programme. Demands made upon the therapist's time by her entire caseload, the limits on the availability of support and the relative urgency of individuals' needs may determine the frequency or duration of contacts. The therapist should analyse the quantity or extent of her interventions against the needs for quality provision and outcome gain. Prioritising needs forms a major part of resource management and requires the therapist's skills in assessment, analysis and negotiation to enable the most crucial needs to be met when resources are limited. In many areas, management procedures have led to the development of priority ratings and therapy protocols to manage interventions in the most efficient and effective way. These should be reviewed regularly to ensure they remain current and meet individuals' needs in light of changing demands and resource availability.

Liaison skills

Good liaison is vital to successful teamwork. Membership of the intervention team will vary in different settings (Fig. 4.4) but should include the people who are most meaningful to the individual – family, friends, neighbours and/or carers. The contribution these people can make towards achieving the individual's wishes and meeting his needs is often vital to the success of the intervention process. Successful teamwork depends upon:

- good communication between team members
- comprehensive identification of needs
- agreed aims and goals by all participating members

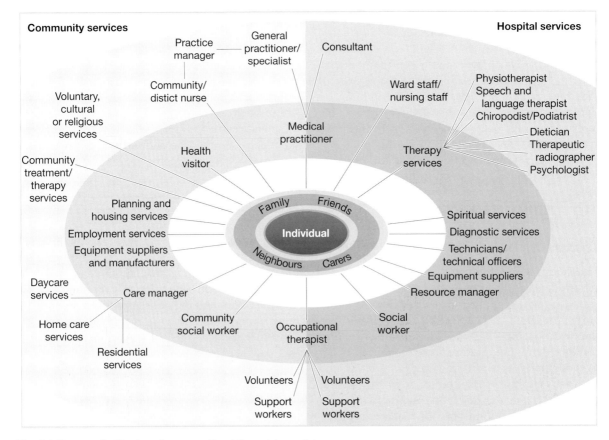

Fig. 4.4 Personnel with whom the occupational therapist may liaise.

- agreed strategies and methods for how aims and goals may be achieved
- respect for, and effective use of, individuals' skills
- clear and agreed understanding of responsibilities
- efficient and effective sharing of information.

Good liaison is important to:

- ensure the programme of intervention is cohesive
- identify the responsibilities of the different team members.

A cohesive programme of intervention. Liaison is a two-way process of giving and receiving information. The therapist should inform herself of other support or treatments the individual is receiving and of the aims and goals of these. She should gain information on frequency and timing of other activities and details of the methods of intervention used. The therapist should also give information on her proposals. Any divergence or overlap should be discussed and outcomes negotiated to achieve optimum benefit for the person and the carers in the most appropriate and efficient format. When face-to-face discussions with other members of the team are not possible, good central notes and records facilitate communication and understanding between team members.

Identifying responsibilities. It is important that all members of the team clearly understand their duties, and that attention to an important area of need is not overlooked or duplicated unnecessarily. This promotes efficiency on the part of the team in terms of time and effort, and the best utilisation of individuals' skills. The clear delineation of responsibilities is likely to encourage a greater sense of duty and desire for achievement, which in turn promotes quality of care.

Discussion on the range of possible solutions with the individual should involve negotiation of his own responsibilities with the therapist. When identifying the responsibilities of the provider – the therapist or carer – the demands these make in terms of skills, knowledge and time should be discussed and agreed.

In some instances there may be role overlap between members of the multidisciplinary rehabilitation team. For efficient management of resources and cohesion of provision, it may be more advantageous for one person to take the care manager or key worker role, thus minimising duplication of effort and preventing confusion. Generic support personnel may also reduce the number of team members. Conversely, in some situations that involve development of a particular skill, repetition by more than one member of the multidisciplinary team may promote or consolidate learning, provided the input is consistent.

Exploration of a wide range of factors and good negotiation with the individual and his carers and other members of the team should enable everyone to understand the intervention proposals. In many cases, intervention will proceed according to the chosen plan. However, there may be unforeseen factors, such as an alteration in the person's health or social situation, or in the facilities or resources available, which will necessitate a change of course. The therapist should use her problem-solving skills and be prepared to modify her plans accordingly. This may be a total reappraisal of the intervention, only a minor modification or a delay or advancement of an activity already included in the programme. The therapist needs to retain a flexible, positive approach to such changes to accommodate the needs of the individual and others in the team, in line with her duties of employment.

EVALUATING OUTCOMES

The importance of this aspect cannot be underestimated both for the benefit of the individual in ascertaining gains or identifying residual problems but also in the context of gathering evidence to appraise and monitor the effectiveness of the intervention and the service provided.

Evaluation comprises skills of analysis and reflection and should be carried out formally through specific tests, measurements and assessments supported by informal observations and discussions with the individual, relatives and carers, and others closely involved with the intervention provided. It should be based on the original aims and goals and considered in the context of the individual's past and present situation, and the interventions used.

A number of tests to measure outcomes are available. Some of these are specific to occupational therapy, such as the Canadian Occupational Performance Measure (COPM) and the Binary Outcome Measure, whilst others are more generic, for example, the Therapy Outcome Measures (TOMs), which is a multidisciplinary measure for use by occupational therapists, physiotherapists, speech and language therapists and nurses. These measures may be used in the clinical and community settings and include issues regarding individuals' emotional well being and satisfaction as well as measures of dysfunction and levels of occupational performance.

WHY EVALUATE?

● **To monitor progess.** Evaluation may be carried out regularly throughout the programme. The therapist should consider the specific goals identified when the intervention was planned as the foundation for determining whether the intervention should be continued or whether a change of activity may be beneficial. The frequency of regular evaluation will be dependent upon the anticipated rate of progress. Where this is expected to be slow, evaluation may be carried out at monthly or longer intervals. Where rapid changes are anticipated, such as in the situation of certain acute orthopaedic hand problems, regular weekly evaluation may be more appropriate.

● **To plan for discharge or referral to others for further intervention.** Evaluation to measure the extent of the progress and any residual deficits that have not been overcome usually occurs in the later stages in relation to the original aims established at the beginning of the intervention. It is usually carried out through a formal measure(s). In some instances this may be the repetition of some or all of the initial assessments performed before planning the intervention. A final evaluation at the end of the intervention provides a valuable record for future reference in the event of the individual's referral to occupational therapy or another discipline at a later date. Information gained may also form part of the basis for the therapist to refer the person to other sources to meet his residual needs.

● **To monitor or measure efficacy.** Information on the outcomes of particular activities or interventions provides evidence of the value of specific techniques or practices. In certain areas, such as long-term or deteriorating conditions, where individuals do not make significant changes in occupational performance but show increased levels of satisfaction, this may be because of acceptance of their situation, which is an equally beneficial outcome and rationale for the therapy provided. Outcome information may also be used to support the justification of therapeutic interventions to clients, other professionals and management. Additionally, it provides a basis on which to design benchmarking criteria, a familiar management quality measure in many service areas. Reflection and analysis of current practices may be based on the outcomes achieved, which may support a need for further investigation and research in the search for greater efficiency and effectiveness in service provision.

Evaluation illustrates the cyclical nature of the intervention process: the earlier stages of analysis of information are returned to, priorities may be re-appraised, and the achievement of aims and goals is quantified.

CONCLUSION

Skills involve the amalgamation of learning and practical experience with inherited abilities and assets. The complex practice of developing, maintaining or improving the occupational performance of others requires considerable flexibility and use of individual personal, professional and practical attributes to facilitate good clinical reasoning, negotiation and decision making. This may be gained through formal learning and practical experience but continuing professional development is necessary to maintain such expertise in order to meet the changing requirements in health and social care provision. Additionally, the intricate nature of societal changes and social and clinical problems adds to these demands.

The process of intervention provides a structure for efficient and effective practice, although this will vary according to the nature of the dysfunction and the diversity of employment settings. Whilst the pressures of time and resources may constrain the totality of the programme, the nature of the problem-solving process remains the same – identifying the problems, prioritising, formulating and implementing solutions and evaluating outcomes. Client-centred practice demands sensitivity and respect for the situation and the personal preferences of each individual in order to collaboratively work together to achieve the desired outcomes.

Managerial skills within multidisciplinary/multiagency service provision require good communication and liaison to facilitate service cohesion and accurate written documentation provides evidence for monitoring practice and audit purposes.

REFERENCES

Canadian Association of Occupational Therapists 1997 Enabling occupation: an occupational therapy perspective. Canadian Association of Occupational Therapy Publications ACE, Ottawa

Christiansen C 1997 Acknowledging a spiritual dimension in occupational therapy practice. American Journal of Occupational Therapy 51(3):169–172

College of Occupational Therapists 2000 Code of ethics and professional conduct. College of Occupational Therapists, London

Crabtree M, Lyons M 1997 Focal points and relationships: a study of clinical reasoning. British Journal of Occupational Therapy 60(2):57–64

de Clive-Lowe S 1996 Outcome measurement; cost effectiveness and clinical audit; the importance of standardised assessment to occupational therapists – meeting these new dimensions. British Journal of Occupational Therapy 59(8):357–362

Dimond BC 1997 Legal aspects of occupational therapy. Blackwell Science, Oxford

Dickinson E 2000 The evidence for evidence. British Journal of Occupational Therapy 63(6):247

Egan M, DeLaat MD 1994 Considering spirituality in occupational therapy practice. Canadian Journal of Occupational Therapy 61(2):95–101

Flemming MH 1991 Clinical reasoning in medicine compared with clinical reasoning in occupational therapy. American Journal of Occupational Therapy 45(11):988–996

Gibbs G 1988 Learning by doing: a guide to teaching and learning methods. Further Education Unit, Oxford Brookes University, Oxford

Hagedorn R 1995 Occupational therapy, principles and processes. Churchill Livingstone, Edinburgh

Hume C 1999 Spirituality: a part of total care? British Journal of Occupational Therapy 62(8):367–371

Johns C 2000 Becoming a reflective practitioner. Blackwell Science, Oxford

Kubler-Ross E 1970 On death and dying. Tavistock, London

Lau RR 1982 Origins of health locus of control beliefs. Journal of Personality and Social Psychology 42(2):322–334

Leonardelli-Haertlein CA 1992 Ethics in evaluation in occupational therapy. American Journal of Occupational Therapy 46(10):950–953

Macdonald EM 1960 Occupational therapy in rehabilitation. Baillière, Tindall & Cox, London

Maslow AH 1968 Towards a psychology of being, 2nd edn. VonNostrad Reinhold, New York

Mattingley C, Flemming MH 1994 Clinical reasoning. Forms of inquiry in therapeutic practice. FA Davis, Philadelphia, PA

Maurer P, Barris R, Bonder B, Gillette N 1984 Hierarchy of competencies relating to the use of standardised instruments and evaluation techniques by occupational therapists. American Journal of Occupational Therapy 38:803–804

Roberts AE 1996 Clinical reasoning in occupational therapy: idiosyncrasies in content and process. British Journal of Occupational Therapy 59(8):372–376

Rogers JC 1983 Clinical reasoning: the ethics, the science and art. American Journal of Occupational Therapy 37(9):601

Rotter JB 1966 Generalised expectancies for internal versus external control of reinforcement. Psychological Monographs 80(1) No. 609, American Psychological Association, Washington DC

Rotter JB 1975 Some problems and misconceptions related to the construct of internal versus external control of reinforcement. Journal of Consulting and Clinical Psychology 43:56–67

Schon DA 1987 Educating the reflective practitioner. Jossey-Bass, San Francisco, CA

Slater DY, Cohn ES 1991 Staff development through the analysis of practice. American Journal of Occupational Therapy 45(1):1038–1044

Spilling R 1986 Terminal care at home. Oxford Medical Publications, Oxford

Trombly C 1995 Occupational therapy for physical dysfunction 4th edn. Williams & Wilkins, Baltimore, MD

5

Assessment

Alison Laver Fawcett

INTRODUCTION

The major goal of occupational therapy is to help people with disabilities to reach their highest levels of skill and function and to enhance, or at least maintain and prevent the deterioration of, their quality of life. Therefore the major goal of occupational therapy assessment is to gain a clear picture of the individual in order to develop an effective intervention plan that will result in improved function and enhanced quality of life.

Assessment has been defined as 'the planned collection, interpretation, and documentation of the functional status of an individual related to the individual's capacity to perform valued or required self-care, work or leisure tasks' (Rogers & Holm 1989 p6). Assessment is an essential component of the occupational therapy process and is used to describe the person's strengths and problems, formulate a prognosis and evaluate the effects of occupational therapy intervention (Law & Letts 1989). Assessment provides the foundation for effective treatment and it is critical to undertake a thorough and reliable assessment at several stages during the occupational therapy process, because without thorough and accurate assessment the intervention selected may prove inappropriate and/or ineffective.

The 1990s saw considerable changes in occupational therapy assessment practice. Historically, therapists have favoured the use of unstandardised assessments, particularly informal interview and unstructured observation of activities of daily living, or have adapted existing standardised tests to suit their clinical environment (Shanahan 1992). There has been a trend towards the development of assessments on an individual department or service basis. This has the advantage that the assessment process can be tailored to the particular client group and to the practice environment. However, a major limitation is that the majority of assessments, which are 'home grown' in individual occupational therapy departments are not rigorously standardised, nor are they backed by research that examines their reliability and validity. In the current environment of evidence-based practice, therapists are being encouraged to use more standardised assessments to ensure that their assessments are as valid and reliable as possible and to enable the measurement of treatment outcomes. Previously, many of the standardised tests that occupational therapists adopted were not developed by occupational therapists and were 'borrowed' from other fields, for example, experimental and clinical psychology (for example, see McFayden & Pratt 1997). A disadvantage of this practice of 'borrowing' tests was that the tests did not always fit well with occupational therapists' philosophy and practice and the use of standardised tests was often rejected because they lacked good clinical utility and face validity. As a result, there was a need for therapists to develop valid, reliable, sensitive and clinically useful assessments of people's functional performance (Fisher & Short-DeGraff 1993). The 1990s saw developments in occupational therapy research that have resulted in an increase in the number of assessments that have been developed by occupational therapists. Therapists now have a much wider choice of suitable standardised assessments from which to select appropriate measures for their client group.

In the past, therapists tended to undertake a formal assessment on referral and then monitor the person's progress informally during treatment. With the emphasis on evidence-based practice, it is no longer sufficient for therapists to undertake one assessment to provide a baseline from which to plan treatment; ongoing evaluative assessment also is required to monitor the effectiveness of intervention in a reliable and sensitive manner.

Assessment is complex and the therapist needs to take many interrelating factors into consideration. Therefore, assessment requires careful planning and conscious decision making to select the optimum assessment strategy for a particular client's needs. No one assessment strategy will be suitable for all people with a particular diagnosis, so the therapist needs to combine the best evidence with a client-centred approach.

This chapter aims to present key issues related to occupational therapy assessment and to describe elements of good assessment practice. The chapter begins with an exploration of the complexity of both occupational therapy assessment and measuring functional outcomes. Clinical reasoning related to assessment is examined, including a description of diagnostic reasoning and the occupational therapy diagnosis. A model for describing levels of function is presented as a tool for framing assessment and, related to this, the pros and cons of the 'top-down' versus the 'bottom-up' assessment approaches are debated. Different methods of data collection are outlined along with consideration of the timing of assessment. Four key purposes of assessment and four levels of measurement scales are defined. Sections on standardised and non-standardised assessments are given, along with definitions for psychometric terms and exploration of the concepts of clinical utility and face validity. The chapter finishes by describing issues related to the selection of assessments.

THE COMPLEXITY OF OCCUPATIONAL THERAPY ASSESSMENT

Occupational therapy assessment is a highly complex skill that combines knowledge, experience, creativity and original thought. From an outsider's viewpoint, occupational therapy assessment might look easy; an observer may think that it does not require a person to hold a degree in order to watch someone get dressed and to say whether he could do it or not.

However, the therapist will be looking at *how* the person gets dressed and identifying *where* and *when* he struggles. The therapist will be hypothesising the *underlying causes* for the problems observed and will be noting how the person responds to different prompts and cues. It is not enough to know that a person can not manage a task, the therapist must also understand *why* in order to plan the appropriate treatment. For example, a person who cannot dress because of spasticity and reduced sensation in one arm needs very different treatment to a person unable to dress because of visual neglect and body scheme deficits, although at first glance the problem may appear similar.

There are several key reasons why occupational therapy assessment is complex. These relate to the:

- nature of occupational therapy practice
- nature of human performance
- influence of the demands of the assessment task
- impact of the familiarity of the task
- effect of the environment in which the assessment is undertaken
- constraints of the practice setting.

THE NATURE OF OCCUPATIONAL THERAPY PRACTICE

Firstly, occupational therapy is both an art and a science. As a result, some aspects of assessment might be standardised, specific and meticulous whilst other aspects might be intuitive, fluid and creative. In addition, a therapist may use both quantitative and qualitative approaches to measurement and will need to find a way in which to incorporate information from both approaches.

Secondly, occupational therapy is a holistic practice in which the therapist is trying to consider the whole person during the assessment process. Therefore, the domain of concern for an occupational therapy assessment is very broad and covers different levels of function from pathophysiology to societal limitation (see p119). A therapist may need to consider the person's environment, family support, roles and values in addition to very specific areas such as range of motion and muscle tone.

Thirdly, occupational therapy is person-centred. This means that each assessment should be individually tailored to that person and should lead to a specific intervention programme. The therapist may be able to draw upon some protocols that are useful for people with similar diagnoses to begin the assessment process but, as the assessment progresses, it should be increasingly targeted towards the specific needs and wishes of the person. The therapist needs to gain a clear picture of the individual, which includes his past life, present situation and hopes for the future, his roles, motivation, locus of control, and his attitudes towards his condition and towards therapy. The therapist uses this information to understand how the medical diagnosis and prognosis may impact upon that person's quality of life. Assessment will cover each person's unique configuration of occupation (broken down into specific activities and tasks) and his physical and social environment (see Chapter 2).

Fourthly, occupational therapists work in a wide range of practice settings, so they need to be able to conduct assessments in varied environments, such as a hospital ward, occupational therapy department, school classroom, nursing home, or a person's home or workplace.

Finally, occupational therapy often is provided within a multidisciplinary context, so the therapist needs to liaise with other professionals. In a team it is important not to have either too much overlap, such that the person is asked the same questions by several members of the team, nor should there be any gaps in the assessment, where members of the team assume that another professional has assessed that area. This means that good communication and a clear understanding of the role of each member of the team is critical for an efficient, effective and thorough multidisciplinary assessment.

THE COMPLEXITY OF MEASURING FUNCTIONAL OUTCOMES

Health professionals are being encouraged to embrace evidence-based practice (EBP). This means that occupational therapists need to measure the effects of their intervention. However, human behaviour is very complex and a person's function may change for many reasons (Fig. 5.1). For example, improvements may be observed as a result of a specific intervention or the success of a combination of interventions. This is important because occupational therapy is rarely the sole intervention and often is provided in a multidisciplinary context. Other factors that might result in observed improvements in function include: a belief or hope that change in function is possible, a placebo effect, a strong sense of locus of control, good coping strategies, high motivation, good rapport with the therapist and feelings of acceptance and support. When undertaking assessment to evaluate the effects of occupational therapy, the therapist needs to define the specific area to be measured and will need to take these confounding variables into consideration.

Function is not static but dynamic. A person's functioning can be influenced by several factors; for example, changing levels of pain, concentration, anxiety, fatigue, response to a drug regimen and the degree of stiffness. Therefore, a single assessment might not present a true and complete picture of the person's ability. Variability in a person's function can be more extreme for certain diagnoses. People with Parkinson's disease, for example, may have very different levels of independence depending on the timing and effects of their medication. A therapist should try to undertake different parts of the assessment on different occasions, varying the time of day and the assessment environment. Test anxiety can impact performance and an individual's performance often improves as the

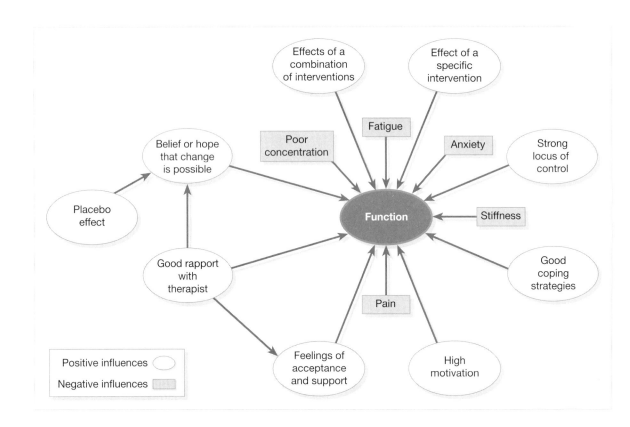

Fig. 5.1 Factors that can influence function.

therapist becomes familiar and good rapport is established.

THE INFLUENCE OF THE LEVEL OF TASK DEMAND

When a person goes to perform a task he firstly obtains factual information about the demands of a task. From these, he develops ideas, insights and beliefs related to the task and then creates strategies to perform the task more efficiently. Performance is affected by how demanding or difficult a task is and by the person's capacity, motivation, experience and knowledge. Occupational therapists need to take these factors into account during assessment. Experience, knowledge and capacity are interrelated. This relationship is complex and subject to individual variation, so these factors are difficult to separate and assess in isolation. How the therapist structures the assessment, and her reasoning and interpretation of assessment data, is critical to her ability to untangle these complex influences upon performance.

A person's capacity, defined in terms of the amount of information that the central nervous system can handle and process, is limited. The brain has limits for the quantity of sensory information (experienced through the visual, tactile, auditory, olfactory, gustatory and proprioceptive systems) that it can process at a time. For example, the auditory system can process only a certain amount of auditory stimulation at a time, which is why it is hard to concentrate on two people speaking simultaneously. All tasks place demands on the capacity of at least some of the body's sensory systems and, consequently, on the brain's ability to process sensory stimulation. The level and quality of a person's performance will be determined by the demands of a task if the demands of that task are within a person's capacity. For example, a person may have the capacity to perform two different tasks, such as eating cereal from a bowl with a spoon and eating a meal using a knife and fork. Although the person can do both tasks, he will eat his cereal with greater ease because it is a less demanding, easier, task. If the person reaches the maximum level of his capacity then performance

will be limited by his capacity, not by the task demands. Capacity alters in relation to both the normal development process and to pathology. In terms of normal development, infants learn to use spoons before they learn to use knives and forks. Capacity can be reduced as the result of an injury or illness. For example, a person who has experienced a stroke and who has associated motor and sensory deficits and a resultant limited capacity in the motor and sensory systems, may be unable to eat using a spoon or using a knife and fork. The difference in task demand is not the issue in this example, because the problems in task performance are related to the person's reduced capacity.

Some assessments take task demand into account and may present assessment items as a hierarchy from the simplest to the most complex task. For example, the Assessment of Motor Process Skills (AMPS; Fisher 1997) provides descriptions for a choice of Instrumental Activities of Daily Living (IADL) that have been calibrated through research to create a hierarchy from easiest to hardest task. Using hierarchies of task demand can save unnecessary testing time for both the therapist and client. For example, the Rivermead ADL Assessment (Whiting & Lincoln 1980) is structured in terms of a hierarchy of items comprising increasingly demanding personal and household tasks. The therapist decides where on the hierarchy to begin testing, based on her hypothesis about which tasks the person may not be able to manage. If the person can perform the selected task then the therapist ensures he can perform the three proceeding tasks and then progresses testing up the hierarchy until he fails to perform three consecutive tasks.

THE IMPACT OF FAMILIARITY ON PERFORMANCE

Familiarity and practice influence performance. When a person practises a task, over time the demands of the task are learned and the person becomes more efficient in the use of his capabilities related to performing that task; the task becomes perceived as being easier. A good example is learning to drive a car. Two adults might have the same capacities but the person who is familiar with driving a car will be better at driving than the person with little driving experience. Therefore, occupational therapists need to be aware of how familiar or novel assessment tasks are to their clients. In addition, following a reduction in capacity, occupational therapists can use practice and repetition to increase a person's task performance and use ongoing reassessment of the task to monitor progress. When repeating an assessment in this way, the therapist must be able to differentiate between changes that result because the assessment is now familiar and changes that have resulted in the person's capacity. Improvements in motor function are an example of this. Therefore, parallel, equivalent forms of an assessment (see p136) might be used, where an unfamiliar task of the same demand and assessing the same capacity is given in place of the familiar assessment task.

THE EFFECT OF ENVIRONMENT UPON PERFORMANCE

The environment in which an assessment is undertaken also may impact upon performance and can have an enabling or constraining effect on a person's function (Law et al 1996). The term 'environment' usually makes people think about the physical elements (including accessibility, architectural barriers and structural adaptations) of a person's setting. However, occupational therapists need to think about the environment in a broader context. A useful definition has been provided by Cooper et al (1995 p56) who state that environment is the 'physical, social, cultural, attitudinal, institutional, and organisational setting within which human function takes place'. The Person–Environment–Occupation Model (Law et al 1996) provides a useful theoretical framework for considering the impact of the environment during occupational therapy assessment. A person, his environment and his occupation (including activities and tasks) interact continually across time and space. The greater the overlap, or fit, between the person, environment and occupation, the more optimal will be the person's function. An intervention that increases the enabling aspect of the environment for an individual and thereby creates a compatible person–environment–occupation fit will increase, or with a progressive condition perhaps maintain, function. For example, if a therapist modifies a kitchen to increase accessibility for a person in a wheelchair then the fit between the person's capacity, the kitchen environment and the activities of meal preparation, washing up and laundry will improve, leading to increased independence.

Familiarity with an environment may influence assessment. For example, people may be more independent within their own kitchens than in unfamiliar occupational therapy kitchen areas. Even if the familiarity of an environment does not impact the final outcome of an assessment, it may affect the speed at which the task is completed. It is quicker to make a cup of tea in your own kitchen because you know where everything is kept. You will still be independent making a cup of tea in a friend's kitchen but it will probably take you longer because you will be searching in an unfamiliar environment for the items and ingredients you need. However, the home environment does not always facilitate function; for example, people may be able to mobilise better on the hard, flat surface of a hospital ward than on the different carpet textures in their own homes.

Occupational therapists are often involved in conducting assessments in people's own home and work environments, as they need to evaluate both environmental barriers and environmental supports to performance. Assessment at home is considered useful because people are more likely to behave and communicate in their normal way in familiar surroundings. The therapist can build a more accurate picture of the person's needs during a home assessment and a home assessment can facilitate access to the views and the needs of the carer. The environment selected for assessment is especially important for people with certain conditions. For example, it is critical to assess the influence of context and environment on the function of a person with dementia (Tullis & Nicol 1999).

Where safety is of concern, it is vital to assess the person in the environment where he will be functioning in order to examine the relationship between potential environmental hazards and the person's ability. Once potential hazards have been identified, changes to the environment can be made to reduce the risks of falls. Some occupational therapy assessments have been designed for use in the home environment. For example, the Safety Assessment of Function and the Environment for Rehabilitation (SAFER Tool; Letts et al 1998) was developed to assess people's abilities to manage functional activities safely within their homes and the Home Falls and Accidents Screening Tool (Home Fast) (Mackenzie et al 2000) was developed to identify hazards associated with falls in the home.

THE CONSTRAINTS OF THE PRACTICE SETTING

The practice setting will influence the therapist's choice of assessment and may serve to enhance or constrain her assessment practice. For example, if a therapist moves to a service that encourages standardised assessment and has a range of published tests available, then her knowledge of different tests and skills in standardised assessment may increase. Conversely, a therapist may be experienced with a particular standardised test but find that it is not available in a new practice setting or that with the demand of her new caseload there is not enough time to administer the test in its entirety. It may not be possible in some settings to assess the client at several different times in varying test environments and cover all the areas of interest within the assessment. Therefore, the therapist needs to use clinical judgement to select the most effective assessment strategy within the physical and political boundaries of the therapy environment. She may be able to conduct only a brief assessment and will need to make decisions about the person's overall ability and prognosis from limited data projections (see p116). This is where the quality of the therapist's clinical reasoning can be critical.

In conclusion, the occupational therapist needs to be like an experienced chef (Fig. 5.2): not sticking rigidly to a set recipe but combining knowledge of different techniques and knowing what ingredients and flavours can be combined in a creative way for each particular situation.

ASSESSMENT AND CLINICAL REASONING

Clinical judgement is 'the ability of professionals to make decisions within their own field of expertise using the working knowledge that they have acquired over time. It is based on both clinical experience and the theoretical principles embedded in their professional knowledge base but it may remain highly subjective' (Stewart 1999 p417). The underlying knowledge base and experience that an occupational therapist brings to an assessment is critical but is not sufficient to address the complexity of assessment. Each assessment also requires the occupational therapist to engage in original thinking. In addition, clinical judgement should be informed by the use of objective, preferably standardised, assessment processes. The therapist needs to address a number of assessment questions. For example, 'What degree of independence does the person have?' 'Why is performance affected?' 'How does the person perform the task?' 'When is the person functioning at his best?'. The specific questions to be addressed will vary from person to person. It is important to recognise the unique conditions that are presented by each person and the assessment should involve careful observations and interpretations in order to identify the optimum strategies for resolving each person's particular problems.

There is a difference between theoretical and clinical reasoning (Mattingly & Flemming 1994):

- **Theoretical reasoning** is learned from sources such as textbooks and lectures and relates to generalities – to what the therapist can predict (Unsworth 1999).
- **Clinical reasoning** occurs as the occupational therapist works to understand the nature of the person's problems and to construct individualised person-centred interventions

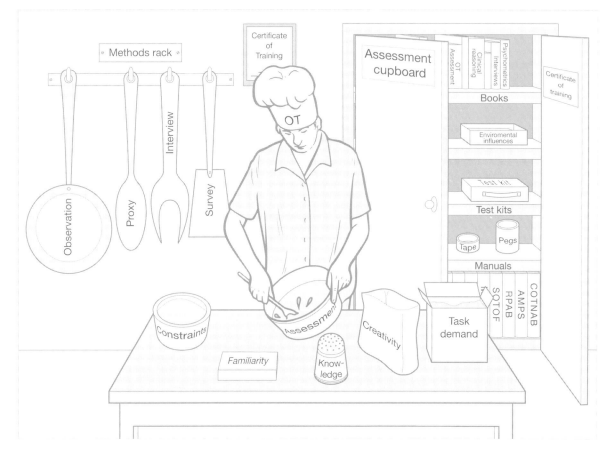

Fig. 5.2 Expertise in assessment is like being a creative and experienced chef.

(Cohn & Czycholl 1991). Clinical reasoning 'is the thinking or cognitive processes and decision making that therapists use to guide their work', it is 'a practical know-how that puts theoretical knowledge into practice' and is concerned 'with deliberating over appropriate action and then putting this in place' (Unsworth 1999 pp45–46).

As part of the assessment process, therapists need to learn about people's individual experiences of their illness or disability. In the philosophy of occupational therapy, every individual is perceived as a unique person. This philosophy needs to be borne out in practice. Therefore, therapists need to take a person-centred approach to understand the unique way in which diagnoses impact the lives of the people who receive occu-

pational therapy. Two people may be of the same age, sex, socio-economic background and have the same diagnosis but their experiences of, and responses to, that diagnosis may be completely different. Therefore, therapists need to engage in assessment and intervention in a phenomenological way. With a phenomenological approach, a person's experience of his body is inseparable from his experience of the whole world and disability is viewed as an interruption or injury to a whole life. So the therapist needs to assess a person in the context of how he did, does and hopes to live his life. Assessment is used to provide an understanding of a person in terms of his daily practices, life history, social relationships and long-term goals and plans that give him meaning and self-identity in life (Mattingly 1994).

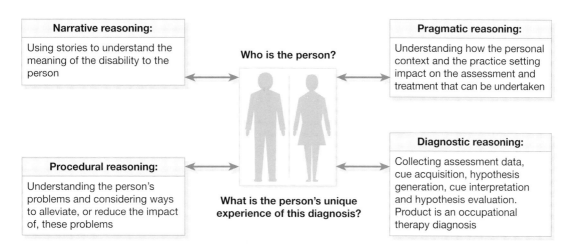

Fig. 5.3 Different types of reasoning used to guide assessment (the definitions used in the figure have been drawn from Mattingly & Flemming 1994, Rogers & Holm 1989, Schell & Cervero 1993, Unsworth 1999).

To obtain this complex image of a person and the impact of the diagnosis on his functioning, therapists need to engage in several types of clinical reasoning during the assessment process. These include narrative, pragmatic, procedural and diagnostic reasoning (Mattingly & Flemming 1994, Unsworth 1999) (Fig. 5.3). Narrative reasoning 'uses storymaking and story telling to assist the therapist in understanding the meaning of disability or disease to the client' (Unsworth 1999 p48). Pragmatic reasoning relates to the therapist's clinical practice setting and personal context. It takes into account organisational, political and economic constraints and opportunities that place boundaries around the assessment and treatment that a therapist may undertake in a particular practice environment (Schell & Cervero 1993, Unsworth 1999). Procedural reasoning is an 'umbrella term that describes a therapist's thinking when working out what a client's problems are and what procedures may be used to reduce the effect of those problems' (Unsworth 1999 p54).

The product of an initial occupational therapy assessment is the formulation of a problem statement. This has been called the occupational therapy diagnosis (Rogers & Holm 1991). The thinking that leads to the occupational therapy diagnosis is referred to as diagnostic reasoning.

Diagnostic reasoning involves creating a clinical image of the person through cue acquisition, hypothesis generation, cue interpretation and hypothesis evaluation (Rogers & Holm 1991). It has developed from scientific reasoning – the process of hypothesis generation and testing, which sometimes is referred to as hypothico-deductive reasoning (Unsworth 1999).

THE OCCUPATIONAL THERAPY DIAGNOSIS

The occupational therapy diagnosis can be viewed in terms of both a process and a product. It has several components (Table 5.1):

- **Descriptive component**: this should describe the specific deficits identified at each level of function that are impacting on the person's ability to engage successfully in their chosen roles and activities.
- **Explanatory component**: the diagnosis should contain an explanatory component that indicates the therapist's hypothesis or hypotheses about the possible cause(s) of the observed functional deficit.
- **Cue component**: this identifies the observed and reported signs and symptoms that led the therapist to (i) conclude that there is a

Table 5.1 Two examples of the components of the occupational therapy diagnosis, showing how the same deficit and pathology can arise from different causes

Component of diagnosis	Example
Example 1 Descriptive	Unable to get dressed independently
Explanatory	Related to: • reduced sensation in left upper limb • reduced active range of motion in left upper limb • spasticity in left upper limb
Cue	As evidenced by: • inability to identify objects through touch in left hand with eyes closed • inability to report temperature or pin prick on left hand and arm on testing • inability to move left elbow, wrist and fingers through full range of motion on command • inability to pick up and manipulate objects in left hand • when left arm is moved through a passive range of movement, full range is present but resistance and increased tone is felt
Pathological	Due to right cerebrovascular accident
Example 2 Descriptive	Unable to get dressed independently
Explanatory	Related: • left unilateral neglect
Cue	As evidence by: • ignores objects to the left of the midline • does not attempt to dress left side of the body • puts both sleeves on right arm
Pathological	Due to right cerebrovascular accident

functional deficit and (ii) hypothesise the nature and cause of the functional deficit.
• **Pathological component**: this provides the pathological cause, if any, of the functional deficit (this part of the diagnosis often relates to, or is drawn from, the medical diagnosis).

In formulating the diagnosis, the therapist also considers the person's strengths, interests and resources, and notes those physical and verbal prompts and cues that appear to facilitate function. So an occupational therapy diagnosis is more elaborate and is broader than the medical diagnosis, as it also encompasses the person's

physical and social environment, motives and values. In addition to a diagnosis, the therapist formulates a prognosis in terms of projecting both the person's likely response to treatment and future functional ability.

The diagnostic reasoning process can be explicated in two ways. First, in terms of the *steps* involved in functional assessment, such as data collection and the analysis and synthesis of that data. Second, in terms of the *principles* and *strategies* that therapists use to collect, analyse and synthesise data (Rogers & Holm 1989). Opacich (1991) has described six key steps, or stages, in an occupational therapy problem-orientated clinical reasoning process:

1. problem setting (context)
2. framing the problem(s)
3. delineating the problem(s)
4. forming hypotheses
5. developing intervention plans
6. implementing treatment.

Diagnostic reasoning is a component of clinical reasoning and primarily occurs during the first four stages of this process.

Problem setting. This stage involves naming the phenomena/constructs that are to become the target of assessment. Rarely in clinical practice do problems present themselves to the therapist as givens. Defined problems are constructed from observed and reported problematic situations that are experienced by clients. These problematic situations can be puzzling, messy and uncertain. The therapist needs to unravel the person's experience of a problematic situation in order to name the problem to be investigated. This involves selecting what will be perceived as the 'things' of the situation. The therapist then sets boundaries to focus the remit of the assessment and imposes upon it a coherence that enables the statement of what is 'wrong' and how the problematic situation needs to be changed (Schon 1983). Box 5.1 provides a case study to illustrate problem setting.

Framing the problem. This stage is where theory and conceptual frameworks play a key role. Framing the problem involves illuminating the problem(s) within a context (Opacich 1991). The problems identified by occupational thera-

---

Box 5.1   Case study: Mr Jones – problem setting

Referral information: Mr Jones was a 76-year-old man living with his wife. He was previously assessed with a diagnosis of progressive aphasia without dementia but his consultant was now querying this diagnosis and his wife was not coping well with supporting him at home.

First home visit/initial assessment: The therapist observed the physical environment and the interaction between Mr Jones and his wife. She conducted an informal interview with the couple. Mr Jones walked across the room and shook the therapist's hand. He sat down in the armchair without any problems. He had dysphasia and was quite hard to understand. He talked mainly about his career and his time as a soldier in the Second World War. He was easily distracted from the therapist's specific questions about current abilities and problems. Mrs Jones reported that her husband could not find things around the house as he reorganised his cupboards and lost things. She told the therapist that she laid-out his clothes in the morning as he got confused deciding what to wear and chose things that did not match, that he had recently given up driving and she did not drive, that he could not remember new dance routines at their dance classes, that he used the wrong tools for gardening tasks, that he had re-cleaned a window he had already cleaned last time he cleaned the windows, that he got out the wrong money when paying for items in shops and that he got confused laying the table for breakfast.

Naming the problems and focusing the assessment: From this first interaction the therapist formed very provisional hypotheses about the problematic situation and used these to name the problems to be investigated. From his wife's report, the therapist hypothesised that Mr Jones had short-term memory problems and was disorientated. She thought that he might have visual object agnosia as he was choosing the wrong clothes, gardening tools and cutlery. These tentative hypotheses related to the cognitive and perceptual systems, so the therapist decided that these systems would be the major focus of the impairment level assessment. At the disability (pp120–121, Table 5.2) level his wife was reporting that Mr Jones had problems with personal ADL (dressing) domestic tasks (laying the table, cleaning the windows) and leisure tasks (dance classes and gardening), so the therapist decided to assess personal and domestic ADL function and leisure interests. At the societal limitation level the couple were restricted by the lack of a car and the referral noted that Mrs Jones was not coping well, so the therapist decided to assess the couple's access to the community and explore whether Mrs Jones was experiencing carer burden.

Setting boundaries: The therapist decided that the motor system appeared to be intact and that mobility was grossly intact, so these areas were not a focus for assessment. Mrs Jones said that Mr Jones was seeing a Speech and Language Therapist and so communication was not a main focus for assessment as this area was being addressed by another professional.

---

pists during assessment are usually framed as problems of understanding; for example, identifying the cause of observed behaviour. The process of framing involves the selection of an initial frame of reference to guide the therapist's reasoning. This is followed by the critique (see p141) and selection of assessment tools designed to address the named constructs. The assessment tools selected should be consistent with the chosen theoretical framework (Rogers & Holm 1991). Assessment should be carefully structured in order to identify specific deficits/constructs. Constructs often are complicated and it can be hard to discern whether dysfunction can be attributed to one or more constructs. This is why the therapist needs to select a frame of reference to structure the assessment and use sensitive, valid and reliable (see pp135–140) assessments to develop and test-out hypotheses about the relationships between dysfunction and underlying deficits/constructs. Box 5.2 gives a case study of

Box 5.2   Case study: Mr Jones – selection of conceptual frameworks

Conceptual frameworks: The therapist needed to understand the underlying causes for the problematic situations described by Mrs Jones. She took a person-centred, also referred to as client-centred, approach (Canadian Association of Occupational Therapists 1991, Sumsion 2000). The therapist drew upon the Model of Human Occupation (MOHO; Kielhofner 1995). She found it useful to consider the person as a dynamic, open system and think about assessment strategies and data in terms of environmental factors and inputs, throughputs, outputs and feedback. In terms of a phenomenological approach, MOHO describes individual constructs of volition (personal causation, values and interests) and habituation (roles and habits) in addition to the mind–brain–body performance subsystem. The therapist prefers to take a top-down approach (see pp120–121) to data collection. With Mr Jones, she planned to begin data collection at the societal limitation and disability levels, then consider functional limitation and impairment level functioning and finally, at the pathophysiology level, weigh-up the evidence to present to the consultant regarding the differential diagnosis (see pp120–121).

Box 5.3 Case study: Mr Jones – selection of assessment methods

Selecting assessments: The therapist decided to start data collection using the Canadian Occupational Performance Measure (COPM; Law et al 1994) for the following reasons: the COPM identifies information about personal ADL, domestic ADL, transportation, shopping, and leisure; it is a person-centred tool that considers the importance of activities to the person and his level of satisfaction with current ability, as well as how well he can do each of the activities discussed. This helps her to prioritise areas for treatment; it is good for evaluating clinical change, so that she will be able to assess the effectiveness of any intervention later on; it is a well-researched measure with published psychometric properties and it can be used as a self-report or proxy-report measure, which will be useful as Mr Jones has communication problems and Mrs Jones appeared a competent informant.

The therapist wanted to supplement interview data with observational data. She chose two assessments that could be undertaken in the home environment and that would simultaneously provide information about ADL functioning and underlying cognitive perceptual functioning. The first assessment was the Structured Observational Test of Function (SOTOF; Laver & Powell 1995). The therapist selected this measure for the following reasons: it provides a structured diagnostic reasoning tool that involves the observation of feeding, pouring and drinking, hand-washing and dressing tasks.

SOTOF gives information at the disability, functional limitation and impairment levels, which involves data about the level of independence, the behavioural skill components of the tasks and the underlying motor, sensory, cognitive and perceptual functioning. SOTOF also allows the therapist to prompt the person and observe responses to any prompts. It is also standardised and has acceptable levels of reliability. The second assessment chosen was the Assessment of Motor Process Skills (AMPS; Fisher 1997). The therapist selected this measure because: it covers the domestic ADL domain; it is well standardised, valid and reliable; it provides data at the disability and functional limitation levels; it takes task demand into account; there is a choice of tasks so it is more person-centred (in that Mr Jones could select tasks that were relevant to him like laying the table, making a cup of tea and re-potting a plant) and, finally, she had been trained to use the AMPS.

To examine carer burden the therapist decided to use a self-report measure, the Zarit Burden Interview (Zarit et al 1980), that Mrs Jones could complete in her own time. She selected this survey because: it was developed to report the burden experienced by the carer in managing a person with cognitive impairment; it considers both emotion-focused stress and demands placed by the physical tasks associated with caregiving; it can be administered either as an interview or as a survey and it is quick to complete and easy to score.

a therapist selecting conceptual frameworks while Box 5.3 illustrates a case study on the selection of assessments.

Delineating the problem. This stage involves the implementation of the chosen assessment methods and strategies. Occupational therapists often use multiple measures of performance and a range of data collection tools (see pp121–126). Once data are collected, they are organised and categorised for interpretation. Standardised assessments should provide clear guidelines for the scoring and interpretation of data (see pp131–133). With non-standardised assessments, the occupational therapist should provide clear details and rationale for how data have been analysed. Box 5.4 provides a case study.

Forming hypotheses. An hypothesis has been defined as a tentative explanation of the cause(s) of observed dysfunction (Rogers & Holm 1991). The delineation of the problem involves the acquisition of cues drawn from the assessment data.

Box 5.4 Case study: Mr Jones – administering the chosen measures

The therapist now administered her chosen measures with Mr Jones and his wife during two home visits. The selected assessments were combined to provide observational, self-report and proxy-report data (pp121–126). This gave the therapist a comprehensive baseline from which to evaluate her provisional hypotheses and generate new, more refined hypotheses. She administered the COPM and SOTOF during one visit. Mr Jones was able to identify problem areas on the COPM but could not manage the ten-point rating scales, so Mrs Jones rated the problems her husband had identified in terms of importance. The therapist then asked Mrs Jones to rate the five most important problem areas in terms of performance and satisfaction. At the end of the first assessment session the therapist left the Zarit Burden Survey with Mrs Jones, for her to complete at her leisure and return at the next visit. At the follow-up home visit, the AMPS was administered and the therapist shared the results of the SOTOF with Mr and Mrs Jones and presented some potential options for treatment related to the identified COPM problem areas.

Box 5.5   Case study: Mr Jones – hypothesis formation

At the end of the two assessment sessions the therapist had a wealth of information and reviewed data from the COPM, SOTOF, AMPS, Zarit Burden Survey and her informal observations of the home environment and Mr Jones' interactions with his wife. From this assessment data the therapist began by generating a list of observed and reported problems. She then considered cues related to these problem areas and developed a series of hypotheses in order to identify the most likely causes of these problems. One overarching hypothesis concerned Mr Jones' diagnosis, which was originally given as progressive aphasia without dementia. During the assessment, the therapist picked up multiple cues that led her to hypothesise that Mr Jones might have dementia. For example, some of the cues that arose from the administration of the AMPS and led to an hypothesis of dementia will be described. Mr Jones could not remember where cutlery was kept: he had difficulty *searching* for the objects he needed in his kitchen and dining room and was unable to *locate* several required objects. He became quite disorientated in his home environment; for example, he kept opening and closing cupboards and drawers in quite a random way and re-looked in places he had already

searched. He forgot which items he needed and did not *gather* all the items needed for both tasks. He was not able to *organise* his space; for example, he could not lay the objects on the table in the appropriate configuration. He forgot to put things away and, when prompted to put things back, could not remember where they were usually kept; in both tasks he did not *restore* all the items and his wife had to assist him with putting things away and the therapist had to prompt him to put the milk back in the fridge.

To interpret these cues and evaluate the hypothesis that Mr Jones had dementia, the therapist chose to use the Clinical Dementia Rating (CDR), a global rating of dementia that takes 'into account both the results of clinician testing of cognitive performance and a rating of cognitive behaviour in everyday activities' (Berg 1988 p637). This helped her by organising the complex and numerous cues into meaningful patterns or groups of cues using the CDR items of: memory, orientation, judgement and problem solving, community affairs, home and hobbies and personal care. These cues were then interpreted in terms of the CDR rating scale (none, questionable, mild, moderate, severe) that equate observed behaviour with signs of dementia.

Cues, in turn, lead to the generation of hypotheses that are then evaluated in the light of cue interpretation. The occupational therapist reflects on the cues acquired and searches previous theoretical and experiential knowledge for recognisable patterns, similarities with other cases and metaphors to direct the formation of hypotheses. Following the formation of a hypothesis, the therapist may conduct further assessment, and subsequent cue interpretation and acquisition is focused on the identification of confirmatory cues. The therapist needs to consider what behaviour would be observed if the hypothesis is true and then plan further assessment to collect this evidence. Care must be taken to be very objective during this process because a person is more likely to see what she expects to see and ignore data that refute her beliefs. For example, the more discrete and targeted the tools and strategies used in the assessment, the easier it is for the therapist to test out these hypotheses and to make valid and reliable clinical decisions (the concepts of validity and reliability are explored on pp135–140). Box 5.5 gives a case study to illustrate how a therapist interprets data to form a hypothesis and then tests-out this hypothesis.

To understand how this clinical reasoning process works in practice it can be helpful to examine several different therapists' reasoning related to specific individuals' circumstances. Detailed examples that outline therapists' thinking during assessment can be found in several chapters in Unsworth's textbook (1999). In addition, Rogers and Holm (1989) provide a useful example that demonstrates cue interpretation and hypothesis evaluation.

DEFINING LEVELS OF FUNCTION

At the stage of problem setting it can be helpful to categorise problems in terms of levels of function and to use the boundaries of a defined level to help focus data collection. The National Center for Medical Rehabilitation Research (NCMRR) drew upon the expertise of a multidisciplinary group to develop a five-level model of function/dysfunction (1992). The NCMRR model's five levels are:

1. societal limitation

Table 5.2 Hierarchy of function/dysfunction (from Laver & Baum 1992, NCMRR 1992)

Level (Level of impact)	Description
Societal limitation (*Society*)	• Restriction, attributable to social policy or barriers (structural or attitudinal), which limits fulfilment of roles or denies access to services and opportunities that are associated with full participation in society • Areas assessed include roles, cultural background, physical and social environment, caregiver issues
Disability (*Individual*)	• Inability or limitation in performing socially defined tasks and activities, within a physical and social environmental context, resulting from internal or external factors and their interplay • Areas assessed include the definition of the activities and tasks the person undertakes related to each of his/her roles followed by the person's level of independence in these identified areas • This includes the domains of personal and domestic activities of daily living, work, leisure/play
Functional limitation (*Function of organs and organ systems*)	• Restriction or lack of ability, resulting from impairment, to perform an action or skill in the manner or range considered normal for stage of development and cultural background • Areas assessed are skill components of tasks • Activity analysis is conducted to break down tasks into their skill components at this level, for example, the ability to reach, grip, manipulate, scan, initiate, recall, sequence, name
Impairment (*Organs and organ systems*)	• Loss and/or abnormality of cognitive, emotional or anatomical structure or function; including all losses or abnormalities, not just those attributable to the initial pathophysiology • Areas assessed include the neuromusculoskeletal, sensory, cognitive, perceptual and psychosocial performance components
Pathophysiology (*Cells and tissues*)	• Interruption of or interference with normal physiological and developmental processes or structures • Usually assessed by the doctor. The therapist needs to understand the underlying pathology to know how the medical diagnosis will translate into functional deficits

2. disability
3. functional limitation
4. impairment
5. pathophysiology.

These are defined in Table 5.2.

'TOP-DOWN' VERSUS 'BOTTOM-UP' ASSESSMENT APPROACH

When the therapist is framing the problem, selecting a theoretical framework and choosing related assessment strategies and tools, an important decision to be made is whether to take a 'top-down' or 'bottom-up' approach to the assessment process. Some assessments simultaneously collect data from several levels of function but usually an assessment tool or strategy focuses on data at one or two levels of function.

The therapist, therefore, has to decide at which level to begin the assessment process. A 'top-down' assessment begins at the levels of societal limitation and disability and 'determines which particular tasks define each of the roles for that person, whether he or she can now do those tasks, and the probable reason for an inability to do so' (Trombly 1993 p253). A 'bottom-up' assessment begins at the levels of pathophysiology and impairment 'focuses on the deficits of components of function, such as strength, range of motion, balance, and so on, which are believed to be prerequisites to successful occupational performance' (Trombly 1993 p253). The 'bottom-up' approach can be associated with a medical model and has been popular in the past. Its advantage is that it provides the therapist with important information about underlying performance component functioning of the individual. However, a disadvantage to the 'bottom-up' approach is that the purpose of the assessment, and ensuing treatment plan, may not be obvious to the person and may, therefore, lack meaning and relevance. In contrast, the 'top-down' approach begins at the level of the person as a whole and starts by investigating past and present role competency and by evaluating the person's current ability to perform meaningful tasks from his previous daily activities. A 'top-down' approach helps the therapist to gain an early understanding of the person's values and needs. When the person experiences a discrepancy between previous and current role and task performance during the assessment process then he can see the need for treatment and will find greater meaning and relevancy in the resultant treatment plan (Trombly 1993). A 'top-down' approach facilitates the development of a partnership between the therapist and individual, in which the person feels valued and understood as a unique individual. Explaining clearly to the person the rationale for both assessment and treatment is essential for joint decision making and the negotiation of goals and is a critical part of person-centred practice (Sumsion 2000). The therapist needs to ensure that the person can make a truly informed choice as to whether to engage with the therapist's proposed assessment and treatment. If he understands and accepts the therapist's rationale, this helps to build trust and rapport and to enhance his motivation to engage with rehabilitation. The 'top-down' approach helps to clarify the purpose of occupational therapy for the individual and also assists the therapist in the formation of an accurate picture of the person and his problem(s), which is critical for the identification of relevant and meaningful treatment goals.

METHODS OF DATA COLLECTION

Assessment involves the use of multiple methods for gathering and organising information that is important to making specific clinical decisions (Hayley et al 1991). A thorough assessment usually involves the application of several data collection methods such as: informal observation, standardised observational tests,

informal interview, standardised interview schedules, review of written documentation and the completion of questionnaires and written tests. Studies have shown that occupational therapists use a variety of assessment methods; for example, in a survey of 50 paediatric occupational therapists (Chia 1996) the following methods of assessment were reported as being used: unstructured observations ($n = 29$; 58%); structured observations ($n = 36$; 72%); interviewing ($n = 49$; 98%); standardised tests ($n = 40$; 80%) and non-standardised tests ($n = 35$; 70%).

The occupational therapist may also collect data from a variety of sources, including the person, his family, other caregivers and members of the multidisciplinary team (Fig. 5.4).

SELF-REPORT

As person-centred practitioners it is very relevant for therapists to collect assessment data from the individual (Law et al 1991, Pollock & McColl 1998). This can be done in the form of an informal or standardised interview or through written data, such as journals and surveys. Table 5.3 gives examples of assessments that use self-report to collect data.

The interview is often chosen as the initial method of data collection and becomes the foundation for building an effective therapeutic relationship. Building good rapport is essential to obtaining a full history from the person. To help put him at ease, it is important for the therapist to provide information at the first contact by ensuring that: she introduces herself, outlines the role of the occupational therapist, explains the purpose of the interview, describes the type of occupational therapy service that is provided in that practice setting and discusses the degree of confidentiality that applies by letting the person know with whom the therapist might share interview information. Therapists need to be aware of how differences or similarities between themselves and the people they are assessing (for example, age, gender and sociocultural background) can serve to either facilitate or hamper the development of rapport and the

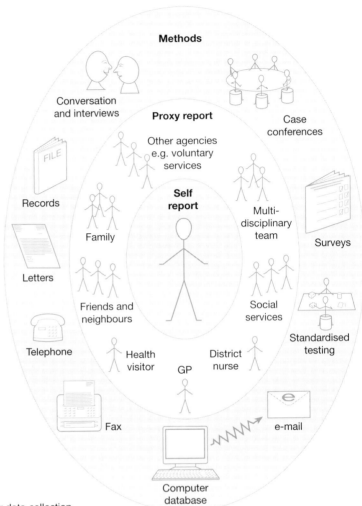

Fig. 5.4 Sources of data and methods for data collection.

establishment of an effective therapeutic relationship. When conducting an interview, therapists should check that the person can hear, comprehend and attend to the conversation. The assessment environment is important and therapists should try to ensure a quiet, private, test environment that is free from interruptions and distractions and neither too hot and stuffy nor too cold and draughty. Where possible, an environment that is familiar to the individual should be used. It is important for the therapists to consider their non-verbal body language and also where they sit in relation to the interviewee. For example, a formal set-up with the therapist

sitting behind a desk might not be conducive to providing a relaxed atmosphere (Fig. 5.5).

When conducting interviews, therapists should take into account a person's cultural background. It can be more difficult to establish good rapport when dealing with language barriers and differences in accepted forms of verbal and non-verbal communication. When the therapist and person cannot communicate directly then a bilingual interpreter, volunteer or family member can be used as a translator. Where possible, try to obtain an outside interpreter. Although family members can be very helpful, they might not always be the best interpreter 'since they may be uncomfortable

Table 5.3 Examples of self-report assessments that can be used with a wide range of individuals

Test	Authors and publication date	Brief description
Canadian Occupational Performance Measure (COPM)	Law et al 1994	Covers: self care, productivity and leisure. The person rates identified occupational performance issues in terms of importance (10 = extremely important to 1 = not important at all) and then rates the most important issues in terms of performance (10 = able to do it well to 1 = not able to do it) and satisfaction with that performance (10 = extremely satisfied to 1 = not satisfied at all). Scales are provided in English and French Note: COPM can also be used as a proxy-report measure with a carer
Life Experiences Checklist (LEC)	Ager 1990	LEC is a quality of life measure designed to gauge the range and extent of life experiences enjoyed by an individual. Covers: home, leisure, relationships, freedom and opportunities. Comprises a 50-item checklist
Occupational Performance History Interview (OPHI)	Kielhofner & Henry 1988	Covers: organisation of daily routines; life roles, interests, values and goals; perceptions of ability and responsibility and environmental influences. Focuses on both past and present for each area. Comprises 39 questions. There is a Life History Narrative Form for summarising data. Scoring uses a 5-point ordinal scale (5 = adaptive to 1 = maladaptive)

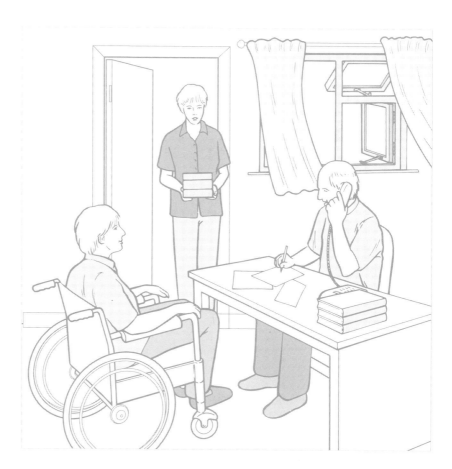

Fig. 5.5 Keep the test environment free from interruptions, distractions and draughts …

interpreting intense personal feelings … or may distort what has been said due to their own interpretations' (McCormack et al 1991 p21). In addition, there might be some information that a person might prefer to keep confidential and not want to discuss in front of a family member. Therapists should try to use interpreters of the same gender and age as the person where possible, because generation and gender differences can affect the interview, particularly when the person is a first-generation immigrant. In addition to language barriers, the occupational therapist should be aware of other factors that could impede the assessment process. These can occur when individuals' backgrounds lead to a distrust of healthcare providers and the healthcare system or when people have a strong sense that the healthcare system does not fit with their cultural traditions (McCormack et al 1991). The therapist's goals for assessment and rehabilitation may need to be adapted if a person comes from a culture where a reliance upon family for care and support following an accident or illness, as opposed to an expectation of a return to independence, exists.

PROXY REPORT

Information can be obtained from a number of other (proxy) sources including the person's primary caregiver (either an informal carer, such as a family member, neighbour or volunteer, or a formal caregiver, such as a warden, nursing home staff or home help), other members of the therapist's multidisciplinary team (for example, physiotherapist, speech and language therapist, psychologist, social worker, nurse, doctor) or other professionals involved with the person's care (such as their general practitioner, health visitor or district nurse). A proxy report may be obtained in person through interviewing the proxy face to face or over the telephone, through case conferences, ward rounds and team meetings or via written data. Written information from family members and neighbours might involve letters and questionnaires. Written information from other professionals might comprise referrals, letters, medical notes and assessment reports. Nowadays, much of this information might be held in an electronic format and could be accessed on a computer database, possibly via the hospital's intranet. Reports and information from colleagues outside the hospital might be sent via fax or e-mail. Table 5.4 gives examples of assessments that use information from a proxy.

The type of information provided by a proxy will vary considerably depending upon the amount of contact the proxy has with the person being assessed, their relationship and their degree of involvement. The therapist needs to be aware of these factors in order to assess the value and reliability of the proxy's report. Sometimes, the therapist might obtain quite different, and even conflicting, information from different sources. In this situation it is helpful for the therapist to develop a series of hypotheses about the individual and his situation and then to examine these hypotheses using all the information available. When interpreting hypotheses using discrepant information from different sources it is helpful to judge the data in the context of the motivations, fears and viewpoints of the people who provided the conflicting opinions. Factors that influence performance, such as pain, fatigue, medication and mood can result in people forming different, yet valid, perceptions about a person's ability. What the therapist might observe a person do in a hospital environment on one occasion may be very different to what the person's family observe him doing regularly at home.

In some cases, where the proxy is an informal carer such as a spouse, parent, sibling or child, the carer may also be the focus of part of the assessment. Where carer burden is identified and support, such as respite, education and counselling, is called for, then the proxy also might themselves require intervention. Where the person has a condition that impacts on his ability to provide an adequate self-report, the relevance of the perceptions and views of the family/caregivers becomes even more critical, for example, when working with children, with people with communication problems (such as following a stroke) and with people with dementia (Tullis & Nicol 1999).

The initial interaction with the person's family/caregiver provides the foundation for building effective partnerships with caregivers to

Table 5.4 Examples of assessments that use proxy report

Test	Authors and publication date	Brief description
Memory and Behaviour Problem Checklist (MBPC)	Original: Zarit et al 1986 Revised: Teri et al 1992	Used with carers of people with dementia. Can be scored through interview or using a self-completion survey format. Covers items such as sleep disturbance, wandering, aggressive outbursts and help needed with self care. Items are scored on a 5-point ordinal scale that measures the frequency and intensity of observed problems (0 = problem has never been observed to 4 = indicates that problem occurs daily or more often)
Pediatric Evaluation of Disability Inventory (PEDI)	Hayley et al 1992	Designed to assess children aged 6 months to 7.5 years. Proxy report can be gained from parents or from educators or rehabilitation professionals who are familiar with the child. Measures capability using a Functional Skills Scale and performance of functional activities using a Caregiver Assistance Scale. A Modifications Scale records environmental modifications and equipment used by the child in routine ADL. Covers: self care, mobility and social functioning
Scale for Assessing Coping Skills	Whelan & Speake 1979	Designed to assess adolescents and adults with learning difficulties. A proxy report can be obtained from either the parents or a professional who knows the person well. Covers three areas: self-help, social academic and interpersonal. Comprises 36 items that are described at five levels of difficulty (a = easiest level to e = most difficult level). Items are scored on two ordinal scales: a 4-point scale of whether the particular ability exists (e.g. 1 = can do without help or supervision, 2 = can do but only with help or supervision, 3 = cannot yet do, 4 = do not know whether he can do this); and a 3-point scale of whether the ability is adequately used or not (5 = uses this ability in an adequate amount, 6 = does not use this an adequate amount, 7 = there is no opportunity to do this)

manage complex issues in the home environment and to integrate the intervention into the person's daily routines at home. An initial interaction with a caregiver can serve several purposes, including the forming of a working relationship, the gathering of information about the client and his environment and the provision of information to the caregiver about the occupational therapist's role, strategies for supporting the individual, available services and caregiver support structures. In some practice settings, the therapist may only have the opportunity to meet the caregiver on one or two occasions, for example, during a home visit. In this case, the therapist may need to interweave both the obtaining of data for assessment and intervention in the form of instruction, advice and support. A study by Clark et al (1995) identified four main types of interaction categories that occur between therapists and caregivers during assessment and treatment:

- **caring interactions** that focused on friendliness and support

- **partnering interactions** that involved seeking and acknowledging input and reflective feedback to help caregivers make changes/modify behaviour or to affirm existing caregiver practices
- **informing interactions** that involved gathering information, explaining information and clarifying information
- **directing interactions** that involved the provision of instruction and advice.

OBSERVATIONAL METHODS

The most reliable form of functional assessment is considered to be direct observation (Law 1993, Skruppy 1993). Occupational therapists are trained in both activity analysis and direct observational skills, so a particular area of occupational therapists' expertise is considered to be 'in assessing clients and drawing inferences based on their direct observation of the client's performance' (Law 1993 p234). Therapists should not just rely upon self- and proxy report for the assessment because some research studies have found discrepancies between reported and observed function. For example, Skruppy (1993) conducted a study in which a sample of 30 subjects were interviewed and then observed performing activities of daily living (ADL) tasks using a standardised test. People without ADL limitations were able to report their abilities accurately. However, Skruppy found that those with limitations in ADL functioning were aware of their difficulties but overestimated their abilities during the interview.

A large proportion of occupational therapy assessments (both standardised and non-standardised) involve the observation of the performance of activities of daily living (ADL). Examples include the Functional Independence Measure (FIM; Granger et al 1993), the Klien–Bell Activities of Daily Living Scale (Klien & Bell 1982) and the Rivermead ADL Assessment (Whiting & Lincoln 1980, Lincoln & Edmans 1990). Another large group of assessments comprise batteries of observational tasks developed to assess functioning at an impairment level. Examples include the Chessington Occupational Therapy Neurological Assessment Battery (COTNAB; Tyerman et al 1986, Laver & Huchinson 1994), the Rivermead Behavioural Memory Test (BMT; Wilson et al 1991) and the Rivermead Perceptual Assessment Battery (RPAB; Whiting et al 1985). A few occupational therapy observational assessments provide data across several levels of function. Examples of observational assessments that examine performance of ADL, at the disability level, and provide information about functional limitations and/or underlying impairment, such as motor and cognitive functioning, include the Arnadottir OT–ADL Neurobehavioural Evaluation (A-ONE; Arnadottir 1990), the Assessment of Motor Process Skills (AMPS; Fisher 1997), the Kitchen Task Assessment (KTA; Baum & Edwards 1993) and the Structured Observational Test of Function (SOTOF; Laver & Powell 1995).

COMBINING METHODS

The most comprehensive way in which to conduct an assessment is to collect data from several sources using a range of assessment methods and then compare the data, looking for similarities and differences in the findings. A major reason why therapists choose to interview people about their function rather than conduct an observational assessment is the time required (Skruppy 1993). The most reliable method is to interview individuals and their proxy about their performance in the full range of their activities and then select a few key activities for observation, as it usually is not feasible to observe all areas of function relevant to an individual. When choosing standardised observational assessments it is helpful to select predictive tests with good predictive validity (see pp138–140). In addition to questioning about level of independence, it can be helpful to consider an individual's perceptions of how important different activities are in their life and also how satisfied they are with their performance (Law et al 1994). This information helps therapists to prioritise areas for further assessment and treatment.

CONFIDENTIALITY

Confidentiality of people's information is critically important. Occupational therapists are both ethically and legally obliged to safeguard confidential information relating to people with whom they work (College of Occupational Therapists 2000). The 'Code of Ethics and Professional Conduct for Occupational Therapists' provides clear guidelines related to confidentiality (College of Occupational Therapists 2000 p3). A therapist might only disclose information (such as a person's diagnosis, treatment, prognosis, personal circumstances or future requirements) under one of three conditions: that the person has given consent; that there is legal justification (for example, by statute or court order); or that it is considered to be in the public interest in order to prevent serious harm, injury or damage to the individual, carer or any other person. The therapist is obliged to keep all information secure and release records only to people who have a legitimate right and need to access that information. Therapists should be aware of local and national policies on electronic notes (which include e-mails, computerised records, letters and faxes) and should adhere to these policies. They should also be aware of other codes of practice, policies and law related to confidentiality issues, such as the Data Protection Act 1998; Human Rights Act 1998; Access to Personal Files Act 1987; Access to Medical Records Act 1988; Access to Health Records Act 1990; and the Patient's Charter 1994 (cited in College of Occupational Therapists 2000).

FACTORS TO CONSIDER WHEN SELECTING AN ASSESSMENT APPROACH

TIMING OF ASSESSMENT IN THE OCCUPATIONAL THERAPY PROCESS

The first factor to consider when planning an assessment approach is the timing of the assessment. On referral, the therapist will need to conduct an initial assessment. This may require several sessions, for example, an initial interview, an informal observation of personal care and the administration of a standardised assessment battery. The initial assessment is used to provide a baseline for treatment planning. Assessment should not stop with the initial assessment but be an integral part of the treatment and assist the therapist's clinical reasoning process as she considers the way in which the person is responding to the treatment plan.

Ongoing evaluative assessment helps with examining progress and monitoring effects of the intervention.

There is a trend towards shorter lengths of stay in hospital, especially in acute care, and occupational therapists play an important role in predischarge assessment. A predischarge assessment provides information about the person's readiness for discharge (including safety and risk factors), the needed and available physical and social supports and any requirements for follow-up therapy (Rudman et al 1998).

The therapist also should conduct a final assessment when the person is discharged from the occupational therapy service. This serves to provide an evaluation of the effectiveness of intervention to date and may also provide new baseline data to be passed on to other colleagues if a person is being referred to another service provider.

PURPOSES OF ASSESSMENT

When selecting a specific assessment or an overall assessment strategy for an individual, it is important for the occupational therapist to consider the purpose for which the assessment information is gathered and how the results or the assessment might be interpreted and used. When undertaking a critique of potential assessments it is vital to consider the intended purpose of the assessments under review because the content, methods, psychometric properties and clinical utility of an assessment should be evaluated against its intended purpose. For assessing an individual, assessments can be grouped in terms of four main purposes (Table 5.5):

- evaluative
- descriptive
- predictive
- discriminative.

Some assessments are developed to address just one of these four purposes. However, many can be used for a combination of purposes.

There are a number of issues to consider when reviewing assessments in terms of purpose. For example, if an evaluative assessment is required, the assessment needs to be sensitive to the appropriate degree of change in performance that is anticipated (see p138). Improvements in function may be small and slow and many assessments lack sensitivity because they do not have sufficient graduations to measure change or because they do not include test items that are the focus of rehabilitation. There is also a paucity of test–retest reliability data for many current assessments.

An issue to consider when selecting a descriptive assessment is the level of data obtained related to the requirements for accurate treatment planning. For example, Activities of Daily Living (ADL) assessment might describe a person's function on a four-point independence

Table 5.5 Four main purposes of clinical assessments (Hayley et al 1991, Law 1993)

Purpose	Description
Evaluative	• Used to detect change in performance over time • Can be used to monitor a person's progress during rehabilitation and determine the effectiveness of the intervention • Should have established test–retest and interrater reliability
Descriptive	• Provides information that describes a person's current functional status or circumstances (e.g. ADL function, home environment) • Often focuses on identifying strengths and limitations • Provides an evaluation at one point in time only • Often used to provide baseline data for treatment planning and clinical decision making • Should have established content and construct validity
Predictive	• Used to classify people into predefined categories of interest • Attempt to predict an event or functional status in another situation on the basis of a person's performance on the assessment. For example, a kitchen assessment in the occupational therapy department might be used to predict whether a person should be independent and safe in meal preparation once discharged home • Should have established predictive validity
Discriminative	• Used to distinguish between individuals or groups • Comparisons are usually made against a normative group or another diagnostic group • Comparisons may be made for reasons such as diagnosis, placement or level of dysfunction in relation to expectations of performance of other healthy people of that age (e.g. to see if a child is developing skills at the expected stage versus has a developmental delay)

See Table 5.11 for description of different types of validity and Table 5.9 for types of reliability.

scale, however this may not provide data on the limiting factors in a person's performance within an activity, nor the reason for any observed deficits. For example, the treatment plan for a person dependent in dressing because of a motor deficit will not be the same as that for a person who is dependent because of apraxia, or visual field deficit or problems within initiation.

When selecting discriminative assessments, the value of the assessment is dependent on the adequacy, and the ability to generalise from, the normative sample or population used to obtain reference data. The lack of normative or comparative test standardisation with a population similar to the specific person restricts the occupational therapist's ability to make accurate and valid comparisons. An example of this is where assessments initially developed and standardised for child populations have been used with adult populations, or where tests developed in one country for a particular cultural group are used in another country without consideration to potential differences.

In addition to individual assessment, occupational therapists may use assessments for other purposes. For example, assessments may be used to evaluate the inputs, processes and outcomes of occupational therapy. If a therapist is undertaking a quality assurance or clinical audit exercise, it is vital to define the goals of the focus of the review so that the outcome measures used for the exercise match the intended goals of the programme/ service/intervention. When measuring outcomes, the therapist explores whether any change has occurred in the person as a result of a specific occupational therapy intervention. It is critical to use objective and sensitive measures because 'any subjective estimate, especially if made by the clinician who has invested time, effort and perhaps more in treating the client, is likely to be unreliable' (de Clive-Lowe 1996 p359). Functional assessments also may be used as outcome measures to address important questions related to service provision, funding issues and healthcare policy. For example, assessment may be used to determine eligibility criteria for a particular service or to evaluate the performance of a service to decide upon future service provision. If occupational therapy services are to be well funded then occupational therapists must carefully select appropriate outcome measures for evaluating and demonstrating the effectiveness of their services.

SCORING SYSTEMS

Many standardised and non-standardised assessments score a person's performance on some sort of scale. It is important for the occupational therapist to be able to recognise the type of scale being used in order to be able to interpret and handle appropriately the person's scores. Stevens (1946, cited in Crocker & Algina 1986) described a four level measurement scale that is still widely used to classify scoring systems today. Stevens' system identified scales that differ in the extent to which their scale values retain the properties of the real number line. The four levels are called:

- nominal
- ordinal
- interval
- ratio.

These levels are defined in Table 5.6.

The majority of scales used in occupational therapy assessments are nominal or ordinal scales. An example of a nominal scale is where gender is coded 1 for female and 2 for male, even though no quantitative distinction between the two genders is implied. The scores indicate that qualitative differences between categories exists and the scores serve as shorthand labels. This can be useful when entering information into a computer database. Nominal scores can be applied to categories such as diagnosis, type of living accommodation, equipment provided and discharge destination.

A frequently used example of an ordinal scale is where scores are assigned to describe levels of independence, such as: 1 = independent, 2 = needs verbal prompting, 3 = needs physical assistance, 4 = dependent and unable to perform activity.

The Fahrenheit temperature scale is an example of an interval scale, in this case, zero does not represent an absence of heat.

Examples of ratio scales include length measured in inches or centimetres, weight measured in pounds or kilograms and age measured in days, months or years since birth.

Table 5.6 Stevens (1946, cited in Crocker and Algina 1986) Four levels of measurement

Level of measurement	Description of level
Nominal	- Numbers are used purely as labels for the elements in the data system, they do *not* have the properties of meaningful order, equal distances between units, or a fixed origin - Any set of numbers may be used - Each unique object or response in the data system must be assigned a different number - Any other set of numbers could be substituted as long as one-to-one correspondence between members of the sets is maintained, this is called ismorphic transformation
Ordinal	- The elements in the data system can be ordered on the amount of the property being measured - The scaling rule requires that values from the real number system must be assigned in the same order - An ordinal scale does *not* have the properties of equal distance between units nor a fixed origin - Scores may be converted to other values as long as the original information about the rank order is preserved, this is called monotonic transformation
Interval	- An interval scale has rank order and the distances between the numbers have meaning with respect to the property being measured - If two scores at the low end of the scale are one unit apart then two scores at the high end are also one unit apart; the difference between two high scores and two low scores represents the same amount of the property - Transformation of values in the scale is restricted and must contain the information in the values of the original scale
Ratio	- A ratio scale has the properties of order, equal distance between units, and a fixed origin or absolute zero point - Once the location of the absolute zero is known, non-zero measurements can be expressed as ratios of one another - Transformation of values is very restricted

The four levels of measurement are in a hierarchy of sophistication, with nominal scales being the least and ratio scales being the most sophisticated level of measurement. In this hierarchy, the more sophisticated scale above contains the properties of the scale below, that is, values meeting the requirements of a ratio scale may be regarded as meeting the requirements for an interval scale and data collected on an interval scale may be regarded as providing ordinal level information. It is very important that therapists do not handle scores in a manner that is inconsistent with the level of measurement used. For example, some assessments, such as the Barthel Index (Mahoney & Barthel 1965) have an ordinal level scale of independence and add scores to provide a total score from the test items. This is dubious because to be independent in one activity, such as in making a cup of tea, does not equal the same level of function as being independent in another activity, such as cooking a meal. Several authors (for example, Hogan & Orme 2000, Murdock 1992) have argued against the use of the Barthel Index because the total score has no real meaning and the same total score does not carry the same meaning for all people with that particular score. In addition, two people might show equal increases in their total scores when retested following treatment but their gains in functional status might be very different (Eakin 1989).

Some assessments do provide scales where the level of difficulty of a task is taken into account and provide a hierarchy that represents level of difficulty, for example, the Assessment of Motor Process Skills (AMPS; Fisher 1997). Another practice to avoid when implementing an ordinal level scale is presuming that an increase in function indicated by moving from needing verbal prompting (score 2) to being independent (score 1) equals the same amount of change as moving from dependence (score 4) to physical assistance (score 3). The presumption of equal change occurring between two scores can be made only when using interval or ratio level scales.

STANDARDISED ASSESSMENTS

In recent years, the provision of health and social care has been exposed to a more market-orientated approach in which organisations who purchase occupational therapy services have become more concerned about 'value for money' and require assurances that the service provided is both cost effective and clinically effective. An emphasis on clinical governance means that therapists are more overtly responsible for the quality of their practice and this is reflected in an increased interest in evidence-based practice. To examine whether an intervention has been effective, therapists need reliable, valid and sensitive outcome measures. Quantifiable data are required to undertake the statistical analyses needed to demonstrate that results obtained from an intervention are significant and not just owing to chance factors (de Clive-Lowe 1996). This has led to an increase in both the development and use of standardised assessments.

If the results of tests given to different people by different occupational therapists, or to the same person by the same therapist on different occasions, are to be comparable then the conditions under which the tests are administered have to be exactly the same. The therapist also wants to be confident that the assessment is accurately measuring the domain of concern. When assessing occupational performance it is virtually impossible to obtain complete accuracy and objectivity but using standardised tests can facilitate objectivity. Assessments can be standardised in two ways: firstly, in terms of procedures, materials and scoring and, secondly, in terms of normative standardisation (de Clive-Lowe 1996). The first method of standardisation involves the provision of detailed descriptions and directions for the test materials, the method of administration, the instructions for administration, the norms, the scoring and the interpretation of scores (Jones 1991) (Table 5.7).

This information usually is provided in a test manual. Standardisation 'extends to the exact materials employed, time limits, oral instructions, preliminary demonstrations, ways of handling queries from test takers, and every other detail of the testing situation' (Anastasi 1988 p25). In addition to basic administration details, other subtle factors might affect a person's test performance. For example, when giving oral instructions 'rate of speaking, tone of voice,

Table 5.7 Factors required for standardisation (from Jones 1991 pp177–178)

Aspect of test	Details required
Test materials	• Exact test materials should be listed • Some tests provide materials as part of a standardised test battery • If the therapist has to collect the materials for the test then precise details of how to construct the test (with exact sizes, colours, fabric of materials, etc.) are required
Method of administration	• Test conditions should be described • Number of people tested at any one time should be detailed (i.e. individual or group assessment, size of group) • Information about time required for administration should be given • Details of any time limits should be provided • Description is needed of how to handle enquiries from the client
Instructions for administration	• Detailed written instructions for the therapist should be provided • Exact instructions to be given to the person being tested • To maintain standardisation, instructions should be followed exactly
Norms	• Norms indicate the average performance on the test and the varying degrees of performance above and below average • Norms should be based on a large, representative sample of people for whom the test was designed • Normative sample should reflect the attributes of the chosen population (e.g. geographical, socio-economic, ethnicity, age, sex, level of education) • The size of the sample used for normative data will vary depending on the nature of the test, the number of test items and the variability in test scores, but in general the larger the sample the more useful the normative data
Scores	• The scoring system should be described clearly • The subject's performance on the test should be evaluated on the basis of empirical data • Scoring methods vary from test to test and may include the use of raw scores that may then be converted to another type of score • Types of scoring include: developmental norms, within-group norms (standard scores, percentiles) and fixed reference group norms • If scores are being added, deducted, etc. then make sure the level of measurement allows the numbers to be handled in that way
Interpretation of scores	• Information to guide the therapist in the interpretation of scores required • A number of factors may influence the person's performance on the test such as test anxiety, fatigue, interruptions, distractions, etc.

inflection, pauses, and facial expression' may all influence how a person responds (Anastasi 1998 pp25–26). For an example of test instructions see Box 5.6.

Standardised assessments can be divided into two main types: norm-referenced or criterion-referenced tests.

NORM-REFERENCED ASSESSMENTS

The performance of any person can be considered in the light of the variable performance that is representative of expected or 'normal' performance. A norm-referenced test, therefore, is an assessment in which a person's test performance is compared with that of a broad group of people (called the normative sample). The normative sample is tested before the assessment is published and the results are often provided in the test manual in the form of tables, which give the distribution, or spread, of scores that the normative group obtained (de Clive-Lowe 1996). Statistical analyses are undertaken to give technical information about the distribution of test scores, such as the average score. These statistics may be presented as a labelled normal curve with specified values attached to standard deviations above and below the mean (Anastasi 1988). The standard deviations from the mean indicate the degree to which a person's performance on the test is above or below average. Some

---

Box 5.6 Example of test instructions (taken from Russell et al 1993, pp41–42)

Lying and rolling

This dimension includes 17 items in the prone and supine positions. These items include the child's ability to:
- roll from prone or supine
- perform specific tasks while maintaining supine or some variation of prone.

Item 1. Supine, head in midline: turns head with extremities symmetrical

0. Does not maintain head in midline.
1. Maintains head in midline 1 to 3 seconds.
2. Maintains head in midline, turns head with extremities asymmetrical.
3. Turns head with extremities symmetrical.

Starting position

Position the child with head in midline and, if possible, the arms at rest and symmetrical (but not necessarily at the side). This will make it easier to determine the appropriate score.

Instructions

Instruct the child to turn his head from side to side or follow an object from one side to the other.
    The child can be instructed to keep his arms still, or, in the case of a younger child who may try to reach for the object, observe whether the upper extremity movements are 'symmetrical' or 'asymmetrical'.
    For a score of 2 (extremities 'asymmetrical') there should be very obvious asymmetry that is dominated by head position.

---

tests provide a cut-off point at which a person's performance is said to be dysfunctional or at which a specific deficit is considered to be present. For example, the Rivermead Perceptual Assessment Battery (RPAB; Whiting et al 1985) provides a graph that profiles scores in relation to expected levels for people of average intelligence and sets a cut-off level of three standard deviations below the mean to indicate a level below which perceptual deficit is presumed.

The standard against which a person is assessed should be what is typically seen for a person of the same age and the process through which the person accomplishes the assessment task must be evaluated against the process for that age and cultural background. It is, therefore,

critical for occupational therapists to understand normal human development, from birth to old age, and to understand the impact of cultural and environmental factors upon performance. To be sure that the data from the normative sample can be generalised to the individuals they are working with, therapists should review the representativeness and sample sizes of the normative data upon which assessments have been standardised. To do this they must consider the characteristics of individuals or groups (such as age, sex, education, sociocultural background) and compare these with the characteristics of the normative sample. The importance of these factors will vary depending on the construct measured. The therapist should consider which characteristics are likely to be relevant to the skills or constructs that the test is designed to measure (de Clive-Lowe 1996). For example, with a paediatric developmental assessment, a child's age will have a profound effect on the motor, language, cognitive and perceptual skills that a therapist would expect a child to have mastered. With an older person, assessed on an Instrumental Activities of Living (IADL) scale, the sex and sociocultural background of the individual and normative sample might have an effect on people's prior experience and performance of specific IADL items; for example, an older woman might not have dealt with the family's finances and an older man might not have dealt with laundry.

CRITERION-REFERENCED ASSESSMENTS

Whereas norm-referenced assessments evaluate performance against the scores of a normative sample, with criterion-referenced assessments performance is examined against predefined criteria. This is useful when examining a person's competence or level of mastery. Criterion-referenced tests are important because therapists are concerned with desired outcomes, such as specified levels of ability in ADL tasks. With a criterion-referenced measure it is essential to have a detailed and unambiguous definition of the criteria against which the person is to be judged. For example, if the desired outcome is independence in getting dressed then the test should describe exactly what the person should be able to do in order to be assessed as being competent in dressing. Depending on the activity to be assessed, different criteria might be necessary for people of different gender, age or cultural backgrounds. In some cases, a time limit might form part of the criteria.

TRAINING AND INTERPRETING STANDARDISED TEST SCORES

It is important to check whether the therapist administering the test has the appropriate knowledge and skill to administer, score and interpret the results of the test correctly. Most published tests require that the person administering the test has obtained certain qualifications and expertise. Some tests require that the test administrator has undertaken specific training on the administration and scoring of the test (de Clive-Lowe 1996). Before using any new test, the therapist should take enough time to 'be fully conversant with the test content, use, reliability and validity before administering the test in order that this is done correctly and that any interpretation of test findings be accurate' (Jones 1991 p179). In addition to reading the test manual and examining the test materials and forms, it can be very helpful to role-play test administration with a colleague to familiarise oneself with the test materials and instructions before using a test with a client.

Most standardised assessments provide a raw or standard score or scores. These scores are not sufficient alone and must be interpreted within the wider context of the specific testing situation and influences of the test environment and the person's current situation and idiosyncrasies (de Clive-Lowe 1996). The therapist needs to pose a series of questions when examining test scores, such as: 'Do I think these scores are a true reflection of the person's function?'; 'If not, did test anxiety, fatigue, motivation, distractions, etc. influence the test results?'; 'How do these scores compare with other data I have collected about this person'? (e.g. through interview, proxy report, non-standardised observations); 'Is there consistency in the data or discrepancies in the picture I am building about this person's ability and needs?'.

It should be remembered that a good test administration is just a beginning and it is critical to document and interpret the results and to share the conclusions drawn from the assessment with that of other relevant personnel. When reporting on standardised test results, the therapist should state the rationale for administering this particular standardised test. In her report, the therapist should also include a description of the person's responses to and behaviour during testing (for example, whether he was anxious, if he complied with requests or was restricted by pain or fatigue). These additional qualitative observations will provide a context for the therapist's hypotheses about the meaning of the test scores (de Clive-Lowe 1996). Table 5.8 suggests some headings for use when reporting the results of standardised tests.

NON-STANDARDISED ASSESSMENTS

Therapists continue to use non-standardised assessments for a number of reasons. For example, therapists report:

- a lack of appropriate standardised assessments
- poor resources (which limit the ability to purchase standardised measures)
- that standardised assessments can be lengthy to administer
- that non-standardised assessments are flexible in terms of procedures, settings and the manner in which the assessment is administered and are, therefore, perceived as being more person-centred
- that non-standardised assessments are seen as useful for observing functional ability in the person's home environment, for addressing the qualitative aspects of performance and for exploring the dynamics between the client and caregiver (Chia 1996, Laver 1994).

Table 5.8 Suggested headings for writing a report on a standardised test administration

Heading	Information to be included
Personal details	Person's name, date of birth, age, diagnoses, address
Date(s) of assessment	It is important to give the date of an initial assessment and any reassessment. If appropriate, also state the time of day. For example, if one test was given first thing in the morning and the reassessment was conducted in the afternoon, fluctuating levels of fatigue or stiffness might influence the test results
Referral information	The name of the person who made the referral and the reason for referral. This should influence the selection of assessment focus/methods and have implications for how the test results are interpreted. For example, the referral might be to assess the person's safety to be discharged home
Relevant background information	Brief information relevant to the selection and interpretation of the assessment. For example, occupational history, hobbies and interests, medication (especially if this leads to varying function), how the person came to be in the present situation. In the example of a home safety assessment, details such as whether the person lives alone would be useful here
Previous assessment results (if any)	Previous assessment might influence the choice of current assessment and will also be useful for comparison to interpret whether the person's function has improved or deteriorated. If no previous assessment data is available, state 'none known'
Test(s) administered	State the title of the test(s) given and provide a brief description of the test and its purpose. This is particularly important if the person reading the report is not familiar with the test(s) used
Behaviour during testing	Describe any behaviour that might have influenced the test results. This information is needed so that anyone reading the report can decide whether the results represent a reliable estimate of the person's ability. Keep descriptions as concise and objective as possible. Include information about apparent fatigue, anxiety, level of cooperation with testing, ability to follow instructions, any distractions or interruptions to the test, etc.
Results	Give a concise summary of the results. If appropriate, attach a copy of the assessment form and/or summary table or graph to the report. If any parts of the test were not assessed, make a note of this and state the reasons for the omission. If using percentile or standard scores, state which norms have been used so that anyone reassessing the person can use the same norms for future comparison (e.g. give date of test manual and the page reference for the table). This is very important where there are several editions of an assessment with updated normative data
Discussion	Consider what the results of the assessment mean, whether the results represent a reliable picture of the person's function and hypothesise about what might account for the results. Relate the discussion back to the reason for referral. Give brief examples of observable behaviour and/or specific test results to justify your reasoning. Also refer back to the 'Behaviour during testing' section if this has a bearing on how the results should be interpreted
Recommendations	These should derive directly from the assessment results and should relate back to the reason for the referral and the person's current situation. If you recommend further intervention give timelines and state an appropriate time for reassessment

A common practice is to take different parts of standardised tests or individual test items and integrate these into a 'therapist-constructed' tailored assessment battery for a specific group or service (Chia 1996). However, once the standard procedure for test administration and scoring has been changed, even in a small way, the reliability and validity of that part of the test or test item can no longer be guaranteed. Therefore, although the test items might have been generated from a standardised test, the ensuing 'therapist-made' assessment cannot be viewed as standardised. A further limitation of this practice, of using test items or parts drawn from standardised tests, is that the original source of, or reference for, the test item is rarely recorded on the tailored assessment and forms. This means that, once the therapists involved in developing the tailored assessment leave the service, new therapists are unaware of the original sources and the rationale for the development of the tailored 'therapist-constructed' assessment battery. Consequently, therapists using inherited 'therapist-constructed' assessments can find it difficult to justify the reasons for carrying out these non-standardised assessments (Chia 1996).

If therapists are to use non-standardised assessments it is critical that they are fully aware of their limitations. The findings from a non-standardised assessment are open to interpretation and are, therefore, much more subjective than the findings gained from a standardised measure. Furthermore, because detailed procedures for administering and scoring the test are rarely available for non-standardised assessments, it is not possible for the therapist reliably to repeat the assessment to evaluate the effects of treatment. The test is even more unreliable if another therapist tries to repeat the assessment with the same person at a later time.

Therapists should not underestimate the consequences of continuing to use non-standardised assessments where standardised measures of the same construct or area of function exist. This has been demonstrated in a study by Stewart (1999), who compared the results of a non-standardised assessment with a standardised measure of severity of disability in a group of elderly people. Stewart's purpose was to examine if there were differences in outcomes and to explore the consequences of these for service entitlement. Her results indicated that the non-standardised measure had 'restricted ability to identify and measure accurately the degree of disability of older people' and 'that because of the limited psychometric rigour of the [non-standardised measure] one consequence for service provision may be that a vulnerable group, elderly frail people, are denied services unnecessarily' (Stewart 1999 p422). Stewart concluded that 'when clinical judgement is based on objective assessment arising from the use of standardized instruments rather than intuitive guesswork, occupational therapists' decision making can be seen to be more rational and consequently defensible'.

In conclusion, many non-standardised 'therapist-constructed' assessments continue to be used in practice and have both strengths and limitations. Therapists should be clear as to the theoretical foundations of all their assessment procedures, including both standardised and non-standardised tests. Where components of standardised tests are used in a 'therapist-constructed' assessment battery, therapists should be able to quote the original source and the rationale for the test item's use in the ensuing non-standardised assessment. In cases where non-standardised assessments are used without such theoretical underpinning or rationale, professional credibility and client welfare can be at risk. Inadequate, and even inaccurate, decisions may be made from non-standardised assessments and can have negative consequences both for the care of an individual and, where the effectiveness of occupational therapy intervention cannot be reliably demonstrated, for service provision as a whole.

PSYCHOMETRIC PROPERTIES

RELIABILITY

It is critical for occupational therapists to consider the reliability of an assessment because the degree of established reliability informs the therapist how accurately the scores obtained from an assessment reflect the true performance of a person on the test (Opacich 1991). The aspects of a person that therapists assess are open to many variables, which may act as 'sources of error' during an assessment. These variables include the person's motivation, interests, mood and the effects of medication. Such variables may influence a person's performance to some degree and can never be completely discounted. Therefore, the therapist needs to know how likely it is that these potential sources of error will influence the results obtained on a test (de Clive-Lowe 1996). This knowledge is produced through studies of reliability in which a test is given by different therapists to large numbers of people at different times and statistical analyses of the similarities and differences in the scores obtained from these various test administrations are calculated. In broad terms, the 'reliability of a test refers to how stable its scores remain over time and across different examiners' (de Clive-Lowe 1996 p359). The therapist should consider several types of reliability (Table 5.9):

- test–retest reliability
- interrater reliability
- equivalent or parallel form
- internal consistency.

A reliability coefficient is used to indicate the extent to which a test is a stable instrument that is capable of producing consistent results. Perfect reliability is represented by a coefficient of 1.0 but in real life this is hardly ever achieved. The therapist, therefore, needs to judge the acceptable amount of error when making clinical decisions from test results. Table 5.10 provides examples of acceptable levels for different types of reliability.

There is no standard for conducting reliability studies and the methods and sample sizes vary widely from test to test. Therefore, in addition to examining the reliability coefficient stated for a test, it is important for a therapist deciding whether the test has acceptable levels of reliability to review the methodology and sample sizes used for examining psychometric properties. This information is usually found in test manuals and

Table 5.9 Types of reliability (adapted from Anastasi 1988, Benson & Clark 1982, Crocker & Algina 1986, Ottenbacher & Tomchek 1993)

Type of reliability	Description
Test–retest	• Therapists need to examine whether their interventions have been effective. Therefore, they administer tests on two or more occasions to monitor changes in function following treatment • Test–retest reliability is the correlation of scores obtained by the same person on two administrations of the same test and is the consistency of the assessment or test score over time
Interrater	• Clients may move between occupational therapy services, for example, from an acute to a rehabilitation ward, from inpatient service to a day hospital or outpatient service. Therefore, an individual might be given the same assessment but by different therapists • Therapists need to know whether any change in a person's performance on a test is caused by a different test administrator or represents a genuine change in the person's performance • Interrater reliability refers to the agreement between or among different therapists (raters) administering the test
Intrarater	• Therapists often use tests that require some degree of observation and/or judgement. They want to know that differences in results obtained for different clients, or for the same person at different times, is not the result of a fluctuation in their own consistency in giving and scoring the test • Intrarater reliability refers to the consistency of the judgements made by the same test administrator (rater) over time
Equivalent (parallel) form	• A parallel form is an alternative test that differs in content from the original test but which measures the same thing to the same level of difficulty • Parallel forms are used for retesting where a learning effect might impact the test results • Equivalent/parallel form reliability examines the correlation between scores obtained for the same person on two (or more) forms of a test
Internal consistency	• Internal consistency refers to whether all the items in a test are measuring the same construct or trait. Items may test the same performance domains and constructs but vary in difficulty • Studies of internal consistency examine both item homogeneity and item difficulty and study the effect of errors caused by content sampling • Items must measure the same construct if they are to be a homogenous item group; a test is said to have item homogeneity when people perform consistently across the test items

Table 5.10 Accepted values for establishing reliability (adapted from Benson & Clark 1982, Opacich 1991)

Type of reliability	Types of test	Procedure	Coefficient
Test–retest	Tests used to evaluate performance over time	Correlation between two administrations of the test to the same people with a defined time interval between the two test administrations	0.70 or above
Interrater	Tests that are administered by more than one therapist	Correlation between the scores recorded by two therapists administering the test to the same person at the same time	0.90 or above
Equivalent forms	Tests that have alternate (parallel) forms	Correlation between two forms of the same test	0.80 or above
Internal consistency	Tests used to infer an underlying construct (includes perceptual and cognitive tests, aptitude tests and personality inventories)	Correlation among items on the same test	0.80 or above

may also be published in journal articles. With interrater reliability, some test developers evaluate the only reliability of the scoring of the assessment through a method that involves different therapists scoring videotaped administrations of a test. For example, the interrater reliability of the Rivermead Perceptual Assessment Battery (RPAB; Whiting et al 1985) was evaluated using the videotaped assessment of six people scored by three occupational therapists, and Matthey et al (1993 p366) suggest that the small 'sample sizes used by the RPAB authors to calculate the reliability coefficients … [make] the reliability data questionable'. The methodology used by Russell et al (1993) to evaluate the interrater reliability of the Gross Motor Function Measure (GMFM) looked at the reliability of testers administering and scoring the test by having three pairs of therapists administer and score the GMFM with a sample of 12 children. Laver (1994) also used pairs of testers, with a total sample of 32 therapists, when evaluating the interrater reliability for both the administration and scoring of the Structured Observational Test of Function (SOTOF; Laver & Powell 1995). The experience of the therapists involved in the studies should also be considered in order to identify whether a newly qualified therapist will obtain consistent results to an experienced senior therapist. In the RPAB manual (Whiting et al 1985) the level of experience of the three therapists used for the

study is not stated. In the study by Russell et al (1993) the six therapists had paediatric experience ranging from 2.5 to 18 years and in the study by Laver (1994) therapists' experience with elderly people ranged from 1 to 15 years.

In addition to therapists' level of experience, some test developers have considered the variation in how lenient or stringent therapists are when judging a person's performance on an observational assessment, this is known as rater severity (Fisher 1997, Lunz & Stahl 1993). For example, therapists wishing to use the Assessment of Motor Process Skills (AMPS; Fisher 1997) are required to attend a rigorous training course so that they can be calibrated for rater severity. Therapists view a series of videotapes of AMPS tasks being administered. Some therapists are found to be more lenient in their scoring and give people higher scores than more severe raters. Knowledge of rater severity scoring the AMPS is accounted for in the determination of the person's ability score, thus reducing the chance of interrater variability confounding the 'true' measure of the person's function (Fisher 1993).

Some test manuals provide details of the standard error of measurement (SEM), which is the estimate of the 'error' associated with a person's obtained score on a test when compared with his/her hypothetical 'true' score. A band of scores can be calculated from this figure, so a manual may say that the therapist can be x (e.g. 95) %

certain that a person's true score lies in the range of the obtained score plus or minus y (e.g. 3).

Therapists also need to consider the specificity and sensitivity of tests. Test specificity is important because therapists want only those people who exhibit a specific behaviour or functional deficit to be identified on a test. A false positive result will occur when someone who does not have a deficit is identified on a test as having the deficit, and a false negative will occur when a person who has a deficit is not shown to have that deficit through his performance on the test. A specific test minimises the number of false positive results that occur when the test is used and will not identify people who do not exhibit the behaviour or deficit being examined (Opacich 1991).

Test sensitivity is important because a sensitive test will identify all those people who show the behaviour or deficit in question. A sensitive test will minimise the chance of a false negative result and can identify what it was designed to test. When using evaluative measures, the therapist should ensure that the test used is sensitive to picking up both the type and degree/amount of change in behaviour or function that is anticipated, or desired, as the result of intervention. This is sometimes referred to as the degree of responsiveness of a test. If a test is not sensitive enough to the target of therapy, then changes that have occurred may be missed and this can be problematic if intervention appears to be ineffective when significant change has actually occurred. For example, The Canadian Occupational Performance Measure (COPM; Law et al 1994) has been developed to measure changes in people's perceptions of their performance and their level of satisfaction with their performance of self care, work and leisure tasks. Studies have a collected reassessment data for 139 people for performance scores and 138 for satisfaction scores. 'Differences in the means between initial and reassessment scores for both performance and satisfaction were statistically significant ($p < 0.0001$). The mean change scores in performance and satisfaction indicates that COPM is responsive to changes in perception of occupational performance by clients' (Law et al 1994 p26).

VALIDITY

Occupational therapists need to know whether an assessment adequately represents the performance domains and/or constructs they are interested in and whether the assessment items address these domains and/or constructs in the correct proportions. This is known as validity. Validation is undertaken by a test developer to collect evidence to support the types of inferences that are to be drawn from the results of an assessment (Crocker & Algina 1986). Occupational therapists should be able to understand several types of validity in order to review test manuals to identify whether psychometric studies have shown the assessment has appropriate levels of validity. Three types of validation, known as content, construct and criterion-related validation are traditionally performed (Crocker & Algina 1986). These three types of validity are defined in Table 5.11.

There is no one recognised measure of validity, so it is usual for researchers to conduct a range of studies to examine its different aspects (Bartram 1990). For example, Baum and Edwards (1993) undertook four analyses to examine aspects of the validity of the Kitchen Task Assessment (KTA). Correlation analysis was used to examine the relationship among the six variables in the measure 'correlation coefficients of 0.72–0.84 suggested that one dimension might exist … and that the cognitive domains selected for the KTA all contribute to the measurement of the cognitive performance of the task' (Baum & Edwards 1993 p433). Factor analysis was undertaken to identify common relationships among the variables, to determine the internal structure of the variables and to establish the KTA as a unidimensional instrument. Correlation analysis was undertaken with other published valid and reliable tests, three neuropsychological and two functional assessments, to determine the construct validity of the KTA. Results indicated that 'the KTA, as a test of practical cognitive skills, is related to the cognitive skills measured by [the other three] neuropsychological tests' (Baum & Edwards 1993 p 435). The fourth investigation involved an analysis of variance to examine per-

Table 5.11 Types of validity (adapted from Anastasi 1988, Bartram 1990, Crocker & Algina 1986, Opacich 1991)

Type of validity	Description
Content validity	• Refers to the degree to which an assessment measures what it is supposed to measure judged on the appropriateness of its content • Relates to the relevance of the person's individual responses to the assessment items, rather than to the apparent relevance of the assessment item content
Construct validity	• A construct is an idea generated from informed scientific imagination to categorise and describe behaviour; it is an abstract quality or phenomenon that is thought to account for behaviour • Construct validity involves the extent to which an assessment can be said to measure a theoretical construct or constructs • Construct validation is needed if the therapist wants to draw inferences from the person's performance on the assessment to performances that can be grouped under the labels of a particular construct (e.g. an item testing an aspect of short-term memory compared to the overall construct of short-term memory)
Criterion-related validity	• Relates to the effectiveness of a test in predicting an individual's performance in specific activities • Measured by comparing performance on the test with a criterion that is a direct and independent measure of what the assessment is designed to predict. Both predictive and concurrent measures can be used to determine criterion-related validity

formance of subjects on the KTA compared to stages of Senile Dementia of the Alzheimer Type (SDAT). Results showed that 'the KTA differentiates performance across all stages of the disease' (Baum & Edwards 1993 p435).

An important type of criterion-related validity is predictive validity. Predictive validation refers broadly to the prediction from the test to any criterion performance, or specifically to prediction over a time interval (Anastasi 1988). This is critical to therapists who often need to make predictions. For example, therapists may need to predict a person's function in a wide range of activities from observation of just a few activities; to predict the person's function in a different environment, such as from a kitchen assessment in an occupational therapy department to the person's level of independence in his own kitchen at home, or to predict functioning in the future, such as upon discharge. Therapists need to be careful that the predictions made from specific test results to other areas of function really are valid. For example, Dunn et al (1990) examined the ability to predict functional daily living skills, as measured by the Community Competence Scale, from neuropsychological tests, as measured using the Halstead–Reitan Battery. They concluded that the neuropsychological tests investigated were moderately predictive of measures of functional daily

living skills but that, while it might be valid 'to make predictions about a patient's global capacity to function independently, predictions [from the neuropsychological test results] regarding specific functional daily living skills may be unwarranted' (Dunn et al 1990 p103).

Face validity

Face validity 'is the dimension of a test by which it appears to test what it purports to test' (Christiansen & Baum 1991 p851). The concepts of content and face validity are similar but should not be confused (Anastasi 1988). 'The difference is that face validity concerns the acceptability of a test to the test-taker, while content validity concerns the appropriateness of the content of the test as judged by professionals' (Bartram 1990 p77). All definitions of face validity agree that the test should be acceptable to the test-taker. However, within the literature, definitions of face validity vary in terms of to who else the test should appear to be acceptable. For example, Bartram (1990 p76), defines face validity as solely the 'degree to which the test-taker sees a test as being reasonable and appropriate'. However, Crocker and Algina (1986 p223) broaden this definition to include 'laypersons or typical examiners', whilst Anastasi (1988 p144) perceives face validity as pertaining to 'whether the test "looks valid" to the examinees who take it, the administrative personnel who decide on its use, and other technically untrained observers'. Therapists need to consider the scope of their service when deciding on the best definition of face validity for their own purpose.

Face validity is not validity in a technical sense and, therefore, it has little direct psychometric importance. However, its evaluation is significant for occupational therapists because if therapists are to be person-centred in their practice then the person's perception of any assessment procedures as being relevant and meaningful is critical. Occupational therapy authors have criticised the use of tests based on items that have little meaning and relevance for the test-taker. For example, Law (1993 p235) notes that 'the client's perspectives, values and efforts are not considered', that assessments 'tend to score performance and emphasize quantity rather than quality of function', that 'few instruments consider client satisfaction' and that 'with most evaluations clients' culture, roles, developmental stages and the environment in which they live are not considered'.

Bartram (1990) has presented several arguments for ensuring good face validity. Firstly, good face validity can have indirect effects on the outcome of a person's performance 'by facilitating rapport between the test and the test-taker which may, in turn, increase reliability' (Bartram 1990 p76). Secondly, engaging a person's motivation to engage in an assessment to the best of his ability is critical to obtaining valid and reliable test results and 'people are more likely to take seriously activities which seem reasonable and which they feel they understand' (Bartram 1990 p76). When reviewing potential tests, therapists may have to conduct their own face validity studies because there is a 'paucity of available research on face validity, despite its probable contribution to prevalent attitudes towards tests' (Anastasi 1988 p145). An example of a face validity study is provided by Laver (1994), who examined the face validity of the Structured Observational Test of Function (SOTOF) with a sample of 40 people following stroke. Following the administration of SOTOF, they were given a structured interview that comprised both open and closed questions. For example, they were asked 'What did you think this assessment was for?' 'Were these tasks something you would normally do?' 'Did you mind being asked to do these tasks?' and 'What did you think of the assessment?'. They were also given questions related to their experience of being tested 'Did you find the assessment … easy, upsetting, enjoyable, difficult, boring, stressful, useful, interesting, relaxing, irrelevant?'. This question format presented the possibility of a negative testing experience and enabled subjects to give an affirmative answer to a negative concept; this is particularly important when conducting research with older populations, who tend to be acquiescent, polite and affirmative in their responses.

CLINICAL UTILITY

Just because a test is well standardised, valid and reliable does not mean it will automatically be useful in the clinical environment. Many an expensive test gathers dust in occupational therapy departments for practical reasons, such as the therapists discovering after purchase that it was too lengthy to administer or too cumbersome to move around. Therefore, it is critical to consider the clinical utility of potential assessments for your service. Clinical utility covers aspects of a test such as cost, acceptability, training requirements, administration time, portability and ease of use (Jones 1991, Law & Letts 1989). These factors are described in Table 5.12.

SELECTING ASSESSMENTS

The decision to use a particular assessment strategy or test should be conscious and the result of informed evidence-based reasoning. There is now a wide choice of tests from which a therapist or occupational therapy service can choose. It is critical that therapists select the most appropriate tests for their service as financial considerations often place limits upon the number of tests that can be purchased for a service. Therefore, careful consideration needs to be given before purchasing a test. Information about different tests can be

Table 5.12 Aspects of clinical utility (adapted from Jones 1991, Law & Letts 1989)

Aspect of clinical utility	Description
Cost	• The initial financial outlay to purchase the test (this might comprise a manual, forms, test materials, etc.) • Equipment, if this is not provided with the test • Training costs, if additional training is required • Any supplies that need to be replaced for each assessment (e.g. food for a kitchen assessment, paper) • The cost of replacement test forms if copyright does not allow these to be photocopied
Time	• The initial time required to learn to administer the test. This might be through attendance on a training course or undertaken individually by reading the test manual and practising test administration • Time required to prepare for test administration each time (setting up the test environment and materials, purchasing supplies, etc.) • Administration time • Time required to score the test and interpret results
Energy/Effort	• The ease with which the therapist can learn to administer the test • The ease of each test administration • Does test administration get easier with practice?
Expertise of rater	• Whether the rater has to have specific qualifications or levels of experience • For some assessment additional training is required
Portability	• Whether it is easy to move the test between potential testing environments • Some materials may be heavy or bulky
Acceptability (this overlaps with face validity)	• Whether the assessment fits with the therapist's philosophy, theoretical frameworks and practice and looks professional • Whether the test is acceptable to the person being tested, including the relevance of the test to him and whether taking the test causes stress and test anxiety • Acceptability to managers and service purchasers • Acceptability to other lay observers, such as the family

obtained in several ways, including reviewing the literature (journal articles and reviews, textbooks, test manuals, CD ROM databases and information on websites), talking to other therapists already using the test and via conference presentations and test training workshops. Some publishers will provide talks and demonstrations and may even provide sample test materials or loan the test for a trial basis. When examining potential tests for your service it is very useful to undertake a detailed test critique. Some critiques already exist in the form of published reviews; for example, Asher (1996) provides an annotated index of many standardised and published occupational therapy assessments. Law et al (1999) have published a CD ROM that provides critiques of 139 pediatric outcome measures. If you cannot find a useful critique of the test already undertaken by another therapist, use the series of questions in Box 5.7 to guide you in this process. Once the critique has been undertaken, summarise your findings into a list of strengths and weaknesses to

---

Box 5.7 Questions for undertaking a test critique

• What is the stated purpose of the test?
• For what population has the test been designed?
• What levels of function does the test address?
• In what environments can the test be administered?
• Is the test standardised?
• Is it a norm-referenced or a criterion-referenced test?
• If norm referenced, is the normative sample representative of the people with whom you will use the test?
• What scoring system is used?
• Does the test have acceptable levels of reliability?
• Has validity been established?
• Does the test have good face validity?
• Does the test have good clinical utility (e.g. time required for administration and scoring, cost of test manual, materials and forms, ease of administration and scoring)?
• What qualifications are needed by the test administrator and is additional training required to administer the test?

---

facilitate a comparison of possible options and help you decide upon final choice of what test to use for your service or specific client.

CONCLUSION

Assessment is of paramount importance to occupational therapy practice because it enables the therapist to:

- Describe the person's functional problems in the form of an occupational therapy diagnosis
- formulate a prognosis
- use the occupational therapy diagnosis and prognosis as a baseline for treatment planning
- monitor the person's responses during treatment
- evaluate the effectiveness of the intervention (Law & Letts 1989).

The practice setting and the nature of the occupational therapy service will place parameters around the type of assessment that is possible. Therapists need to be pragmatic in their choices but should also lobby for improvements when restrictions place unacceptable limitations on the quality of the assessment that can be undertaken; a rushed, one-time assessment is rarely a sufficient baseline from which to plan effective treatment. No assessment of human functioning can be entirely objective and therapists need to make careful observations, hypotheses and judgements that could be open to some degree of error. Therefore, in order to ensure that their assessments are as valid and reliable as possible, occupational therapists should endeavour to use standardised assessments where available.

In the future, the profession needs to achieve a shift from the use of non-standardised 'therapist-constructed' assessments to well-researched, clinically useful, standardised measures. In a political environment that places increasing emphasis on quality, clinical governance and evidenced-based practice, a greater use of standardised assessments should assist therapists to present more objective and precise findings and to evaluate their interventions in a reliable and sensitive manner. Therapists need to make time to critically examine all non-standardised assessments used within their service. Where these non-standardised assessments are found to be unsuitable for future practice, therapists need to review and trial potential standardised measures to replace them.

When selecting assessments for a service, care should be taken that a potential test has good face validity and clinical utility, in addition to thorough standardisation, established validity and acceptable levels of reliability. It should be remembered that a good test administration can be rendered useless if the results are not documented adequately and the results are not shared with the client and other relevant personnel so, when planning an assessment, sufficient time should be allowed for scoring, interpretation, report writing and feedback. Finally, assessment should never be viewed in isolation, for *it is not an end in itself*. Assessment always should be at the heart of the initial interaction with a person and should then be interwoven as an important component of the whole intervention process, right through to a final evaluation when the person is discharged from the occupational therapy service.

ACKNOWLEDGEMENTS

This chapter is dedicated to the memory of the man who inspired the 'Mr Jones' case studies, and who died suddenly whilst I was finishing the work and whose name was changed to maintain anonymity.

I would like to acknowledge the important influence that two occupational therapy colleagues have had in shaping my occupational therapy practice and research. As a novice clinician, my Head Occupational Therapist at Bolingbroke Hospital, Julia Gosden, and District Occupational Therapist for Wandsworth Health Authority, Beryl Steeden, taught me about the importance of standardised assessment, funded me

to attend the College of Occupational Therapists 'Assessment Techniques and Psychological Testing' course and encouraged me to engage in research to develop a standardised assessment – to them both I will always be grateful.

On a personal note, I would like to thank my husband, Alexander Fawcett, and our family and friends who have given me so much encouragement and support during the writing process. In particular, I am grateful to John and Dee Fawcett and Christine and Vic King who looked after our baby son, Lucas, on numerous occasions to give me time to write in peace!

REFERENCES

Ager A 1990 The Life Experiences Checklist (LEC). NFER-Nelson, Windsor

Anastasi A 1988 Psychological testing, 6th edn. Macmillan, New York

Arnadottir A 1990 The brain and behaviour: assessing cortical dysfunction through activities of daily living. CV Mosby, St Louis, MO

Asher I 1996 Occupational therapy assessment tools: an annotated index. American Occupational Therapy Association, Bethesda, MD

Bartram D 1990 Reliability and validity. In: Beech JR, Harding L (eds) Testing people: a practical guide to psychometrics. NFER-Nelson, Windsor, ch 3, pp 57–86

Baum CM, Edwards DF 1993 Cognitive performance in senile dementia of the Alzheimer type: the kitchen task assessment. American Journal of Occupational Therapy 47:431–436

Benson J, Clark F 1982 A guide for instrument development and validation. American Journal of Occupational Therapy 36(12):789–800

Berg L 1988 Clinical dementia rating (CDR). Psychopharmacology Bulletin 24(4):637–639

Canadian Association for Occupational Therapists 1991 Occupational therapy guidelines for client-centred practice. Canadian Association for Occupational Therapists, Toronto

Chia SH 1996 The use of non-standardised assessments in occupational therapy with children who have disabilities: a perspective. British Journal of Occupational Therapy 59(8):363–364

Christiansen C, Baum C (eds) 1991 Occupational therapy – overcoming human performance deficits. Slack, NJ

Clark CA, Corcoran M, Gitlin LN (1995) An exploratory study of how occupational therapists develop therapeutic partnerships with family caregivers. American Journal of Occupational Therapy 49(7):587–594

Cohn ES, Czycholl C 1991 Facilitating a foundation for clinical reasoning. In: Self-paced instruction for clinical education and supervision (SPICES). American Occupational Therapy Association, Rockville, MD

College of Occupational Therapists 2000 Code of ethics and professional conduct for occupational therapists. College of Occupational Therapists, London

Cooper B, Rigby P, Letts L 1995 Evaluation of access to home, community and workplace. In Trombly CA (ed) Occupational therapy for physical dysfunction, 4th edn. Williams & Wilkins, Baltimore, MD, ch 5, pp 55–72

Crocker L, Algina J 1986 Introduction to classical and modern test theory. Holt, Rinehart and Winston, Fort Worth, TX

de Clive-Lowe S 1996 Outcome measurement, cost-effectiveness and clinical audit: the importance of standardised assessment to occupational therapists in meeting these new demands. British Journal of Occupational Therapy 59(8):357–362

Dunn EJ, Russell Searight H, Grisso T, Margolis RB, Gibbons JL 1990 The relation of the Halstead–Reitan neuropsychological battery to functional daily living skills in geriatric patients. Archives of Clinical Neuropsychology 5:103–117

Eakin P 1989 Problems with assessments of Activities of Daily Living. British Journal of Occupational Therapy 52:50–54

Fisher AG 1997 The assessment of motor process skills, 2nd edn. Three Star Press, Fort Collins, CO

Fisher AG 1993 The assessment of IADL motor skills: an application of many faceted Rasch analysis. American Journal of Occupational Therapy 47(4):319–329

Fisher AG, Short-DeGraff M 1993 Improving functional assessment in occupational therapy: recommendations and philosophy for change. American Journal of Occupational Therapy 47:199–201

Granger CV, Hamilton BB, Linacre JM, Heinemann AW, Wright BD 1993 Performance profiles of the Functional Independence Measure. American Journal of Physical Medicine and Rehabilitation 72(2):84–89

Hayley SM, Coster WJ, Ludlow LH, Haltwanger JT, Andrellos PJ 1992 Pediatric Evaluation of Disability Inventory: development, standardization and administration manual. New England Medical Center, Boston, MA

Hayley SM, Coster WJ, Ludlow LH 1991 Pediatric functional outcome measures. Physical Medicine and Rehabilitation Clinics of North America 2:689–723

Hogan K, Orme S 2000 Measuring disability: a critical analysis of the Barthel Index. British Journal of Therapy and Rehabilitation 7(4):163–167

Jones L 1991 Symposium on methodology: the standardized test. Clinical Rehabilitation 5:177–180

Kielhofner G 1995 A model of human occupational: theory and application, 2nd edn. Williams & Wilkins, Baltimore, MD

Kielhofner G, Henry AD 1988 Development and investigation of the Occupational Performance History Interview. American Journal of Occupational Therapy 42:489–498

Klien RM, Bell B 1982 Self-care skills: behavioural measurement with Klein–Bell ADL scale. Archives of Physical Medicine and Rehabilitation 63(7):335–338

Laver AJ 1994 The development of the Structured Observational Test of Function (SOTOF) Unpublished Doctoral Thesis, University of Surrey, Guildford (held at the College of Occupational Therapists library).

Laver AJ, Baum CM 1992 Areas of occupational therapy assessment related to the NCMRR model of Dysfunction. In: Laver AJ 1994 The development of the Structured Observational Test of Function (SOTOF). Unpublished Doctoral Thesis, University of Surrey, Guildford, 185–186, 191

Laver AJ, Huchinson S 1994 The performance and experiences of normal elderly people on the Chessington Occupational Therapy Neurological Assessment Battery (COTNAB). British Journal of Occupational Therapy 57(4):137–142

Laver AJ, Powell GE 1995 The Structured Observational Test of Function (SOTOF). NFER-Nelson, Windsor

Law M 1993 Evaluating activities of daily living: directions for the future. American Journal of Occupational Therapy 47(3):233–237

Law M, King G, Mackinnon E et al 1999 All about outcomes – pediatrics. Slack, NJ

Law M, Cooper B, Strong S, Stewart D et al 1996 The Person–Environment–Occupation Model: a transactive approach to occupational performance. Canadian Journal of Occupational Therapy 63(1):9–23

Law M, Baptiste S, Carswell-Opzoomer A et al 1994 Canadian Occupational Performance Measure, 2nd edn. CAOT Publications ACE, Toronto.

Law M, Letts L 1989 A critical review of scales of activities of daily living. American Journal of Occupational Therapy 43:522–528

Letts L, Scott S, Burtney J et al 1998 The reliability and validity of the Safety Assessment of Function and the Environment for Rehabilitation (SAFER) Tool. British Journal of Occupational Therapy 61(3):127–132

Lincoln NB, Edmands JA 1990 A re-validation of the Rivermead ADL Scale for elderly patients with stroke. Age and Ageing 19:19–24

Lunz ME, Stahl JA 1993 The effect of rater severity on person ability measure: a Rasch model analysis. American Journal of Occupational Therapy 47(4):311–317

McCormack GL, Llorens LA, Glogoski C 1991 Culturally diverse elders. In Kiernat JM (ed) Occupational therapy and the older adult. Aspen, Gaithersburg, MD

McFayden AK, Pratt J 1997 Understanding the statistical concepts of measures of work performance. British Journal of Occupational Therapy 60(6):279–284

Mackenzie L, Byles J, Higginbotham N 2000 Designing the Home Falls and Accidents Screening Tool (Home FAST): selecting the items. British Journal of Occupational Therapy 63(6):260–269

Mahoney F, Barthel D 1965 Functional evaluation: the Barthel Index. Maryland State Medical Journal 14:61–65

Matthey S, Donnelly SM, Hextell DL 1993 The clinical usefulness of the Rivermead Perceptual Assessment Battery: statistical considerations. British Journal of Occupational Therapy 56(10):365–370

Mattingly C 1994 Occupational therapy as a two-body practice. The lived body. In: Mattingly C, Flemming MH (eds) Clinical reasoning: forms of inquiry in a therapeutic practice. FA Davis, Philadelphia, PA, ch 4, p 64

Mattingly C, Flemming MH 1994 Clinical reasoning: forms of inquiry in a therapeutic practice. FA Davis, Philadelphia, PA

Murdock C 1992 A critical evaluation of the Barthel Index, Part 1. British Journal of Occupational Therapy 55:109–111

National Center for Medical Rehabilitation Research (NCMRR) 1992 Report and plan for medical rehabilitation research to Congress. NCMRR, US Department of Health and Human Services, National Institutes of Health, Bethesda, MD

Opacich KJ 1991 Assessment and informed decision making. In: Christiansen C, Baum C (eds) Occupational therapy – overcoming human performance deficits. Slack, New Jersey, ch 14, pp 355–372

Ottenbacher KJ, Tomchek SD 1993 Reliability analysis in therapeutic research: practice and procedures. American Journal of Occupational Therapy 47:10–16

Pollock N, McColl MA 1998 Assessment in client-centred occupational therapy. In: Law M (ed) Client-centered occupational therapy. Slack, New Jersey

Rogers JC, Holm MB 1989 The therapist's thinking behind functional assessment I. In: Royeen CB (ed) AOTA self study series assessing function. The American Occupational Therapy Association, Rockville, MD, lesson 1

Rogers JC, Holm MB 1991 Occupational therapy diagnostic reasoning: a component of clinical reasoning. American Journal of Occupational Therapy 45:1045–1053

Rudman DL, Tooke J, Glencross T et al 1998 Preliminary investigation of the content validity and clinical utility of the predischarge assessment tool. Canadian Journal of Occupational Therapy 65(1):3–11

Russell D, Rosenbaum P, Gowland C et al 1993 Gross motor function measure manual. Neurodevelopmental Clinical Research Unit, McMaster University, Hamilton, Ontario

Schell BA, Cervero RM 1993 Clinical reasoning in occupational therapy: an integrative review. American Journal of Occupational Therapy 47:605–610

Schon DA 1983 The reflective practitioner – how professionals think in action. Averbury, Aldershot

Shanahan M 1992 Objective and holistic: occupational therapy assessment in Ireland. Irish Journal of Occupational Therapy 22(2):8–10

Skruppy M 1993 Activities of Daily Living evaluations: is there a difference in what the patient reports and what is observed? Physical and Occupational Therapy in Geriatrics 11(3):13–25

Stewart S 1999 The use of standardised and non-standardised assessments in a social service setting: implications for practice. British Journal of Occupational Therapy 62(9):417–423

Sumsion T 2000 A revised occupational therapy definition of client-centred practice. British Journal of Occupational Therapy 63(7):304–309

Teri I, Truax P, Logsdon R, Uomoto J, Zarit S, Vitaliano PP 1992 Assessment of behavioural problems in dementia – the revised Memory and Behaviour Problems Checklist. Psychology and Aging 7(4):622–631

Trombly C 1993 Anticipating the future: assessment of occupational function. American Journal of Occupational Therapy 47:253–257

Tullis A, Nicol M 1999 A systematic review of the evidence for the value of functional assessment of older people with dementia. British Journal of Occupational Therapy 62(12):554–563

Tyerman R, Tyerman A, Howard P, Hadfield C 1986 The Chessington OT Neurological Assessment Battery (COTNAB). Nottingham Rehab, Nottingham

Unsworth C (ed) 1999 Cognitive and perceptual dysfunction: a clinical reasoning approach to evaluation and intervention. FA Davis, Philadelphia, PA

Whelan E, Speake B 1979 Scale for assessing coping skills. In Whelan E, Speake B (eds) Learning to cope. Souvenir Press, London

Whiting S, Lincoln N 1980 An ADL assessment for stroke patients. Occupational Therapy February: 44–46

Whiting S, Lincoln N, Bhavnani G, Cockburn J 1985 The Rivermead Perceptual Assessment Battery (RPAB). NFER-Nelson, Windsor

Wilson B, Cockburn J, Baddeley A 1991 The Rivermead Behavioural Memory Test. Thames Valley Test Company, Suffolk

Zarit SH, Todd PA, Zarit JM 1986 Subjective burden of husbands and wives as caregivers: a longitudinal study. Gerontologist 26(3):260–266

Zarit SH, Reever KE, Bach-Peterson J 1980 Relatives of the impaired elderly: correlates of feelings of burden. The Gerontologist 20(6):649–655

6

Activity analysis

Marg Foster   Joanne Pratt

INTRODUCTION

One of the core beliefs of occupational therapy is in the value and use of purposeful and meaningful activity to minimise limitations and achieve goals in occupational performance. If activities are to be used for this purpose they must be analysed to ascertain their meaning and component elements so that the requirements for successful participation and their potential therapeutic value to maintain or improve occupational performance can be determined. Synthesis of the findings enables the therapist to correlate the needs of the individual with the demands and potential of the activity.

The therapist's skills in activity analysis and synthesis are essential to enabling her to utilise activities with purpose and precision. Llorens (1993) defined activity analysis as a 'process by which properties inherent in a given activity, task, or occupation may be gauged for their ability to elicit individual motivation and to fulfil patient needs in occupational performance and performance components'. Such analysis is a complex and lengthy process but it is vital to identify the component elements in order to evaluate them in relation to the individual's problems and needs. Analysis enables the therapist to:

- Understand the meaning and relevance of activity in the context of quality of life and occupational performance.
- Understand the numerous elements of the activity, the essential component tasks and

parts that combine to create successful performance.

- Identify the skills required to perform each element of the activity. This enables the therapist to relate these to an individual's performance levels in order to understand why particular elements are proving difficult for them, or the potential of the task or activity to develop or maintain particular skills.
- Assist in considering service needs in terms of determining the capital and running costs for viability for use as a therapeutic medium. This may include such issues as:
  - the space required to perform the activity
  - the cost and availability of tools, equipment and other resources
  - the time for preparing the activity and achieving potential outcomes
  - any specific health and safety requirements
  - staff expertise and training needs.
- Look at the demands of the activity in relation to the individual's skills levels. This requires consideration of the functional areas included in the performance of the activity, the basic skills of the individual concerned and his occupational performance limitations. It also includes the potential of the activity to be broken down into component tasks and graded according to the individual's requirements.

This chapter will consider the meaning and relevance of activity in occupational performance, outline different methods of activity analysis and describe a systems approach, with macro and micro levels, to use as a framework to understand the role of activity analysis in work performance.

MEANING AND RELEVANCE OF ACTIVITY IN OCCUPATIONAL PERFORMANCE

The central component of occupational therapy is an understanding of occupational perform-ance. Occupations are made up of a combination of different activities, for example, homemaking includes cooking, cleaning, laundry, home maintenance, shopping and childcare. Each of these activities consists of a number of different tasks. Laundry involves collecting and sorting washing, using the washing machine (a task made up of a number of different component elements), hanging washing on the line or using a tumble dryer and ironing and folding clean garments. To successfully maintain the role of homemaker, an individual must:

- have basic skills in physical, psychological, cognitive, sensory and other areas of performance to complete the task to an acceptable level
- have the ability to sequence these elements appropriately in a logical order within the task
- be able to combine the tasks together in a meaningful pattern for successful completion of the activity
- be able to carry out the activity to a satisfactory level for successful occupational performance as part of the homemaking duties.

Humans are essentially active beings. Some activities, such as getting out of bed, are regular elements of daily living and are carried out as part of a personal routine. Other activities relate to the roles individuals hold – those of home-maker, worker, carer, student, and so on – and the performance of tasks and activities within these roles will be dependent on the individual's per-ceived requirements of the role. The significance placed on these activities and the standards to which they are carried out will frequently relate to the perceived value and importance of the role. Activities also reflect the person's culture and social status. The very choice of activity, as well as the way in which it is performed, may be influenced by cultural norms or the expectations of the individual or relevant others within the social or environmental setting (Table 6.1). Henderson et al (1991) stated that the purpose and meaning of activities are attributes of people rather than of the activities themselves. Golledge

Table 6.1 Cultural influences on performance (after Christiansen & Baum 1991)

Influence	Factors affecting performance
Geographical	Place of origin: its dialect, colloquialisms and/or main language; climate, natural resources and staple diet
Community	Environmental strengths and weaknesses as an urban or rural area: its economy, social and health issues, including housing and the dominance of one kind of tenure over others; the population and its ethnicity
Family	Structure: whether there is a set role structure and how strictly this is enforced; style of living and balance of productivity, leisure, self care
Oneself	Work ethic and use of time: sense and definition of personal space; coping mechanisms; ways of expressing emotions; role selection

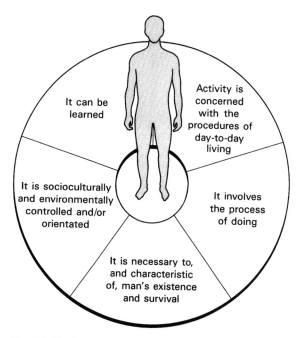

Fig. 6.1 The importance and relevance of activity in daily life.

(1998) discussed different definitions and meanings of occupation, purposeful activity and activity in relation to occupational therapy practice. Wilcock (1998) explored the relationships between occupation and health and concluded that 'health and wellbeing result from being in tune with our "occupational" nature. For health and wellbeing to be experienced ... engagement in occupation needs to have meaning and be balanced between capacities, provide optimal opportunity for desired growth in individuals and groups, and be flexible enough to develop and change according to context and choice'. Cynkin and Robinson (1990) stated that activities 'distinguish both our shared humanness and our individuality', and summed up the distinctive features of activity as (Fig. 6.1):

- a series of operations carried out as part of the procedures of day-to-day living
- involving a process of doing
- characteristic of and necessary to human existence
- socially regulated
- able to be learned.

If therapists are to use meaningful and purposeful activities in their interventions then they need to be aware of the value of the activity to the individual concerned, its importance in the individ-

ual's pattern of living and the specific tasks, techniques and levels of performance that the individual wishes to achieve. Hagedorn (2000) suggests the use of a spider diagram or mind map to identify individual meaning and purpose. The activity is placed at the centre of the diagram and, through asking questions such as 'What's in it for you?', 'Why do you do it?', the therapist and the individual produce a spider diagram with personal reasons and purposes at the end of each limb.

When considering the therapeutic use of activity, the therapist should also be clear of the purpose of using an activity; is it to fulfil the individual's self-care needs, role duties or quality of life, or is it to be used specifically to address a particular area of dysfunction, through graded specific actions, tasks or behaviours?

Therapists need to be able to analyse activity to identify the tasks involved, how the tasks can be carried out, the essential skills required for successful performance and how the tasks combine in the total activity pattern. Synthesis of these findings with personal meaning, relevance and the individual's situation and needs assists the matching process between the person and the activity. Nelson (1996) stated that 'the use of occupational synthesis to encourage therapeutic occupation is the process that best distinguishes the occupational therapy profession from other professions'. It is therefore a fundamental and vital skill that is used frequently throughout all stages of the intervention, assessment, planning, intervention and evaluation. The therapist uses her assessment skills to identify what activities are involved in the individual's roles. Her understanding of the tasks that make up these activities and the skills required to complete these tasks successfully will be used in conjunction with her specific assessment of the individual's strengths and weaknesses to determine where the performance problems may occur. A functional assessment of the task may provide further information on performance levels. Understanding the importance of the activity in the individual's life and his individual skill levels will provide the basis for planning and prioritising. Intervention aims to address the task demands so that the activity can be carried out successfully by the individual or appropriate others. Achievement in specific tasks may produce success in activity and be an end in itself by attaining a satisfactory level of performance for an individual. However, tasks and activities may also be used as means to developing specific attributes that will contribute to many different activities. These attributes may be developed through specific graded means according to the demands of the task and the individual's functional deficit. To do this, the therapist should have identified the individual's level of functional performance and be conversant with the specific demands of the stages of the task in terms of anatomical, physiological, psychological, sensory and cognitive skills. From this information, the task may be graded to improve the level of the individual's performance and changed according to increased levels of attainment or, in cases of progressive disease, tasks may be modified to maintain successful outcomes by accommodating functional deterioration (Fig. 6.2).

ACTIVITY ANALYSIS MODELS

There are a number of models of activity analysis. A simple basic analysis considers the essen-

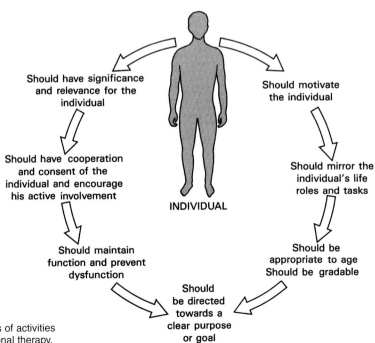

Should have significance and relevance for the individual

Should motivate the individual

Should have cooperation and consent of the individual and encourage his active involvement

Should mirror the individual's life roles and tasks

INDIVIDUAL

Should maintain function and prevent dysfunction

Should be appropriate to age
Should be gradable

Should be directed towards a clear purpose or goal

Fig. 6.2 Specific characteristics of activities appropriate for use in occupational therapy.

tial purpose of the activity and how and where it may be carried out. More complex detailed analyses explore the specific skills required to carry out each individual task and consider the variations that can occur and how these might modify or change the basic skill requirements. Hagedorn (2000) refers to this format as 'demand analysis'. Additionally, analysis may be used to consider the specific application of the activity to the individual's needs or for therapeutic purposes – 'applied analysis'. Therapists use all forms of analysis at different times, depending upon the situation. If considering introducing the activity to a particular unit, the therapist will need to consider the requirements for the activity, in terms of materials and equipment, and the specific potential of the activity in terms of what skills it can offer, and relate these to the needs of the individuals she may be working with, the purpose of her interventions and the frames of reference, approaches and techniques that could be used. The following section will consider a simple and a more complex form of analysis, and culminates by considering applied analysis in practice.

BASIC, SIMPLE ANALYSIS

This form of analysis considers basic questions regarding the essential purpose of the activity. It is frequently the forerunner to more detailed analysis of the specific components of an activity. It forms the basis for consideration of the potential of the activity for therapeutic purposes. Issues considered in this simple form of analysis concern the what, why, where, when, how and who of the performance of the activity (Table 6.2):

- **What** is the activity? Does it relate to other activities, if so how? Is it a simple or a complex activity? Can it be broken down into specific tasks?
- **Why** is the activity done? What is its essential purpose? What is the objective of carrying it out? Is it essential to daily occupations or is it suitable for specific therapeutic gain?

Table 6.2 Basic, simple analysis of making a cake

Question	Possible answers
1. Does the activity relate to other activities – how? Is it simple or complex? Can it be broken down into specific tasks?	Links to other cooking activities Depends on type of cake – relatively complex in most cases Yes – it has a number of different stages that can be done separately (see 'How is it done? below)
2. Why is the activity done? What is its essential purpose? Is it a daily occupation? Can it be used for therapeutic gain?	Relates to role in life, daily living activity, work, pleasure To make a cake to eat or serve to others Domestic task for housewife, work for a cook, social skill Provides opportunity for achieving goals in physical, psychological, cognitive, cultural and social demands of person's role
3. Where is it carried out? What location needed? What tools/materials are needed?	In the kitchen Suitable kitchen location to simulate person's needs Cooker, cooking utensils, recipe book, ingredients
4. When does it occur? Is it a regular activity? Is it occasional but necessary?	No specific time of day Cooks do it regularly, homemakers less regularly Not essential for housewife – could buy cake – but provides satisfaction in role. May have a social meaning when entertaining
5. How is it done?	Choose recipe, purchase ingredients, switch on oven to correct heat, weigh ingredients in appropriate amounts into separate containers, mix ingredients in a relevant order, transfer mixture to cake tin/s, put into oven for correct time, remove from oven to cool, wash-up utensils, transfer cake to serving plate. Optional = icing
6. Who is involved?	Can be done alone or in a group as a shared or parallel activity. Can be done by any age group, gender, culture Does not need more than one person to complete

- **Where** does it take place? Is the activity usually carried out at a specific location? Will the choice and suitability of environment significantly affect its success? Is a suitable environment easily accessible for practice with appropriate tools and materials?
- **When** does it usually take place? Is it a regular activity carried out at a particular time of day or week? Is it an occasional but necessary activity? Are any specific actions necessary before or after the activity for successful completion?
- **How** is the activity carried out. What are the essential tasks, stages and sequences within the activity? How long does the activity usually take to complete and is it a continuous process or are there natural breaks or rest periods? What specific personal attributes are essential to success – motor, sensory, cognitive, psychological, and so on? Are there any specific safety hazards inherent in the activity?
- **Who** is involved in carrying out the activity? Does the activity require only one performer or are other performers needed to achieve success? If others are necessary, what part do they play in the performance of the activity and do they also require specific skills?

DETAILED ANALYSIS MODELS

These are described in many texts and vary only according to the preference of the author and the focus of the text. Detailed analyses itemise the demands of the activity or task in terms of the sequences and component elements necessary for satisfactory completion. These include the physical, sensory, cognitive, social, emotional and cultural demands of the activity. An example of such a detailed analysis is given in Box 6.1.

Analysis may be based on a particular method of carrying out the task but, where there are likely to be variations in techniques, such detailed analyses should also consider how these variations change the basic component requirements. For instance, when analysing getting in or out of the bath, the motor and coordination demands will be significantly different depend-

ing upon whether the individual steps over the edge of the bath in a standing position, holds onto a handgrip in the bath or sits on the edge of the bath and swings their legs over into the water. Similarly, the performance of the activity, and its meaning and relevance, can vary significantly according to factors such as gender, age or culture. Cynkin and Robinson (1990) refer to these as 'actor variations'. They should form an essential part of any activity or task analysis in order to understand unique individual methods and meanings, and minimise bias or judgemental opinions regarding right or wrong techniques or values.

Detailed demand analysis provides an understanding of the complexity of the task or activity and forms the basis for consideration of the application of the activity for therapeutic purposes. By comparing the demands of the tasks with a person's attributes or weaknesses it also provides the therapist with an understanding of why specific activities or tasks may pose particular difficulties for certain individuals.

APPLIED ANALYSIS

This considers the application of the activity for therapeutic purposes. Applied analysis should utilise the simple and detailed analysis together with the environmental setting of the service, the needs of the service users and the preferred models and frames of reference used in the practice setting. Common factors which apply in almost all situations when considering the therapeutic application include (Table 6.3):

- The environment in which the activity does or could take place, including space and equipment, and its availability for use. Similarly, the therapist needs to consider the environment the activity creates, that is, the relevance, value, emphasis, priority created by or given to the activity by an individual or his sociocultural group. The environment can also play a part in shaping and directing an activity, for example, interaction with particular settings, negotiation of the layout of the environment and the equipment within

---

Box 6.1 Detailed demand analysis

Having identified the purpose, sequence and duration of the performance of the activity, and the space, tools and materials required, it may be necessary to ask any of the following questions and to identify how, when and where within the activity or task any particular skills or changes in demands and requirements are needed.

Physical skills

Position
- What is the starting position when carrying out the activity – sitting, standing, lying?
- Any changes that occur during the sequence of performance of the activity.

Movements
- Which joints are involved and what movements are required?
- Which muscle groups are involved at specific stages?
- What ranges of specific movements are required at each joint?
- Is the action unilateral or bilateral?
- Is the movement required:
  - active, static or passive?
  - repetitive, assisted or resisted?
  - fast or slow, smooth or irregular?

Strength
- Does the activity require a high, moderate or low level of muscle strength?
- Is the effort continuous or intermittent?
- Does the activity require high, medium or low levels of stamina and endurance?

Coordination
- Does the activity require gross or fine motor coordination?
- Is the coordination unilateral or bilateral?
- Where does the coordination take place – hand/hand, hand/eye, lower limbs?

Hand function
- Does the activity require grip – cylinder, ball, hook, plate, pincer or tripod grip?
- What levels of manipulative or dextrous movements are needed?
- Are any precise actions needed?
- Are both hands required equally?

Sensory and perceptual skills
- Does the activity require vision – short and/or long distance, colour recognition?
- Auditory – is hearing necessary to identify particular sounds, tones or volume?

- Gustatory – does the activity involve the ability to identify or discriminate between tastes?
- Olfactory – is the ability to identify or discriminate between smells necessary?
- Touch – does the activity require gross or fine sensation?
- Is the ability to distinguish shapes, textures or temperatures necessary?
- Are stereognosis, proprioceptive or vestibular skills required?

Cognitive skills
- Is the level of thinking concrete or abstract?
- What level of concentration does the activity require – is it constant or changing?
- Is short-term, long-term or procedural memory required?
- Are organisational skills needed – logical thinking, planning, decision making, problem solving?
- Are specific levels of numeracy or literacy required?
- Does the activity involve time recognition and time management skills?
- What levels of responsibility and control does the activity involve?
- Are there opportunities for use of imagination, creativity or improvisation?

Social interaction skills
- Is the activity carried out with others?
- Is the interaction formal or informal, cooperative, competitive, in parallel or compliant?
- What forms of communication are involved:
  - receptive: listening and interpreting?
  - expressive: verbal, written, technological?
  - non-verbal, touch?
- Does the activity involve attention to others through debate or negotiation?

Emotional skills
- Does the activity require insight or ability for self-expression?
- Are attitudes and values inherent in the activity?
- Is the activity likely to demand conflict, handling feelings, testing reality or role identity?
- Does the activity require patience, managing impulses or self-control?

Cultural demands
- Is the activity specific to certain cultural groups in terms of gender, ethnicity, class or age?
- What is the sociocultural symbolic meaning of the activity?
- Does the activity require particular cultural values, approaches or techniques?

---

it, or familiarity with its orientation and demands.
- The emotions the activity can evoke. How does the activity motivate an individual and is this likely to contribute to personal

effectiveness? Is the activity likely to evoke negative feelings, which will impede progress with certain individuals? How does the activity relate to a person's interests, roles and values?

Table 6.3 Factors to consider in applied analysis

Factor to consider	Issues to consider
Environment of activity	Availability, relevance, impact on activity/individual
Emotions generated by activity	Motivation, contribution to personal effectiveness, negative feelings, links to interests, roles and values of individual
Appropriateness	Age, developmental stage, gender, sociocultural background Individual's needs – personal and dysfunctional needs
Adaptability	Modification and/or grading opportunities Use with different models/frames of reference/approaches
Occupational value	Use as part of self care, role duties, leisure Transferability of skills gained
Cost implications	Equipment, materials, training Cost to individual of continuing activity after treatment
Safety	Hazards, levels of risk, safety and risk management
Time	Time for completion by individual Level of supervision required by therapist/others

- The appropriateness of the activity to the chronological age and developmental stage of the individual, regardless of his problems, to enable him to learn or relearn age- and role-appropriate skills and behaviours.
- The appropriateness of the activity to the person's gender. This will be dependent upon the sociocultural background of the individual – are certain activities considered gender specific within his culture or social group or is there an accepted wider, more flexible approach to participation in specific activities.
- The adaptability of the activity. This is very important if optimum use is to be made of it. Can the activity be modified or graded to meet a broad range of individual occupational performance requirements? Can it be used with a number of different models, frames of reference and intervention approaches (Table 6.4). Is it suitable for both individual interventions and group work?
- The degree of occupational application of the activity. The potential use of the skills acquired in self care, role duties or social and leisure activities, and their transferability to different uses.

Table 6.4 Applied analysis – an illustrative example of the use of a gardening activity with three different approaches

Activity	Task	Approach	Objective/goal
Transplanting seedlings in a greenhouse	Carrying tray of seedlings to greenhouse bench	Biomechanical	Improving muscle strength and range of movement
		Neurodevelopmental	Improving balance and bilateral upper limb use
		Cognitive	Sequencing and spatial awareness in finding way to greenhouse bench from verbal instructions
	Pricking-out seedlings into pots from tray	Biomechanical	Improving pinch and gross handgrip
		Neurodevelopmental	Improving standing balance bilateral hand activity
		Cognitive	Sequencing and numeracy counting seeds and pots
	Watering seedlings in tray	Biomechanical	Grip strength – holding watering can and pouring
		Neurodevelopmental	Balance while pouring Use of both hands Controlling pouring
		Cognitive	Decision making on how much water to pour and where to pour

- The cost implications of the activity to the service and the service user. Intervention must be cost effective and efficient in relation to staff time and service resources. Factors to consider include whether suitable equipment and materials are available at reasonable prices, whether a completed article is produced, the time available for individuals to pursue the activity, and the cost implications for the individual pursuing the activity either in the therapeutic setting or elsewhere, for example, at a sports club.
- The safety of the activity. Whilst in almost every activity there is an element of risk, under the health and safety regulations the person receiving occupational therapy should expect this to be minimised, that is, the environment must be as hazard-free as possible and intervention techniques must be safe for the individual and the therapist. However, the situation will vary according to the intervention venue. Legislation and regulations will determine the different safety precautions in each specific setting.
- The time required to complete the whole activity. The therapist should analyse the time factor for completion of the whole activity and the time for specific elements and tasks. In locations where early discharge is anticipated, some activities may not be appropriate because of the short time for which the individual may be receiving therapy. Identification of specific needs and prioritisation should be considered when determining the appropriateness of particular tasks or activities for individuals or groups.

Grading tasks and activities

In many instances, part of the application of the activity to individual needs will involve grading. Grading of activity to gradually increase or decrease the demands on the individual in its execution enables the therapist to adjust the activity to the person's maximum capability, specific needs and particular circumstances. The activity must remain relevant and practical, and the adjustments should be made to motivate the person to continue participation, maintain improvement or adapt the task to cope with deterioration. The therapist should consider whether the grading method is activity-centred, where the task itself is graded to meet a particular need, or person-centred, in which case the person's range of movement, cognitive skills, and so on, are gradually altered in order to perform the task. Whatever form of grading is used, the therapist should adhere to the following rules:

- the task must encourage and maintain a good working posture and position
- the modification must comply with health and safety regulations
- the individual must know and understand why he is required to perform the activity in a specific way, which may differ from the norm
- modification or adaptation must maintain a positive rather than a negative effect on the individual
- the therapist must consider the time required for modification, the supervision required when carrying out the activity and the maintenance of any adapted activities.

Grading techniques

A number of different techniques are employed to grade activity, depending upon the required area of change.

Positioning

By altering the position of the person in relation to the activity and its accessories, specific requirements regarding range of movement and balance may be modified. Positions may be changed to gradually extend the range of a specific movement or to facilitate changes in balance. Changes from a sitting position to a standing posture will significantly alter balance requirements and the extension of the active work area, either vertically or horizontally, will add to the range of movement demands for the upper limb joints.

Resistance

Altering the resistance to an activity changes the demand on muscle strength. Natural resistance occurs through the gradual use and manipulation of heavier equipment or tools, or through the increased resistance offered by the materials used, for example, sawing or planing hard wood or mixing a fruit cake offers greater resistance than planing soft wood or stirring a sponge mixture. Gradual reduction of gravity-assisted support and the application of artificial resistance through the addition of brakes, weights or springs against which the individual has to work to carry out the task progressively increases demands on muscle strength for successful performance.

Endurance

Careful gradation in this aspect builds up activity tolerance. This may be done in a number of ways. Starting with light activities, the programme may be gradually upgraded until the person is able to manage heavier work appropriate to his needs. Increasing the length of time spent in the activity also builds up activity tolerance, as does increasing the number of sessions in a given timescale. This form of grading is frequently used to build up endurance to meet employment needs.

Dexterity

Increasing the manipulative requirements of the activity enables the development of increased dexterity. Activities that involve progressively finer movements demand precision and control. Computer and keyboard activities, as well as a number of remedial games, may be used specifically to develop fine grip and finger dexterity. Timing of these fine manipulative activities not only demands the usual levels of dexterity but can also be used to increase speed.

Coordination

Along with improving dexterity, the gradual increase in the demand for fine movements and decrease of gross movements encourages motor control. Dependent upon the needs of the individual in relation to his daily occupations, it may be necessary gradually to reduce the activities that focus on gross motor skills and increase those with fine motor demands.

Mobility

This may commence with the introduction of transfer skills from one sitting position to another, for example, from bed to chair, and chair to toilet. As balance and lower limb muscle strength improves, standing and walking skills may be introduced and graded, possibly in conjunction with physiotherapy activities. Increase in the time spent standing and decrease in the support provided either by a chair or perching stool will promote weight bearing through the lower limbs. This may be upgraded to transferring weight from foot to foot, as in reaching objects across a table or bench, before introducing activities that involve walking from place to place. Later upgrading could extend the distance to be covered when walking, introduce the use of steps and stairs or, where appropriate, could include walking over uneven surfaces such as gravel paths, grass or gardens.

Sensation and perception

Although these two attributes are very different, the methods of grading may be similar. Grading to improve sensory awareness could be carried out by starting with items that are clearly different and gradually reducing the difference. For example, the therapist might start with materials of very different textures and, as sensation improves, the similarity between the materials is increased so that the person has to use finer sensory skills to identify differences. Similar techniques can be used in the development of perceptual skills, particularly in areas such as form constancy, figure ground discrimination and colour recognition.

Developmental grading

In certain areas it might be necessary for grading to occur in line with the sequences of normal development; for example, the person should be able to sit upright before standing, and stand before walking. This is important for people with neurological deficit, who might have to learn or relearn normal movement patterns.

Cognitive skills

These may be graded through the use of activities that demand increased levels of application of cognition. In addition to tasks that demand specific attributes in numerary or literacy, they also include activities that involve attention, memory and concentration. These can be upgraded from simple memory exercises to more complex recall activities. Cognitive skills may also be upgraded through activities that involve increasing amounts of selection and choice, where individuals have to evaluate options to make judgements and decisions. Planning and organising skills are included in this area where activities might include such aspects as logical sequencing. Problem solving involves not only evaluation of the existing factors, identifying causes, relationships and effects, but also creative thinking and imagination and, in some instances, consideration of improvisation could be appropriate.

Social interaction

The individual might begin by working alone and progress to working with one other person before being integrated into a small group. Demands within the task for communication and cooperation with other group members can be increased gradually, and the introduction of different levels of responsibility as a group member broadens and adds to the complexity of social skill requirements. Responsibility for initiation of a particular group activity, or added obligations for either the task or the group, furthers the need for interpersonal communication, negotiation and social skills.

Complexity of the task

This involves the selection of activities that increasingly require greater skill in specific areas as the person's abilities increase. Increasing the number of stages involved in the completion of

the task, or introducing more complicated procedures to a particular stage, will add to the overall complexity of the task.

In all aspects of applied analysis it is important that the therapist assesses the person's skill levels regularly to ensure the grading is appropriate to his individual needs and progress. It is also important that the reason for the grading is understood by both the therapist and the individual. Successful completion of an easier task provides a sense of achievement, which could be lost when attempting an upgraded task unless the positive reason for upgrading to increase demands and maintain progress is understood by the individual.

ACTIVITY ANALYSIS AND WORK

Activity analysis is a vital skill when individuals experience difficulty in occupational performance at work. It is a skill that combines knowledge of human performance across such diverse areas as physiology, psychology, ergonomics, ageing and medical conditions with the ability to ask appropriate questions. In this section of the chapter a systems approach, with macro, meso and micro levels, will be used as a framework to understand the role of activity analysis in work performance.

The questions occupational therapists seek to ask in this area of practice range from the impact on an individual worker to the company's recruitment policy and practices, which will affect a number of people. Examples of questions to be asked include: What are the effects on the individual of changing his shift patterns now that he has to inject insulin?' 'What impact will a change of seating have on seamstresses in a garment factory?' 'What reasonable accommodations can be made to an assembly-line task to mitigate the effects of the ageing process on eyesight, hand function or stamina?' 'How will the employer's plans for increased efficiency through, for example, longer but fewer shifts per week, be managed on the shop or office floor?' 'Is there a relationship between the employer's policy on the payment of overtime wages, which can prolong the working day by up to 3 hours, and the injury statistics in an industrial laundry?' 'What changes are needed to the company's recruitment strategy to make it more compliant with the Disability Discrimination Act?' 'What is the best way to regrade a worker's return to his job following a period of extended sick leave?'.

ACTIVITY ANALYSIS AT A MACRO LEVEL

Work, and especially paid employment, within any society is influenced by social, cultural, historical, legislative and economic factors. Increasing technology in the worksite and the globalisation of a number of industries also means that the nature of work has to be continually redefined. For example, how is the job of a mail courier described when the speed of communication has shrunk from weeks by post at the beginning of the 20th century to seconds by e-mail in the 21st century? The occupational therapist needs to develop a dynamic understanding of the nature of work in the community within which she practices to ensure that her interventions are relevant and effective.

To begin this process, activity analysis can be used at a macro level to seek information about the context of work in the local community. Key questions at this level include:

- what is considered work in this village, town, city or country?
- what type of work do people do?
- is there a division between 'women's' work and 'men's' work?
- what status is attached to particular jobs and what is the reason for this?
- how long is the working week?

In the United Kingdom, for example, the Department for Education and Employment suggests that the workforce has increased steadily and will reach 27 million people by the year 2006, but some trends are particularly notable:

- service industries will continue to grow and there will be a further decline in primary and manufacturing industry, although this will be at a slower rate than in the 1980s and 1990s. This may mean that the occupational make-up of employment will continue to change in favour of white collar, non-manual occupations, especially those that require higher-level qualifications
- female employment and part-time working is expected to grow, largely in response to these changes in the nature of work. The male activity rate is expected to continue to decline
- self-employment is expected to grow at four times the overall employment rate
- small firms of less than 50 employees now account for 99% of all firms and for 50% of non-government employment
- the proportion of the workforce who have full-time, permanent work is falling
- the labour force is ageing and, as employers will need to employ older workers to remain competitive, it is hoped that age discrimination will decrease
- ethnic minorities form an increasing proportion of the labour force but have a younger age profile and a higher proportion of the 16–24 age group in education than the white population
- the position of people with disabilities in the labour market is expected to change now that the key provisions of the Disability Discrimination Act (1995) are in force.

Within a particular company, activity analysis at a macro level could mean that the therapist has to understand the nature of the company's business, that is, is it a service provider or a manufacturer? What does it produce and/or sell? What is its mission statement and objectives for the year? Who are its clients? The answers to these questions can be used to inform strategies that are used for embedding occupational therapy services within the business.

ACTIVITY ANALYSIS AT A MESO LEVEL

While the trends mentioned earlier reflect a national picture, it is important that therapists supplement this knowledge with local information. Communities are increasingly diverse and it is important to try to understand the dimensions of this diversity, by age, gender, sexual orientation, religion, race, ethnicity and disability. A community profile (Box 6.2) can be compiled, using activity analysis skills to create a rich, useful resource. Following on from this, if the therapist is working for a particular business or the department provides services to a range of industrial clients, it could be very useful to obtain or compile a profile of the workforce along these dimensions. The information could be useful in many ways, for example, targeting under-represented groups for recruitment, anticipating health needs and the services likely to be required.

Box 6.2   Community profile

Define and describe the community
- The geographical boundary of your area.
- The urbanisation of the area by proportion with rural areas.
- The population of this area by age, gender, race, religion, ethnicity, level of education.
- The economy of the area, what is it based on?
- Number, type and size of employers.
- The history of employment patterns in the area.
- How people in the area spend their leisure time, which activities are currently or traditionally popular.
- Transportation systems in the area.
- The number and type of training opportunities in the area.
- Access to child- or elderly-care facilities.
- Local rehabilitation providers and/or competitors.
- Occupational health resources.

Collect the data by using multiple sources and contacts
- Local newspapers.
- The telephone book.
- Local schools, training colleges, vocational training programmes.
- Social survey results.
- Tourist office.
- Local development agencies.
- The Department for Education and Employment.
- The Internet.
- Retired workers.
- Employers.
- Community centres.

Analyse the data
- Create categories for information.
- Use written evaluation and interpretation.
- Use descriptive statistics.
- Use survey results.

Compile the profile
- Use box or drawer files.
- Produce a summary report.
- Use written and/or software versions.

Use and disseminate the findings
- To develop plans for your service.
- When producing client/employer education or awareness leaflets.
- When marketing your service.
- When making presentations.

ACTIVITY ANALYSIS AT A MICRO LEVEL

Therapists work at a micro level within a system when assessing and planning intervention for the individual employee of a company. The Northern Ireland Committee of the College of Occupational Therapists (1992) distinguished work skills, work behaviours and work tolerance, which largely relate to the psychological and social aspects of an employee role. In addition to these elements, the therapist must understand the individual's capacity to meet the demands of a specific job. Activity analysis skills at this level are used to assess the individual's functional capacities, the job requirements at a task level and how well these two areas are matched. Fleishman and Quaintance (1984) have defined ability categories as part of the process of describing human tasks. These have been put into categories below and, depending on the level of skill involved in a job or task(s), the occupational therapist may have to explore or assess any number of them with the individual worker:

- **Neuromotor**: control precision; multi-limb coordination; response orientation; rate control; reaction time; arm–hand steadiness; manual dexterity; finger dexterity; wrist–finger speed; speed of limb movement; static, dynamic, explosive and trunk strength; extent and dynamic flexibility; gross body coordination and equilibrium; stamina, speech clarity.
- **Sensory/perceptual**: spatial orientation; visualisation; perceptual speed; selective attention; time sharing; near and far vision;

visual colour discrimination; night, peripheral and depth vision; glare sensitivity; general hearing; auditory attention; sound localisation; speech hearing.

- **Psychological/cognitive**: oral comprehension, written comprehension, oral or written expression, fluency of ideas, originality, memorisation, problem sensitivity, mathematical reasoning, number facility, deductive and inductive reasoning, information ordering, category flexibility, speed and flexibility of closure.

One area where a great deal of work has been done is in the development of *functional capacity assessments*. A number of commercial systems have been devised based on international engineering standards, which in turn are based on anthropomorphic data. These come from size and velocity of movement measurements of large numbers of humans to determine average and modal ranges. Such assessments, which can incorporate simple work-related tasks of pushing, pulling, lifting and carrying varying sizes and weights of objects, can provide objective measurements of an individual's performance against industry standards. The advantages of such assessments are said to rest on their objective measurement of performance and they are increasingly being used in the United Kingdom for medicolegal purposes. The disadvantage of such assessments is that they may have limited resemblance to an actual job or to the work conditions in which an employee is expected to perform.

Functional capacity assessments are often combined by therapists with *job simulation*. This involves the re-creation or imitation of the tasks or demands of the client's actual job, usually in the rehabilitation setting or department. Effective job simulation is based on the therapist's skill in activity analysis, whereby she breaks down job requirements into their main tasks and, subsequently, into the component parts of the task. The client is encouraged to attempt and then improve performance through practice of these tasks. Job simulation is used both as a form of assessment of the client's functional status and as an intervention as part of a larger programme of work hardening or rehabilitation.

A *job analysis* combines activity analysis skills with the assessment of job requirements. A job analysis may involve one or all of the following steps: review of the company's job description of the role, interview with the employee's line manager or supervisor, visit to the worksite to observe workers performing the job tasks, assessment of the ergonomics of the workstation and their 'fit' to the individual worker, assessment of job demands – physical, cognitive or social – in terms of the frequency and duration of each of the tasks viewed as essential and/or necessary in the job description. Where an employee with a disability has been hired for a job or an existing employee has acquired a disability, *a job site analysis* may be undertaken to determine access and egress for each of the job's tasks, and to the worksite in general.

The occupational therapy case studies in Boxes 6.3 and 6.4 serve to illustrate the previous discussion of the ways in which activity analysis underpins the entire occupational therapy process. Table 6.5 summarises the roles occupational therapy can play within systems. Macro, meso and micro levels of activity analysis for both employee and employer are highlighted.

Table 6.5 Activity analysis within the macro, meso and micro systems of employment

System level	Employee	Method of activity analysis	Employer	Method of activity analysis
Macro (societal)	Describing 'work' within a particular society in terms of its social, cultural, historical contexts	History of and current legislation National employment patterns and changes Surveys of social trends	Company's mission and objectives	Mission statement Identification of service and client base Legislation: national requirements, standards and guidelines European Union Directives on workplaces and practices
Meso (group)	Dimensions of diversity: gender, age, disability, religion, ethnicity	Community profile (see Box 6.2)	Work practices within the business The business' site(s) Risk assessment for injury prevention to reduce liability and litigation Disability management in the workplace	Workforce profile Workforce audits of health/ sickness/injuries/compliance with legislation requirements Policies and procedures manuals Ergonomic assessment of worksite to include noise, temperature, light, vibration, tool use and work station design
Micro (individual)	• **Work skills**: (i) physical demands; (ii) worker functions in relation to people, data and things; (iii) temporal demands • **Work behaviours**: (i) work attitudes; (ii) work habits; (iii) work traits • **Work tolerance**: ability to meet job requirements	Interview Identification of employee's perceptions of job role Observation/measurement of the components of occupational performance, i.e. neuromotor, psychological/social, physiological, cognitive Job simulation Functional capacity assessments	Job requirements Risk assessment	Observation Interview Job description Job analysis Worksite assessment of physical, social, cognitive job demands Access audit Injury prevention mechanisms

Box 6.3 Case study: Darren M.

DATE OF BIRTH
3 November 1970.

DIAGNOSIS/DISABILITY
Head injury, unconscious for 6 days, severe facial injuries requiring facial reconstruction and plastic surgery, right shoulder weakness and pain as a result of impact injury following motor vehicle accident.

DATE OF ASSESSMENT
Visit to the workplace to look at alternative duties and to discuss role of rehabilitation provider took place 24 November 1998.

PURPOSE OF ASSESSMENT
To assess the duties and work layout in relation to Darren's injuries and physical limitations.

ASSESSMENT USED
Interview, observation, video analysis.

SUMMARY OF FINDINGS
Darren worked as a truck-driver and garbage collector for a waste disposal company. The worksite that was assessed was the company garbage collection depot. Present at the visit were Darren's employer, Darren (the injured worker), Darren's girlfriend and the occupational therapist.

Prior to the injury, Darren was working on a casual basis, working approximately 20–25 hours a week. He performed both functions – truck-driver and garbage collector.

There are two types of trucks, a smaller truck that is a one-person operation, and the larger truck, which is a two-person operation. In a two-person team there is a driver and an offsider. Usually, these two will swap places. Most of the bins are of the wheelie bin variety. These are pulled manually towards the truck, where they are connected to the lifting device (this involves some lifting into place), which then empties the bins. The empty bins are replaced and the worker jogs on to the next bin. However, there are still bins of the old variety, which need to be lifted manually into the back of the truck. This lifting involves the worker lifting to the end of reach, with upper arms fully extended.

Darren worked shifts of 6–8 hours.

ISSUES IDENTIFIED
- Darren's shoulder is not yet strong enough to return to the full duties of garbage collector, and will need a strengthening programme.
- Darren has not yet had a clearance to return to driving and so is unable to return to truck-driving at this stage.
- Darren is a qualified mechanic and would be able to work on small engines in the workshop. A stool on wheels would enable him to work in a position where his arm is not in elevation.
- Referring to the physical assessment report, Darren would be advised to avoid activities involving repetitive arm and shoulder movements until his shoulder has recovered strength and is pain-free.

RECOMMENDATIONS
The table below illustrates the occupational therapist's analysis of the task requirements for the main activities available to Darren at work.

Main activities	Task requirements
1. Service small equipment for company	Sitting on stool Bilateral hand skills, including coordination and dexterity Possible kneeling and crouching Intact perceptual and cognitive skills
2. Assist in tidying workshop	Standing Walking Some sweeping Bending Picking up light objects
3. Assist in servicing vehicles	Bilateral hand skills, including coordination and dexterity Bending Some reaching, depending on size of the vehicle engine
4. Answering telephones	Upper limb dexterity Coherent speech Writing messages

continued

Box 6.3 *continued*

5. Washing/polishing vehicles

Upper limb dexterity
Full range of motion at shoulder
Ability to maintain arm in an overhead position
Ability to undertake repetitive (e.g. scrubbing, wiping, polishing) arm activities

6. Garbage collection

Bilateral hand skills, coordination, dexterity and strength
Full range of motion at shoulder and upper arm
Upper limb and upper body strength
Ability to undertake overhead lifting of up to 30 kg
Repetitive lifting
Ability to pull wheeled bins weighing up to 60 kg
Excellent cardiovascular fitness
Cognition intact
Running
Balance, when riding on the back of the trucks

7. Driving garbage truck

Cognition intact
Medical clearance
Approval to resume driving
Sitting

The first four identified duties appear to be within Darren's current physical abilities. However, duties 5, 6 and 7 should not be introduced until Darren has completed a physical upgrading and strengthening programme and has received clearance to undertake repetitive lifting and to resume driving.

It is recommended that, when medically cleared:

● Darren initially returns to work on selected duties not involving repetitive lifting or shoulder activity and on limited hours
● Darren's return to work is monitored by the Rehabilitation Service and upgraded as appropriate, in consultation with the treating practitioner
● a gym strengthening programme is arranged as soon as practicable
● Darren has his driving assessed in the near future.

Box 6.4 Case study: Ms S.

DATE OF BIRTH
17 February 1961.

DIAGNOSIS/DISABILITY
Neck and left shoulder pain.

DATE OF ASSESSMENT
9 September 1998.

PURPOSE OF ASSESSMENT
To assess the duties and work layout in relation to Ms S.'s injury and physical limitations.

ASSESSMENT USED
Interview, observation, photographs.

BACKGROUND
Ms S. has been working in law firms providing administrative support for most of her working life. She has been employed with her current employers, A&B Solicitors, for approximately 5 years. On 18 February 1997, Ms S. reports that a heavy folder or book fell against the back of her neck; she was subsequently affected by neck and left shoulder pain.

SUMMARY OF FINDINGS
Ms S. works as a full-time paralegal secretary/administrative support to a Solicitor and partner. She provides administrative support to the solicitors. This can involve telephone calls, word processing, customer service, data entry and research.

continued

Box 6.4 *continued*

Two main work areas were assessed during the worksite visit:

- Ms S.'s office, incorporating an L-shaped desk
- a typewriter workstation at the front of the office shared with other workers. Ms S. faces the screen when she uses the typewriter and writes on a work surface that is at a 90-degree angle to the typewriter area. She has a footrest, an ergonomic keyboard with inbuilt wrist rest and an adjustable chair.

Present at visit were Ms S. (the injured worker) and the occupational therapist. They agreed that Ms S. should avoid activities that involved her in:

- maintaining static postures of the neck and shoulder, particularly when these postures varied from the midline
- flexion of the neck, particularly for prolonged periods
- heavy lifting, or activities requiring force or strength at left shoulder
- overhead reaching, particularly for extended periods.

Ms S. is able to pace the physical demands of her work and takes regular breaks to move around and to vary her position.

RECOMMENDATIONS

The table below illustrates the occupational therapist's analysis of task demands of the main activities performed by Ms S. Her considerations and recommendations appear in the right-hand column.

Main activities	Task demands	Considerations/recommendations
Prolonged periods of writing	Neck flexion Static grip, right hand	Trial of sloped writing surface to minimise neck flexion
Data entry and keyboarding	Neck flexion as screen is too low Static postures for prolonged periods Increased neck flexion as fatigue affects neck muscles and posture	Screen should be raised by 50 mm Consider trial of biofeedback with worker Trial of high back support for use in worker's car Trial of saddle chair
Customer service on telephone	Sometimes worker holds telephone receiver with a combination of neck flexion and rotation	Provision of a telephone headset

The occupational therapist identified issues and made the following recommendations to the employers regarding their responsibility under Occupational Health and Safety legislation:

- Lighting levels in both the assessed work areas were well below that recommended for clerical workstations. (Fluorescent light tubes lose efficiency after 1–2 years and should be replaced regularly. It was noted that several lights were not working at all and these should be replaced.)
- Consideration should be given to replacing fluorescent tubes over 2 years old to increase light to appropriate levels for clerical work. A follow-up assessment of the lighting levels is recommended.
- The typewriter is part of a system that shows the type on a screen to the right of the operator. The operator faces the typewriter but must work with their head facing to the side for prolonged periods. This work position significantly increases the risk of developing or aggravating neck pain.
- Apparently there is a way that the writing can appear on the typewriter, rather than a screen to the right of the operator. I have suggested to Ms S. that she use this facility to ensure that she maintains a forward-facing posture. While I understand that staff without neck issues may be unwilling to change, I feel it is important that the risks involved are explained to them so that they are making an informed choice and take the necessary steps/exercises to avoid injury in the future.
- The chair is not height adjustable, nor adjustable for lumbar support; the desk is also not height adjustable. A multi-user workstation requires, as a minimum, a height-adjustable chair and a footstool.
- Provision of adjustable ergonomic chair and footstool.

It is suggested that the following be incorporated into the rehabilitation plan for Ms S. as they are specific to her injuries:

- provision of a headset for use at the telephone
- typewriter screen to be raised and trialed at this height
- a trial of biofeedback, trial of a high back support for the car and a trial of a saddle chair all recommended.

It is further suggested that the employer undertake the following as Occupational Health and Safety considerations that will benefit any worker in the firm:

- Fluorescent tubes not working to be replaced. Consideration to be given to replacing tubes over 2 years old to increase light to appropriate levels for clerical work. A follow-up assessment of the lighting levels is recommended.
- Education of the staff regarding posture, work pauses and avoiding occupational overuse injuries.
- Provision of adjustable ergonomic chair and footstool for the typewriter work area.

ACKNOWLEDGEMENTS

Grateful thanks is expressed to Mandy Richardson of Commonwealth Rehabilitation Services, Australia who provided the case studies and to Dorothy Ferguson and Lesley Whyte, Dept. of Nursing and Community Health, Glasgow Caledonian University, who shared their ideas on community profiling.

REFERENCES

Cynkin S, Robinson AM 1990 Occupational therapy and activities health. Little Brown and Co. Boston, MA

Fleishman E, Quaintaince M 1984 Taxonomies of human performance: the description of human tasks. In: Christiansen C, Baum C (eds) 1991 Occupational therapy: overcoming human performance deficits. Slack Inc., NJ, pp 461–464

Hagedorn R 2000 Tools for practice in occupational therapy. Churchill Livingstone, Edinburgh

Henderson A, Cermak S, Coster W, Murray E, Trombly C, Tickle-Degnen L 1991 The issue is: occupational science multidimensional. American Journal of Occupational Therapy 45:370–372

Llorens LA 1993 Activity analysis: Agreement between participants and observers on perceived factors in occupation components. Occupational Therapy Journal of Research 13(3):198–211

Nelson DL 1996 Therapeutic occupation: a definition. American Journal of Occupational Therapy 50(10):775–782

Northen Ireland Committee of the College of Occupational Therapists 1992 Employment assessment and preparation. College of Occupational Therapists, London.

Wilcock A 1998 Occupation for health – keynote lecture at the 22nd Annual Conference of the College of Occupational Therapists. British Journal of Occupational Therapy 61(8):340–345

FURTHER READING

American Association of Occupational Therapists 1993 OT for the injured worker. American Occupational Therapy Association Inc., Rockville, MD

Argyle M 1990 The social psychology of work. Penguin Group, London

Callahan DK 1993 Work hardening for a client with low back pain. American Journal of Occupational Therapy 47(7):645–649

Canelon MF 1995 Job site analysis facilitates work reintegration. American Journal of Occupational Therapy 49(5):461–467

Golledge J 1998 Distinguishing between occupation, purposeful activity and activity. Part 1 Review and explanation. British Journal of Occupational Therapy 61(3):100–105

Harvey-Kefting L 1985 The concept of work in occupational therapy: a historical review American Journal of Occupational Therapy 39(5):301–307

Jacobs K 1985 Ergonomics for therapists. Butterworth-Heinemann, Newton, MA

Labour Market and Skill Trends 1997/8: SEN ISSN 1365–7399 Download 4/9/99 from http://dfee.gov.uk/skillnet

McCormack GL 1988 Pain management by occupational therapists. American Journal of Occupational Therapists 42(9):582–590

Pratt J, Jacobs K (eds) 1997 Work practice – international perspectives. Butterworth-Heinemann, Oxford

USEFUL CONTACTS

http://www.ergonomics.org.uk is the website of the Ergonomics Society in the UK. It contains general information about ergonomics, conference and approved courses.

http://www.ergoweb.com is a website which offers a number of useful case studies describing ergonomic interventions for specific jobs, their effectiveness and costs.

continued

7

Tools for living

Cath Doman   Pauline Rowe
Liz Tipping   Annie Turner
Elizabeth White

INTRODUCTION

Annie Turner

The ultimate aim of intervention by the occupational therapist is to facilitate the occupational performances identified as important by a person with limitations. The abilities, roles, functions and skills required to perform these occupations develop throughout life and their development is facilitated by biological, psychological, social, cultural and environmental factors.

de Kleijn-de Vrankrijker et al (1998, cited in McColl & Bickenbach 1998) consider that such abilities develop in both a qualitative and a quantitative way as we grow and mature. We become aware that abilities can be judged both from outside, as a result of external measurements of our performance, as well as by ourselves from within. Throughout life we are constantly judged on our performance and abilities. Academic examinations, swimming certificates, driving tests, being complimented on a meal well cooked, getting a sticker for being 'brave' at the dentist, are all examples of how our abilities are judged and rewarded by others. However, we also judge our abilities from within. At what point, and on what basis, for example, do we consider that we can speak French, ride a horse or consider ourselves to be a good team worker? What happens to enable us to judge our abilities as a wallpaperer or a cyclist to be less than average?

Judging our abilities is integral to our self-concept and self-image. Performance of occupations to a level of self-satisfaction or expectation is an essential part of our self-esteem and identity. Anything that challenges these abilities also challenges our own, and others', ideas of who and what we are. It is important, then, that activities are performed to a level that meets our self-image and expectations

deKleijn-de Vrankrijker et al (1998, cited in McColl & Bickenbach 1998 p17) contend that any 'complex ability is executed in mutual relationship with a person's physical, social and cultural environment, with use of the means and equipment that is present in that environment'. Use of tools or equipment is seen as a normal part of the execution of many occupations. We use a kettle to boil water, a spoon to eat soup, a telephone to communicate and a bath to keep clean. Where the task or environment are particularly challenging, specialist tools are required. A climber may use crampons, communicating in another language may require an interpreter, crossing rough terrain can only be undertaken in a specialist vehicle. Tools to help us with our daily living are the norm, as are specialist tools for particular challenges. Such is the case for those with limited functional skills.

Much has been written about the different philosophies related to the restrictions experienced by people with limited physical abilities. McColl and Bickenbach (1998) summarise five of these major viewpoints as follows:

- **Biomedical perspective**: this sees disability in the light of illness and impairment and looks at it as a medical phenomenon based on what the individual is unable to achieve. The 'patient' is seen as needing help from a health professional in order to 'get better'. Long-term disability is, therefore, seen as a failure for both the individual and the health service. This perspective does not generally accept the person as he is.
- **Philanthropic perspective**: the inability to perform is seen as a human tragedy in which the person is a victim in need of permanent sympathy and charity. The person, or group of people similarly categorised, may be the focus of fund-raising events. Those who grow

up as the recipients of this philosophy may see themselves as helpless and lacking a locus of control. This perspective assumes people remain in this state and expects that they will be actively grateful for help received.

- **Sociopolitical perspective**: difficulties that arise are seen as being caused by social attitudes and environments. For example, the inability to access a building is seen as being caused by poor design rather than the person's level of ability. The central belief is that social and political environments can be modified to accommodate people with different levels of abilities. This perspective is seen as empowering the individual as it accepts him as he is and requires social and environmental changes to accommodate him.
- **Sociological perspective**: the inability to perform is based on social norms and expectations and is, therefore, a social construction. People with differing abilities are seen as outside social norms, that is, they are 'abnormal', thus reinforcing the idea of them as outsiders. It is seen as the job of the providers to 'normalise' people's behaviours and abilities so that they fit in to society. In this perspective, therefore, the onus is on the individual to change.
- **Economic perspective**: this sees a person's inabilities as having a social cost caused by the need for additional resources, both human and financial, to support those who are less productive. This perspective leads to limitations of resources available to disabled people.

These are complex and often unconscious views perpetrated through actions of those working for, and driven by, laws, services and institutions. However the therapist feels personally, she must acknowledge the attitudes and perspectives that drive services and service provision. She may reflect on how these can appear to be perpetrated in different sections of this chapter.

A person may need assistance to interact with the environment to perform desired or required occupations. Whatever philosophical perspective the individual sees as driving the problem, there is no doubt that complex issues impinge upon the solution. It may, for example, be ideal to change an environment to assist occupational performance but time, legislation and funding can inhibit this. It might be sound reasoning to suggest that a person drives an adapted car but his self-esteem, expectations and family attitudes may make this unfeasible. Notwithstanding, when deciding on a solution, actions should follow a hierarchy, with the simplest and least intrusive being considered first. The solution should be driven by needs. Whilst it will inevitably be tempered by policies and procedures, it should not be confused with wants and desires.

This chapter explores some of the principles that the therapist may adopt when considering the provision of tools available to facilitate a person's occupational performance. Necessarily, it addresses functional performance, thus focusing on issues and tools related to occupational mobility within indoor and outdoor environments. Section 1 – Management of the environment – considers the home as a tool for living and how changes can facilitate occupational performance. Section 2 – Principles of orthotics – examines how orthoses act as tools to facilitate function. Section 3 – Moving and handling – discusses the context and processes that surround the need to help a person transfer themselves as part of desired occupations and explores some of the tools, in the form of techniques, human assistance and mechanical and other equipment, required to facilitate this. Finally, Section 4 – Aids to mobility – considers the tools available to facilitate a person's mobility so that they can execute their occupational performance.

MANAGEMENT OF THE ENVIRONMENT

Cath Doman

INTRODUCTION

Occupational therapy aims to enable individuals to achieve their maximal occupational performance by restoring function or compensating for functional deficits. The physical, emotional and sociocultural environmental contexts in which this takes place have powerful influences on human functioning and must therefore be central considerations in the occupational therapist's assessment.

This section introduces the impact the physical, social and emotional environments have on life and the role the occupational therapist has in empowering and advising individuals with disabilities to achieve independence and function in the face of this.

PRINCIPLES

HUMAN INTERACTION WITH THE ENVIRONMENT AND ITS IMPACT ON FUNCTION

The environmental context in which we exist has a fundamental impact on occupational behaviour. Kielhofner (1992) states that 'the human body and mind are in constant interaction with the physical and sociocultural environment'. Humans act on, and react to, their environment constantly. When physical dysfunction is present, either from birth or from trauma or pathology occurring at any stage in life, it has an impact on the individual's ability to interact with his environment. Equally, the environment imposes different and additional pressures. The occupational therapist's role is to facilitate performance by adapting the task to reduce its complexity or by adapting the physical environment to enable the person to interact with it.

THE PHYSICAL ENVIRONMENT

The physical environment includes all inanimate, non-human and natural aspects in the world around us (Hagedorn 1992). It is where every activity of daily living takes place and therefore has an enormous impact on human life. Most interactions are carried out without thought or difficulty, for example, opening a door, climbing stairs, crossing a road, getting dressed or going to the toilet. Activities such as these are habitual and generally do not challenge us when physical function is unimpaired. Other activities are more challenging, requiring a higher level of concentration, attention and physical dexterity, for example, driving a car or skiing a slalom course.

The physical environment can easily challenge or prevent our ability to interact with it – a door may be locked or a zip may break on a garment while dressing. The routine, habitual approach is interrupted and the individual has to adapt to the challenge the environment has presented him with by approaching the task in a different way.

The man-made, built environment has, until recent years, been designed around standard anthropometric dimensions to meet the needs of the average person. An airline seat, for example, will fit only a small percentage of people who fall within the average human shape. The tall, overweight or pregnant individual will not fit so easily. Goldsmith (1984 p117) states:

It is hazardous to make design decisions on the basis of catering for the average man or woman. In a representative sample of a population, 50 per cent of measures will be greater than the average and 50 per cent will be less. Dimensions based on the average will therefore best satisfy only 50 per cent of potential users.

People with full physical functional ability have the capacity to adapt to many everyday challenges the environment presents. When an individual has a physical disability, compensatory techniques need to be adopted, changing the environment to a state that allows the person with a disability to interact with it. Alternatively, when the environment cannot be changed, the technique itself must be adapted.

Compensatory approach

The built environment can create physical barriers to achieving occupational performance, thus preventing the individual from interacting with his environment. The occupational therapist's role is to work in partnership with the individual to enable him to achieve daily living tasks by removing either the barriers or the effect they have. This is achieved by analysing the activity and the environment to establish which component(s) is inhibiting performance. Intervention can then be focused on removing or compensating for that component.

Disabling environments and attitudes

The social model of disability postulates that it is the environment (sociocultural and physical) that causes disability, rather than pathology or the individual's physical function. For example, a person cannot access a building because of various steps and narrow, heavy doors. The design of the building is the cause of the access problem, rather than an individual's disability.

Attitudes towards disability are also a source of barriers. For example, a wheelchair user is denied access to a cinema because the manager deems him to be a fire hazard. With appropriate access and procedures in the event of an emergency evacuation to assist people unable to help themselves, the potential hazard is managed effectively. Under the Disability Discrimination Act 1995, such a refusal is now illegal.

Legislation

The 1995 Disability Discrimination Act in the United Kingdom also addresses architectural barriers, requiring all businesses and organisations to ensure their goods and services are accessible to all people, regardless of disability.

In the USA, The Americans with Disabilities Act (ADA) 1990 (cited in Reed 1993), requires all new buildings to be wheelchair accessible and has detailed architectural specifications for guidance. It also extends to public transport. Such legislation aims to prevent attitudinal and physical barriers to access.

EMOTIONAL AND SOCIOCULTURAL ENVIRONMENTS

The emotional value a person places on his environment must be taken fully into account when considering an adaptation. Places, and the people and memories in them, hold specific values, emotions and associations. To one person, the family home is a place of warmth, comfort and security; to another it may be a place of anxiety and distress.

The values attached to a place can also change due to life events. For example, a person experiencing an increased number of falls at home may change from feeling safe and secure at home to feeling frightened and anxious that they will fall, sustain an injury and not be able to summon help. The occupational therapist's intervention may be to assist the person to change elements of their home to reduce the risks, thereby enabling safe interaction with their home environment and regaining a feeling of security.

Alternatively, for another individual, changing the environment may be an entirely inappropriate approach that will emotionally incapacitate them further. The occupational therapist must be careful not to make assumptions about these factors, leading to incorrect interventions. Box 7.1 provides a case study to illustrate this.

Box 7.1   Case study: Considering emotional needs during environmental adaptation

An elderly lady with terminal breast cancer returns home from hospital. She lives alone in a house with three bedrooms upstairs and a living room, kitchen and bathroom with toilet downstairs.

She is unable to climb the stairs and has very limited mobility. She is in great pain and quickly becomes exhausted by exertion.

Her occupational therapist suggests that she convert the living room into a bed-sitting room so that she has all the necessary facilities to hand.

The lady is adamantly opposed to this and becomes very distressed at the idea. On further investigation, it becomes apparent that she associates this arrangement with the illness and death of her father, which in turn exacerbates her fears about her own illness.

Through understanding this particular emotional context, the lady is assisted to consider her options for living at home. She chooses to live upstairs. Toileting is managed with a commode and a care package is provided to assist with personal care and meal preparation.

Rather than seeing the house as a collection of rooms with predetermined and unchangeable uses, the house is approached as a tool for living in. Thus it meets the lady's specific physical and emotional needs, preserving her dignity and choice. She is able to end her days in comfort, without additional, unnecessary emotional distress.

The sociocultural environment refers to all aspects of the human environment the individual interacts with now, in the future and in the past. The social groupings that occur naturally through families, friendship, culture, religion and locality influence people's roles, attitudes and how they perceive themselves.

The physical, emotional and sociocultural environments interlink and overlap. The occupational therapist must consider all these aspects in the assessment to ensure that their influences on function are fully understood. When assessing an individual with a physical disability, it is likely that the physical environment will have the most significant influence on function and compensatory techniques will need to be employed to overcome performance deficits. However, the therapist should not automatically assume that this is the case and must take care to consider the social, cultural and emotional aspects of the environmental context of the individual.

PROCESS

APPROACHES TO ENVIRONMENTAL ASSESSMENT

Detailed assessment, taking into account the physical barriers, emotional associations and the social situation is fundamental to approaching an individual's functional problems.

An assessment for an adaptation or equipment should always be led by the needs of the person rather than by the resources available. The temptation is to link presenting problems with preset solutions, for example:

Difficulty climbing = installation of a
the stairs   stairlift

or

Difficulty getting in = an automatic bath
and out of the bath   seat

By approaching the presenting problem in this manner, the true impact of the dysfunction on the person's occupational behaviour can be missed or misinterpreted. The same solution cannot be applied repeatedly to the same problem regardless of the individual's personal circumstances.

The assessed needs should be addressed in a hierarchical manner, considering the simplest option first before moving on to more complex options (Box 7.2).

The potential solutions develop in terms of level of need, cost and disruption. Generally, the greater the need, the more likely the solution is to be costly and complex.

Identification of the individual's needs provides the foundation for proposing solutions. The occupational therapist and the individual concerned must be clear as to the nature of the problem to be solved before solution options are considered.

A process of option appraisal ensures that the identified needs are matched to the most appropriate option. It places the individual's unique experience in the centre of the assessment process and prevents the occupational therapist from making assumptions about the impact the particular dysfunction has on the individual's life. It facilitates a creative, problem-solving approach (Fig. 7.1).

The process ensures that the full impact of occupational dysfunction on the person's life is understood by the occupational therapist. It

---

Box 7.2 Hierarchical consideration of options for environmental adaptation

Occupational dysfunction
A person has increasing difficulties climbing the stairs due to deteriorating mobility caused by multiple sclerosis. He cannot access the bathroom, toilet, his bedroom or his children's bedrooms.

Options:
1. Install a banister rail
2. Reconfigure the use of the rooms in the house, to avoid having to use the stairs
3. Install a stairlift
4. Install a through-floor lift
5. Extend the ground floor of the property to provide the full range of accessible accommodation
6. Move to a more appropriate property

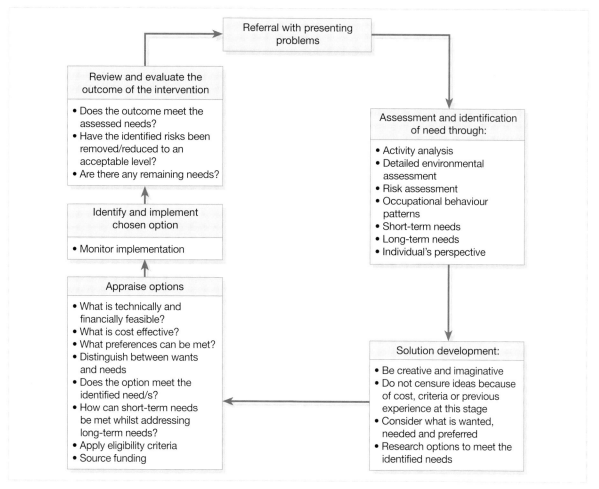

Fig. 7.1 The optional appraisal process to environmental adaptation.

allows the occupational therapist to apply her knowledge without making assumptions about the needs of the individual. It encourages a step-by-step approach to problem solving by considering the simplest ideas first before moving onto more complex solutions.

The occupational therapist must have a full understanding of the individual's occupational behaviour, including his roles and habits, to begin to identify a means of accommodating or resolving the dysfunction. Without extensive, assessment-based knowledge about the impact of the physical dysfunction on the person's occupational behaviour, the degree of risk and the short- and long-term needs, the chosen course of action could prove to be unsafe, inappropriate or only meet a short-term problem.

ASSESSMENT OF NEED IN THE CONTEXT OF PRIORITISATION AND ELIGIBILITY CRITERIA

A cash-limited culture is reality in contemporary health and social care service delivery. This is managed in two ways, enabling therapists to target spending on those most in need and at greatest risk:

1. **Eligibility criteria:** local authorities use eligibility criteria to target and ration the services they provide (Mandelstam 1998). These will make explicit the type of circumstances to which the local authority has a legal responsibility to respond and the extent of that response.

2. **Prioritisation:** when demand for a service exceeds the number of staff and the time available to provide it, it is necessary to set clear priorities as to which needs or problems have to be dealt with immediately and which can be dealt with later, without the individual experiencing undue risk. The person with the most pressing clinical need must be seen before those with less emergent problems.

Working with prioritisation and eligibility criteria

The occupational therapist has a professional responsibility to work within her employer's published criteria. Having assessed the person's needs, the occupational therapist must then overlay the criteria to identify which needs fall within the authority's remit and what priority the need must take. The service will become inconsistent if occupational therapists and their colleagues do not practise within the authority's criteria and some people will receive more extensive services than others.

The practical implications of this approach are that disabled people will have their needs assessed but may not be eligible for service provision. This is illustrated in Box 7.3. The box highlights an apparent conflict between the occupational thera-

---

Box 7.3   Case study: Reconciling need and criteria

Referral synopsis: Mr G. requests provision of a ramp to access his house.

Assessment synopsis: Mr G. is mainly wheelchair dependent. He cannot manage the doorstep. He leaves the property a few times a year when his son takes him out.

Typical local authority criteria regarding access: access adaptations to a person's property will be funded if they attend a day centre, a day hospital or have regular medical appointments to attend.

Assessment outcome: the occupational therapist agrees that a ramp is a safe and appropriate way to resolve the problem. However, under the current criteria, this cannot be funded by the local authority. Advice is given regarding ramp design to enable Mr G. to fund the construction of a suitable ramp, should he wish to do so.

---

pist's professional assessment and the eligibility criteria operated by her employer. The solution may not lie in the employer's scope and the occupational therapist's intervention may take the form of enabling the person to take action themselves on the advice they have been given.

In seeking funding for specialised equipment or adaptations to meet the assessed need of an individual, the occupational therapist must provide evidence through a process of clinical reasoning, justifying the decision in relation to the agreed eligibility criteria and providing evidence to establish the priority afforded to the individual's needs.

PRACTICAL TECHNIQUES AND INFORMATION SOURCES

With experience, the occupational therapist will develop an extensive battery of knowledge on adaptation options, building techniques, architectural information and on the huge range of compensatory equipment available. Regardless of this, however, the primary role of the occupational therapist is to assess an individual's needs. Once the needs have been identified, and the activity analysed, there are many texts and other resources, such as Disabled Living Centres or the Disabled Living Foundation, which provide detailed technical information on equipment and adaptations. These resources will enable the occupational therapist to match the person's need to the specification of the adaptation or piece of equipment.

It is important that the occupational therapist remains focused on the needs of the individual, to prevent reliance on product knowledge that soon becomes outdated and potentially inappropriate. In a community occupational therapy service, the referral type is very wide-ranging and does not fall into neat diagnostic categories that the therapist can become extremely knowledgeable about. A focus on clear identification of need is therefore of paramount importance.

The occupational therapist cannot intervene effectively to facilitate performance unless both the occupation and the environmental context it is occurring in are fully understood (Kielhofner & Forsyth 1997).

PRINCIPLES OF ORTHOTICS

(WITH SPECIFIC REFERENCE TO THE HAND)

Pauline Rowe

INTRODUCTION

An orthosis, or splint, can be defined as an externally applied device used to control or support a body part. The terms can be used synonymously but, traditionally, practitioners refer to appliances for the upper limb distal to the elbow as splints. Here, the terms will be used interchangeably without this connotation.

When considering tools for living to assist occupational performance, the role of orthoses in this area may not be immediately apparent as, by their nature, orthoses immobilise or at least limit range of movement in some joint or body part. However, it must be remembered that the ultimate aim is to achieve an optimum position and physiological state, thereby maximising functional ability and maintaining the balance of the hand. This in turn will facilitate the individual's occupational performance.

Some orthoses are prescribed to enable increased function during their use and may have the added benefit of helping to prevent deterioration of the condition or secondary involvement and deterioration of other structures. With some orthoses, which are holding the affected body part in a fixed position, the increase in functional ability may not occur during the wearing of the orthosis but will result following its prescribed use. For example, the potential use of orthoses following a median nerve lesion, as described by Callahan (1984, cited in Malick & Kasch 1984), serves to illustrate these points. Callahan describes how a thumb opposition splint, which positions the thumb in abduction and opposition to the second and third digits, can provide major assistance in activities of daily living by assisting thumb function for prehension. This orthosis also prevents contracture of the first

web space. If the person prefers to use his hand without an orthosis (relying on lateral pinch and substitution patterns to provide sufficient thumb function), a thumb web spacer needs to be worn at night and careful passive range of motion carried out on a regular basis to prevent contracture occurring. Such measures will clearly enhance occupational performance by either compensating for, or adapting, the person's functional ability.

It is important to understand what part an orthosis can play in the total intervention programme. This applies to the overall treatment of an individual in addition to how the orthosis contributes to the occupational therapist's interventions.

Orthoses may be used for a variety of conditions and with different aims, depending on the particular circumstances. Although orthotics is based in biomechanical principles – an external force being applied to some body part – it also relies on knowledge of anatomy and physiology. Orthoses are not only used within the biomechanical approach, but also within rehabilitative/compensatory and sensorimotor/neurodevelopmental approaches. Their use within the latter is particularly open to debate, especially the use for conditions of spasticity.

Depending on the reasons for prescribing, an orthosis may be static or dynamic. Static orthoses, as the name suggests, are ones that have no moving parts. Dynamic orthoses have a fixed or static base to which sections are attached to produce or assist movement. It is important for the therapist to have a sound grounding in the principles of orthotic design and this knowledge is usually first focused on static orthoses. These same principles apply to the construction of the static base of dynamic splints, with added principles for the manufacture and application of the dynamic portions. This section intends to provide an overview of some of the basic principles.

ASSESSMENT

Occupational therapy is a profession that considers each individual holistically and assessment of physical, psychological and social factors is important in orthotic provision. This determines the individual's particular needs under the umbrella of the clinical features common to the presenting condition. These points of general and specific information enable the therapist to begin the problem-solving process and determine which treatment aims may be statisfied or supported by the provision of an orthosis and which specific design and material would be the optimum choice.

PHYSICAL FACTORS

It is important to have clinical knowledge of the diagnosis, its clinical features and prognosis, because these will have implications for the aims of the orthosis, its design and the materials chosen. Although basic decisions can be made on the basis of the diagnosis, it is only by specific assessment of the individual that exact information on the current state of that person can be obtained. Features of relevance to orthotic provision include:

- skin condition
- the presence of oedema
- range of movement
- the extent of any deformity.

Skin condition

This may be affected by pathology or by medication. Assessment has to be made not only of the skin covering the part(s) directly involved but also those areas over which the orthosis will extend for purposes of leverage, pressure reduction and strapping. Relevant observations include colour, texture, integrity and the position of scars and nodules. Assessment should ascertain the temperature of the skin and the extent of any sensory loss. If an orthosis is supplied to a person with sensory impairment it is particularly important to protect him from warm materials while fabricating the orthosis and he must be instructed to check for early signs of pressure or skin irritation when wearing the device.

Oedema

Oedema may be present as a sign of a clinical condition but the volume of even a healthy hand may change during any 24-hour period. In addition, the wearing of an orthosis may result in some immobilisation of the limb, which in turn, through reduction in the pumping action of skeletal muscles, will decrease venous return and therefore produce oedema. Conversely an orthosis may reduce oedema and prevent sequelae of tissue damage and contracture (Coppard & Lohman 1996).

Whatever the cause, oedema may be transient and therefore regular fittings must be arranged. Where possible a design should be chosen to incorporate the potential for adjustments to accommodate fluctuations in size.

Comparison with the unaffected side can be of help in determining whether all oedema has subsided. However, when comparing the upper limbs allowance should be made for the possibility of differences between the dominant and nondominant sides.

Range of movement

The alignment and range of active and passive movement at relevant joints should also be assessed. Range of movement may be limited by a variety of factors, such as pain, oedema and soft tissue or bony deformity. Conversely, movement may extend beyond a joint's normal range as when ligaments are lax.

Deformity

The body part may be at risk of being placed in a position of deformity by the disease process, as in plantar flexion of the ankle in Duchenne muscular dystrophy, or as a result of trauma suffered, as in the case of a peripheral nerve lesion. Assessment needs to be made of the current extent of any deformity and how fixed this is.

PSYCHOLOGICAL, PERSONAL AND SOCIAL FACTORS

The principles of person-centred, holistic, empathetic occupational therapy practice are applicable to the orthotic aspect of intervention. Two people with the same diagnosis and clinically at the same stage may have very different psychological reactions. These, along with personal, social and work-related interests and needs, add to the complexity of issues. By effective communication the therapist can learn from the individual what impact they feel the condition has had on them. This may include their family role(s) and other aspects of their life, including work and hobbies. Interrelated issues, such as their economic status, and social and emotional well-being, also need to be discussed and considered.

The active involvement of the person in the assessment of their priorities will help ensure a greater potential for compliance with the orthotic regimen. If the therapist strives to understand the person's perspective on his condition and its impact on his life, the clinical aim(s) of orthotic provision may be better matched with those the individual hopes the orthosis will achieve. Similarly, if the person is made aware of the functions and limitations of the orthosis he may be more likely to wear it as prescribed than if he has unrealistic expectations, and hence sees it is an encumbrance or a miraculous cure.

THERAPEUTIC USE OF ORTHOSES

Upon completion of an holistic assessment, one or more orthoses may be designed to meet the specific and often interdependent aims of treatment.

POTENTIAL AIMS OF ORTHOSES

The following list of potential aims gives one example of when an orthosis may be applied:

- pain relief – carpal tunnel syndrome
- facilitation of healing – ligament repair following whiplash injury
- prevention of development of soft tissue deformity or contractures – burns
- maintenance of improvements achieved by other forms of treatment – control of contractures between passive stretching
- protection of joint integrity by immobilisation – rheumatoid arthritis
- improvement or maintenance of joint alignment – ulnar deviation in rheumatoid arthritis
- assistance of weakened muscles – peripheral nerve lesion

- substitution for lost muscle power – muscular dystrophy and peripheral nerve lesion
- protection of vulnerable anatomical structures – meningomyelocele cyst.

In general, orthoses may be protective, supportive or corrective (Malick 1980). In the case of static orthoses, these aims are achieved by using one of three positions as a base: rest, function or immobilisation. Dynamic splints use a static base from which appropriate forces are applied to assist, resist or produce movement.

POSITION OF REST

A position of rest is based on the natural position the healthy body part assumes with normal muscle balance between antagonistic muscle groups. A prime objective when orthoses are constructed for the axial rather than appendicular regions is to achieve postural symmetry. In the case of the hand, the position of rest as described by Malick (1980) is when the wrist is in 10 to 20 degrees of extension, the thumb is in partial opposition and forward, and the distal and proximal interphalangeal and metacarpophalangeal finger joints are slightly flexed (Fig. 7.2). Whilst at rest, the fingers adopt this flexed pattern because the flexor muscles are stronger than the extensors.

Symptoms may be alleviated by providing rest to the affected body parts and can subsequently reduce inflammation, as in rheumatoid arthritis, or facilitate healing following a whiplash injury.

POSITION OF FUNCTION

According to Malick (1980) the position of function of the hand can generally be described as similar to that which it adopts when holding a

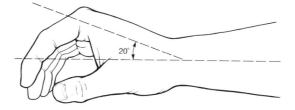

Fig. 7.2 Neutral or resting position of the hand (adapted from Malick 1980 with kind permission of Harmarville Rehabilitation Center, Pittsburg, PA).

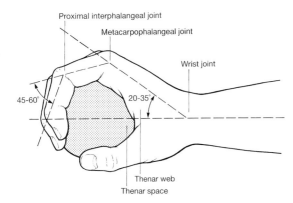

Fig. 7.3 Functional position of the hand (adapted from Malick 1980 with kind permission of Harmarville Rehabilitation Center, Pittsburg, PA).

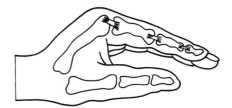

Fig. 7.4 Position of prolonged immobilisation (collateral ligaments of finger joints are taut) (Lister 1993).

ball (Fig. 7.3). The wrist is in 20–30 degrees of extension, the thumb is abducted and opposed. The transverse arch at the level of the metacarpal heads is increased in curvature and the amount of flexion in the fingers is approximately 30 degrees at the metacarpophalangeal joints and 45 degrees at the proximal interphalangeal joints.

Orthoses based on this position can enhance the function of the hand by maintaining the 20–30 degrees of wrist extension needed for full flexion of all the joints of the fingers and powerful prehension or grip. It can also prevent deterioration of structures (including the more proximal joints of the upper limb, which provide a wide range of hand positioning) which can result when the hand is not used.

POSITION OF IMMOBILISATION

It may be necessary to immobilise the hand to allow healing to occur. As this process may continue for a long period, it is important to maintain stretch on soft tissues to prevent contractures. An optimal position of immobilisation for the hand is illustrated in Figure 7.4. In this position, where the metacarpophalangeal joints are flexed to 90 degrees and the proximal and distal interphalangeal joints are extended, the collateral ligaments are taut. This ensures that if adhesions form in the ligaments during immobilisation of the hand, they will not restrict non-extensible ligaments in a shortened position that in turn would prevent movement of the fingers.

PRINCIPLES OF ORTHOTIC DESIGN

There are texts, such as Salter and Cheshire (2000), which outline the orthotic management of specific conditions and give more detailed information on the principles to be applied. The actual treatment protocol being followed by the team may also affect the provision of orthoses in terms of exact type and the timing of their use. There are many anatomical, biomechanical and social factors to be considered when designing orthoses. The following points identify some of the key, generic principles. Particular reference will be made to the hand to illustrate points.

BIOLOGICAL AND BIOMECHANICAL PRINCIPLES

A detailed description and application of biomechanical principles can be found in Bowker et al (1993). They outline how external forces such as gravity and internal forces of muscle contraction and the tension of ligaments are constantly acting on the body. Following disease or injury, the body's ability to produce appropriate forces across joints may be adversely affected or lost, as in flaccid paralysis of muscles following peripheral nerve lesion with antagonist muscle groups still producing normal muscle tone, or lax joint capsules and ligaments in rheumatoid arthritis. By considering the body as a system of levers, with the joints being the fulcrums, orthoses can apply support to counteract the imbalance caused by trauma or pathology, or the effects of gravity, to provide rest to damaged structures while they heal.

ANATOMICAL LANDMARKS

If an orthosis is to fit correctly and position the body part in correct alignment, the therapist must have a sound knowledge of the normal anatomy, functional anatomy and lines and patterns of movement of the region. Surface anatomy is also used to ensure individualised fitting. These individual features may be used as points of reference when making a pattern, adjusting an orthosis during manufacture, or modifying a pre-formed, 'off-the-shelf' orthosis.

Examples of this are illustrated with reference to the hand, which has three arches – the distal and proximal transverse arches and the longitudinal arch (Fig. 7.5). These arches are an essential consideration in orthoses if undue pressure and discomfort are to be avoided. The curvature of the arches changes as the hand is used. Observation of the hand during movements such as precision or power grip shows how, along with these changes of curvature, the soft tissues (such as the musculature of the thenar eminence) could easily be impinged upon by an orthosis. Skin creases on the palmar surface, such as the digital, palmar, thenar and wrist creases, lie in relation to

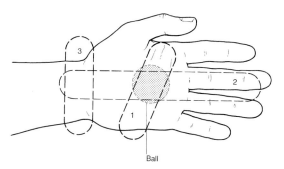

Fig. 7.5 Arches of the hand: palmar view, left hand. 1, Distal transverse arch; 2, longitudinal arch; 3, proximal arch (adapted from Malick 1980 with kind permission of Harmarville Rehabilitation Center, Pittsburg, PA).

underlying joints (Fig. 7.6) and can be used to determine the position and boundaries of orthoses. Creases must be included within an orthosis if it is intended to immobilise the joint. Conversely, to allow movement at a joint, the corresponding creases must not be impinged upon.

PRINCIPLES OF PRESSURE REDUCTION AND MANAGEMENT

It is inevitable that pressure is exerted on the body parts covered by the orthosis. This has to be

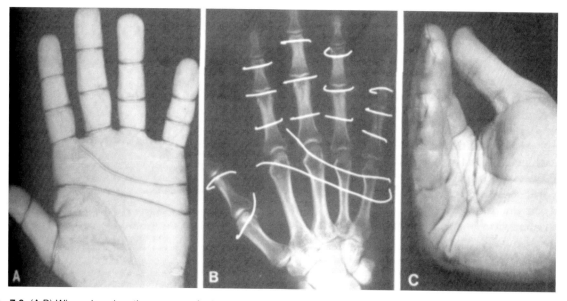

Fig. 7.6 (A,B) Wires placed on the creases of a hand that was subsequently examined radiographically to reveal the relationship of those creases to the various joints. Note in particular that the proximal digital creases do not correspond to any joint and that a line joining the ulnar end of the distal palmar crease to the radial end of the proximal palmar crease most closely approximates to the metacarpophalangeal joints. (C) Flexion of the metacarpophalangeal joints illustrates that their corresponding 'skin joints' are the proximal and distal palmar creases (adapted from Lister 1993 with kind permission).

sufficient to achieve the desired positioning of the body part(s) but not so great as to cause damage to the underlying structures by impairment of blood supply or lymphatic circulation, or by skin or nerve impingement. This is achieved by the pressure being evenly distributed over as large an area as possible. Thus, in orthoses designed to support the hand and wrist in a functional position, the material extends proximally two-thirds up the forearm and forms a gutter, the height of which is half the depth of the arm. Removing the orthosis for set periods of time can also be helpful in pressure management but checking of pressure exerted by the orthosis during wear is still crucial (see p179).

Pressure may be localised by indentations in the material if sufficient expertise and care are not applied during manufacture. Any segments made with thermoplastic materials can be spot heated to correct this. Areas with minimal soft tissue or sites of bony prominences can also be potential sites of increased pressure and damage to the skin can easily result. This pressure can be avoided either by padding the area around the bony prominence during manufacture and then removing this padding, so the material is then raised in the region of the prominence, or by padding around these areas to lift off the pressure.

Another aspect where skin and underlying soft tissues could be damaged is at the edges of the orthosis adjacent to joints that are to be moved during wear. Here it is advisable to roll back the orthotic material to ensure a rounded, smooth edge.

COSMESIS, COMFORT AND COMPLIANCE

The appearance of an orthosis is important. It should be professionally finished with neat edges, no ink or marks on the material and be as unobtrusive and low-profile as possible.

The cosmesis, weight and size will have an effect on whether an orthosis is worn. The fact that wearing the orthosis can feel restricting in terms of movement and function, and hence seem uncomfortable, can deter the person from wearing it. Therefore the person's understanding of the benefits and limitations of its use and the

consequences of lack of use or misuse are crucial factors in compliance.

In construction, the individual's priorities need to be incorporated into the design whilst still striving for optimum clinical aims. Clinical knowledge and problem-solving skills within a person-centred, holistic approach can facilitate the production of an orthosis that attains these goals. As Bowker et al (1993) state, 'It may be necessary to compromise bio-mechanical effectiveness in order to make the orthosis acceptable. Better a partly effective compromise solution that is used than a technically brilliant one that lies in the cupboard under the stairs'. Coppard and Lohman (1996 p3 and p17) support this when they state 'splint design must be based on scientific principles, and splint fabrication requires creative problem solving because each patient and splint may be different ... Splint design is limited only by a person's creativity'.

MATERIALS

There is an ever-changing range of materials available as companies continue to improve their qualities. The majority of materials are thermoplastics, that is, they become malleable when exposed to dry, wet or steam heat. Each company will supply details of the required temperature and form(s) of heating that can be used for each of their range of products. Other materials react when ingredients are mixed together or when they come into contact with the air.

Properties of the materials that will need to be considered in the process of orthotic design include conformability, rigidity (resistance to bending), strength (resistance to fracturing), strength to bulk ratio, elasticity, shrinkage, memory, setting time and whether the material can be reheated/remoulded. In addition, therapists will learn useful tips on how to emphasise or reduce certain properties. The most common example of this is the adjustment to the self-adhesive property of some materials. This can be increased for the attachment of straps or eliminated altogether for orthoses where the material is wrapped over itself, as in bracing. Another example is the prestretching of selected parts of the orthosis to increase the ability to curve the material, as is needed for moulding around the web space of the thumb.

Although some materials may seem expensive, the potential of earlier discharge along with improved occupational performance can out-weigh the initial cost of the orthosis. However, the cost is still an important factor to consider. This is not always as simple as the price per unit area. If one material is reheatable and can there-fore be adjusted as required, as in serial splinting, then it may be more cost effective than one that is less per square metre but cannot be remoulded.

Some materials are available in a range of colours that can allow choice and thus enhance compliance. The selection of materials should incorporate individual preferences whilst still striving for optimum clinical aims.

MANUFACTURE OF ORTHOSES

Many therapists will make an individual pattern to meet the particular clinical and personal needs of each individual. Although this may seem time consuming to the neophyte therapist it can, with experience, be completed quickly. Templates or 'off-the-shelf' orthoses require adjustments to ensure correct fit and can be equally, or more, time consuming. A personalised pattern can enable an orthosis to be moulded in one fitting, which eases the person's discomfort and anxiety. Although adjustments may still need to be made, for example if the material is very elastic, these should be minor and can often be carried out during the working time of the material thus avoiding the need to reheat.

Once made, the orthosis must be checked for correct fit and points of excessive pressure. An orthosis that fits correctly may leave a red area when it is removed, but this will disappear within seconds. If the redness lasts longer this is an indication of a pressure point, which can occur over a bony prominence. Adjustments must be made to correct this and experience will help decide whether to spot heat or reheat and mould the whole orthosis. As Coppard and Lohman (1996) state 'the activity of the therapist re-heating and adjusting one spot often affects the adjacent area, thereby producing another area requiring adjustment'.

The orthosis must also be evaluated in terms of it achieving the identified aims, being cosmeti-cally pleasing and as unobtrusive as possible. The methods of assessment will be selected from the range used in current practice and can be quantitative or qualitative.

The wearer or key carer responsible for the person must be instructed on how and when to use the orthosis and how to check for such things as pressure and skin deterioration. All users should have a means of contacting staff to answer any queries or discuss concerns.

Table 7.1 summarises some of the questions to be asked and issues to be considered. It is not meant as a prescriptive, nor exclusive list, but is hopefully a helpful starting point.

CONCLUSION

There is a need for flexibility in orthotic design and fabrication in order to meet individual needs but the design and construction have to arise from a solid base of researched evidence rather than custom and practice. Relevant journals contain current work and membership and newsletters of groups such as the Clinical Interest Group in Orthotics Prosthetics and Wheelchairs (CIGOPW) are useful for keeping up to date. CIGOPW, a specialist section of the College of Occupational Therapists, has produced standards and guidelines on occupational therapy in the practice of orthotics (1998) to provide a frame-work for effective and safe practice and the main-tenance of a high quality of service provision.

Critical appraisal of research papers is central and is 'not just about finding the research evi-dence which supports what you do, but also about challenging our beliefs and assumptions' (Jerosch-Herold 1998a). Evidence-based practice, the integration of current best evidence with individual clinical expertise when making deci-sions about the care of individuals (Sacket et al 1996, cited in Jerosch-Herold 1998b), linked with a problem-solving approach, may assist in further development of orthotic provision and enhance current good practice.

Table 7.1 Summary of points to consider and questions to ask yourself during the design and construction of an orthosis

Timing	Questions to ask	Points to consider
Before manufacture	*Clinical perspective* Why would I make an orthosis?	What aims of treatment would it achieve? identified from diagnosis clinical features prognosis Are these aims being achieved by other aspects of treatment? Would an orthosis improve on this?
	Current clinical features	Skin condition Pain Deformity Range of movement Motor loss Sensory loss Skin condition Scars, open wounds Oedema
	Wearer's perspective What is his response to the condition?	Positive mental attitude Anxious Pain tolerance
	What are his priorities?	Regain function: work social pursuits ADL Appearance: of limb/body part? of orthosis?
	What does he expect the orthosis to achieve and in what timescale?	
	Is he aware of the limitations imposed by wearing the orthosis?	
	Does he understand the consequences of not wearing the orthosis?	
When manufacturing	Which orthosis design should I choose?	What parts need to be supported? What positioning needs to be achieved? What anatomical landmarks are to be used? Which is the least obtrusive design pattern, precut or off-the-shelf? What are the relative costs of the options? What are implications of individual's preferences/priorities?
	What material properties are needed?	Rigidity (resistance to bending) Conformability Strength (resistance to fracturing) Strength–bulk ratio Elasticity Shrinkage Memory Method of heating if thermoplastic Method of application Setting time Colour – person's preference
	Safety precautions	Temperature of the materials Comfort of individual when positioning

continued

Table 7.1 *continued*

Timing	Questions to ask	Points to consider
After manufacture	*Evaluation of the orthosis*: Before patient leaves the department	Is the positioning of the limb/body part correct? Does it incorporate only the anatomical structures it needs to? Does it fit: are there any pressure points? red areas on skin? indentations in the material? Does the orthosis look professional: smooth edges? no pen marks? securely fitted straps? Does the person/carer know: how and when the orthosis is to be worn? what to check for during use? who to call if any concerns? when the follow-up appointment is?
	Ongoing evaluation	How will I assess if the orthosis is achieving its aims? When and how will progress be recorded?

MOVING AND HANDLING

Liz Tipping

INTRODUCTION

Loss of independent mobility can have wide-ranging consequences for people, whether it is as a result of a short-term problem, such as a minor injury following trauma, or a long-term problem, such as a progressive neurological condition. It can severely limit a person's activities and affect the way he is able to cope with everyday occupations. Even the most basic tasks can become time consuming and arduous, and assistance may be needed from the occupational therapist to enable the person to move and transfer either independently or with help.

At one end of the scale, independence may mean autonomous mobility, whilst at the other end of the continuum it may refer to a state in which the person decides where when and how he wishes to be moved. For many, the long-term reality is a state somewhere between these two. It is the task of the occupational therapist to facilitate how this can be achieved in order to best serve the person's occupational needs. However, where possible, the overall aim should be for independence, with the therapist taking a hierarchical approach to the solution, starting with the least intrusive measure. Initially, the person should be encouraged to move themselves with help from verbal prompts, or a piece of equipment may need to be introduced to allow independent transfers, for example, a sliding system or transfer board. If help from carers is required, then equipment, such as a hoist, that reduces the amount of force needed to carry out the manoeuvre with minimal risk may be necessary. Ultimately, the task may need omitting altogether by adapting the person's routine on enviroment for example, or by providing equipment which eliminates the need for transfer.

Occupational therapists have both professional and legal responsibilities towards individuals, carers and others to ensure safe moving and handling practice. Statistics show that injuries as a result of manual handling tasks are very high within the health and social care sector and that sprains and strains to the back are the most commonly reported (Health and Safety Executive 1998). The therapist therefore needs to be aware of relevant legislation and have sound knowledge of the principles of back care.

LEGISLATIVE FRAMEWORK

The Health and Safety at Work Act 1974 (HMSO 1992) was implemented to protect people in the workplace and sets out clear duties for employers and employees. However, the scale of accidents resulting from manual handling and the resultant loss of productivity and increased costs have led to further regulations, which supplemented this legislation. These regulations were much more prescriptive in order to improve health and safety in general and, more specifically, to improve manual handling practice (Back Care 1999).

The Management of Health and Safety at Work Regulations 1992 introduced the philosophy of risk assessment. They state that every employer is required to make suitable and sufficient assessment of any hazardous tasks within the workplace and to remove or reduce those risks to a reasonably practicable level. This applies to all hazardous situations but, where this assessment highlights risks from manual handling tasks, the Manual Handling Operations Regulations 1992 (HMSO 1992) need to be applied. Regulation 4(1)(a) states that: 'Each employer shall, so far as reasonably practicable, avoid the need for employees to undertake any manual handling operation at work which involves a risk of their being injured' (Health and Safety Executive 1998 p9).

The regulations introduce some key terms, which are defined in Box 7.4. Box 7.5 outlines the responsibilities of both employers and employees under the Manual Handling Operations Regulations 1992 (HMSO 1992). Employers are required to take a clear hierarchical approach when assessing and reducing the risk of manual handling injuries. Employees are obliged to comply with any safe systems of work that have been introduced to reduce the risk of injury. This duty is absolute and, if breached, could result in disciplinary proceedings.

Box 7.4 Definition of terms used within manual handling

- Hazard – an event or condition that has the potential to cause harm
- Risk – the likelihood of it happening
- Reasonably practicable – the cost of preventive steps weighed against the benefits

---

Box 7.5 Employers' and employees' responsibilities under the Manual Handling Operations Regulations 1992 (from Health and Safety Executive 1998, with permission)

Employers' responsibilities
- **Avoid** hazardous manual handling operations so far as is reasonably practicable
- **Assess** any hazardous operations that cannot be avoided
- **Remove or reduce** the risks of injury
- **Review** if conditions change
- **Provide information/training** to employees about loads

Employees' responsibilities
- **Take reasonable care** of their own health and that of others
- **Cooperate** with their employers on health and safety issues
- **Comply** with any safe systems of work that have been introduced to reduce the risk of injury
- **Undertake** appropriate training offered by the employer

Although no formal employer/employee relationship exists, the occupational therapist none the less has a duty of care to teach carers and family members how to handle safely, taking into account their levels of competence. She must ensure that she has the necessary skills to give competent instruction in order to guard against claims of professional negligence (Dimond 1997). This is particularly relevant when working with individuals within their own homes, where care may be given by a wide variety of paid and unpaid carers and other professionals. Effective communication is vital to ensure safety and consistency of handling procedures. Written care plans, which include details of moving and handling procedures, should be available to everyone and ideally a copy should remain in the person's home.

PRINCIPLES OF BACK CARE

The occupational therapist needs to apply her knowledge of the anatomy of the spine and the biomechanics of human movement to the principles of back care. The natural curves of the spine give it stability and strength. If they are not maintained during handling then the risk of a back injury is increased (Fig. 7.7A). The spine is also subject to compression and shearing forces, which, if excessive, can result in damage. For example, lifting a heavy load while bending and twisting will increase these forces and may lead to a prolapsed intervertebral disc. Lifting with a stooped or rounded back with the load held away from the body (Fig. 7.7B) increases the stresses on the intervertebral discs and the small muscles of the back have to exert large forces to counterbalance not only the weight of the trunk but also the weight of the load being moved. These safer handling principles are summarised in Box 7.6.

Box 7.6 Back care principles for safer handling

- **Maintaining** the natural curves of the spine
- **Flexed hips and knees**, using the large muscle groups to apply the force
- **No twisting**, bending or awkward postures
- **No excessive force** for pulling, pushing, lifting or lowering
- Maintaining a **stable base** of support
- Keeping the **load close** to the body
- **Avoidance of repetitive tasks** – the cumulative effects on joints, ligaments and discs can also lead to damage

---

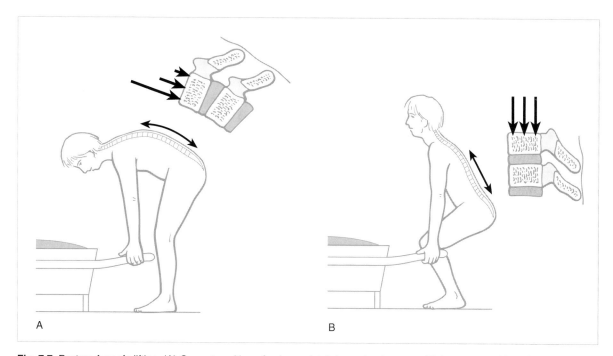

A   B

Fig. 7.7 Posture for safe lifting. (A) Correct position of spine maintaining natural curves, (B) incorrect position of spine in which natural curves are flattened.

RISK ASSESSMENT

The Guidance on the Regulations (1998) requires that an ergonomic approach is taken to remove or reduce the risk of manual handling injuries (Health and Safety Executive 1998). The first step is to analyse the situation using the key components of a risk assessment (Box 7.7).

With their understanding of the effect of the environment on occupation and their skills in activity analysis, occupational therapists are ideally placed to recognise hazardous manual handling situations. Assessment forms based on Figure 7.8 (Health and Safety Executive 1998) can be found in health and social services departments and are used to identify the problem areas that need to be addressed. It must be emphasised, however, that the risk assessment process is not just a paper exercise and action must be taken to implement changes. The occupational therapist must look at ways of effectively removing or reducing the risk of injury. Again, using the TILE categories as a guide can help the ther-

apist to identify methods of reducing the level or risk and ensure compliance with the regulations (Box 7.8).

Whatever the solution used to reduce the levels of risk, the way the therapist approaches the introduction of a new technique or piece of equipment is vital if it is to be accepted. Careful assessment and a sensitive approach, taking into account the needs and wishes of the individual and the family, and involving them in the discussions, can help to allay concerns and fears.

However, if the person is unable to assist with the move and appropriate equipment is not available, then the option of not moving him may need to be considered. There may be conflict between the wants and needs of the person and the carers who are assisting him. The risk assessment in this instance must be clear. There are very few, if any, circumstances where it is right for carers to risk permanent damage to their backs by undertaking such manoeuvres and it is important that the occupational therapist is aware of the procedures open to her in these circumstances.

Box 7.7   Key components of risk assessment (TILE)
• Task • Individual • Load • Environment

HANDLING TECHNIQUES

A very small number of basic techniques is described and illustrated here, and it must be emphasised that they are designed to be used where the person requires assistance. The person

---

Box 7.8   Principles and techniques to reduce levels of risk

TASK
- Does the task need to be done? Avoid if possible
- Plan manoeuvre carefully
- Can equipment be used effectively?
- Avoid repetitive handling
- Incorporate rest breaks/variety

LOAD
- Assess person/load – can they assist?
- Ensure the person fully understands the manoeuvre – planning
- Are more helpers required?
- Use handling aids where appropriate
- Change technique – use equipment

INDIVIDUAL
- Plan manoeuvre carefully – give clear instructions
- Avoid restrictive clothing or unsuitable footwear
- Be aware of own limitations
- Is training required to improve technique, posture, risk awareness?

ENVIRONMENT
- Plan the move – keep distances to a minimum
- Create as much space as possible
- Ensure correct heights for transfers
- Consider installation of appropriate ramps, rails, etc.

Manual Handling of Loads: Assessment checklist

Section A – Preliminary: *Circle as appropriate

Job description: Factors beyond the limits of the guidelines?	Is an assessment needed? (i.e. is there a potential risk for injury, and are the factors beyond the limits of the guidelines?) Yes/No*

If 'Yes' continue. If 'No' the assessment need go no further.

Operations covered by this assessment (detailed description): Locations: Personnel involved: Date of assessment:	Diagrams (other information)

Section B – See over for detailed analysis

Section C – Overall assessment of the risk of injury?   Low/Med/High*

Section D – Remedial action to be taken:

Remedial steps that should be taken, in order of priority:
1
2
3
4
5
6
7
8
Date by which action should be taken:
Date for assessment:
Assessor's name: Signature:

TAKE ACTION ... AND CHECK THAT IT HAS THE DESIRED EFFECT

Fig. 7.8 An example of a risk assessment form (Crown copyright material reproduced with the kind permission of the Controller of Her Majesty's Stationery Office).

Section B – More detailed assessment, where necessary:

Questions to consider:	If yes, tick appropriate level of risk			Problems occurring from the task (Make rough notes in this column in preparation for the possible remedial action to be taken)	Possible remedial action (Possible changes to be made to system/task, load, workplace/space, environment. Communication that is needed)
	Low	Med	High		
The tasks – do they involve: • holding loads away from trunk? • twisting? • stooping? • reaching upwards? • large vertical movement? • long carrying distances? • strenuous pushing or pulling? • unpredictable movement of loads? • repetitive handling? • insufficient rest or recovery? • a work rate imposed by a process?					
The loads – are they: • heavy? • bulky/unwieldy? • difficult to grasp? • unstable/unpredictable? • intrinsically harmful (e.g. sharp/hot)?					
The working environment – are there: • constraints on posture? • poor floors? • variation in levels? • hot/cold/humid conditions? • strong air movements? • poor lighting conditions?					
Individual capability – does the job: • require unusual capability? • hazard those with a health problem? • hazard those who are pregnant? • call for special information/training?					
Other factors: Is movement or posture hindered by clothing or personal protective equipment?	Yes/No				

Fig. 7.8 *continued*

must be weight bearing and be able to contribute to the move. If the carers are having to compromise their posture or use excessive force, then alternative techniques and equipment must be used:

1. Sitting to standing independently using verbal prompts (Fig. 7.9)
2. Sitting to standing with assistance (Fig 7.10):
   - Ask the person to shuffle forward in the chair, or assist him to do so. Ensure correct positioning of his feet.
   - The carer stands to the side of the person, facing the same direction, and places the near side arm around his waist. A handling belt may help the carer to grip more easily and allow for an upright posture.
   - With the other arm, the carer supports the person, using a palm to palm grip.
   - If only one carer is needed, the person is asked to push down on the arm of the chair with his other hand.
   - The command to stand is agreed, for example, '1,2,3, stand'. It may be helpful to rock gently on the counts and, at the command, the person pushes up into a standing position.

- This assist allows the carer to maintain an upright stance and a wide base of support. She transfers her weight from the back leg to the front one, and, moving in the same direction, is able to remain close to the person.
- The carer then stays close to the person while they gain their balance, before collecting any aids.

Figures 7.11 and 7.12 illustrate a selection of basic techniques designed to be used where the person requires assistance from one or two helpers sitting up in bed and moving up the bed. Figure 7.12 shows the use of a sliding sheet, which has been placed under the person's buttocks and heels to facilitate the move up the bed. A number of sliding systems, of varying designs, is available on the market and prescription will depend on individual assessment.

Figures 7.13 and 7.14 illustrate some examples of unacceptable techniques which do not comply with current standards and regulations and should, therefore, not be used. Further examples can be found in The National Back Pain Association's 'The Guide to Handling Patients' (1997).

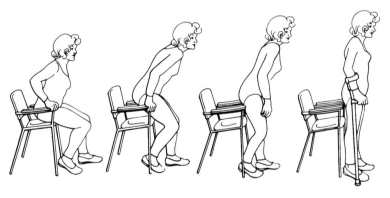

Sit well forward on the chair with both feet on the floor and the weight taken through the stronger (rear) foot – if this is applicable. Hold the arms of the chair firmly. Keep the head up.

Push up with the hands and feet, with the head well forward.

Transfer weight evenly onto both feet, and adjust balance.

Collect aids

Fig. 7.9 Transfer from sitting to standing.

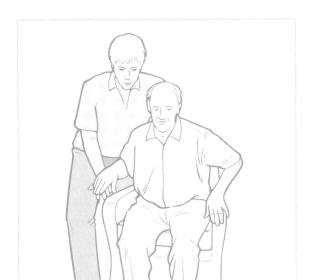

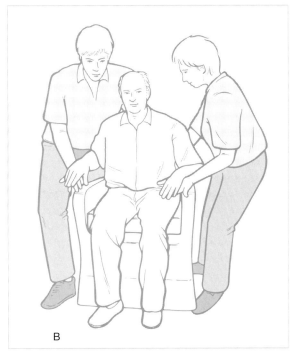

A

B

Fig. 7.10 Sitting to standing with assistance. (A) Assistance from one helper, (B) assistance from two helpers.

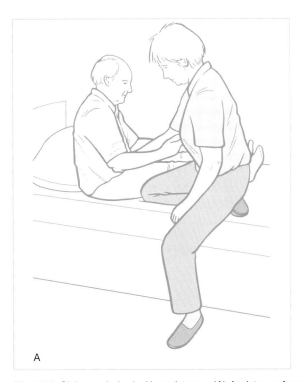

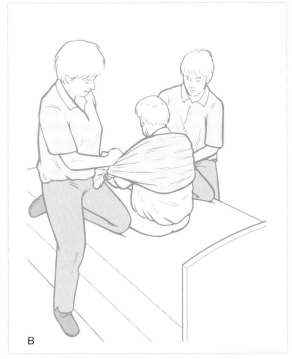

A

B

Fig. 7.11 Sitting up in bed with assistance. (A) Assistance from one helper, (B) assistance from two helpers.

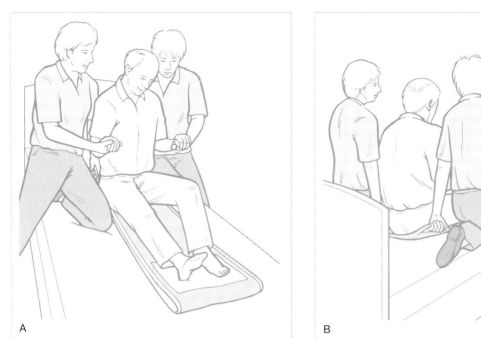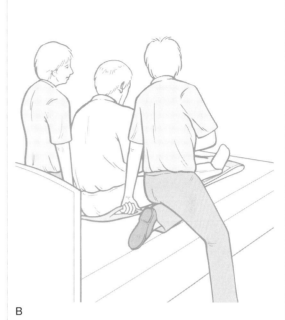

Fig. 7.12 (A) Moving a seated person up the bed using a sliding sheet with two helpers, (B) using a sliding sheet.

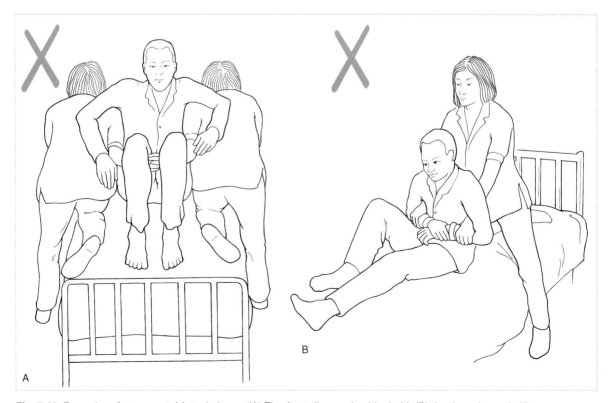

Fig. 7.13 Examples of *unacceptable* techniques. (A) The Australian or shoulder hold, (B) the through-arm hold

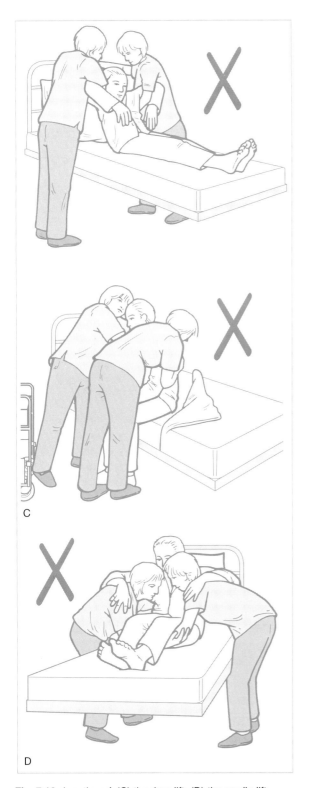

Fig. 7.13 (*continued*) (C) the drag lift, (D) the cradle lift.

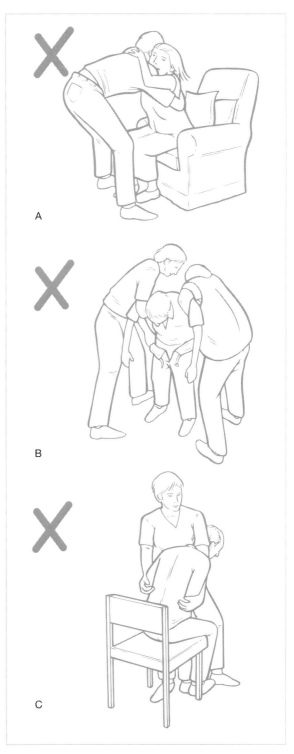

Fig. 7.14 Examples of *unacceptable* techniques – front transfers. (A) The pivot lift, (B) the elbow hold, (C) supporting a person while attending to personal care.

CONCLUSION

When selecting a technique to help a person move, it is important that the person's abilities and the level and availability of assistance required are fully assessed. Numerical guidelines indicate that maximum weights or forces for lifting and lowering are 17 kg for women and 25 kg for men where loads are held close to the body at an optimum height (Health and Safety Executive 1998). It must be noted that the combined maximum weight for two people is two-thirds of their combined capacity (National Back Pain Association 1997). However, these are guidelines only. Individual risk assessments are needed for each circumstance.

Where possible, normal patterns of movement should be encouraged during the manoeuvre, so as to give the person the opportunity to give his maximum assistance. When selecting a technique the carer must also try to ensure she is able to maintain the correct posture throughout the move or transfer. She should consider the consequences should something go wrong, for example, should the person's legs give way during the manoeuvre. If the carer and individual were 'attached', as in the case of a pivot lift (see Fig. 7.14A), then this could easily lead to injury.

Some basic techniques have been illustrated, together with some examples of unsafe practice; however, there are no 'recipes' to cover every situation. The risk assessment process for each circumstance is the key to avoiding or reducing the level of risk. Adequate training must be given and maintained to ensure that techniques and equipment are used safely and appropriately.

Where the occupational therapist is treating people in the rehabilitation setting, as when working in the person's home, the risk assessment still applies and any risk must be reduced to a reasonably practicable level. Accurate recording of the assessment and the remedial action are essential. The occupational therapist must comply with the law and the standards of the profession. She will need all her skills to ensure that any changes of technique or introduction of equipment is accepted both by the carers and by the individual themselves.

AIDS TO MOBILITY

Elizabeth White

WALKING AIDS

The selection of an appropriate walking aid is vital to preserve and promote independent mobility. The underlying function of any walking aid is to increase stability for people with poor balance, muscle weakness or lack of confidence (Richardson 1995) or to reduce pain or the fear of falling (Cochrane & Wilson 1991). Some walking aids may assist upright posture and can improve the user's gait and walking speed (Disabled Living Foundation 1998a). By enlarging the supported base of the user it becomes easier for the person to maintain their centre of gravity when upright and, by transferring part of the weight bearing to the arms, loading is removed from the legs, pelvis and lower spine.

PROCUREMENT OF WALKING AIDS

In the United Kingdom the majority of walking aids are provided on free loan from the National Health Service via acute or community services. Walking aids may also be obtained from the user's local Social Services Department when a daily living need can be demonstrated (Mandelstam 1993). Other sources of supply include voluntary services, such as the Red Cross, or private purchase from mobility shops or mail order catalogues.

ASSESSMENT FOR WALKING AIDS

Assessment for a walking aid is usually undertaken by a physiotherapist but recognition of need may be identified by other professionals, such as nursing staff or occupational therapists, particularly in community settings. Mobility assessment must consider whether the need is temporary or permanent and whether the user has a stable or deteriorating condition. Recognition that all walking aids have advantages and disadvantages according to individual need (Richardson 1995) means that priorities and expectations must be discussed with the user and any involved carers in order to ensure appropriate selection, and this must include the environment in which the walking aid is to be used.

ENSURING APPROPRIATE FIT

The walking aid must be at the correctly set height for each individual user to provide optimum support and effectiveness. Handgrip height is established by measuring from the ulnar styloid to the floor when the user is standing up and wearing appropriate shoes. This allows a few degrees of elbow flexion to be included so that the mobility aid is at the correct height when the elbow is extended during walking. A range of handgrips is available, with alternative shapes allowing contouring for improved grip and different weight-bearing abilities within the hand.

ENSURING SAFE USE

The user must always be instructed in the appropriate method of using the equipment supplied and be made aware of who to contact for repairs or replacement. Walking aids without wheels should be fitted with rubber tips or ferrules to reduce the possibility of slipping and to improve grip. Regular maintenance should be undertaken to identify signs of wear or to replace ferrules when these wear smooth. Walking frames with wheels require checking to keep the wheels moving freely and to maintain the recommended pressure in pneumatic tyres.

WALKING STICKS

A walking stick is an effective aid for balance and confidence for the person who has a sufficient level of upper limb strength (Cochrane & Wilson 1991). Walking sticks are available in wooden or aluminium construction and must be cut or adjusted to suit the individual user. A variety of shaped handgrips offers the option to provide an effective and contoured grip; a straight handle is more comfortable to hold, while a crook handle can be hooked over the arm when not in use.

Walking sticks may be supplied singly or in pairs. When one stick only is used, it should be held in the opposite hand to the weak leg to offer a good supportive base and to reduce limping. A four-point gait provides the maximum stability from walking with two sticks, moving one foot then the opposite stick followed by the alternate foot and second stick.

A major disadvantage of walking sticks is their instability when not in use, and a strap may be required to secure the stick to the user's arm or wheelchair. Some sticks are sectional or telescopic and can be folded to fit into a bag or pocket.

TRIPODS AND QUADRUPODS

Tripods and quadrupods (Fig. 7.15) provide greater stability than a standard walking stick due to the increased number of points of contact with the ground. Different size bases are available. The larger the base, the more stable the walking aid will be but it will take up more space and may not fit on a stairtread. Handgrips are either straight or swan-necked, the latter transferring the user's weight directly over the base.

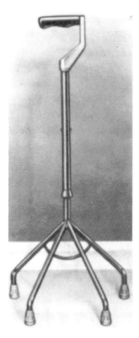

Fig. 7.15 A quadrupod.

The use of tripods and quadrupods may be contraindicated for some rehabilitation treatments (Disabled Living Foundation 1998a) and this must be considered when selecting an appropriate mobility aid.

CRUTCHES

Crutches (Fig. 7.16) offer more support than walking sticks and may be preferable for people with reduced grip strength. They also allow a partial or non-weight-bearing gait. It is recommended that crutches should only be used following a therapist assessment (Disabled Living Foundation 1998a) as there is a variety of different walking patterns that may be adopted, according to the individual needs and abilities of the user.

Crutches are divided into two types:

● Elbow crutches have an open or closed cuff that allow some weight to be taken through the forearm; the handle height should be adjusted appropriately for each user. A number of handgrip types is available, including a gutter trough (see Fig. 7.16B),

which may suit the needs of a user with painful hands or elbow contractures (Cochrane & Wilson 1991).
● Axilla crutches have a padded top that rests between the upper arm and the chest wall. The pad should not press into the armpit as this may cause nerve or blood vessel damage. The majority of the user's weight is taken through the handgrip and greater energy expenditure is required to use this type of crutch than elbow crutches, although walking may be quicker.

WALKING FRAMES

A large variety of walking frames (Fig. 7.17) is available and these are mainly recommended for elderly people or those with poor balance as they offer a large base within which to maintain the centre of gravity. The therapist must instruct the user in the correct use of the frame to ensure safe mobility and transfers. It may be necessary for the user to have two frames so that one can be kept upstairs, and the size of frame must be considered to ensure it can be accommodated within the home.

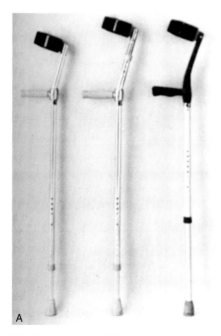 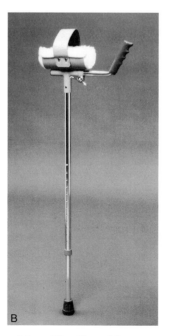 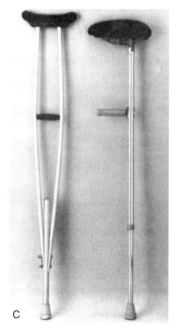

Fig. 7.16 Crutches. (A) Elbow crutches, (B) gutter crutches, (C) axilla crutches.

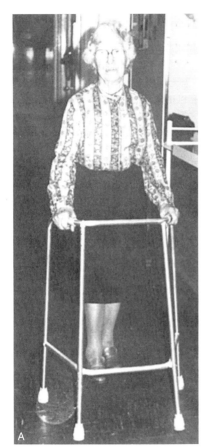

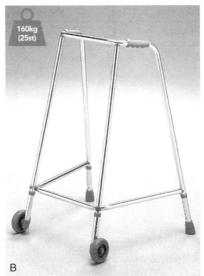

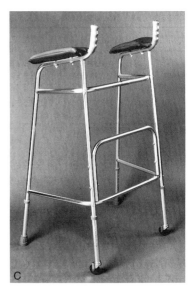

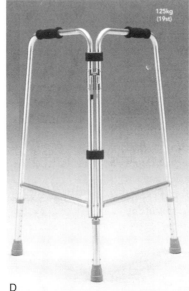

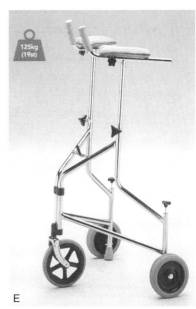

Fig. 7.17 Walking frames. (A) Non-wheeled zimmer frame, (B) wheeled zimmer frame (reproduced by kind permission of Days Medical Aids Ltd), (C) gutter frame, (D) triangular frame (reproduced by kind permission of Days Medical Aids Ltd), (E) three-wheeled walker (reproduced by kind permission of Days Medical Aids Ltd).

Walking frames are divided into two types:

- Non-wheeled frames are frequently known as zimmer frames and are often prescribed to fulfil the indoor mobility needs of elderly people. Although stable, their use interferes with the normal gait pattern.
- Wheeled zimmer frames allow a more normal walking pattern and provide good support, although they are difficult to manoeuvre and the wheels can be hazardous when negotiating thresholds.

Within the two categories of walking frames, many variations exist including gutter frames for people with poor grip, triangular frames, which can be accommodated in small areas, reciprocal frames to encourage a normal gait and frames with integral seats.

The therapist should be aware of the types of frame that are available for supply from the local equipment store, although alternative models may be considered if a user's clinical need cannot be fulfilled by a standard model.

With all walking aids, the weight of the user should be considered during the selection process and reference made to the manufacturer's instructions if there is any doubt concerning the suitability of the product for the individual user.

HOISTS

The use of hoists is rising due to the increasing awareness of risk to healthcare staff, users and carers from poor handling techniques. The Manual Handling Operations Regulations (Department of Health 1992) give clear guidelines of measures to reduce the risk of injury to employees who are manoeuvring individuals. Not only is lifting the whole weight of the person not recommended, but care must also be taken when supporting the person's weight. Risk assessments are increasingly commonplace and assessment of an individual's needs and abilities should be undertaken by nursing and/or therapy staff (see pp184–186).

Cassar and Costar (1998, p7) stated that selection of manual handling equipment should: 'reduce the manual load of staff, be easy to operate or use, be capable of dealing with the client in safety, be capable of being used in the intended location, be in sound condition and properly maintained'.

ASSESSMENT FOR A HOIST

A number of assessments should be included when selecting the appropriate hoist and slings for each individual user. These include:

- user's height and weight
- the diagnosis and prognosis
- the level of functional ability
- the level of postural support
- the manoeuvre that is planned

- the frequency of hoisting
- lifestyle factors and user expectations
- the environment for hoist use
- carers' needs and abilities
- user's comfort and personal preference.

PROCUREMENT OF HOISTS

Hoists are now widely used in hospitals and nursing homes and in the management of disability at home. Within the community, hoists are normally supplied on free loan from the local National Health Service or Social Services Department equipment store following a request from a nurse or therapist. Hoists may also be privately purchased or loaned by a voluntary organisation.

TYPES OF HOISTS (Fig. 7.18)

A variety of hoists can be supplied to fulfil the individual needs of the user, their carer and their home circumstances (Fig. 7.18):

- Mobile hoists may be battery operated, hydraulic or manually wound up and down. Their main use is in assisting a carer to transfer a person from one piece of furniture to another, for example from a bed to a wheelchair or commode. They are not suitable for transporting people for any distance. A wide range of mobile hoists is available and selection of an appropriate model must include assessment of the weight and sitting ability of the user, the space in which the hoist is to be used and the height of clearance that will be available when transferring. It is also essential to consider the needs of the carer who will be operating the hoist and the different furniture that is necessary to access by hoist.
- Wall-mounted hoists allow short distance transfers and can be used where there are space restrictions that prevent the use of a mobile hoist. They can be swung through a 90 degree arc and are most appropriate for bed to chair or commode transfers.
- Ceiling track hoists run on a permanently fixed track that is attached to the ceiling.

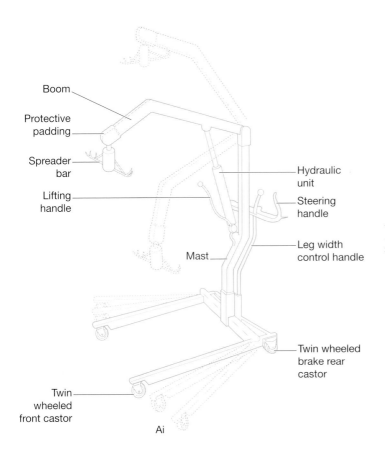

Boom

Protective padding

Spreader bar

Lifting handle

Hydraulic unit

Steering handle

Leg width control handle

Mast

Twin wheeled brake rear castor

Twin wheeled front castor

Ai

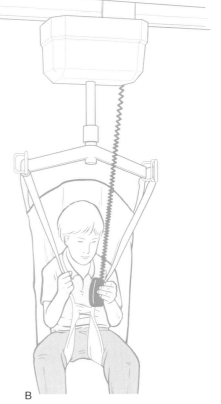

B

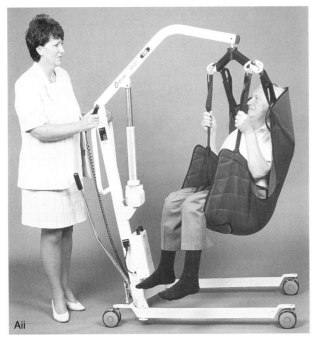

Aii

Fig. 7.18 Hoists. (Ai) Mobile hoist (reproduced by kind permission of the Disabled Living Foundation), (Aii) mobile hoist in use with a universal sling (reproduced by kind permission of Sunrise Medical), (B) ceiling track hoist (reproduced by kind permission of the Disabled Living Foundation).

They may allow the user to be transported from one room to another, although structural adaptations may be needed to the property to accommodate this. Ceiling track hoists can be operated by the user, thus allowing independent transfers between different pieces of furniture such as bed, wheelchair and commode.

- Overhead hoists may be used when the property is unsuitable for the fixing of a ceiling-mounted hoist or when the user is excessively heavy. A hoist operated by one or two electric motors is mounted on an overhead track, supported at either end by an 'A' frame with free-standing legs.

HOIST SLINGS

Selection of the correct sling is essential in achieving the best outcome from the equipment provision and Beresford (1998) considered that selection of the appropriate sling played a vital role in the user's willingness to accept the equipment. Consideration must be given to the user's physical abilities, comfort and level of support required and to the interventions that are to be carried out by hoisting. Slings come in different sizes to suit individual needs and are frequently colour-coded for easy identification of size. It is important to use a sling that is recommended by the manufacturer for compatibility with the hoist in question.

SLING TYPES

- Toiletting slings (Fig. 7.19A) allow wide access to the user for personal hygiene activities. They are easy to position but require the user to have good upper body strength as they give little trunk support.
- Hammock slings (Fig. 7.19B) are appropriate for more severely disabled people, offering full support and a high level of comfort. However, they are difficult to position, except in lying, and provide little access for hygiene management.
- Universal slings (Fig. 7.19C) give good support and comfort and may incorporate head support. The leg bands can be used in a

variety of ways to suit transferring or toileting requirements.

- Two-piece band slings are generally not recommended as they provide little support and can allow the user to slip between the bands. However, the Disabled Living Foundation (1998b) considers that, on occasion, band slings may be the best option, particularly if they allow independent transferring.

If a person's clinical needs cannot be fulfilled by a standard hoist sling, the manufacturer may be approached to make a sling for an individual's specified requirements.

WHEELCHAIRS

Responsibility for the provision of wheelchairs in England and Wales transferred to the National Health Service in 1991, following the recommendations of the McColl Report (McColl 1986). The requirement for wheelchair services was defined as being: 'to meet the basic need for short-range mobility of people of all ages who have serious and permanent difficulties in walking' (McColl 1986 p6).

In recent years, the demand for wheelchairs has been growing due to the increase in the elderly population (Dudley & McMahon 1994), advances in medical technology, which have resulted in the survival of many people with severe levels of trauma, disease or birth injury (Pope 1996) and the rising expectation of user groups (McCreadie & James 1995). It is estimated that there are now over 700 000 users of wheelchairs in England (College of Occupational Therapists 1993–6).

PROCUREMENT OF WHEELCHAIRS

The majority of wheelchairs in the United Kingdom are supplied on free loan to eligible people by National Health Service wheelchair services. Short-term provision may be made by hospitals for a short-term need such as hospital discharges or by voluntary agencies such as the Red Cross. Private or charitable funding may be

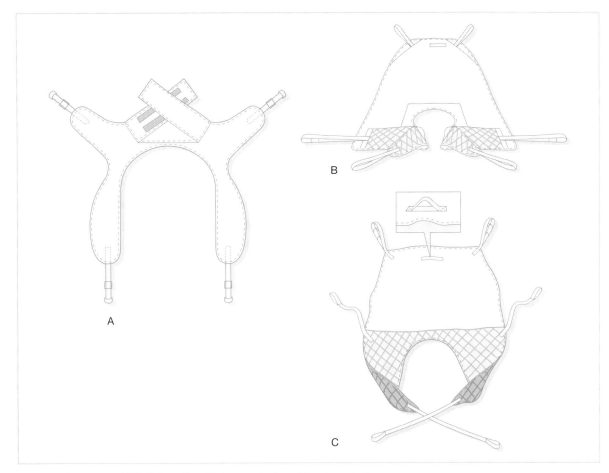

Fig. 7.19 Sling types. (A) Toileting sling, (B) hammock sling, (C) universal sling.

used for wheelchairs outside the criteria for National Health Service funding.

Wheelchair voucher scheme

The wheelchair voucher scheme was introduced in 1996 to give wheelchair users more choice in the provision that was available to them (National Health Service Executive 1996b). The scheme offers three options:

1. To accept the National Health Service wheelchair prescribed to fulfil basic clinical need.
2. Partnership option – to contribute to the cost of a more expensive chair of the user's choice from a range specified by the wheelchair service, which would continue to own and maintain the chair.
3. Independent option – to contribute to the cost of a more expensive chair of the user's choice from an approved supplier. The user would own the chair and be responsible for its maintenance.

The voucher scheme was intended for manual wheelchairs only in the first instance and it was expected that the average voucher period would be 5 years, subject to the user's clinical condition.

REFERRAL AND ASSESSMENT

Most National Health Service wheelchair services use individually designed referral forms, which provide information regarding the wheelchair applicant and their needs. Basic models may be prescribed from this information alone, while therapist assessment is available for people with more complex needs.

Effective wheelchair selection includes a broad spread of assessment issues. These include:

- the user's height and weight
- the primary diagnosis, prognosis and any secondary disabilities
- the level of functional ability
- the anticipated frequency and environment of wheelchair use
- lifestyle factors and user expectations
- psychosocial needs
- postural and pressure management issues
- the carers' needs
- the user's comfort and personal preference.

IMPLICATIONS OF POOR WHEELCHAIR SELECTION

McColl (1986) found that inadequate assessment contributed to many disabled people using unsuitable wheelchairs, which affected their ability to lead independent lives. Table 7.2 lists the implications.

WHEELCHAIR PRESCRIPTION

Following the assessment procedure, the selection of an appropriate wheelchair can be made. The development of high performance and modular wheelchairs, and the increasing range supplied by National Health Service wheelchair services, have enabled wheelchair users to have their individual needs met more closely, increasing independence and minimising the effects of disability (Disabled Living Foundation 1993).

TYPES OF WHEELCHAIRS

Self-propelling wheelchairs

Self-propelling wheelchairs (Fig. 7.20A) have large rear wheels with handrims to allow users with sufficient upper limb strength and stamina to manoeuvre themselves independently, both

Table 7.2 Implications of inaccurate wheelchair selection

Problem	Implication
Seat too wide	Unstable sitting position Difficulty in accessing the self-propelling wheels Environmental barriers
Seat too narrow	Discomfort in sitting Risk of developing pressure sores Difficulty in transferring
Seat too long	Restriction to lower limb circulation Discomfort behind the knee Poor postural support
Seat too short	Insufficient seating support Increased pressure loading on supported area
Seat too high	Difficulty in accessing the wheelchair May be unable to use standard table Reduces efficiency of self-propelling
Seat too low	Poor sitting support Reduces efficiency of self-propelling
Armrests too high	Elevates shoulders Reduces access to self-propelling wheels
Armrests too low	Reduces support leading to poor posture Restricts respiration
Footplates too high	Discomfort in hips and knees Reduces supported sitting area
Footplates too low	May catch on kerbs or pavements Encourages poor posture by altering pelvic positioning

indoors and outdoors. Many carers also find large-wheeled chairs easier to push, although they may be heavier or more bulky to lift into a car.

Transit or attendant-propelled wheelchairs

Transit or attendant-propelled wheelchairs (Fig. 7.20B) have small rear wheels and are pushed by a carer. They may be selected for the user with a physical or cognitive disability that prevents them from safe or effective handling of a self-propelling model. Such chairs generally fold into a compact size for car transportation and most have removable armrests and footplates to reduce the lifting weight and facilitate transfers.

Standard self-propelling and transit wheelchairs still form the bulk of National Health Service wheelchair service provision. Table 7.3 details features of these standard models.

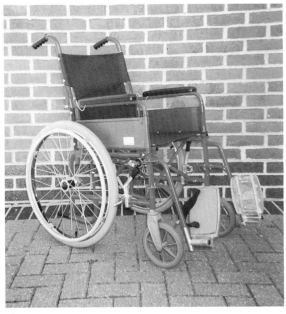

A

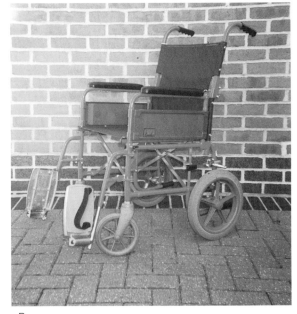

B

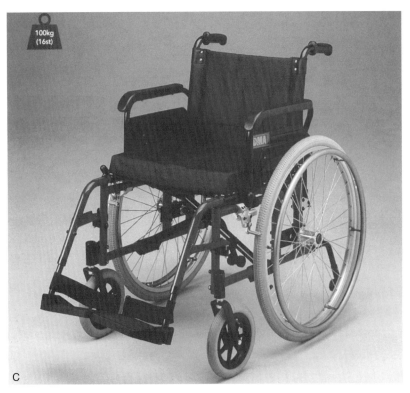

C

Fig. 7.20 Types of wheelchairs. (A) Self-propelling wheelchair, (B) transit chair, (C) lightweight chair, (D) indoor powered chair, (E) indoor/outdoor powered chair, (F) scooter. (A, B, C, F reproduced with kind permission of Days Medical Aids Ltd.)

Fig. 7.20 D–F see opposite

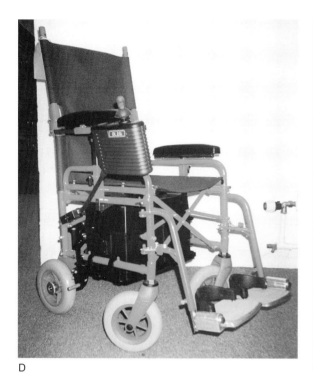

D

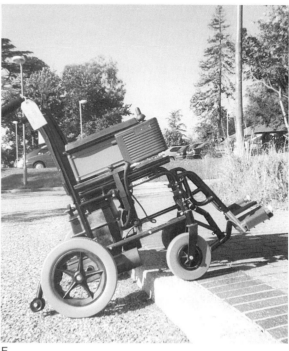

E

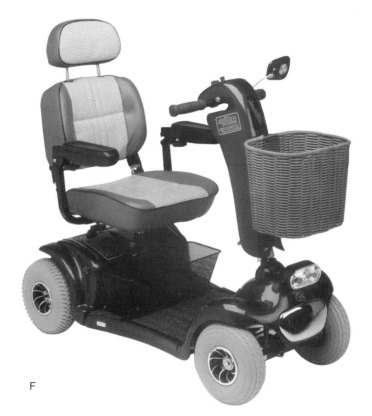

F

Fig. 7.20 D–F.

Table 7.3 Standard NHS wheelchairs

Model name	Type	Seat size W × D (cm)	Rear wheel diameter (cm)	Weight (kg)	User weight limit (kg)
8L	Self-propelling	43 × 43	56	18.5	101
8BL	Self-propelling	41 × 41	51	17.0	101
8LJ	Self-propelling	38 × 43	56	18.0	101
9L	Transit	43 × 43	32	15.4	101
9LJ	Transit	38 × 43	32	15.4	101

Children's wheelchairs and buggies

There is a wide range of buggies and manual and powered wheelchairs available for children with ongoing mobility difficulties. McColl's recommendation (1986) was that wheelchair services would not make provision to children under 30 months. However, exception may be made where the level of disability requires special seating for postural management. Assessment procedures are similar to those of adults but adjustability to accommodate growth or changing needs must be included. Suitability of the wheelchair for transport to and from school may also be a consideration.

High-performance and lightweight wheelchairs

For the full-time or active wheelchair user, the provision of a lightweight or high-performance wheelchair (Fig. 7.20C), adjusted to suit the user's functional abilities, can significantly enhance independent mobility and lifestyle. Additional assessment factors must include the user's ability to balance the wheelchair, transferring ability and transportation needs.

Features available on high-performance wheelchairs include:

- range of wheel and castor sizes and models to enhance manoeuvrability and handling
- quick release wheels
- adjustable wheelbase length and seat angle
- cambered wheels to improve turning ability, though this widens the wheelbase
- adjustable height backrest
- tension-adjustable seat and back canvases
- rigid frame for added strength and improved performance
- footbars or flip-up footplates

- anti-tip bars to prevent the chair from tipping backwards.

Special wheelchairs

For the user with a specific clinical need which cannot be met from within the standard range of chairs, alternative options may be considered. These include:

- extended rear axle model for bilateral above-knee amputees
- one-arm drive chairs for the user with functional ability only in one arm
- recliner wheelchairs for people who cannot sit upright or lack hip flexion
- tilt-in-space chairs, which allow adjustable positioning while maintaining the angle between the seat and backrest
- elevating seat models to enable the user to access different height furniture
- stand-up wheelchairs to allow the user to achieve an upright position from sitting.

Indoor powered wheelchairs

Indoor powered wheelchairs (Fig. 7.20D) are supplied by National Health Service wheelchair services to people whose mobility is so restricted that they can neither walk nor self-propel a manual wheelchair sufficiently to achieve indoor independence. Controls are normally mounted on the armrest of the chair but if the user has insufficient hand function to operate a standard control knob, alternative options include controls operated by chin, head or suck/blow tube. Provision of an indoor powered wheelchair would be expected to improve the level of functional ability of the user. These chairs are compact and manoeuvrable although their short wheelbase and smooth tyres mean they are not suitable for use on uneven ground.

Indoor/outdoor powered wheelchairs

Funding for indoor/outdoor powered wheelchairs (Fig. 7.20E) was only made available to National Health Service wheelchair services in 1996 (National Health Service Executive 1996a), with the intention of enhancing powered provision for severely disabled people. These models are sufficiently manoeuvrable for indoor use but robust enough for limited outdoor use. Some models have kerb-climbers, which allow shallow kerbs to be mounted, although descent must be undertaken backwards. Distance of travel on each battery charge is dependent on the capacity of the batteries and is affected by the weight of the user and the terrain on which the chair is used.

Outdoor powered wheelchairs

Outdoor powered wheelchairs are large, robust models, generally insufficiently manoeuvrable for indoor use but suitable for rough ground, slopes and kerb-climbing. Such models are normally obtained through charitable or private funding, or may be obtained through the Motability scheme (Disability Information Trust 1994).

Attendant-controlled powered wheelchairs and power packs

When the wheelchair user cannot self-propel and the carer has a medical condition that prevents them from pushing a manual wheelchair, an attendant-controlled powered chair may be supplied, with the controls mounted on the wheelchair push-handles.

Power packs are clip-on units with rechargeable batteries, which can be attached to some manual wheelchairs to provide assistance on slopes or hills. It is essential to confirm compatibility between the wheelchair model and power pack unit.

Scooters

Scooters (Fig. 7.20F) are available either for pavement use (Class 2 vehicle) or for road use (Class 3 vehicle). Any disabled person who has the physical and mental ability for safe handling and control may use a scooter. These are not supplied by wheelchair services and are usually purchased by private or charitable funding. Advice on the most suitable model may be obtained from Mobility Centres.

ASSESSMENT FOR POWERED WHEELCHAIRS

Additional assessment issues must be considered when a powered chair is requested. Functional ability must be observed and cognitive ability and eyesight recorded. Information about the user's home circumstances, space for operation of the wheelchair and charging facilities must be established, including suitable access when an indoor/outdoor model is requested. If the chair is for a child or person with learning difficulties, an extended assessment period may be needed to ensure safe handling of the chair is understood. Ramps must be of a gradient that is compatible with the wheelchair manufacturer's recommendations while the weight of the chair is a factor when a vertical lift is fitted. Although some powered wheelchairs can be dismantled for car transportation, the components are very heavy and a hoist or ramp may be required.

WHEELCHAIR ACCESSORIES

A wide range of wheelchair accessories is available to allow a wheelchair to be tailored to suit individual needs. Care should be taken to select accessories which are compatible with the chosen wheelchair model. Accessories include:

- 2-inch or 3-inch vinyl seat cushion
- back cushions
- pelvic straps and harnesses for postural support
- extended backrest
- head and neck supports
- thoracic pads for lateral support

- meal tray
- amputee stump support
- elevating leg rests
- mobile arm supports.

WHEELCHAIR CUSHIONS

The range of wheelchair cushions available is increasing due to the rising number of wheelchair users and greater emphasis on the management of pressure needs. There are three main reasons for prescribing wheelchair cushions: comfort and positioning, pressure relief and postural management (White 1999a). Assessment for appropriate wheelchair cushions includes:

- diagnosis and prognosis
- user's weight
- the type of wheelchair in use
- time spent in the chair
- presence of existing pressure sores
- sitting posture
- continence
- sensory impairment
- transferring method
- functional ability
- transportation needs
- comfort.

Assessment tools include numerical risk indicators such as the Waterlow score (Waterlow 1985) or a pressure mapping system (Fig. 7.21).

Wheelchair cushions may be made of different densities of foam or a variety of gel types. Air flotation and battery-operated alternating pressure cushions offer a higher level of pressure relief, while a contoured shape gives improved postural management. Many wheelchair cushions are very expensive and are available subject to local eligibility criteria.

SPECIAL SEATING

Special seating is supplied to people who lack the ability to sit unsupported in a standard wheelchair. Aims of special seating are to:

- maintain a balanced and symmetrical seating position

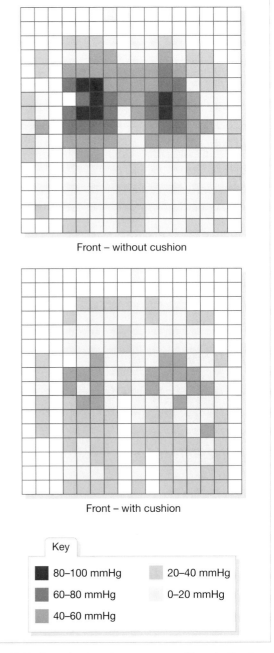

Front – without cushion

Front – with cushion

Key

■ 80–100 mmHg ▨ 20–40 mmHg
■ 60–80 mmHg ░ 0–20 mmHg
■ 40–60 mmHg

Fig. 7.21 Example of seating pressures with and without a suitable cushion (reproduced by kind permission of Sumed International (UK) Ltd).

- reduce susceptibility to pressure sores
- improve functional ability
- reduce spasticity, deformity and discomfort

- improve general health
- reduce the care load.

Assessment includes establishing the user's postural and functional ability, their symmetry and load bearing in sitting, and the presence of fixed deformities. Lifestyle and carers' needs must be included, alongside psychosocial needs and comfort (White 1999b).

Types of wheelchair special seating include fixed format seating systems, adjustable seats, modular seats and customised seats (British Society of Rehabilitation Medicine 1995). The seating unit may be interfaced with a buggy, manual or powered wheelchair in order to fulfil postural, mobility and lifestyle needs (Fig. 7.22).

The case studies in Boxes 7.9 to 7.13 show how the principles of wheelchair prescription are applied when selecting an appropriate wheelchair.

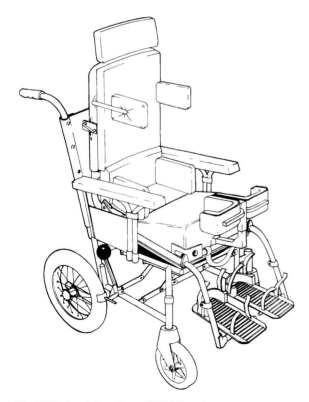

Fig. 7.22 Special seating – CAPS II seating system, (reproduced by kind permission of Active Design Ltd).

Box 7.9 Case study

Mr Jones, a 76-year-old man, had a diagnosis of peripheral vascular disease resulting in a left below-knee amputation. He weighed 12 stone, was 5 feet 8 inches tall and his occupational therapist referred him to the local Wheelchair Service for the provision of a self-propelling wheelchair due to the permanence of his disability.

A model 8L wheelchair with left stump-board was prescribed and delivered to the hospital to give Mr Jones independent mobility. The hospital occupational therapist supplied a 2-inch thick gel and foam cushion for use in the acute stage, which met Mr Jones's pressure needs, provided stability for his residual limb and gave a suitable height to facilitate bed and toilet transfers.

In the preprosthetic stage, occupational therapy included self-care activities and upper limb strengthening, while Mr Jones walked with the Ppam-aid in the parallel bars in the physiotherapy gym. During early limb use, Mr Jones undertook donning and doffing of his limb as part of dressing practice, and was able to interchange the use of the stump-board with the standard wheelchair footplate to match his level of limb use. Once he was able to transfer independently and walk with a zimmer frame, Mr Jones was discharged home.

Following outpatient therapy, Mr Jones achieved a two-point gait using walking sticks, or walked with a trolley when undertaking kitchen activities. The wheelchair was retained for outdoor use and car transportation; a standard 2-inch seat cushion was issued and the stump-board was subsequently returned to the Wheelchair Service.

OUTDOOR TRANSPORT

Changes in society and the expectations of disabled people have resulted in an increase in demand for access to outdoor transport. The issue of indoor/outdoor powered wheelchairs by National Health Service wheelchair services (National Health Service Executive 1996a) has allowed many previously housebound people to go out independently in their locality. Public transport is becoming more accessible to people with mobility problems, with the introduction of wheelchair-accessible buses, trains and taxis and special arrangements for air travel (Department of Transport 1996). The mobility component of the Disability Living Allowance, available to

Box 7.10 Case study

Laura was referred to the Wheelchair Service at the age of three. She was severely affected by spinal muscular atrophy and was unable to sit or stand without support. She could not raise her arms against gravity and wore a spinal brace to aid her support. Her initial referral was for a supportive buggy to fulfil transit needs and to give symmetrical positioning in sitting.

A further referral was received when Laura was four for an indoor powered wheelchair to enable her to achieve independent mobility within her home, as she was unable to walk and could not self-propel in a manual wheelchair. Due to her need for postural support, a seating system was supplied to interface with the powered wheelchair base. Laura's hand function was weak and a centrally mounted touch-sensitive controller was fitted to operate the wheelchair. Two trays were supplied. One had a cut-out for the control switch to enable Laura to support her arms when accessing the controls; the second had a high mounting to facilitate independent feeding. Laura quickly

proved herself a competent driver and her independent mobility enabled her to keep up with her younger brother, who had just learned to walk.

A referral was made to the Social Services and wheelchair access to Laura's home was planned as part of a more major adaptation, which was likely to take up to 2 years to complete.

Laura commenced mainstream education and required powered mobility for independence within the school environment. Due to the lack of wheelchair access at home, her National Health Service powered wheelchair could not be transported to and from school. The Education Department therefore funded a similar model of chair from the same wheelchair supplier and Laura's seating system was used on both chairs.

Once the planned home adaptations are completed, Laura will be assessed for an indoor/outdoor powered wheelchair to extend her independent mobility into her local outdoor environment.

Box 7.11 Case study

Mr Duncan was a 59-year-old man who had suffered from a stroke, resulting in a dense left hemiplegia with no active movement in his arm or leg.

Mobility in the early stages of rehabilitation required the use of a transit wheelchair, which allowed no independence, but excessive use of Mr Duncan's right arm resulted in increased tone in his hemiplegic side. Five months after his stroke, Mr Duncan remained unable to mobilise independently and he was referred to the Wheelchair Service for assessment in an indoor powered wheelchair.

Wheelchair assessment included both Mr Duncan's mobility needs and his postural support. He had a marked pelvic obliquity and was unable to maintain a symmetrical upright sitting posture. An initial assessment in a powered wheelchair revealed a neglect of his left side, which caused difficulties with accurate handling of the wheelchair. Further training in the use of the powered chair as part of Mr Duncan's occupational therapy programme was unable to resolve this problem sufficiently to allow safe unsupervised handling of the chair.

Mr Duncan was discharged to a nursing home with his mobility needs fulfilled by a 9L transit wheelchair. A posturally supportive cushion with additional insert to correct his pelvic obliquity, and a shaped back support with thoracic supports, were fitted to the wheelchair to control his posture. A shaped armrest pad provided support for his hemiplegic arm. Mr Duncan was transferred by hoist and the occupational therapist carried out training for the care staff to ensure that Mr Duncan would be positioned properly in his wheelchair.

Box 7.12 Case study

While diving on holiday, 32-year-old Jane had had an accident resulting in an incomplete lesion of her spinal cord at the level of C6. Following extensive rehabilitation, she was discharged to a ground floor flat and wished to resume an independent lifestyle, including returning to work as a secretary.

Jane's upper limb function was weak but she was able to transfer herself, using a straight sliding board, between her wheelchair, the bed and the driving seat of her car. The car had been adapted to hand controls and Jane obtained a very lightweight wheelchair through the Voucher Scheme, which she was able to dismantle while sitting on the driver's seat and lift the parts of the chair into the car. At work, she had a designated parking space adjacent to the office entrance and, on arrival, called one of her colleagues from her mobile phone to save the energy requirement of unloading the wheelchair herself.

At home, Jane had been assessed by the Social Services Department occupational therapist and adaptations carried out to her flat to facilitate her independence. These included lowering her kitchen work surfaces, adapting her bathroom to a flush-floor shower room and installing a level access with adjacent covered car-port so that she could access her car easily whatever the weather.

Box 7.13   Case study

Mrs Bailey had been diagnosed with multiple sclerosis when she was 38 years old. Her condition gradually deteriorated and, due to her altered abilities, her need for mobility and transfer equipment also changed.

By the time she was 53 Mrs Bailey had become unable to walk and used an indoor powered wheelchair for independent mobility around her home. A ceiling track hoist was mounted over her bed, to enable her carers to transfer her from the bed to the wheelchair for mobility, or to a Mayfair commode for personal hygiene activities. Mrs Bailey had good head control but weak trunk muscles, so a hammock sling was used for safe transfers. She was rolled onto the sling when she was ready to get out of bed and the sling was removed once she was positioned in her wheelchair.

At one time, Mrs Bailey was able to undertake a standing transfer from her wheelchair to the car, aided by a turning disc. When she became unable to weight-bear on her legs, she needed to be transported in her wheelchair. She received the higher level mobility component of the Disability Living Allowance and used this to purchase a vehicle with ramped rear access. A winch mechanism was installed in the vehicle to assist access in her powered wheelchair, then this was clamped using a four-point webbing harness. A separate lap and diagonal seat belt was used to secure Mrs Bailey safely.

severely disabled new claimants between the ages of 5 and 65, may be used to meet the additional costs of outdoor transport or can be used to purchase a car or outdoor powered wheelchair through the Motability scheme (Disability Information Trust 1994).

DRIVING

A person with a disability who wishes to learn to drive, or to return to driving having become disabled, must be as competent as any other road user. Any acquired or worsening disability must be reported to the Driver Vehicle Licensing Authority, who will require a medical report to establish whether a driving licence will be permitted (Disabled Living Foundation 1999).

Mobility Centres offer advice to drivers and passengers with disabilities. They can undertake assessments, which include driving ability, cognitive functioning, concentration levels and reaction times, and visual acuity. Specially trained driving instructors are available to teach people

with disabilities to drive motor vehicles or powered wheelchairs. Recent advances in technology have meant that driving has become a realistic option for many disabled people and perceptual problems or poor concentration are more likely to result in an inability to drive than a physical disability alone.

PASSENGERS

A disabled passenger may not be safely seated in a motor vehicle using a conventional lap and diagonal seat belt and a range of special harnesses and child safety seats is available for use on car, minibus or coach seats.

While recommended safe practice suggests that the safety of passengers is greatest if they can be transferred to a vehicle seat (Medical Devices Directive 1992), some severely disabled or heavy people may need to be transported in their wheelchair (see below). The Blue Badge Scheme, introduced throughout the European Community in January 2000, allows parking concessions for both drivers and passengers who have severe mobility difficulties or are registered as blind (Disabled Living Foundation 1999). This scheme replaced the previous Orange Badge scheme.

TRANSPORTATION OF OCCUPIED WHEELCHAIRS

Suitable access to motor vehicles includes a range of ramps or tail-lifts. Either option must be designed to accommodate the combined weight of the wheelchair plus occupant, while the gradient of any ramp must comply with the wheelchair manufacturer's recommendation for stability of the chair. An increasing number of wheelchair models is being crash-tested for use within a vehicle and each manufacturer's recommendations regarding clamping must be followed. Four-point webbing straps are commonly used, which allow some flexibility in use and do not damage the wheelchair frame, although special seating systems may require additional strapping. The user must be separately secured with a lap and diagonal seat belt. Standard wheelchair pelvic belts are not suitable for this purpose. Occupied wheelchairs must face forwards or backwards, with the chair either placed against a vehicle bulkhead or with headrest fitted to prevent injury in the case of sudden braking.

TRANSPORTATION OF UNOCCUPIED WHEELCHAIRS

An unoccupied manual wheelchair can be transported in the vehicle or car boot. Dismantling is recommended to reduce the lifting weight, while all parts must be secured safely to prevent injury or damage. When the disabled person is the driver, wheelchair selection should include choosing a model that he can lift independently into the car; alternatively, an automatic car roof storage system or hoist can be fitted. Many powered wheelchairs can be dismantled but the weight of their components limits effective car transportation unless suitable ramps or hoisting equipment are available.

While access to outdoor transport is increasing the options available to people with mobility problems, there is little funding available for car conversions and wheelchair lifting equipment. Increasingly, wheelchair services are receiving requests for lightweight models as many users expect to transport or travel with their wheelchairs, and the increasing number of carers who are themselves elderly has underlined this need (Smith et al 1995).

REFERENCES

BackCare 1999 Safer handling of people in the community. BackCare, Middlesex

Beresford SA 1998 Equipment to enable safe patient handling. British Journal of Therapy and Rehabilitation 5(10):13–15

Bowker P, Condie DN, Bader DL, Pratt DJ, Wallace W (eds) 1993 Biomechanical basis of orthotic management. Butterworth Publishers, Boston, MA

British Society of Rehabilitation Medicine 1995 Seating needs for complex disabilities. British Society of Rehabilitation Medicine, London

Bull R 1998 Housing options for disabled people. Jessica Kingsley Publishers, London

Callahan A 1984 Nerve injuries in the upper extremity. In Malick MH, Kasch MC (eds) Manual on management of specific hand problems. American Rehabilitation Educational Network, Harmaville Affiliate, Pittsburg, PA

Cassar S, Costar S 1998 Patient handling aids: prescribing guidelines. British Journal of Therapy and Rehabilitation 5(10):7–9

Chronically Sick and Disabled Persons Act 1970 HMSO, London

CIGOPW 1998 Occupational therapy in the clinical practice of orthotics: standards and guidelines. College of Occupational Therapists, London

Cochrane GM, Wilson AK (eds) 1991 Walking aids, 2nd edn. Disability Information Trust, Oxford

College of Occupational Therapists 1993–6 National prosthetic and wheelchair services report. Department of Health, London

Community Care (Direct Payments) Act 1996. HMSO, London

Coppard BM, Lohman H 1996 Introduction to splinting: a critical thinking and problem solving approach. Mosby, St Louis, MO

Department of Health 1992 Manual handling operation regulations. HMSO, London

Department of Transport 1996 Door to door: a guide to transport for disabled people, 5th edn. HMSO, London

de Kleijn-de Vrankrijker MW, Heerkens YF and van Ravensburg CD 1998 Cited in McColl MA, Bickenbach JE 1998 Introduction to disability. WB Saunders, London

Dimond B 1997 Legal aspects of occupational therapy. Blackwell Science, Oxford

Disability Information Trust 1994 Outdoor transport, 7th edn. Disability Information Trust, Oxford

Disabled Living Foundation 1998a Equipment for positioning, standing and walking. Hamilton Index, part 2 section 8. Disabled Living Foundation, London

Disabled Living Foundation 1998b Manual handling, hoists and lifting equipment. Hamilton Index, part 4 section 20. Disabled Living Foundation, London

Disabled Living Foundation 1999 Transport. Hamilton Index, part 1, section 1. Disabled Living Foundation, London

Disabled Living Foundation 1993 Wheelchair information. Disabled Living Foundation, London

Dudley NJ, McMahon M 1994 The changing pattern of wheelchair provision. Clinical Rehabilitation 8:70–75

Goldsmith S 1984 Designing for the disabled, 3rd edn. RIBA Publications Ltd, London

Health and Safety Executive 1998 Manual handling operations regulations 1992. Guidance on the regulations. HMSC, Norwich

HMSO 1992 Manual handling operations regulations. HMSO, London Housing Grants, Construction and Regeneration Act 1996. HMSO, London

Jerosch-Herold C 1998a Evidence-based practice – how to do a literature search. British Journal of Hand Therapy 3(1):21–23

Jerosch-Herold C 1998b Evidence-based practice – how to critically appraise a research paper. Part II Interpreting the findings and their applicability to practice. British Journal of Hand Therapy 3(3):8–9

Kielhofner G 1992 Conceptual foundations of occupational therapy. FA Davis, Philadelphia, PA

Kielhofner G, Forsyth K 1997 The model of human occupation: an overview of current concepts. British Journal of Occupational Therapy 60(3):103–110

Lister G 1993 The hand: diagnosis and indications, 3rd edn. Churchill Livingstone, Edinburgh

McColl I 1986 A review of artificial limb and appliance centre services. Department of Health and Social Security, London, vol 1

McColl MA, Bickenbach JE 1998 Introduction to disability. WB Saunders, London

McCreadie MJ, James R 1995 An audit of wheelchair service provision in three regions. British Journal of Therapy and Rehabilitation 2(9):465–472

Malick MH 1980 Manual on static hand splinting, 4th edn. Harmarville Rehabilitation Centre, Pittsburg, PA, vol 1

Mandelstam M 1993 How to get equipment for disability, 3rd edn. Jessica Kingsley and Kogan Page for the Disabled Living Foundation, London

Mandelstam M 1998 An A–Z of community care law. Jessica Kingsley Publishers, London

Medical Devices Directive 1992 Safety guidelines for transporting children in special seats. Medical Devices Directive Report MDD/92/07 Medical Devices Directive, Blackpool

National Assistance Act 1948. HMSO, London

National Back Pain Association 1997 The guide to the handling of patients, 4th edn. National Back Pain Association, Middlesex

National Health Service Executive 1996a Powered indoor/outdoor wheelchairs for severely disabled people HSG(96)34. Department of Health, Wetherby

National Health Service Executive 1996b Wheelchair voucher scheme HSG(96)53. Department of Health, Wetherby

NHS and Community Care Act 1990. HMSO, London

Pope P 1996 Postural management and special seating. In: Edwards S (ed) Neurological physiotherapy. Churchill Livingstone, New York, ch 6

Richardson B 1995 Out and about – solving problems of mobility. In: Bumphrey E (ed) Community practice. Prentice Hall/Harvester Wheatsheaf, London, ch 12

Richardson B 1997 The inter-professional curriculum for back care advisors. College of Occupational Therapists, London

Sacket DL, Rosenberg WMC, Muir Gray JA, Haynes RB, Scott Richardson W 1996 Evidence based medicine: what is it and what isn't it. British Medical Journal 312:71–72

Salter M, Cheshire L (eds) 2000 Hand therapy principles and practice. Butterworth–Heinemann, London

Smith C, McCreadie M, Unsworth J 1995 Prescribing wheelchairs: the opinions of wheelchair users and their carers. Clinical Rehabilitation (9):74–80

Waterlow J 1985 A risk assessment card. Nursing Times 81:48–55

White EA 1999a Wheelchair cushions: assessment and prescription. British Journal of Therapy and Rehabilitation 6(2):76–81

White EA 1999b Wheelchair special seating: need and provision. British Journal of Therapy and Rehabilitation 6(6):285–289

FURTHER READING

Disability Information Trust 1998 Manual wheelchairs: a practical guide. Disability Information Trust, Oxford

Disability Information Trust 1998 Powered wheelchairs and scooters: a practical guide. Disability Information Trust, Oxford

Disability Information Trust 1998 Wheelchair accessories. Disability Information Trust, Oxford

Green EM, Mulcahy CM, Pountney TE 1992 Postural management theory and practice. Active Design, Birmingham

Ham R, Aldersea P, Porter D 1998 Wheelchair users and postural seating. Churchill Livingstone, New York

Heywood F 1994 Adaptations: finding ways to say yes. SAUS Publications, Bristol

Heywood F 1996 Managing adaptations: positive ideas for social services. Policy Press, Bristol

Mandlstam M 1997 Equipment for older or disabled people and the law. Jessica Kingsley Publishers, London

Mayall JK, Desharnais G 1995 Positioning in a wheelchair, 2nd edn. Slack Inc., Thorofare, NJ

Mountain G 2000 Occupational therapy in social services departments. A review of the literature. College of Occupational Therapists and Centre for Evidence-based Social Services, London

Munroe H 1996 Clinical reasoning in community occupational therapy. British Journal of Occupational Therapy 59(5):196–202

Nocon A, Chesson R 1997 'Until disabled people get consulted …': the role of occupational therapy in meeting housing needs. British Journal of Occupational Therapy 60(3):115–122

continued

8

Professional context

Sue Griffiths   Donna Schell

INTRODUCTION

At all levels of practice, management is an integral component of occupational therapy and therefore relevant to all practitioners. The following definition of management illustrates how each practitioner is involved in management at some level:

Management is a set of activities (including planning and decision making, organising, leading and controlling), directed at an organisation's resources (human, financial, physical and information) with the aim of achieving organisational goals in an efficient and effective manner.

(Griffin 1993 p5)

Occupational therapists are involved with planning interventions and work schedules, providing input to team, departmental or organisational plans and decision making. Organising other people and resources to put plans into action is a routine activity; likewise setting up and fulfilling policies and procedures. Leading activities incorporates motivating people and communication, as well as leadership, and, as such, the therapist will be involved at treatment and team levels. Controlling activities refers to setting standards, measuring performance and monitoring resources.

Underpinning successful management of practice needs a clear understanding of the context in which it takes place. This context includes the organisational philosophy of health and social care, the strategic direction of its provision and the subsequent structures and systems supporting delivery of that care. Both national and local

* A logo in the margin will identify at which 'level' an issue is being discussed:

I = Individual
S = Service
O = Organisation
N = National.

politics will influence it. The occupational therapist needs to be aware of the context in which she works for the following reasons:

- By understanding the philosophy and thinking behind policy, she can recognise current trends in service delivery and anticipate its future direction. Subsequently, the occupational therapist can be more proactive in determining service delivery. This is particularly important in the constantly changing environment of health and social care in which policies and organisations are frequently reconfigured.
- Occupational therapists are working increasingly in an environment of multi-agency service provision, determined by local needs and the local mix of services available. Traditional professional roles and responsibilities are changing rapidly, several professions will be able to achieve the same health gain but possibly via different routes. Within an atmosphere of cooperation and collaboration, the occupational therapist in the 21st century needs to be aware of the political agenda of reducing professional boundaries and to consider the subsequent impact (positive and negative) on the care of individuals and on the profession.
- The well-informed occupational therapist will have increased professional credibility, which may open up opportunities for influencing health and social care delivery locally.

LEVELS OF PROFESSIONAL CONTEXT

To help structure thinking about professional context, this chapter will look at issues at four levels or from four perspectives (Fig. 8.1).*

Individual occupational therapist level

This level is concerned with the immediate issues of the care of people, workload management, and of personal and professional development. From this position the occupational therapist can consider the other three levels.

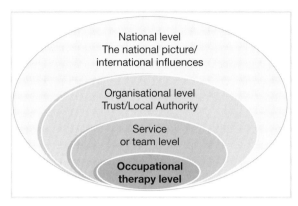

Fig. 8.1 Levels of professional context.

Service or team level

This level relates to service delivery for a specific group or a specific professional service offered. The occupational therapist needs to be aware of the purpose of the service provided to groups of people, commissioning agency requirements, service agreements, monitoring measures as well as routine operational policies and procedures, for example, health and safety policies, record keeping, discharge planning and caseload prioritisation.

Organisational level

As a service provider, the occupational therapist needs to have an idea of the organisation's strategic vision, likely mergers, alliances, changes, provision of services and commissioning requirements. It is useful to understand the planning process and the organisations involved both in planning and delivering health and social care. For example, in the United Kingdom a general understanding of the area's Health Improvement Plan (HImP) and specific requirements for a service area will provide an overview of services planned or available, a service expectation to work to and a framework in which to plan service improvements.

As an employee, the occupational therapist needs to be aware of the organisation's employment conditions, resource allocation skill mix, education/training opportunities and research/development initiatives.

National level

The occupational therapist needs to be aware of what is happening in national health and social care policy in order to understand current service provision and be able to anticipate future needs. Professional journals, newsletters and circulars at work, as well as radio, television and newspapers, are all sources of current information. Likewise, the Internet can provide instantaneous updates on policy development through government websites.

The purpose of this chapter is to present a range of management issues relevant to the student and practising occupational therapist. Profession-specific information will be provided in greater detail than generic management information (to which the reader will be directed in the Further Reading section p251). The chapter comprises three sections:

- policy and professional bodies (it should be noted that the examples of policy are drawn from the United Kingdom, and predominantly from England and Wales)
- employment and professional legislation
- practice.

POLICY AND PROFESSIONAL BODIES

HEALTH AND SOCIAL POLICY CONTEXT IN THE UNITED KINGDOM

The purpose of this section is to put practice into current context, with a short backward glance to health and social care development and an exploration of current trends. A detailed investigation of the development of health and welfare services can be traced through other textbooks identified in the Further Reading section (p251).

Prior to the 'welfare state', the voluntary sector initiated and provided a wide range of social services from which most state provision can trace its origins. The first National Health Service (NHS) Act (HMSO 1946) promoted the establishment of a comprehensive health service to address the needs of people with physical and mental health problems by providing care, advice and treatment (free at the point of delivery). In 1948, healthcare was divided into hospital services, teaching hospitals, community health (run by local authorities) and independent contractors. This cumbersome service remained in operation until 1974, when local authority health services were embraced by the NHS and a new management structure was established. In 1983 a review of the management of the NHS was commissioned, which resulted in introducing general management principles.

While one upheaval in the NHS followed another, local government was not without its share of change. The 1948 National Assistance Act (HMSO 1948) established the welfare role of local authorities; for example, residential care for elderly people and services for those with long-term and permanent disabilities. The Local Authority Social Services (LASS) Act 1970 (HMSO 1970b) heralded new 'welfare' organisations – social service departments within local government. The Chronically Sick and Disabled Persons Act 1970 (HMSO 1970a), the forerunner of virtually all 'disability' legislation in the UK today, provided specific services for people in the community. In addition, provisions made by housing departments, public and environmental health departments and education authorities had a far-reaching impact on personal social services.

In the 1980s it was generally recognised that demand for both health and social care had exceeded supply. There were no clear guidelines for prioritising care or rationing services according to greatest need. There was a lack of parity in the provision of health and social care across the nation and also between care groups. Informal social care through voluntary and private sectors was available but not coordinated and potentially haphazard. Concurrently the philosophy of community care had infiltrated thinking with the intention of treating and maintaining people in their own homes, by providing care and support in the community (as opposed to hospital) to facilitate maximum independence.

Radical changes to address these issues were implemented through the 1990 NHS and Community Care Act (HMSO 1990). The Act separated the purchasing of healthcare from its provision and created an internal market through which purchase and provision was agreed and monitored. This trend was seen to a lesser extent in local authorities, where social services became purchasers and coordinators of mixed economy care packages and less involved in providing social care. The intention was to make greater use of the private, independent and voluntary sectors.

Management responsibility was devolved to smaller units of organisation, for example the newly created self-governing healthcare trusts, and clinical accountability across the professions was introduced through a system of clinical audit. Market forces were used to encourage competition between providers, thereby driving down the cost of healthcare.

A change in government in 1997 led to a change in policy, which discarded competition through an internal market and instead encouraged collaboration and commissioning. The White Papers 'The new NHS: modern, dependable' (HMSO 1997) and 'A first class service' (HMSO 1998a) outlined a number of changes, which became statutory through the Health Act of 1999. GP surgeries were grouped together into Primary Care Trusts (PCTs) (Fig. 8.2) with a remit to promote the health of their local population, reduce inequalities in healthcare provision and develop both primary care and community services. An infrastructure was developed to improve the quality of service delivery with national bodies to issue guidelines for clinical interventions (National Institute for Clinical Excellence; NICE), set standards for service delivery (National Service Frameworks; NSF) and monitor local quality measures (Clinical Governance) in trusts and Primary Care Groups/Trusts (PCTs) through the Commission for Health Improvements (CHImP). These are discussed further from page 245 onwards.

CURRENT TRENDS IN HEALTH AND SOCIAL CARE

The following trends have been drawn from a wide range of health, social care and management sources. They represent the professional

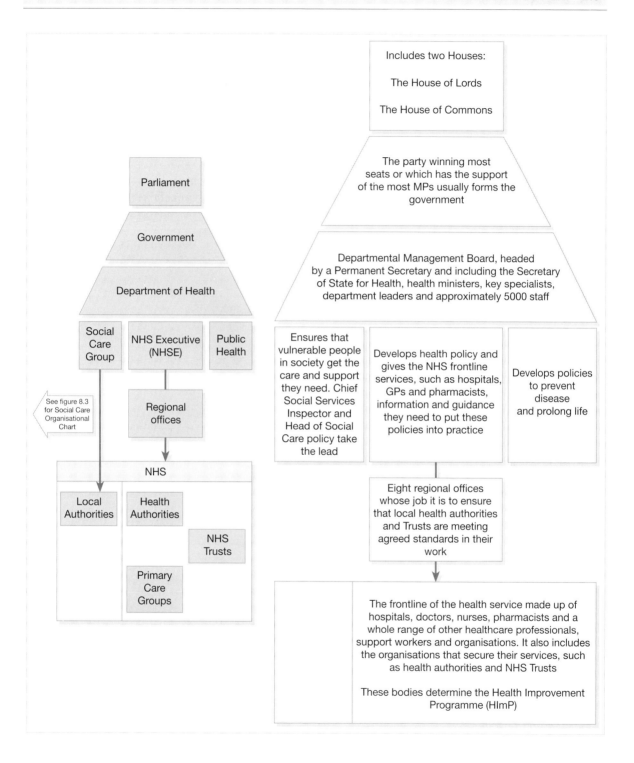

Fig. 8.2 Organisation and key responsibilities of the Department of Health and NHS, 2001.

context at time of publication. Some may stand the test of time, others may not and should therefore be tested against current literature.

Person-centred care

There is an increasing transfer of resources into primary care to fulfil the concept of community care, with a concurrent devolvement of responsibility for healthcare to the individual. The user is increasingly better informed through service information, the media and the Internet. Consequently, he is more proactive in determining health and social care options. Organisational structures are being reconfigured to facilitate greater user involvement in commissioning service provision and influencing person-centred service delivery. There is a move towards greater transparency in clinical decision-making, for example discussion of healthcare options as opposed to prescription, user access to patient records and copies of letters between professionals. The regular use of user focus groups, the consultation process for the National Health Service Plan, national patient and user experience surveys, the potential use of citizens' juries (Lenaghan et al 1996) and lay involvement in research and development programmes (Oliver 1996) are all indicative of the rising power of the user's voice. Health and social care delivery is subsequently user-focused and less professionally directed or dominant.

Collaborative and integrated care

Collaboration, or working together for the benefit of the individual, is encouraged in local and national policy. At a national level, a 'duty of cooperation' is required within the NHS and between the NHS and local authorities with statutory mechanisms for strategic planning, pooled funds, integrated provision and 'operational flexibilities' (HMSO 1999). At an organisational level, it is evident in joint planning and commissioning through the HImP; joint working ventures with local authorities; the independent and charitable sectors.

At service delivery level, integrated care (Box 8.1) expects services to be arranged around

Box 8.1 Definitions of types of care (adapted from Abreu et al 1996, Hitchens 2000, McDonald 1999, National Health Service Executive 2000b)

Primary care
Refers to community-based care. It is usually a person's first contact with healthcare and includes services provided by GPs, nurses and other professions (occupational therapists, physiotherapists, counsellors) employed or contracted by GP surgeries. Dentists are also included.

Secondary care
Refers to hospital-based or specialist care. Entry to secondary care is through GP referral, self-referral and Accident and Emergency departments.

Intermediate care
Refers to temporary residential care for patients whose needs are beyond the capacity of the primary care team (or the carer) but who do not need the services of a district general hospital. It may include rehabilitation or just provide 'recovery' time.

Continuing care
Refers to 'care provided by the NHS beyond the acute phase of illness and rehabilitation, in whatever setting is most appropriate: hospital, nursing home or the patient's own home' (McDonald 1999). The criterion for continuing care is a need for continuous or frequent medical or specialist nursing intervention.

Integrated care
Is where organisations, funding and professional boundaries are overcome to arrange health and social care services around the needs of the individual.

Critical or care pathway
Is the route through a continuum of care for a given health condition, where all the procedures and services are identified and anticipated within a time frame. The contribution of each member of the multidisciplinary team is identified and standards for service delivery agreed

the needs of the individual as opposed to organisational or professional boundaries. Critical or care pathways (Box 8.1) (tools originally intended to anticipate and cost packages of care) are being used to evaluate a person's experience through an episode of care and overcome professional or organisational boundaries where necessary. Interprofessional working is expected, requiring an understanding of each team member's role and a willingness to share common professional tasks to allow optimum use of the skill mix available. Specialised assessments, treatments and skills will remain the domain of individual professions. Career paths are less likely to follow traditional progression through professional grades and are more likely to be flexible, following clinical rather than professional specialisation.

Lifelong learning

Lifelong learning is encouraged for all staff, and the maintenance of a licence to practice through professional re-registration will be dependent on this (Health Profession Council p222). Professional self-regulation is mandatory but clinical accountability is taken beyond personal responsibility to being watchful of fellow team members.

Recognition of 'talents'

There is an increasing recognition in management of the value of people, in particular 'talents' or people with special skills, imagination, dreams, innovation and charisma. 'A Health Service of all the Talents' (2000a) draws on a commercial world concept that a company is as good as its 'talents' (Chowdhury 2000). There is therefore a need to identify or attract talents because they have the potential to stimulate others, share knowledge and encourage a culture of excitement.

People-friendly management

There is a move towards people-friendly management (Chowdhury 2000), promoting mutual respect and care that is consistent with the co-operation and collaboration theme. Working towards a common vision goes beyond cascading management's goals to capturing emotional commitment and corporate imagination.

Evidence-based and knowledge-based cultures

The evidence-based movement seeks to base practice decisions on the best research evidence available. Knowledge-based decision making has also come into the arena from social care origins. It draws on a broader set of information, incorporating user research and practitioner perspectives. Such concepts, in conjunction with endeavours to achieve parity of health and social care provision,

have led to setting national standards and guidelines for service delivery and interventions (see p246). Quality in health and social care is now expected and the focus of that quality has moved beyond access and information to effectiveness of practice.

POLICY MAKING AND INFLUENCING THE POLITICAL AGENDA

The Department of Health is one of a number of government departments charged with responsibilities relating to health and social care in the United Kingdom. Its structure and relationship with the NHS and local authorities is illustrated in Figures 8.2 and 8.3. The Department of Health and the three groups (i.e. Social Care, National Health Service Executive (NHSE) and Public Health) are responsible for national policy making in health and social care and creating a system that lives up to expectations. The Department of Health obtains profession-specific and care group advice from its own staff, for example, the Occupational Therapy Officer, NHS and LASS employees, who join inspection teams and task groups as required.

The Occupational Therapy Officer establishes a robust relationship with the professional association, the British Association/College of Occupational Therapy and attends all BAOT/COT Council meetings to enable two-way communication (Fig. 8.4).

A basic understanding of political systems is important when a profession wishes to influence policy and strategy. Members of the profession are encouraged to speak out and assert views in a local or national arena. Attracting media attention to aspects of practice is another method of influencing opinion and understanding. Promoting a better understanding of practice and its potential for health gain is critical for future professional success. Lobbying MPs can be effective at all levels and demands differing degrees of formality. The College of Occupational Therapists (COT), our professional body, lobbies MPs and ministers on our behalf, attempting to promote the principles we believe in as a profession. Equally, approaching one's own MP can be

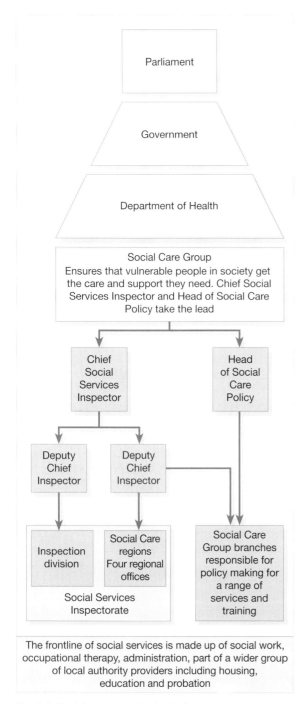

The frontline of social services is made up of social work, occupational therapy, administration, part of a wider group of local authority providers including housing, education and probation

Fig. 8.3 Social care organisational chart.

another route to communicate our views and needs.

It is useful for occupational therapists to understand the procedure for the making of policy and legislation, in order to take opportunities to influence. Figure 8.5 gives an outline of this process.

If occupational therapists are to influence the political agenda of the day, they must investigate opportunities where there is potential for evidence of gain through their intervention and where there are available funds invested. More emphasis remains on prevention rather than cure and, consequently, there is evidence of more investment of government funds into early intervention work. Government priorities are described in their manifesto and in more detail in specific plans they develop. In the UK, 'The NHS National Plan' (2000b) currently provides a clear description of areas in which extra funding is to be invested – it is these areas that have to attract our attention as a profession if we want to be 'heard'. 'Dependence' costs the nation dearly and occupational therapists are in an opportune position to effect change in this area.

PROFESSIONAL BODIES

Professional bodies have responsibility for the promotion of good practice and the prevention of malpractice. They are concerned that occupational therapists achieve and continuously maintain high standards of competence. An occupational therapist is personally accountable for actively maintaining their professional competence and familiarising themselves with current issues affecting practice.

The British Association of Occupational Therapists (BAOT) and the College of Occupational Therapists (COT)

The profession of occupational therapy in the United Kingdom is administered, represented and regulated by a body consisting of two interlinked companies:

- British Association of Occupational Therapists (BAOT)
- College of Occupational Therapists (COT).

The BAOT is the 'parent' organisation and includes Union membership. This Union will

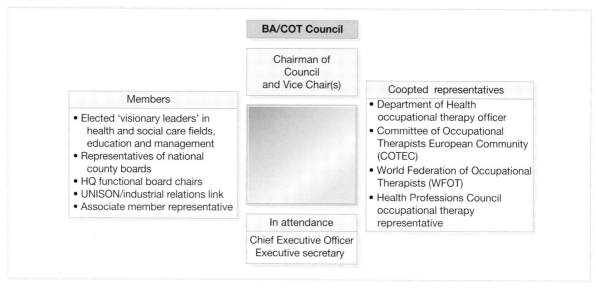

Fig. 8.4 BAOT/COT Council organisational structure, 2000.

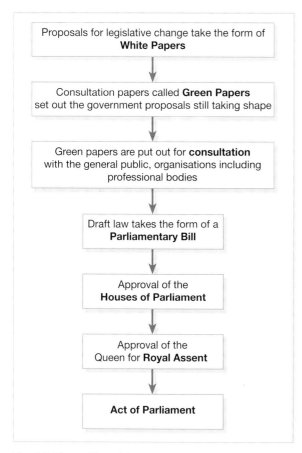

Fig. 8.5 The making of the law in the UK.

provide a series of services to its members, related to employment conditions and rights. It will:

● negotiate improvements to pay and terms and conditions of employment, locally and nationally
● provide support and/or representation for members facing problems at work
● enable members to influence issues affecting them at work and in the wider community
● provide mechanisms for members to determine policy on issues specific to the profession
● provide a range of specially negotiated benefits that can save money.

The COT deals with the professional standards and educational aspects of occupational therapy, together with the development of research activity, evidence-based practice and continuing professional development for its members. The COT represents the profession at a local, national and international level. Its advisory role is crucial in influencing all government policies and procedures affecting the practice of occupational therapy. Box 8.2 presents the mission statement for the BAOT/COT current at the time of publication.

Council is the policy-making forum of the organisation. Council members are mainly elected from their local representative group of members and from the Board of Directors of the

---

Box 8.2 The BAOT/COT's mission (College of Occupational Therapists 2000b)

'Members First' is the vision statement produced by the Council. This statement contains the purpose of the organisation and within that its commitment to its members. It states:

'The College of Occupational Therapists aims to provide a clear identity for all its members through the provision of the highest standard of expert, professional opinion and advice informed by research, scholarship, innovation and promotion of excellence in practice.

The College will provide timely, responsive, specialist support for all members to encourage the personal and intellectual development of confident, competent occupational therapists and support staff.

The College values the contribution of all members and will build upon the trust of its members by establishing an accountable, responsive, learning professional organisation, managed with integrity, probity and sound financial stewardship.

The College is concerned with the achievement of healthy outcomes through occupation and will actively support the provision of efficient, reliable and effective services which benefit all users of occupational therapy.'

BAOT (see Fig. 8.4). The organisation has elected Boards, responsible to Council, which set the work agenda and priorities for the corresponding Groups at headquarters. The work of these Boards broadly falls into the three categories shown in Figure 8.6.

Occupational therapists and support workers are encouraged to participate in activities to support and develop their profession at a national, regional and local level. Members can participate in committees and groups that repre-

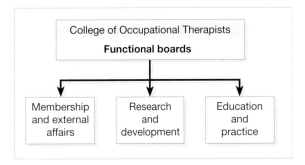

Fig. 8.6 BAOT/COT Boards and Groups.

sent their locality or they can focus on specialist fields of practice, for which in the United Kingdom there are a number of active specialist sections and special interest groups.

CODE OF ETHICS AND PROFESSIONAL CONDUCT

The BAOT/COT produces a public statement of the values and principles used in promoting and maintaining high standards of professional behaviour in occupational therapy. The purpose of the Code of Ethics (College of Occupational Therapists 2000a) is to 'provide a set of principles that apply to occupational therapy personnel at all levels, including students'. Provided to all BAOT members, this document does not impose a legal obligation on practitioners but it does set out a framework for ethical practice, which COT stipulates that members should adhere to. Employers may incorporate the phrase 'adherence to one's professional code of conduct' within the contract of employment, thereby establishing a contractual obligation.

The Code provides essential guidance and information concerning client autonomy and welfare, services to clients, personal and professional integrity, professional competence and standards.

PROFESSIONAL COMPETENCIES

The ability of an individual to work to an agreed standard of professional practice relies upon the foundation of sound theoretical knowledge and subsequent development of increasing, advanced clinical skills. Individuals gain a level of expertise and competence throughout their basic training in order to qualify and register. It is their responsibility to maintain and further advance this level after registration (College of Occupational Therapists 2000a, 5.1.1). Indeed, current expectations now demand evidence of one's continued competence to practice in order to fulfil regulatory standards. This particularly applies to those who take breaks in service.

Employing authorities require their employees to work to a specific level of competence and describe this in an employee's job description. Expectations exceeding this level of competence must be met by appropriate training. Interviews are often designed around these expectations of competence and applicants are invited to provide evidence that they have or can work to the required level. Staff with supervisory responsibilities must delegate within the skill and competence of the staff member and provide adequate supervision whilst retaining overall responsibility for the delegated task.

During the late 1990s, the United Kingdom introduced national occupational standards for professional activity in health promotion and care, designed to be applied to a range of health professions. The occupational standards provide a description of competent professional performance to achieve high quality services. They cover activities in three broad areas (Box 8.3). Each of these three broad areas is then divided into 'key roles', within which units of competence describe good practice. Elements, the basic building blocks of standards, then provide the detailed descriptions of competent performance. An example of an occupational standard applicable to occupational therapy is provided in Figure 8.7.

The standards define functions and outcomes in clear, precise and measurable terms. In the same way that service providers can use the standards to describe the services they offer, commissioners can use them to specify the services they require. Many public sector organisations in the United Kingdom are using occupational standards to support the reshaping of services, procedures and skill mix.

Locally, managers of occupational therapy services are using the standards to compile job descriptions for all grades of staff, to establish training and development plans, for recruitment purposes and to ensure staff work within their boundaries and levels of competence. Individuals can benefit from the logical description of what is required of them, knowing that they have a sound evidence base and comparability with their colleagues.

PROFESSIONAL AND EMPLOYMENT REGULATION

This section considers the mechanisms in place to regulate both professional practice and employment. Although these are national edicts, it is vital for the individual occupational therapist to be aware of these regulations, which guide and safeguard the practitioner, user and employer.

REGISTRATION

Registration is each therapist's licence to practice, aiming to guarantee competence to treat, monitor performance, hold individuals accountable and restrict the use of professional titles, such as 'occupational therapist'. It is the public's guarantee of protection. A therapist's professional framework for practice commences with a recognised pre-registration course in occupational therapy. These courses must be approved, meet statutory and professional practice requirements, and ensure that standards are enforced so that occupational therapists are safe, competent practitioners.

REGULATING PRACTICE

Government legislation places paramount importance on the need to have stringent mechanisms in place to regulate practice. In 'The New NHS: Modern and Dependable' commitments to 'strengthen the systems of self-regulation, by ensuring they are open, responsive and publicly

---

Box 8.3 Broad areas of occupational standards (Department of Employment and Education 1997)

The foundations of professional activity
Basic competencies upon which professional practice is built, such as ethics and practice, self- and team development, communicating, working with colleagues and other agencies.

The context of professional activity
Describes the context in which services are being delivered: describes policy development, research commissioning services, projects and activities and managing services.

The range of professional activities
Deals with activities that may be engaged in to optimise health and social wellbeing.

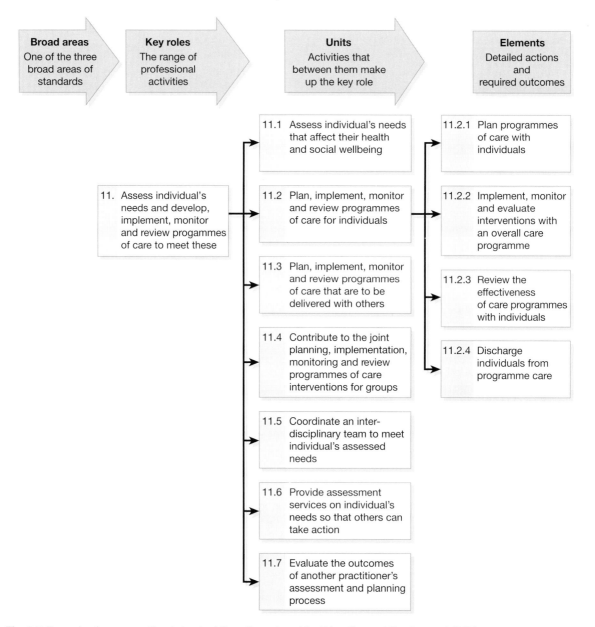

Fig. 8.7 Example of an occupational standard (from Department for Education and Employment 1997).

accountable' (HMSO 1997) are evidence of this. References in the Health Act 1999 further support this priority by ensuring that standards of professional self-regulation are rigorous and in line with the valid expectations of patients' (HMSO 1999).

THE UK'S REGULATION BODY

Regulatory systems in the United Kingdom are established and monitored by the Health Professions Council (HPC), arising from the Health Act 1999. It has four statutory committees (Box 8.4) each with different responsibilities.

Box 8.4 Health Professions Council committees

Investigating committee
Permanent, with representation from professional bodies, peer and lay members.

Health committee
Powers to investigate where a registrant is unable to practise due to ill-health, where suspension rather than disciplinary action is more appropriate.

Professional conduct committee
Will hold a range of powers to reprimand, suspend, re-educate, fine and 'strike off'.

Education committee
Concerned with pre- and post-registration education and ongoing professional competence.

The HPC establishes UK-wide standards of training, professional conduct and competence for each profession, for the protection of the public and the guidance of employers. This is underpinned by accountability of practitioners for maintaining safe and effective practice wherever they are employed. Measures will be in place to deal with individuals whose continuing practice presents an unacceptable risk to the public.

(HPC Draft consultation document, DOH 1999)

The HPC incorporates a Professional Advisory Panel, which represents all professions. It is responsible for promoting high standards of professional education and professional conduct. It prepares, maintains and publishes a register with separate parts for each profession. The HPC approves training courses, the professional qualification and the educational institutions. It imposes restrictions on individuals using registered titles, so restricting unqualified individuals from referring to themselves as 'occupational therapists'.

The HPC introduces mechanisms to measure individuals' competence to practice. This requires practitioners to demonstrate evidence of continued competence at agreed intervals. A comprehensive record of personal and professional development activities is integral to this evidence and all practitioners should be active in maintaining a professional portfolio throughout their career. The COT provides guidelines on continuing professional development portfolios to support this. To ensure these regulatory safeguards are fully beneficial, it is a legal requirement that public sector employees are registered and maintain this registration. Registration should be checked by employers upon appointment and annually thereafter.

LITIGATION IN THE UNITED KINGDOM

The upsurge in litigation in health and social care in recent years has resulted in the need for occupational therapists to raise their awareness and knowledge concerning their practice and how it relates to the law. The following summarises legal issues relevant to the practice of occupational therapy. However, the issues are complex and the reader is advised to explore these issues further through the Further Reading section (p251).

Negligence

Litigation refers to proceedings in the civil courts, which include claims of negligence. Negligence can be implied only in circumstances where harm has been caused and it may take two forms:

- negligence by act relates to an action that ought not to have been undertaken
- negligence by omission relates to an action that was not undertaken but should have been.

Dimond (1997) identifies four components to negligence:

- duty of care
- breach of the duty of care
- causation
- harm.

Duty of care

'Occupational Therapists have a duty of care to take reasonable care for clients whom they accept for treatment/intervention' (College of Occupational Therapists 2000a p3, 2.2). A duty of care is the therapist's professional responsibility to ensure that her actions or omissions do not cause reasonably foreseeable harm to an individual. The issue is complex in terms of how far the duty of care extends and when a practitioner is absolved of her duty of care if, for example, a client refuses treatment or advice.

Breach of duty of care

To determine a breach in duty of care, the required standard of care has to be established (Dimond 1997). This is done by identifying the standard of competencies and skills expected of an ordinary practitioner with the same level of training, years of experience following the accepted, approved standard of care.

However, there are exceptions: the law accepts that people do make mistakes. Therefore, the therapist acting 'in good faith' who makes 'an error of judgement' may not be seen as in breach of her duty of care. It is vital, none the less, that staff are able to justify their choice and method of intervention according to current practices.

Causation

Causation is concerned with the claimant showing that there was a breach of duty of care and that the breach caused actual and 'reasonably foreseeable harm'.

Harm

Actual harm in the form of personal injury, death and loss or damage to property has to be established before compensation can be considered.

Vicarious liability

An employer is usually liable for harm wrongfully caused by employees and damages may be awarded against him or her if an employee is negligent. According to the concept of vicarious liability 'provided you are acting within the agreed responsibilities of your job, then your employer accepts that damage caused during the course of your legitimate duties is his responsibility' (British Association of Occupational Therapists 1990). However, if a staff member causes damage to a third party whilst acting outside her legitimate duties she will be said to be 'on a frolic of her own'. The employer can then refuse to accept vicarious liability and the individual could become personally liable. Therefore, it is wise for practitioners to have professional indemnity, such as that offered by the BAOT.

Referrals for treatment

Following acceptance of the referral, a duty of care to that individual will have been initiated. Therefore, any intervention must be accepted practice and at least to a basic standard and level of service. If for any reason these basic standards cannot be met, occupational therapy staff should not accept a referral or commence treatment (College of Occupational Therapists 2000a section 3.1).

Acceptance of treatment

Underpinning acceptance of treatment is the recognition and respect of the individual's autonomy and involvement in the treatment decision-making process (College of Occupational Therapists 2000a section 2). An individual participates in treatment by consent. His participation in an activity is an implicit acceptance of any risk involved, provided that the activity has been explained and the risks are comprehended. Under common law, an individual has the right to give, or withhold, consent prior to examination or treatment. Exceptions include urgent or life-saving treatment, statutory requirements to examine individuals under Public Health legislation and detention under certain sections of the Mental Health Act 1983. People are entitled to receive sufficient information, in a manner they understand, about the proposed treatments, any alternatives and any substantial risks, so that they can make a balanced judgement. Care should also be taken to respect an individual's wishes.

Consent to treatment may be 'implied' or 'expressed'. It is implied by compliant actions, for instance attending for assessment or offering an affected hand for the fitting of an orthosis. In express consent the individual confirms his agreement in explicit terms, orally or in writing. Oral consent may be sufficient for the vast majority of contacts with clients, by a profession such as occupational therapy. Written consent should be obtained for any procedure or treatment that carries any substantial risk or has a significant side-effect. Both types of consent should be recorded in clients' notes.

Issues of professional competency are covered on page 220 and supervision on page 234.

EMPLOYMENT

As health and social care is delivered by a widening range of providers, so the diversity of potential employers of occupational therapists increases (Fig. 8.8). Public sector occupational therapy staff may be employed either on nationally agreed remuneration scales and conditions or on those agreed locally. In addition there will be local policies and procedures, which an employing authority has set within national guidelines. These concern, for example, accident reporting, fire policy, grievance and disciplinary procedures, and health and safety.

The practical implementation of employment is covered in the section on human resources (pp226-234), whilst the regulatory structure is detailed below. Most of the framework for managing human resources is still provided by legislation, current national management and staff-side agreements plus a wide range of health and local authority circulars. A number of the key Acts are summarised in Table 8.1.

Grievance and disciplinary procedures

These procedures, which form part of the contract of employment, exist to ensure fairness, consistency, equity and to facilitate the management process. They aim to establish particular standards of performance and to assist in the management of difficult situations. Public sector employers issue all employees with a copy of the organisation's procedures. In the event of a grievance, such as level of grade or behaviour towards the employee, an employee formally takes up an issue of concern

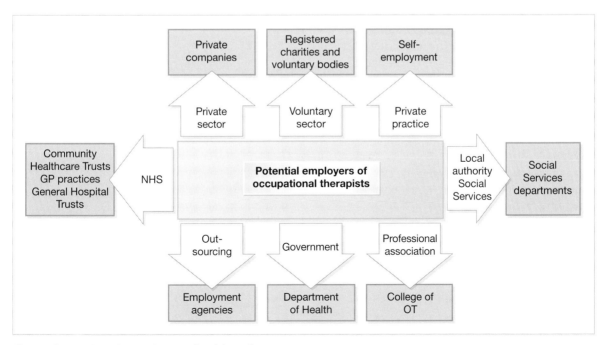

Fig. 8.8 Potential employers of occupational therapists.

Table 8.1 Employment law relevant to the practice of occupational therapy

Act	Key provision	Act	Key provision
The Health Act (1999)	State registration of therapists employed in the public sector	Race Relations Act 1976 (amended 2000)	Ensures that no employee receives less favourable treatment on grounds of gender, race, marital status, disability through the recruitment, training or promotion process
Health and Safety at Work Act (1974)	Safe working systems and safe working conditions	Sex Discrimination (1975/86) and Race Relations (1976)	Unlawful to discriminate against anyone on grounds of race, sex and marital status
Employment Protection (1975)	Protects employees from unfair dismissal	Disability Discrimination 1995/99	Provision for disabled people to access public services without discrimination. Further addition in 1999 to provide for the employment of disabled people

with her line manager. A disciplinary procedure is a formal process for improving the employee's performance and/or behaviour, which is judged inadequate for the job. This procedure includes verbal and written warnings to ensure employee compliance with the organisation's rules. There will be penalties for misconduct and poor performance, including summary dismissal for certain offences such as theft.

To ensure consistency, equity and fairness these procedures must:

- be agreed between management and the staff side as legitimate and written down
- promote consistency in similar situations
- define the authority of the individuals operating them
- structure, and therefore clarify, the relationship between managers as delegated power holders of the organisation and the agreed appeals system
- be logical, that is, follow proper procedural stages
- enshrine and legitimise employees' rights to representation
- eliminate victim isolation.

PRACTICE

RESOURCES AND SYSTEMS

Organisational goals

The definition of management given in the introduction identified a set of activities 'directed at an organisation's resources with the aim of achieving organisational goals' (Griffin 1993). An organisation should have a strategic vision for its future with goals identified to achieve that vision (see Box 8.5 for terminology). The vision, mission and goals should be corporate and ideally owned by each member of staff, working towards the vision. Although the organisation's goals may be broad, it behoves smaller units (departments, teams or services) to translate them in to their own specific goals. It is helpful for a team to consider its specific vision, mission, values and goals for its part of the service.

The organisation's resources involved in achieving the corporate goals can be divided up into human, financial, facility and information resources. This section will consider some of the resource management systems of routine use to the student or newly qualified occupational therapist.

HUMAN RESOURCES

The most valuable and costly resource to any health or social care organisation is its staff or its 'human' resource. This section looks at providing human resources at a national level through

---

Box 8.5   Terminology of strategic planning

- **Vision** – a picture of the organisation's future success.
- **Mission** – a statement of purpose.
- **Values** – the organisation's guiding principles and beliefs.
- **Goals** – identified action to achieve the vision.
- **Strategies** – approaches and methods to achieve goals.

workforce planning, then staffing a service at an organisation or service level and finally it considers employment issues at the individual level, where the occupational therapist is the human resource.

Workforce planning

To understand the staffing levels and skill mix available in your service area, it is helpful to consider who determines the number of health and social care workers available, the mix of professions and level of skill. Health and social services rely upon there being sufficient staff available with the right skills to offer a comprehensive and efficient service. The process of workforce planning was radically changed through recommendations outlined in 'A Health Service for All The Talents' (HMSO 2000a). This suggested mechanisms for determining skill mix (Fig. 8.9) to ensure:

- integration between workforce plans, service and financial plans

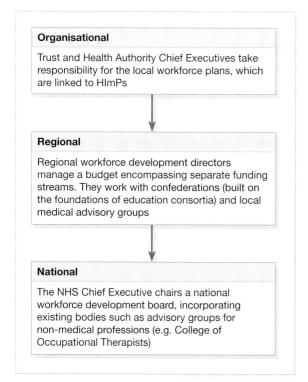

Organisational

Trust and Health Authority Chief Executives take responsibility for the local workforce plans, which are linked to HImPs

Regional

Regional workforce development directors manage a budget encompassing separate funding streams. They work with confederations (built on the foundations of education consortia) and local medical advisory groups

National

The NHS Chief Executive chairs a national workforce development board, incorporating existing bodies such as advisory groups for non-medical professions (e.g. College of Occupational Therapists)

Fig. 8.9 Proposed workforce planning arrangements (adapted from HMSO 2000a).

- a holistic, flexible approach to workforce planning across primary, secondary and tertiary care and across staff groups
- responsiveness to service change
- ability to support multidisciplinary working.

In practice, the flexible approach described in the second entry in the list above can be seen in the evolution of nurse prescribing and nurse consultant posts to alleviate workload pressures on medics. Likewise, therapist consultant posts, generic practitioners and assistants show increased speciality for some areas and generic working for others, according to service need. Consequently, the structure and delivery of education for health and social care is included in the reforms to meet the changing needs of the workforce.

In the past, the role of the allied health professions has often been undervalued and misunderstood. However, in the consultation document 'Meeting the Challenge: A Strategy for the Allied Health Professions' (HMSO 2000) their value is reinforced and the commitment extends to ensure skills are used flexibly and creatively to benefit clients.

The effective management of staff in public sector services is critical to the success and modernisation of these services (National Health Service Executive 2000). Of particular importance is their availability, suitability, competence and motivation to work. To guide effective management of staff, the National Health Service Executive's Publication 'Human Resource Performance Framework' (ibid) has been issued, giving NHS Regional Offices the leäd responsibility to ensure national targets are met for three performance objectives:

- improving working lives
- working together
- developing the workforce.

These objectives are expanded in Box 8.6.

Another national scheme to promote investment and development of staff is the Investors in People Standard. Organisations (public sector and private) can apply for accreditation through meeting, or exceeding, the minimum standard for investing in its workforce. The Investors in People Standard incorporates four main principles:

Box 8.6   Human Resources Performance Framework (National Health Service Executive 2000a)

Improving working lives	**Working together**	**Developing the workforce**
The Improving Working Lives campaign was launched in 1999. The standard aims to create a well managed flexible working environment that supports staff, promotes their welfare and development and provides a productive balance between work and life outside work.	Working Together – securing a quality workforce for the NHS – was launched in 1998 and marked the beginning of a process aimed at improving the standards of human resource (HR) management. The targets included: • employers have training and development plans for the majority of health professional staff • employers meet the criteria to use the employment service disability symbol • employers have plans to meet the three 'equality aims' • reducing the incidents of violence to staff, accidents at work and levels of sickness.	Region-wide initiatives to maximise the number of nurses and health professions employed and to tackle shortages. The Regional Offices will work with confederations and other bodies to plan for the priority services, to agree targets for vacancy, turnover rates and return to employment.

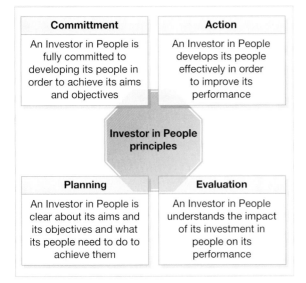

Fig. 8.10 Principles of the Investors in People accreditation standard.

commitment, planning, action and evaluation (Fig. 8.10). The identification and communication of organisational aims and objectives and the process of individual performance review (see p231) are both integral to the award's standards.

Staffing a service

In the past, an occupational therapy service was staffed according to its establishment, that is, a specified number of employees by grade for which the service was provided with a pay budget. Increasingly, the trend is to staff a service within a cash-limited, agreed budget, which must allow for staff salaries, travelling and subsistence, study leave, uniform (NHS), any allowances, equipment, materials and publications. Within this framework, the manager has to provide a staffing structure, that is, the ideal skill mix to accomplish the service's objectives and undertake the daily workload. The manager will thus utilise her resources flexibly, continually weighing service demands against both staff and non-staff resources at her disposal. To provide the most cost-effective, high-quality service, a manager needs to plan, modify and/or develop her human resource requirements. Workforce planning at this level involves assessing skill mix, that is, identifying the balance needed between state registered occupational therapists, other qualified and trained staff and those who hold no formal qualifications. Managers should review the skill mix continuously, as client needs and service delivery change with time.

It is essential that a structured and well-planned approach to recruitment is adopted. This will ensure that the most suitable person is recruited and the legal requirements met. The process starts with the job specification and ends with the successful candidate being inducted to the post; it is outlined in Figure 8.11.

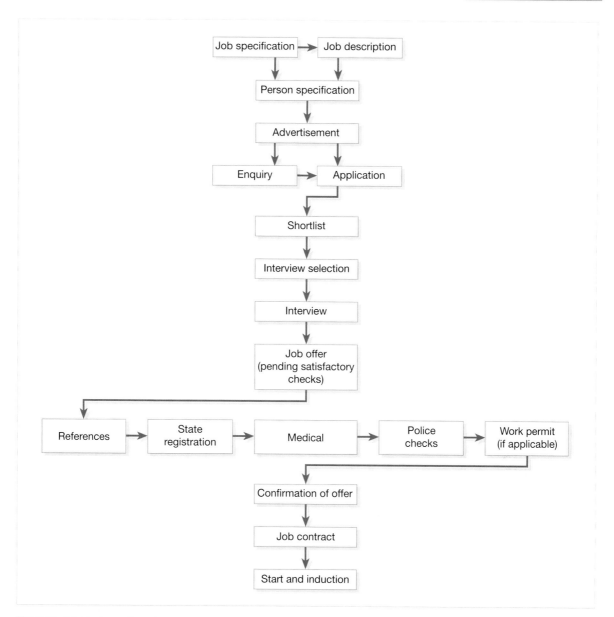

Fig. 8.11 A typical recruitment process.

The therapist as an employee

Seeking employment that suits the therapist's needs and career aspirations is a challenge, which many find complicated and stressful. The compatibility of 'postholder with post' is paramount in meeting the needs of the employing authority and the individual therapist. This section reviews the process of securing a post from the perspective of the therapist and looks at areas of good practice, which she will need to undertake when developing a career pathway.

Advertisements

One of the first sources of information available is in an advertisement. This 'broadcast' of the employer's requirements is crucial in attracting the right applicant. A good advert is aimed at the right audience, gives an adequate description of the post, presents the right image and is in the right publication at the right time.

Specifications and job description

The job and person specifications are the 'blueprints' against which the most suitable candidate can be matched. They are valuable sources of information for prospective applicants to determine job suitability. The job specification provides information on the overall purpose of the job, why the job exists and the key tasks or activities of the position. The person specification outlines the qualities required in the successful candidate, divided into essential and desirable categories. It provides a measure against which selection, on paper and in interview, will take place. The job description provides basic information on the overall purpose of the job and jobholder's accountabilities. Typical headings are shown in Box 8.7.

Application

When the time comes to 'put pen to paper', preparation is the key to success. It is wise to produce drafts of the application form to ensure the finished article is neat, sequenced and presentable. Written work should be grammatically correct and all spellings should be accurate. Applicants are often asked to attach a curriculum vitae (CV) to a completed application form; this should be in summary form unless a detailed version has been requested. It is advisable to complete the application and CV with the job and person specification in mind, given that these are the criteria against which the application will be assessed. The application, together with a brief covering letter, should reach its des-

---

Box 8.7   Job description headings

- Job title
- Reporting to
- Responsible for
- Definition of overall purpose
- List of principal accountabilities, key tasks or duties

---

tination – usually a human resources department – by the date given.

The curriculum vitae (CV)

A well-written and organised CV provides the right level of easily retrievable information and projects a professional image. Good CVs stand out in the crowd. The following presents a brief guide (see also the Further Reading section, pp251–252):

- Compile a general CV and then adjust and add to it for the particular job you are applying for. This ensures the CV emphasises the information most important to the job.
- Keep the CV brief and relevant; two sides of A4 is ideal for junior positions where applicants may have little career history. Longer career histories need to be summarised to avoid lengthy, irrelevant material, which may be distracting. Bullet points are useful and make quick reference easy.
- The order of elements in the CV should be logical and helpful to the reader. The most important information should be presented first.
- CV templates can be found in books and in word processing packages for ideas.

The interview

The key to a successful interview is thorough preparation. Researching the post can make the difference between success and failure. A candidate who knows what the interviewer wants has more chance of giving the astute answers, right impression, showing motivation and providing evidence of competence.

Applicants are sometimes asked to prepare a presentation. This is seen as an opportunity to promote oneself. It can build confidence but requires thorough preparation to be successful.

Job offers

Job offers may come by phone or by letter. They are usually provisional, dependent upon satisfactory references, medical, police checks and state registration checks. It is important for the applicant to receive a job offer in writing before handing in her notice to her current employer.

Job contract

The terms and conditions of the post are often summarised at interview but in many cases they follow in the job offer letter, with the detail in the job contract. The latter is a legal document by which the employer and employee agree to enter into a formal contract of employment. Responsibilities are held by both parties. Information in the job contract will include title and grade of position, salary and methods of payment, holiday entitlement, sickness procedures, benefits, supervisory responsibility, accountability, lines of reporting, grievance and disciplinary procedures (p225).

In the event of the post not being offered, it is worth asking for feedback for future reference. Constructive criticism, when combined with some encouraging comments, can be very helpful in considering how to manage future job applications.

Induction

In advance of starting a new post, it is advisable for a prospective employee to enquire about the planned programme of induction she is likely to follow. For the employee and employer to negotiate the exact programme is helpful, as it provides an opportunity to tailor the process according to individual need.

Career pathways

Deciding how long to stay in a position and how to plan one's career pathway can be complex. Factors to be taken into consideration when contemplating a career move include remuneration, conditions of working, recognition of efforts, achievements, motivation, clarity of role, support, direction and delegated authority. A working environment that nurtures motivation, recognition, support, reward and is flexible to working

patterns is to be appreciated. Developing clinical specialist and/or management skills, with advancement in responsibility, are usually determining factors. Personal circumstances will often dictate an individual's flexibility to move geographically.

Individual performance review

The purpose of an individual performance and development review (IPR) is to allow each individual to contribute towards the objectives of the organisation and to receive regular feedback about their performance and development (Fig. 8.12). It is widely accepted that people perform most effectively when they:

● understand their role and their contribution to the organisation and know what is expected of them
● receive regular feedback about how they are doing in their role.

The process for conducting these reviews varies across employing authorities. One example is illustrated in Figure 8.13.

Advance preparation is integral to the success of the procedure. Employees can make best use of this review by completing preparatory forms in good time, keeping records of training/development opportunities taken up throughout the year and being familiar with organisational goals

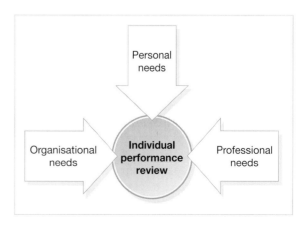

Fig. 8.12 Individual performance review elements.

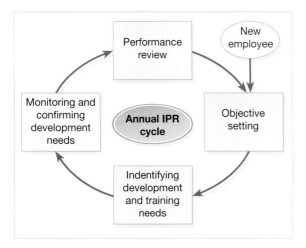

Fig. 8.13 Annual IPR cycle.

and service objectives. Feedback should be provided on both successes and any problem areas. The meeting should be a two-way dialogue and there should be equal involvement from both participants.

The first part provides opportunity to discuss the extent to which the employee has achieved the targets and objectives set the previous year. In the absence of objectives, the central focus should be upon the job description. In the second part, discussion should explore professional development, for example, new areas of interest, further skills, experience or training that would benefit both the individual and the organisation. This will be based upon what is needed in order to perform the job effectively, meet personal aspirations and any legal or professional obligations that apply.

The last part involves setting objectives and targets for the forthcoming year. These should follow the SMART model (Box 8.8). The discussion will take account of the objectives and plans for the service in which the employee is working and the previous discussions relating to performance. At the end of the objective setting, the objectives should be recorded.

Throughout the year, the manager will need to monitor the progress towards objectives, with particular emphasis on those areas that cause the employee difficulty. This may form part of the professional supervision process or be held with

the line manager responsible for conducting the IPR.

Through an established IPR system incorporating all staff grades, a manager can identify the following: the key tasks required by grade, competencies expected after specific time periods and the knowledge and skills required to develop within a grade or to progress to the next level. From this standpoint the service manager is able to plan, systematically and objectively, a strategy for formal or informal staff education to meet identified needs.

Continuing professional development and education

Continuing professional development (CPD) involves the ongoing maintenance and advancement of professional knowledge, expertise and competence. It should be planned through individual performance review, supervision and critical appraisal to benefit both individual and organisation (Fig. 8.14).

How do managers and staff meet identified CPD needs? Traditionally, courses have been considered the mainstay of continuing education but experience demonstrates that there are other, more effective means to develop skills, knowledge and expertise, such as:

- on-the-job coaching by mentoring staff
- job rotation (particularly in the case of junior therapists and helpers)
- working alongside or shadowing a more experienced colleague
- reading professional journals – this can be encouraged and enhanced through journal clubs (see p244)
- undertaking research
- undertaking one-off workplace projects

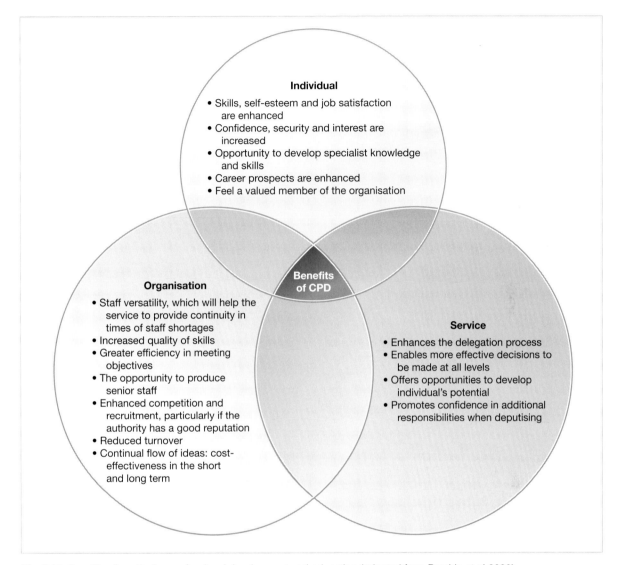

Fig. 8.14 Benefits of continuing professional development and education (adapted from Brechin et al 2000).

- utilising opportunities offered by the Open University and other organisations
- using self-development or learning packages developed in the service
- experiential learning, which provides new experiences in a practical setting.

Advances in health and social care, new technology and changing systems bring about the need for constant re-education and reassessment of our competence to practice. 'Fitness to practice' and our 'fitness for purpose' are terms used to reflect the importance of professional accountability. With the expectations concerning professional regulation and maintenance of state registration through evidence of continued competence, it is imperative that the practitioner records her professional development.

The COT has produced a number of helpful publications designed to support good practice in CPD. These include a professional portfolio,

CPD diaries and postgraduate directories of training and education.

Portfolios

A record of professional development has become a much-valued tool in mapping one's career pathway. The use of portfolios is not new, students in training have been encouraged to use portfolios for many years. Postgraduate practitioners are now reaping the benefits of maintaining portfolios to enable them to structure and formalise opportunities for development and reflective practice. The COT has developed an integrated system for professional development. Professionals are encouraged to maintain entries of annual performance reviews, objectives, CVs and professional development events in an 'active' file on paper or on disk. Portfolios are used as tools to support systems for professional supervision and can accompany a practitioner throughout her career. Expectations concerning regulation and evidence of ongoing competence to practice suggest the growing trend and importance of maintaining portfolios as evidence of continued competence.

Supervision

The term supervision can loosely be used to describe a number of approaches from overseeing someone else's performance at work to enabling a person to reach their full professional potential through reflection of practice.

From the therapist's perspective, to have an opportunity to discuss one's practice with a more experienced member of the same profession can assist in developing more advanced professional skills. Effective professional supervision encourages the practitioner to reflect upon practice, in particular critical incidents, identify antecedents, evaluate performance and consider more effective approaches. Adherence to professional standards of practice can be monitored through the process of supervision.

Line management supervision is concerned with the monitoring of performance against required standards, ensuring the individual manages her workload and meets predetermined outcomes. It provides the opportunity to identify stressors and negotiate boundaries. Professional supervision and line management supervision is often combined in posts below head occupational therapist level.

Whilst the combined approach can be efficient in terms of time and energy, it may present conflicts, for example, how much disclosure should a practitioner make, given her manager's involvement in her career progression? Equally, in a separate system, the bond of confidentiality can place undue pressure on a supervisor if they feel the line manager should be made aware of factors affecting an individual's performance.

The opportunity to shadow other practitioners is invaluable in developing professional skills and familiarising oneself with new client groups. The supervisor, in these cases, need not be the person's line manager but a practitioner identified as having an appropriate level of relevant experience.

Peer group supervision can also be mutually beneficial. People with similar levels of responsibility or clinical fields come together to reflect on practice through case study presentation or critical incident analysis. This may identify shared learning needs and subsequent action through, for example, journal clubs, peer group teaching and bringing in other experts.

Responsibility for the success of the supervision relationship lies with both parties. Each has a part to play and should be an active participant throughout. Bringing issues to the supervision meetings is part of this expectation. Box 8.9 provides some guidelines for productive supervision (see also Further Reading, pp251–252).

FINANCIAL RESOURCES

National level. Financing health and social care is a problem common to most countries (Levitt et al 1999). In developed countries, it is usually financed by a mixture of state funding, insurance and some direct payments from the user. In the United Kingdom general taxation is the main source of funding for the NHS, with National Insurance contributions and some

---

Box 8.9   Guidelines for productive supervision

- Suitably qualified supervisor
- Regular occasions to meet
- Accessibility of supervisor
- Listening skills
- Allocated time, without disruptions
- Conducive environment, relaxed and quiet
- Clear structure to discussions, where the supervisor listens and reflects what is said
- Reference to national guidelines for standards
- Problem-solving skills
- Sound theoretical skills
- Supervisor to have knowledge of subject or have knowledge of who to refer individual to
- Clear and concise records to assist progression and refreshing memories

---

Box 8.10   Glossary of financial terms

Budget: total amount of finance allocated to a budget holder/manager to run a service for a period of time

Budget holder: person delegated the management responsibility for a service's budget

Capital expenditure: sums paid for acquisition of assets (e.g. a new building or piece of equipment)

Cost centre: accounting centre to which costs are attributed and identified, e.g. ward, occupational therapy

Establishment: total number and grades of staff in a particular service

Recurring expenditure: costs (not for capital assets) occurring throughout the year, e.g. salaries, utilities

Incremental drift: cost associated with staff in post receiving annual salary increments, causing workforce cost to rise each year

Invoice: documentation for revenue or expenditure, usually incorporating a request for payment

Non-pay budget: all expenses of a service, except staff salaries

On-costs: additional costs of staff over and above salaries, i.e. employer's contributions to employee national insurance and superannuation

Pay budget: budget to cover staff salaries, including on-costs

Petty cash: money available to cover small and incidental expenditure

Revenue: day-to-day income of a service

Top slicing: taking first call on allocation of financial resources prior to distributing budgets

Whole time equivalents (WTE): hours allocated to a post expressed as a proportion of full-time, e.g. half time would be expressed as 0.50 WTE

---

direct charges as well. Local authorities are funded by revenue support grants, supplemented by significant amounts of local taxes and service charges. In the independent sector, income is generated through direct user payments, insurance and contracts with the public sector. 'For profit' organisations pay out surpluses to stakeholders, whilst 'not for profit organisations' reinvest surplus in the organisation or associated charities. Voluntary organisations may receive grants and finance through fund raising.

Organisational.   Whether an organisation is self-funding (e.g. NHS Trusts) or operating with a devolved budget (e.g. LASS, with additional local income) the expectation is a balance of income against expenditure. The organisation allocates budgets to services, enabling each to carry out their duties and responsibilities.

Team or service.   Budgets are allocated on an annual basis and divided into pay and non-pay (Box 8.10). The financial year for the public sector in the United Kingdom runs from 1 April to 31 March. To monitor expenditure against the budget, monthly budget statements are issued to the budget holder. Budget adjustments may be required to account for service changes (e.g. grant monies, additional staff, pay awards) or organisational edicts (e.g. 'efficiency measures' where the organisation needs to reduce expenditure to break even).

Individual level.   The occupational therapist needs to be aware of her own responsibility in keeping to the budget allocated by:

- utilising materials and equipment prudently
- using appropriate systems for ordering materials and equipment (there may be cost parameters for independent orders and procedures for seeking permission for expenditure over a specified limit)
- submitting expense forms by the required time, for example, monthly monitoring of travel expenses facilitates better budgetary control than infrequent high expense claims

- recognising the implications of efficiency measures on service delivery and identifying appropriate action with supervisor. For example, part of a service may be withdrawn or specific pieces of equipment may not be routinely provided
- recognising individual responsibility in keeping utility costs down.

FACILITY RESOURCES

Facilities includes any building, the utilities within the building (heat, light, water, electricity), communication systems (telecommunications, IT), equipment (patient related, non-patient, literature) and materials and disposables (ingredients, craft items).

Service or team. The manager has a duty to ensure that the workplace, its facilities and the equipment under their responsibility meet with health and safety regulations through routine risk assessments. Equipment should meet appropriate standards of safety and facilities should be adequately resourced and safe for practice.

INFORMATION RESOURCES

Information resources have grown significantly since the early 1980s with the increasing availability and capability of information technology. Correspondingly, the management of such resources has taken an increasingly important role in any organisation. Health and social care organisations routinely collect a wide range of information (Fig. 8.15), which can be divided into care-related (user information, quality and knowledge) and organisation-related information (human resources, health and safety). Common to each segment is the need to provide information for monitoring, evaluation and planning purposes.

Individual occupational therapist level

Occupational therapists are required to 'accurately record all information related to professional activities' (College of Occupational Therapists 2000a 3.4), including those directly and indirectly related to intervention, professional development and organisational procedures. Dimond (1997) provides principles to follow concerning written documentation (Box 8.11) and the COT has issued standards for occupational therapy record keeping (College of Occupational Therapists 2000a). These provide a framework for setting and auditing standards locally. With the increased use of computers for recording and storing information, making computer back-ups needs to be a routine procedure. It is good practice to keep signed and dated copies of important documentation, including, where necessary, printed e-mails.

Confidentiality of user records. Confidentiality is clearly laid out in the profession's code of ethics (College of Occupational Therapists 2000a. Section 2.3) and should be included in the employer's standards of practice. This is in concordance with the Data Protection Act (HMSO 1998), which outlines the following principles for data protection

User information	Quality information	Human resource information	Financial information	Health and safety	Facilities information	Knowledge R&D EBP
Profile Record of care outcomes	Standards Audits	Skill mix E & T Annual leave WTE	Income Expenditure Budgetary	Risk assessment	Room booking Equipment Maintenance	Library and internet sources Guidelines
Policies and procedures						
Information collected for quality assurance/audit/clinical governance purposes						
Activity information related to user contact						

E & T, Education and Training. WTE, Whole Time Equivalent. R&D EBP, Research and Development Evidence Based Practice.

Fig. 8.15 Types of information collected.

Box 8.11 Principles to follow in record keeping (after Dimond 1997 with kind permission of Blackwell Science Ltd)

Records should:

* be made as soon as possible after the events which are being recorded (i.e. within 24 hours)
* be accurate, comprehensive and clear
* be written legibly and be jargon free
* avoid opinion and record only the facts that were observed
* be signed by the marker
* not include abbreviations, unless commonly used and understood
* not be altered, unless the changes are made so that the original entry is clearly crossed out but still readable and any change should be dated and signed

---

Box 8.12 Application of data protection (adapted from Data Protection Act 1998, Department of Health 1994a, National Health Service Executive 2000)

Access of records
The individual can access records (manual and electronic, NHS and LASS) whenever they are made. Organisations will have their own procedure for access and a small fee will be attached.

Protection from illegitimate disclosure
Personal health and social information is confidential to an individual and can only be disclosed to others if required for the following reasons:

* planning and implementation of treatment
* if required for clinical audit
* public health and social information – to monitor and inform planning
* research, subject to ethical approval
* statutory statistics
* organisation's administration
* restricted access

Storage
* Records must always be kept securely. When a room containing records is left unattended it should be locked
* The movement of records should be recorded, so that they can be traced to the new location

Disposal
* Statutory minimum retention periods for both clinical and administrative records should be adhered to. The length of retention depends upon the type of record but should be reflected in organisational policies and procedures
* Disposal after the expiry of the retention period may involve transfer of data to another form, e.g. microform, or destruction, i.e. shredding, pulping or incineration

---

required of anyone processing personal data. Personal data covers fact, opinions and intended interventions for the individual. It must be:

* fairly and lawfully processed
* processed for limited purposes
* adequate, relevant and not excessive
* accurate
* not kept longer than necessary
* processed in accordance with data subject's rights
* secure
* not transferred to countries without adequate protection (HMSO 1998).

The individual has statutory rights of access to clinical information and protection from illegitimate disclosure and the data controller (any staff involved in creating or using personal data) has requirements for storage and disposal of data (Box 8.12).

Organisational level

The organisation will have policies and procedures for ensuring both the security of confidential information and the dissemination of public information.

National level

New information technology capability and more universal availability is opening the information highway for new methods of recording and sharing information:

* Electronic Patient Records and Electronic Social Care Records enable health and social care staff to access and share information with colleagues on or off site, 24 hours a day (NHS Information Strategy 1999 in National Health Service Information Authority 1999, Department of Health 2000d).
* Integrated information systems provide management with the most current and accurate information available. However, information may be open to misinterpretation without input from those involved in generating it.
* Electronic bibliographic databases and electronic journals all increase the individual

practitioner's access to current, worldwide literature.

- User-friendly health and welfare knowledge is available on the Internet for anyone to access. Medical advice can be sought on the Internet, over the telephone (e.g. NHS Direct), on local radio and on digital television.

However, although the potential is considerable, there are significant issues that need to be considered:

- Maintaining the confidentiality of information through secure storage and protected access. With increased joint working, a wider range of agencies (e.g. the housing department, the police) may have legitimate access to people's records. Some portions of a record will be restricted and some information may be considered to require a higher level of confidentiality (Austin 1996). Policies are required to identify which individuals are permitted access and at what level. Rigorous procedural systems should allow legitimate access only.
- Measures to assure the security of data need to be in place to reduce loss; for example, routine back-up procedures, protection and detection of viruses, as well as procedures to minimise data loss in the event of power failure.
- The lack of consensus in clinical terminology and acronyms within the profession (Brewin 1996) and between professions is a source for concern in shared records. However, national and international work is underway to address this issue.
- The wide availability of data to managers who have no understanding of the context in which it was generated or the purpose of data capture may lead to limited interpretation and poorly informed decision making.
- The quality of information reported is only as good as the quality of information provided by practitioners. Therefore inconsistent or inaccurate data collection will have repercussions in the reports and decision making generated on the basis of data provided.
- There are a number of ongoing costs associated with increased information

---

Box 8.13 The Garner Report (Garner 1999)

'Information management is concerned with how information is generated, interpreted, used and distributed.'

The report recommends:
1 Formalising links with the NHS Information Authority
2 Investing in a centre of excellence for professions allied to medicine
3 Making information more meaningful
4 Undertaking further work on record structures, in particular, clinical terms, definitions and headings
5 Providing support, information and advice about the development of the electronic patient record
6 Developing an information literate, competent and confident workforce
7 Supporting the National Electronic Library for Health

---

technology. In addition to the initial outlay for hardware and software, the ongoing costs include staff training, IT support and upgrading as technology inevitably advances.

The Garner Report.   The Garner Report (Garner 1999) was a joint venture between the Chartered Society of Physiotherapists and the College of Occupational Therapists. It made recommendations for future information management (Box 8.13).

SELF-MANAGEMENT

This section looks at how the individual occupational therapist manages herself, with particular reference to time management strategies and the management of an occupational therapy workload. Underpinning effective self-management is an appreciation of one's role in the organisation and the systems available to support that role. It may be helpful to ask 'What am I employed to achieve?' and 'What are the most important components of my job?'. Such questions should be informed by the job description and clarified through supervision and individual performance reviews.

Time management strategies

The following presents four simple time management strategies. A wide range of literature is available for a more comprehensive coverage (see Further Reading, p252):

1. size up the task
2. know yourself
3. prioritise
4. plan and control.

Size up the task

Whether the task is a one-off project or the provision of occupational therapy to a service area, it is important to assess the size of the task, clarify what is required and ask yourself whether you are equipped for the task. Time parameters need to be agreed: for example, response time to referral, project monitoring and project completion times. Objectives need to be clarified with the supervisor or project commissioner to ensure all parties are working towards the same goal. The balance between the challenge of the task and the individual's perceived skill to meet it is delicate but vital to successful completion (Csikszentmihalyi & Csikszentmihalyi 1988). If the challenge outweighs the individual's perceived ability to achieve it then stress, procrastination and non-performance results. Breaking a task down into small achievable parts helps to target progression and reduce procrastination. Setting realistic time frames for each part enables you to check that the whole task can be completed by the deadline and it encourages you to start sooner rather than later. Concern about one's ability to meet the challenge can be addressed through supervision and continual professional development. The section on workload management (p241) includes a tool to help assess the manageability of a caseload.

Know yourself

Productivity fluctuates throughout the day according to an individual's biorhythms. Figure 8.16 presents a chart in which peak, medium and low performance times can be identified and used to maximise performance. Peak performance times (for many between 10.00 a.m. and 12.00 noon) should be used to do the most demanding tasks of the day (e.g. complex assessments, important report writing) whilst low times should be used for routine administration, answering e-mails and making non-demanding telephone calls. Recognising your body's need for physical and mental breaks enhances performance. Time management experts (Godefroy & Clark 1990, Seiwert 1989) suggest that performance is sustained for longer with regular short breaks (up to 10 minutes).

Identifying personal strengths and limitations is an essential part of time management. The old adage 'it is better to underpromise and over-deliver' holds true but can be difficult for those who want to please. Judging what is achievable within a time frame is a skill that may need nurturing through supervision or discussion with colleagues.

Prioritise

The ability to prioritise is an essential skill in today's work environment. It is necessary to distinguish between that which is important and that which is urgent. An urgent activity is not necessarily important but needs to be dealt with immediately, whilst an important activity

	7.00	8.00	9.00	10.00	11.00	12.00	13.00	14.00	15.00	16.00	17.00	18.00
Peak												
Medium												
Low												

Fig. 8.16 Levels of performance during the working day.

will generally require more thought and hence more time to complete. The following are general guidelines in identifying and setting priorities: (caseload prioritisation is addressed on p241):

- list the tasks requiring attention including both regular and one-off responsibilities
- identify which tasks are urgent, important, short-term, long-term, routine, regular, interesting, dull
- allocate timescales, checking with other parties involved
- establish whether any tasks can be delegated and to whom
- establish whether any tasks can be simplified or eliminated
- set aside specific peak time for important activities and schedule time in the diary for the remaining activities
- be proactive as well as reactive by keeping an eye on the longer term goals and scheduling some time for them.

Plan and control

Having sized-up the tasks and identified the priorities, daily and weekly diary planning is required to maximise use of peak performance times and ensure effective use of other times. Inevitably, other considerations from users and colleagues will complicate the planning process but the above strategies can be used as guiding principles when providing options for appointments. In planning, it is helpful to schedule breathing space between commitments to deal with urgent telephone calls, queries, record keeping, seeking advice, etc. For jobs that involve several roles it is worth planning chunks of time to each role to avoid a continually shifting mindset. It is good practice to schedule regular time for continuing professional development (see p232) but this may need to be negotiated with the line manager to be in line with organisational policy.

Planning time is not enough, the actual use of time needs to be actively controlled to keep time robbers at bay (see Box 8.14). The therapist needs to identify what comprises lost time and how that time was lost. The following may help to minimise time robbers.

- Concentrate on one task at a time. Where possible, complete one task before going on to the next. It is better to have completed three out of six tasks than to have half done six. If a task cannot be completed in one sitting, list the remaining action and schedule it in the diary. File completed work.
- Restrict interruptions by setting aside periods of time for specific tasks and informing

---

Box 8.14 Time robbers (after Mike West, Sunley Management Centre, University College Northampton)

The following checklist can be used to both identify time robbers and to discuss strategies to reduce their impact.

	Regular problem	Often a problem	Seldom a problem
Planning			
Unclear about priorities			
No planned work schedule			
Half finished tasks			
No self-imposed deadlines			
Attempting to do too much			
No planned administration time			
Continual crisis management			
Organising			
Cluttered work environment			
Looking for misplaced items			
Duplication of effort			
Controlling			
Drop-in visitors			
Telephone interruptions			
Inability to say no			
Lack of self-discipline			
Lack of motivation			
Coping with change			
Doing jobs others could do			
Perfectionism			
Communication			
Failure to listen			
Under-/over-communicating			
Too many meetings			
Long, rambling meetings			
Decision making			
Snap decisions – not thought out			
Indecision/procrastination			
Excessive fact-finding			
Others			

colleagues of this arrangement. The answerphone may help further control interruptions for a short period of time.

- Plan the content of telephone calls (before phoning) to focus on objectives and minimise time wastage.
- Prepare for meetings in advance (read through minutes and other paperwork, identify issues to raise) and reduce rambling meetings by introducing a time frame for each agenda item.
- Influence the work environment and work around its constraints. For example, by using the library or the line manager's office in order to write an important report the distractions of working in an open plan office are minimised.
- Handle paper as little as possible. Use one of four options: act on it immediately, file it (noting further reading in the diary if required), pass it on or dispose of it.
- Write the next day's action plan at the end of the day.

Workload management

Workload may be measured or viewed from different perspectives. It is worth noting that there is a difference in understanding in workload terminology between the United Kingdom and North America, therefore definitions are given where appropriate.

Individual occupational therapist level

The occupational therapist will be concerned about how to manage a workload and what is a reasonable workload to bear. An individual occupational therapist's workload is illustrated in Figure 8.17. It may include all activities associated with the caseload plus other organisational activities (e.g. team meetings, quality assurance, planning and developing) and professional activities (supervision, education and promotion).

Caseload can be defined as the number of current cases for whom an occupational therapy team or service has taken clinical responsibility. Caseload also refers to the clinical component of

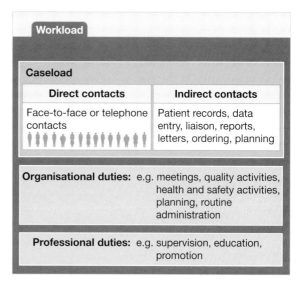

Fig. 8.17 The occupational therapist's workload.

the occupational therapist's overall workload. Tools have been developed to help occupational therapists assess and monitor their caseload but few have been published. Fortune and Ryan (1996) developed a caseload weighting system (based on the work of Haylock and McGovern (1989)) for community occupational therapists, which could be applied to other settings.

Fortune and Ryan's tool (Box 8.15) is subjective but it reflects the therapist's perceived complexity of the case and perceived capability to treat the individuals referred. It can help identify a caseload appropriate to the level and skill of the individual and may be negotiated through supervision. It can be used to track progression for the newly qualified occupational therapist. When accepting new cases it can be used to identify what type of case there is room for; it may also be used to protect the occupational therapist from working with more cases than she can safely cope with.

When faced with a number of new referrals what other principles should guide selection?

- Degree of risk for the individual in terms of vulnerability (e.g. immediate discharge or living alone), condition (e.g. pressure sores). There may be service policies with criteria to guide risk assessment.

Box 8.15   Categories for Caseload Weighting Tool (Fortune & Ryan 1996)

Following an initial occupational therapy assessment, the therapist allocates a numerical value (1, 2 or 3) to each case according to the complexity and length of intervention required. Numerical values are based on the categories below. Totalling all the values for each case in the caseload produces a figure that can be used to assess and compare the complexity of the caseload. The tool takes into consideration the clinical reasoning processes required in the treatment process.

Simple (quick) – 1	Simple (long) – 2	Complex – 3
Follow a set procedure	Assessment and intervention plan quickly completed, but procedural tasks take time	The problem(s) is not readily identified
Minimal liaison required	Specialist equipment is awaited for trial and issue	The problem(s) is identified but not readily resolved. May require specialist expertise
Minimal documentation	Time delays due to involvement of other agencies	Trial period required for solutions and appraisal
The person's problems are readily recognised with simple solutions		There are problems in interaction, developing rapport and trust. Additional time is required
The person's occupational difficulties are limited to discreet tasks		There are changing conditions which makes consideration of the present and future difficult/complex
The person is satisfied with the intervention plan		Multi-agency liaison is required Inevitably complex cases require complex documentation

In the UK, weighting refers to perceived difficulty or complexity; in North America, it refers to the quality of contact, e.g. individual or group contact.

- Impact of occupational therapy on the user – does he require core occupational therapy skills or skills another health professional could give?
- The consequences of not receiving occupational therapy, for example, what damage may result from not receiving education in joint protection.
- Length of time waiting – how long has a person had to wait? Is it within the quality assurance standard?
- Do I have the appropriate skills and facilities or should the person be referred on to someone else?

Service or team level

Workload management is concerned with ensuring that the team or department's work is covered by the most appropriate or best skill mix available. A good team or departmental manager should monitor her staff's individual workload through supervision to ensure they are able to meet the load whilst monitoring activity levels (number of contacts), quality standards and outcomes to ensure service agreements or commissions are met.

Time sampling may be a statutory or organisational requirement and provide a baseline for audit, staff development bids, total service or individual performance review. It involves recording work activity at regular intervals through the day (10 or 15 minutes) to provide data to analyse staff use of time.

Organisational level

Information from departments is used to monitor the service provided and to supply data for planning, development and commissioning purposes. It is used to control spending to ensure break even in business terms.

National level

At a regional and national level, information is required for future workforce and resource planning, determining trends and future healthcare needs (p227).

EFFECTIVE PRACTICE

Individual level

The terms effective practice and clinical effectiveness are used routinely in current policy and literature. But what do they mean and why are they important to the individual occupational therapist? Clinical effectiveness was defined by the National Health Service Executive (NHSE) as 'The extent to which specific clinical interventions, when deployed in the field for a particular patient or population, do what they are intended to do, i.e. maintain and improve health and secure the greatest possible health gain from the available resources' (Department of Health 1996 p45). The focus is on the person. The responsibility lies with the therapist to identify the most appropriate intervention to ensure maximum health gain within the resources available. In both health and social care within the United Kingdom there are frameworks to encourage effective practice in the form of Clinical Governance (NHS) and the social services Quality Framework (p245).

The occupational therapist can employ a number of strategies to increase the effectiveness of her intervention:

- keep the person at the centre of practice
- ensure practice is evidence-based wherever possible
- maintain currency of professional knowledge
- routinely reflect on and evaluate interventions
- appraise methods of measuring health gain
- ensure consistent effective communication
- partake in quality assurance activities
- be open to change.

By being person-centred and looking at practice through the eyes of the user, the practitioner can identify professional and organisational barriers to effectiveness. For example, is it in the user's best interests to have a visit from one practitioner who then refers the individual to a number of other professionals who subsequently make appointments? This is time consuming for both user and practitioners. User involvement in both treatment planning and evaluation will lead to a greater understanding of need and a more user-sensitive service. The use of critical pathways and user guidelines for service delivery will further contribute to clinical effectiveness.

There are a number of ways of ensuring practice is evidence based wherever possible. Although the evidence base for occupational therapy is sporadic at present, research evidence is increasing and evidence-based guidelines are available through professional and other bodies (see p247). Where guidelines are absent, the occupational therapist may need to search and appraise the best evidence available herself. There are a number of excellent textbooks and journal articles providing a practical guide through the process (see Further Reading p252). Because of the wide range of methodologies used in occupational therapy research, it is worth consulting literature that is written for occupational therapists or other professions with similar research paradigms.

Currency of professional knowledge can be maintained by keeping abreast of current literature and so being aware of recent research developments. Literature reviews, systematic reviews and meta-analyses provide a useful collation of research. Whilst a literature review will provide an overview of literature on an issue (not necessarily all research based), a systematic review will appraise research studies addressing a specific research question. A meta-analysis collates the data from a number of studies addressing one specific research question. Although such secondary research studies can potentially provide evidence for practice, they should be read carefully and appraised using a checklist (see Further Reading p251).

A regular habit of reading professional journals will undoubtedly contribute to clinical effectiveness. The instigation of a journal club within a team can be an effective and enjoyable means of reading and appraising articles relevant to shared client groups or current clinical issues. The concept underpinning a journal club is a mutually recognised need to learn and keep up to date. Effective journal clubs run on democratic lines, where everyone is an equal and valued participator. Providing food enhances informality and enjoyment of the experience. Journal clubs can take a range of formats (Box 8.16).

Developing and maintaining the currency of professional skills contributes to clinical effectiveness. As well as internal and external training or education, shadowing a more experienced colleague or secondment to a more specialised service area may provide hands-on continuing professional development.

Reflection is a skill for life. To facilitate reflection, students are encouraged to keep reflective diaries and this process should continue throughout the therapist's career. Verbalising ideas and thoughts through writing or talking helps the occupational therapist develop critical thinking. Supervision, case presentation and peer audit all provide excellent opportunities to take a step out of the situation to evaluate (see p234).

It is reasonable to expect that interventions should be evaluated and show some health or functional gain. However, although the gain may appear self-evident, it is not always easy to measure. When considering how to measure health gain or outcome, the occupational therapist needs to identify precisely what 'gain' is expected, who is involved in the process and at what level it is best measured. For example, increased functional performance in self-care activities following a knee replacement could be the result of the occupational therapist and physiotherapist providing graded opportunities for mobilisation, advice and practice in routine self-care activities, as well as rekindling the individual's confidence. It could also be said that it is the result of the whole multidisciplinary team working with the client pre- and postoperatively.

In measuring health and functional gains, the following need to be taken into consideration:

- what gain is expected for any individual or group?
- who requires information on outcome and for what purpose?
- who is involved? Is it a discrete outcome to occupational therapy or is the whole team involved?
- what is the individual's perspective of gain – are the practitioners, individual and carer considering the same issues?

Having addressed these issues, the question of how to measure is raised. A number of practical articles and textbooks are recommended in the Further Reading section (p251). Where outcome measures are already incorporated into practice it is worth appraising how accurately they measure gain and what contribution they make to assessing clinical effectiveness. You may want to explore the basis on which the measure(s) was selected

---

Box 8.16 Some journal club formats (adapted from Sackett et al 1997)

Scenario-based
A three-staged process where each week a scenario is presented and search terms agreed. The following week, resumés of selected research studies are presented, from which one or two articles are selected for critical appraisal the following week.

Client group
Research studies are selected because they address issues, treatments or treatment strategies relevant to a specific client group.

Treatment techniques
Research studies are selected to look at efficacy or intervention environment of specified treatments.

Methodology focus
Studies are selected to broaden understanding of a range of research methodologies. To appreciate methodological strengths/weaknesses different studies could be selected addressing the same issue.

Profession-based
Selecting articles exploring role from a range of professional journals can be used in a multidisciplinary (MD) team to increase understanding of member's contribution. Journal clubs in MD teams naturally provide an opportunity for clarifying role and contribution. The MD team could look at research studies on interprofessional working to stimulate ideas for more effective team working.

and consider its currency in the light of recent developments.

The last strategy to increase clinical effectiveness involves an 'open to change' mindset. There are continual developments both in the interventions used and the context in which service is delivered. Therefore the content of clinical effectiveness is dynamic and, by its very nature, always changing. To be open to change, to be willing to look at practice objectively and to be able to accept constructive criticism, will all contribute to increasing clinical effectiveness.

Team, service and organisational levels

At the team, service and organisational levels, effective practice should be facilitated through clinical governance (NHS) and the quality service framework (social services). Both create a structure to integrate a range of quality activities through continuous quality improvement schemes, with clear lines of responsibilities and adequate policies and procedures. Figure 8.18 outlines activities incorporated in clinical governance.

Quality culture

Underpinning effectiveness is a corporate attitude or culture of quality. Quality refers to the degree of excellence that is measurable against a set of requirements. The concept of quality has changed over time, from controlling the outcome to looking proactively at every part of the organisation to meet tomorrow's expectations and needs (Box 8.17). Continuous quality improvement is seen as a state of mind and should be everybody's concern.

Fundamental to quality issues are standards. Standards refer to written statements specifying the minimum level of performance expected in any area of the intervention process. This may include access, assessment, delivery, evaluation, documentation and other forms of (formal) communication. Standards should not be confused with policies and procedures (Box 8.18).

Methods for assessing and improving quality

Clinical audit, critical pathway analysis, quality circles and benchmarking are a few of the current methods available.

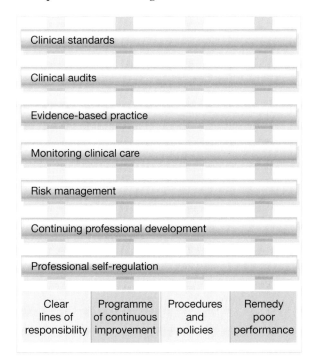

Fig. 8.18 Clinical governance framework.

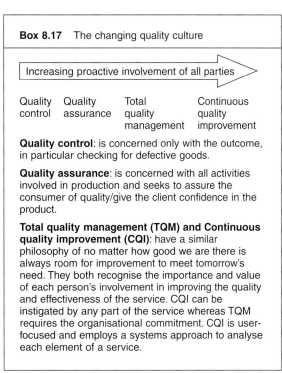

Box 8.17 The changing quality culture

Increasing proactive involvement of all parties

Quality control — Quality assurance — Total quality management — Continuous quality improvement

Quality control: is concerned only with the outcome, in particular checking for defective goods.

Quality assurance: is concerned with all activities involved in production and seeks to assure the consumer of quality/give the client confidence in the product.

Total quality management (TQM) and Continuous quality improvement (CQI): have a similar philosophy of no matter how good we are there is always room for improvement to meet tomorrow's need. They both recognise the importance and value of each person's involvement in improving the quality and effectiveness of the service. CQI can be instigated by any part of the service whereas TQM requires the organisational commitment. CQI is user-focused and employs a systems approach to analyse each element of a service.

Box 8.18   Guidelines, standards, policies and procedures (College of Occupational Therapists, 2000c)

Clinical guidelines outline the nature and level of intervention that is considered best practice for specific conditions in specific populations ... They are systematically developed statements which assist the occupational therapist and user in making decisions about appropriate health and social interventions for specific condition or population. They are sets of recommendations ... based upon the best available evidence. In social services they are sometimes referred to as service guidelines.

Standard: a written statement specifying the minimum level of performance expected in any area of intervention.

Policy: a written statement explaining the departmental/organisational belief or intention on a given issue. It may include a number of procedures to be undertaken in specific circumstances.

Procedure: a set of actions to be undertaken in specified circumstances.

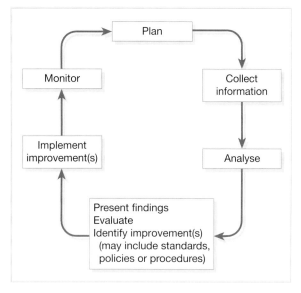

Fig. 8.19 The audit cycle.

Clinical audit.   The term clinical audit means different things to different people, probably because it is a broad term manifest in diverse activities. It can be defined as 'a clinically led initiative which seeks to improve the quality and outcome of patient care through structured peer review whereby clinicians examine their practices and results against agreed standards and modify their practice where indicated' (Department of Health 1996 p2). Audit should form part of routine practice with the aim of improving the quality of care. It should be instigated by practitioners, informed by the user view and involve all relevant stakeholders (DOH 1994b).

Audit may be used as part of the initial standard-setting process (Sealey 1999) or at a later stage to monitor and review the efficacy of existing standards. An audit may focus on one element of a service but highlight a number of interrelated issues. For example, an audit of people who did not attend their appointment at an outpatient service may raise issues of user understanding of the purpose and value of treatment, accessibility of service in terms of location and timing, people's previous experience of the service (the welcome they received, how valuable they perceived the treatment to be) as well as monitoring non-attendance and cost to the service.

The process of audit (audit cycle) follows a similar format (Fig. 8.19), although different authors may take a slightly different focus, reflected in minimal variations. The planning process is crucial to the success. It involves:

- identifying the area of service for audit (criteria include risk, potential cause for concern, complaint, recognised ineffectiveness)
- identifying all relevant parties (including users, where possible) and agreeing level of involvement
- agreeing the purpose of audit and subsequent objectives
- selecting and appraising relevant literature (research, recent audits on issue, guidelines and standards)
- designing an audit that incorporates appropriate methods to capture and analyse indicative, real and relevant data
- allocation of tasks and timeline.

Critical pathway analysis.   This can be used to track a person's route through all services involved in an episode of care. Areas where the service could be improved through better integration, liaison or reconfiguration are identified and the action agreed.

Quality circles. A quality circle involves similar issues but tackles them from a grass roots service delivery level. The whole team meets regularly to consider what areas of the service need improving and how those improvements might be made. The underlying principle is equality and value, that is, the whole team is included and each person's contribution is valued.

Benchmarking. This provides a means for comparing one's own service with recognised services of excellence to identify the potential for improvement.

National level

At a national level there are institutions to support and monitor clinical effectiveness.

Guidelines

Both professional and government bodies support clinical effectiveness by the production of guidelines (Box 8.19), which outline the most effective intervention or options for specific conditions (Sealey 1999). A number of guidelines are available regarding service delivery

---

Box 8.19 Examples of organisations in the UK that produce health and social care guidelines

- College of Occupational Therapists – profession-specific guidelines.
- National Institute of Clinical Excellence (NICE) produces guidelines on clinical interventions.
- National Service Frameworks (NSF) produces guidelines on service delivery.
- Social Care Institute for Excellence (SCIE) produce guidelines on best practice in social care.
- Social Services Inspectorate.
- Scottish Intercollegiate Guidelines Network (SIGN).
- NHS Research and Development Programme – produces guidelines on technology assessments.
- Centre for Reviews and Dissemination – produces high quality systematic reviews and maintains the Database of Reviews and Abstracts of Effectiveness (DARE).
- Centre for Evidence-based Social Services, University of Exeter.
- Promoting Action on Clinical Effectiveness (PACE) – a King's Fund Project committed to seeing research put into practice through/using guidelines.
- Cochrane Collaboration – a worldwide network of researchers producing rigorous systematic reviews, which can be used for guidelines.

---

to specific groups and those for specific occupational therapy interventions continue to increase. These guidelines have a number of positive features (Eccles & Grimshaw 2000):

- they improve the quality of care
- they promote treatments of proven benefit and discourage those of proven ineffectiveness
- they provide a standard of care and improve the consistency of care
- well publicised guidelines raise public awareness and enable users to make informed choices.

However, as Eccles and Grimshaw (2000) point out, one needs to exercise some caution:

- not all guidelines are evidence-based, some may be derived from consensus, conference or expert opinion
- there may be human error in the appraisal process
- there may be a paucity of good-quality evidence
- there may be other political agendas influencing considered best practice.

It is advisable to appraise guidelines, in particular the procedures involved in their development. They should be seen as a guide, not a prescription. They are to inform the therapist and, as such, should be included in the clinical reasoning process of identifying with the individual the best treatment options.

A number of specific journals and Internet sites focus on publishing the results of systematic reviews (see Further Reading).

Clinical effectiveness and adherence to standards is monitored at a national level through professional, governmental and consumer organisations. Those involved in the UK include:

- Health Professions Council (p222)
- The Council for Health Improvements (CHImP)
- The National User Performance Survey
- The Social Services Inspectorate
- The Audit Commission.

MANAGING CHANGE

The occupational therapist is constantly facing change in a range of contexts. In some contexts,

> **Box 8.20**   Glossary of terms (Burnes 1992, 2000)
>
> **Radical change**
> Involves 'large-scale, organisation-wide transformation programmes involving the rapid and wholesale overturning of old ways and ideas and their replacement by new and unique ones'.
>
> **Incremental change**
> Involves small-scale localised projects designed to deal with one problem and one goal at a time for part of the organisation.
>
> **Continuous transformation**
> Involves an ongoing process of change necessary to survive in a constantly changing environment.

the therapist is adapting to change and in others she is facilitating change. For instance, national changes in policy may be reflected at organisational and service delivery levels and may result in radical restructuring or incremental modifications (Box 8.20). The succession of changes in the NHS and social services have required a continuous transformation process. At team level, continuous quality improvement schemes may involve a number of localised modifications in service delivery. Changes in work role through service or professional development may bring about overt or subtle changes in expectation and performance. Helping people adjust to radical, incremental or continuous changes in health status involves the practitioner as a change facilitator or supporter.

To manage change, in whatever context, it is helpful to understand the form and processes involved. Change may arrive in different forms – it may be:

- thrust upon you: the most difficult form to manage, as you have no choice and may feel disempowered
- anticipated and expected: you may have been involved in the consultation process but not in the decision making. You may or may not feel some ownership of the change
- desired or even instigated by yourself: you feel at one with the change and able to be proactive in the process.

The process of organisational change has been described through various models, most of which

are based on the work of Kurt Lewin (Lewin 1958), who identified three stages of change:

- Unfreezing: recognising the need to change (external imposition or internal conviction)
- Moving: discarding old practice and changing to new practice
- Refreezing: consolidating new practice.

These concepts are reflected in the Action Research model (Box 8.21), which integrates collaborative

> **Box 8.21**   Action Research Model of Change (Robbins 1993)
>
> **Action Research** is: 'a change process based on the systematic collection of data and then selection of a change action based on what the analysed data indicate.' (Robbins 1993)
>   It involves five steps in an ongoing spiral (Fig. 8.20).
>
>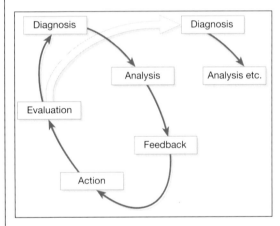
>
> **Fig. 8.20** The spiral of change in the Action Research Model.
>
> Diagnosis involves gathering data about the problem or change issue from all relevant stakeholders (internal and external, who may be affected by the issue of concern). There is usually a change agent to act as a catalyst and ensure comprehensive data collection.
>
> **Analysis** of data leads to identification of primary concerns, problem areas and possible outcomes. This is **fed back** to the stakeholders who together clarify the problem/change and agree a course of **action**. Action includes method(s) of **evaluation** and monitoring or reporting schedules. Final evaluations of both the change process and 'product of change' are presented to the group and completion or continuation of process is decided.

change management with a systematic research methodology to evaluate the changes made.

Change can evoke a mixed response from anger, anxiety, uncertainty and stress to excitement, creativity, heightened awareness and relief. The negative aspects are usually the focus of concern and there is a wealth of literature available (see Further Reading). Of interest to the occupational therapist is the link made between change, stress and self-esteem (although the concept of self-efficacy might be more accurate). Carnall (1999) shows how performance initially increases with stress but after a while plateaus and then decreases (Figure 8.21). Carnall links self-esteem with performance and change with stress, identifying a potential threshold beyond which behaviour becomes volatile and unpredictable. He describes a

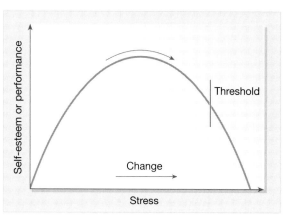

Fig. 8.21 The relationship between performance and stress (from Carnall 1999 by kind permission of Prentice Hall Europe).

coping cycle that reflects concepts of grief whilst demonstrating potential changes in performance and self-esteem (Box 8.22).

Box 8.22 The coping cycle (after Carnall 1999 by kind permission of Prentice Hall Europe)

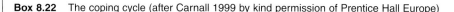

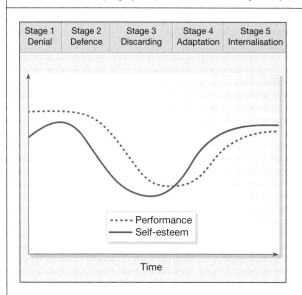

Stage 2: defence
As the realities of change become clearer with new roles or tasks imminent, there may be feelings of frustration (imposition of change) and depression (loss of the familiar). Underpinning this may be fears of inadequacy where the challenge outweighs the perceived skill. As a result defensive behaviour may ensue related to job role and territory.

Stage 3: discarding
Moving away from the past into the future may require opportunity to experiment with new practice and as old practice is superseded and discarded. The crisis of change creates tensions for all involved. It can be both frightening and exciting, challenging one's identity which is reflected in changes to self-esteem.

Stage 4: adaptation
Considerable energy is required in trying out new practice, evaluating and modifying. At times, there may be feelings of frustration and anger as systems are not operational or fault free and performance is not up to pre-change level. However, esteem rises with commitment to new practice and experience of coping.

Stage 5: internalisation
New practice and new relationships are tried, tested and accepted. Confidence in practice increases performance.

Carnall notes that progression through each stage is neither neat, predictable nor continuous. It is possible to be stuck in a stage and not move on.

Stage 1: denial
There is a tendency for an individual to deny the validity of change and suddenly find value in their current situation, questioning the need for any form of change. Carnall suggests an increase in self-esteem at this stage, but no change in performance. However, if the change is sudden and radical it may overwhelm and immobilise reason and action.

As change is inevitable, and yet also potentially detrimental and disempowering, how can it be managed to minimise damage whilst maximising desired effect? Five components to effective change management are outlined below:

Communication. At every stage in the process, intelligible two-way communication is vital to ensure all parties understand and sign up to the need for change, the processes involved in changing and the implications that the changes will have on working practices.

Time. Time is needed to take on board new concepts, to think through what the change will mean to the individual and to adjust. However, time is often at a premium and may not be available, therefore strategies to hasten the process may be required. For instance, anticipating likely change through an understanding of current policy making (see p217), using staff meetings and supervision to discuss potential change and its practical implications. Lastly, having a mindset seeking continuous quality improvement facilitates flexible thinking and openness to change.

Opportunity to experiment. Change is more easily accepted if there is opportunity to experiment or pilot elements of the proposed change. This provides occasion to rehearse, evaluate and modify, as well as creating confidence and ownership of new practice.

Support. Support is required throughout the process in diverse forms: professional support in terms of discussion, advice and endorsing ability; resource support in possibly additional staff time, equipment and materials; supervisory support; and team support.

Self-awareness. Being aware of personal reactions to change through reflection of previous experiences of change can help the individual anticipate potential sources of stress and conflict, and thereby inform the planning process. Issues may be identified for discussion in supervision or team meetings.

CONCLUSION

It is fitting to conclude the chapter on Professional Context with a section on managing change. With the escalating rate of change, the twenty-first century occupational therapist needs to be alert, equipped and proactive in taking on the new challenges our professional context is sure to bring.

REFERENCES

This chapter has been informed by a range of articles from the *Health Service Journal, British Journal of Occupational Therapy, American Journal of Occupational Therapy, Australian Journal of Occupational Therapy, Canadian Journal of Occupational Therapy* and *Occupational Therapy News* (published by the British Association of Occupational Therapists).

Abreu BA, Seale G, Podlesak J, Hartley L 1996 American Journal of Occupational Therapy 50:417–427
Austin C 1996 Confidentiality, clinicians and computers. British Journal of Occupational Therapy 59:62–64
Brechin A, Brown H, Eby MA 2000 Critical practice in health and social care. Sage and Open University, London
Brewin M 1996 The occupational therapy terms project: the final report on its development and outcomes. British Journal of Occupational Therapy 59:381–384
British Association of Occupational Therapists 1990 Position statement on professional negligence and litigation. British Association of Occupational Therapists, London
Burnes B 1992 Managing change. Pitman Publishing, London
Burnes B 2000 Managing change: a strategic approach to organisational dynamics. Financial Times – Prentice Hall, Harlow

Carnall C 1999 Managing change in organisations. Prentice Hall Europe, Hemel Hempstead
Chowdhury SEA 2000 Management 21C. Financial Times, Prentice Hall, Harlow, UK
College of Occupational Therapists 2000a Code of Ethics and Professional Conduct for Occupational Therapists. College of Occupational Therapists, London
College of Occupational Therapists 2000b Members first. College of Occupational Therapists, London
College of Occupational Therapists 2000c The production of college documents: position statements, standards for practice and clinical guidelines. College of Occupational Therapists, London
College of Occupational Therapists 2000d Standard for record keeping. College of Occupational Therapists, London
Csikszentmihalyi M, Csikszentmihalyi I 1988 Optimal experience: psychological studies of flow in consciousness. Cambridge University Press, Cambridge
Department for Education and Employment 1997 Occupational standards: professional activity in health promotion and care. DFEE, London
Department of Health 1994a Confidentiality, use and disclosure of personal health information, issued for consultation. HMSO, London

Department of Health 1994b The evolution of clinical audit. HMSO, London

Department of Health 1996 Promoting clinical effectiveness: a framework for action in and through the NHS. National Health Service Executive, Leeds

Department of Health 1997 The New NHS: Modern and Dependable. HMSO, London

Department of Health 1998a A first class service. HMSO, London

Department of Health 1999 Modernising regulation. The New Health Profession Council. HPC Draft consultation document

Department of Health 2000 Information for social care: a framework for improving quality in social care through better use of information and information technology. Department of Health, London http://www.doh.gov.uk/scg/information.htm

Department of Health 2000a A health service of all the talents: developing the NHS workforce. HMSO, London

Department of Health 2000b The NHS National Plan. HMSO, London

Department of Health 2000c Meeting the challenge: a strategy for the allied health professions. HMSO, London

Dimond B 1997 Legal aspects of occupational therapy. Blackwell Science, Oxford

Eccles M, Grimshaw J 2000 Clinical guidelines: from conception to use. Radcliffe Medical Press, Abingdon, Oxford

Fortune T, Ryan S 1996 Applying clinical reasoning: a caseload management system for community occupational therapists. British Journal of Occupational Therapy 59:207–211

Garner R 1999 Garner project, scoping information management needs in occupational therapy and physiotherapy. College of Occupational Therapists, London

Godefroy CH, Clark J 1990 The complete time management system. Piatkus, London

Griffin RW 1993 Management. Houghton Mifflin Company, Boston, MA

Haylock S, McGovern J 1989 A method of caseload management. British Journal of Occupational Therapy 52:380–382

Hitchens B 2000 Health Service Journal, 110.

HMSO 1946 The National Health Service Act. HMSO, London

HMSO 1948 The National Assistance Act. HMSO, London

HMSO 1970a The Chronically Sick and Disabled Persons Act. HMSO, London

HMSO 1970b The Local Authority Social Services Act. HMSO, London

HMSO 1983 Mental Health Act. HMSO, London.

HMSO 1990 The National Health Service and Community Care Act. HMSO, London.

HMSO 1998b Data Protection Act. HMSO, London http://www.doh.gov.uk/dpa98/

HMSO 1999 The Health Act. HMSO, London

Lenaghan J, New B, Mitchell E 1996 Setting priorities: is there a role for citizens' juries. British Medical Journal 312:1591–1593

Levitt R, Wall A, Appleby J 1999 The re-organised National Health Service. Stanley Thornes, Cheltenham

Lewin K 1958 In: Swanson GE, Newcomb TM, Hartley EL (eds) Readings in social psychology. Holt, Reinehart and Winston, New York

McDonald A 1999 Understanding community care: a guide for social workers. Macmillan Press, London

National Health Service Executive 2000a Human resources framework. National Health Services Executive, Leeds http://www.doh.gov.uk/hrstrategy/index.htm

National Health Service Executive 2000b Availability and patterns of secondary care services affecting entry, primary/secondary care interface http://www.doh.gov.uk/ntrd/rd/psi/priority/first/18.htm

National Health Service Executive 2000c Data Protection Act (1998). Department of Health, London http://www.doh.gov.uk/coinh.htm

National Health Service Information Authority 1999 The information for practice. NHS Information Authority, London http://www.enablingpp.exec.nhs.uk

Oliver S 1996 The progress of lay involvement in the NHS research and development programme. Journal of Evaluation in Clinical Practice 2:273–280

Robbins SP 1993 Organisational behaviour. Prentice Hall International, New Jersey

Sackett DL, Richardson WS, Rosenburg W, Haynes RB 1997 Evidence based medicine and how to teach EBM. Churchill Livingstone, Edinburgh

Sealey C 1999 Clinical governance: an information guide for occupational therapists. British Journal of Occupational Therapy 62:263–269

Seiwert LJ 1989 Managing your time. Kogan Page, London

FURTHER READING

Health and social policy

Baggott R 1998 Health and healthcare in Britain, 2nd edn. Macmillan Press Ltd, Basingstoke

Bushfield J 2000 Health and healthcare in modern Britain. Oxford University Press, Oxford

Ham C 1999 Health policy in Britain: the policies and organisation of the National Health Service, 4th edn. Macmillan Press Ltd, Basingstoke

Policy making

http://www.parliament.uk

Professional regulation/legislation

College of Occupational Therapists 2000 Legal briefing pack. College of Occupational Therapists, London

Sterry M 1998 Personal injury litigation and the College of Occupational Therapists' code of ethics and professional Conduct. British Journal of Occupational Therapy 61:263

Human resources

Alsop A, Ryan S 1996 Making the most of fieldwork education: a practical approach. Chapman and Hall, London

Hughes L, Pengelly P 1997 Staff supervision in a turbulent environment: managing process and task in front-line services. Jessica Kingsley Publishers, London

Jackson AL 1999 Prepare your curriculum vitae. National Textbook Company, USA

Ledgerd R 2000 On your marks! College of Occupational Therapists, London

Marler M 1995 Job interviews made easy. National Textbook Company, USA

Wheelan SA 1999 Creating effective teams. Sage Publications Inc, CA

Information resources

National Health Service Information Authority 1999 The information for practice. NHS Information Authority, London http://www.enablingpp.exec.nhs.uk

National Health Service Executive 2000 Data Protection Act (1998). Department of Health, London http://www.doh.gov.uk/coinh.htm

Time management

Lomas B 2000 The easy step by step guide to stress and time management. Rowmark Ltd.

Williams P 1995 Getting a project done on time: managing people, time and results.

Workload management

Fortune T, Ryan S 1996 Applying clinical reasoning: a caseload management system for community occupational therapists. British Journal of Occupational Therapy 59(5):207–211

Haylock S, McGovern J 1989 A method of caseload management. British Journal of Occupational Therapy 52(10):380–382

Evidence-based healthcare and currency of knowledge

Texts with an * include critical appraisal checklists.

British Journal of Occupational Therapy 1997 Evidence based practice issues in occupational therapy. Special issue 60(11)

* Bury T, Mead J 1998 Evidence-based healthcare: a practical guide to therapists. Butterworth-Heinemann, London

College of Occupational Therapists 2000 Position statements, standards for practice and clinical guidelines. College of Occupational Therapists, London

Eccles M, Grimshaw J 2000 Clinical guidelines from conception to use. Radcliffe Medical Press, Abingdon, Oxfordshire

Evidence-Based Practice Forum. Ongoing series in American Journal of Occupational Therapy from 1999 volume 53(5), p537. Edited by L.Tickle Degnan

* Greenhalgh T 1997 How to read a paper – the basics of evidence based medicine. BMJ Publishing Group, London

Mountain G 2000 Occupational therapy in social services: a review of the literature. College of Occupational Therapists, London

Muir Gray JA 1997 Evidence based healthcare. Churchill Livingstone, Edinburgh

* Taylor MC 2000 Evidence-based practice for occupational therapists. Blackwell Science, Oxford

Measuring health gain

Austin C, Clark C 1993 Measuring outcomes: for whom? British Journal of Occupational Therapy 56(1):21–24

Bowling A 1993 Measuring health – a review of quality of life measurement scales. Open University Press, Buckingham

Bowling A 1995 Measuring disease. Open University Press, Buckingham

de Clive-Lowe S 1996 Outcome measurement, cost effectiveness and clinical audit: the importance of standardised assessment to OTs in meeting these new demands. British Journal of Occupational Therapy 59(8):357–362

Jeffrey L 1993 Aspects of selecting outcome measures to demonstrate the effectiveness of comprehensive rehabilitation. British Journal of Occupational Therapy 56(11):394–400

Quality issues

Lugan M, Secker-Walker J 1999 Clinical governance: making it happen. The Royal Society of Medicine Press, London

Pacham G 2000 Quality assurance and clinical audit: information and equipment provision. British Journal of Occupational Therapy 62(6):278–283

Managing change

Broome A 1998 Managing change. Macmillan Press, London

Carnall C 1999 Managing change in organisations. Prentice Hall Europe, Hemel Hempstead

---

USEFUL CONTACTS

Bandolier (EBM Journal)
http://www.jr2.ox.ac.uk:80/Bandolier

CASP – Critical Appraisal Skills Programme
http://www.his.ox.ac.uk/casp/index2.html

Centre for Evidence-Based Medicine
http://cebm.jr2.ox.ac.uk/

Cochrane Library http://www.update-software.com/ccweb/cochrane/cdsr.htm

Guidelines on line http://www.guidelines.co.uk

Links to Evidence Based Medicine and Practice Websites
http://www.wolfson.tvu.ac.uk/learn/links/evid.stm

NHS Centre for Reviews and Dissemination
http://nhscrd.york.ac.uk/

Principles for practice

SECTION CONTENTS

9

Psychosocial perspectives in person-centred practice

Hilary Johnson

INTRODUCTION

This chapter aims to provide a basic understanding of some of the leading psychosocial frameworks and perspectives underpinning person-centred practice in the treatment of people with physical dysfunction. The chapter begins by tracing the origins of humanistic psychology in phenomenology, paying particular attention to the influential theories of Abraham Maslow and Carl Rogers, and then briefly considers the wider impact of these ideas on service delivery and changing perceptions of disability. Following this, the benefits and limitations of the humanistic approach in present-day clinical settings, and its implications for practice in treating people from a variety of ethnic and religious backgrounds, are explored. A further section deals with lifespan development through childhood, adolescence and adulthood, highlighting some of the difficulties commonly faced by those who are disabled. The next section looks at the nature of change and loss, describing the ways in which people adapt to major life events. The chapter ends with a brief summary of the work of Elisabeth Kubler-Ross on death and dying.

PHENOMENOLOGY, HUMANISTIC PSYCHOLOGY AND THEIR INFLUENCE ON PRACTICE

WHAT IS PHENOMENOLOGY?

Phenomenology is an approach to the understanding of the world we live in. In recent years it has come to permeate almost every sphere of human thought, from philosophy, religion and the social sciences to the higher physics. In philosophical terms, phenomenology abolishes the distinction between objective and subjective existence; reality both transcends individual (and social) experience and is constructed by it. In the physical sciences, it acknowledges how the material under investigation is affected and changed by the very act of observation. We can never know reality 'as it is', but only as it is perceived through our senses, ordered by our minds, shaped by political and cultural bias and described in language. Impartiality, once the acclaimed hallmark of the historian, has been consigned to the academic wastebin; literary texts are deconstructed; and the claims of medical science and psychology to some kind of enduring, objective 'truth' have come under increasing scrutiny. This is not to say that all objective approaches should now be set aside; quantitative methods, especially necessary in outcome measurement, and the traditional 'scientific' frameworks remain vitally important for the therapist who is more likely to 'think simultaneously in two blurred frames: phenomenological and biomedical' (Finlay 1999). The multidimensional therapist with a two- or even three-track mind is now definitely 'in' (Finlay 1999, Mattingly & Fleming 1994).

The convergence (some might say confusion) of subject and object that lies at the heart of phenomenology has led researchers to place an increasing emphasis on the importance of qualitative methods that attempt to describe and interpret human behaviour from the standpoint of the individual or groups who are being investigated. This approach has carried over into clinical practice, with the therapist making a conscious effort to bracket her own presuppositions and, through a premeditated act of empathy, attempting to gain a deeper insight into an individual's life-experience or 'story'. One result of this is likely to be a shared understanding, or 'therapist–client story', which combines the therapist's technical knowledge with the unique experience of the person. In the case of a person who has sustained a disabling physical trauma, it would mean examining its impact from the viewpoint of the disabled person himself, discovering and taking into account his personal framework and what is meaningful and relevant to him. If the person receiving treatment were from a different culture, it would mean assessing the lifestyle and problems of the person from the perspective of his own values, beliefs and cultural norms. Clearly, such an approach sits well with the traditional emphasis of occupational therapy on treating the whole person.

WHAT IS HUMANISTIC PSYCHOLOGY?

Humanistic psychology may be understood as a subset of phenomenology. In the early 1960s, when a group of American psychologists (including Abraham Maslow and Carl Rogers) founded the Association of Humanistic Psychology, phenomenological ideas were much 'in the air'. They formed the intellectual background or *Zeitgeist*, the springboard for exciting new developments. The importance of phenomenology to Maslow and Rogers was the value it placed on the individual's own interpretation of his environment and life events. It enabled them to move away from the deterministic models of psychoanalysis and behaviourism, and the godlike role of the doctor or therapist, towards a more 'human' model, which found the locus of control and the pathway for treatment within the person himself.

The writings of both Maslow (1970) and Rogers (1967) show the human personality as innately good. The person is regarded as a worthwhile being, inwardly motivated towards growth, maturity and the fulfilment of his higher needs and potentialities. Rogers called this drive the actualising tendency. In Maslow's terminology the pinnacle of fulfilment is self-actualisation.

Maslow: the hierarchy of needs

Figure 9.1 shows how Maslow groups human needs into categories or key areas, which are then arranged in a hierarchy. He states that the needs at each successive level of the hierarchy must be at least partially satisfied before those at the next level can be properly addressed. For example, someone who feels insecure and unsafe, particularly in childhood, may have difficulty in giving and receiving love; and a person who is unable to see to his basic biological and self-care needs may have very limited self-esteem. However, it would

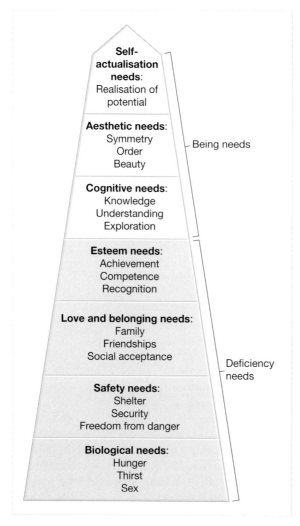

Fig. 9.1 Maslow's hierarchy of needs (adapted from Maslow 1970).

be a mistake to think of the hierarchy as a kind of ladder – a case of 'if I don't climb the next rung, then I can't progress further' – or worse, a series of therapeutic hoops that must be negotiated in the right order as part of a treatment programme. As we shall see when we come to consider the importance of balancing independent living needs against other, sometimes more pressing needs higher up the scale, there can be considerable overlap and fluidity between the different levels.

More firmly demarcated are the boundaries between what Maslow called *deficiency* needs, consisting of the four lower levels of the hierarchy, and *being* needs, which occupy the upper three levels. Individuals who are engaged in a struggle to meet deficiency needs will have little energy remaining to devote to the satisfaction of being needs. A homeless person sleeping under a bridge and dependent on charity for his next meal is unlikely to spend his periods of inactivity discovering beauty in the urban landscape. People whose early lives have been shrouded in abuse and neglect find it more difficult to become self-actualisers, while those whose deficiency needs have been met in childhood are likely to have a firmer base on which to develop a strong, secure, healthy sense of self. But even Maslow's distinction between deficiency and being needs, useful as it may be, is not to be taken in an absolute sense. We all know or have read about cases where people have achieved great things against seemingly overwhelming odds. There are opportunities to grow and develop whatever our experience of life has been. We must always beware of putting limits to the human spirit.

Rogers: the concept of self and person-centred therapy

Carl Rogers focused specifically on issues of self-concept, autonomy and self-direction. When looking at the ways in which we perceive ourselves, Rogers made a distinction between the *ideal self* – the person we would like to be – and the *real self* – the person we actually are. The greater the congruence between the two aspects of self, the more emotionally stable, the happier and more fulfilled the person is likely to be. A child brought up with *unconditional positive regard*, that is to say, one who is being valued for himself as a growing human being, is more likely to develop a *congruent* self-concept; his sense of what is required of him and of the kind of person he wants to be is generally in agreement with the sense of who he is. The child reared with *conditional positive regard*, being valued for 'good', 'correct' behaviour, thinking and feeling, is more likely to distort his sense of self, his ideal self consisting of a long series of 'I shoulds', impossible to achieve. Such a child may have difficulty growing into a mature, self-actualised adult.

Rogers, however, never applied his theories to people in a way that would seem to limit their potential. He believed that humans have the capacity to reflect on life and make positive changes for themselves. Relating this to clinical practice, he held that the individual is always the person best qualified to decide in which direction growth (i.e. the route to self-actualisation) will take place.

It should be borne in mind that, as a psychotherapist, Rogers developed his ideas within the context of mental health. Central to his thinking was the notion of 'person-centred' psychotherapy, in which he saw the client/therapist relationship as a partnership, with the therapist acting as a sounding-board for the individual, helping him to work through his problems and reach his own decisions about the future. According to Rogers, the therapist and individual are both specialists in their own right and both have specialist knowledge. The therapeutic relationship allows a sharing or exchange of that knowledge in an adult-to-adult way without the individual experiencing any loss of status or autonomy. It is up to the therapist to give unconditional positive regard. This does not mean that she must personally approve of all and every kind of behaviour. Rather, she must refrain from making negative or destructive criticisms, while drawing out and affirming whatever is capable of positive development. Thus, she supports the person's self-esteem so that he can explore his problems and the options open to him without fear of being 'judged'.

Wider impact of the humanistic approach

As phenomenological principles caught hold and began to influence wider service delivery, they naturally met with resistance and began to be challenged. A frequent criticism was that the qualitative research methods to which they gave rise lent themselves less easily to clear measurement of outcomes. This was important, as it could affect funding programmes and threaten the continued existence of services. It has been pointed out that the history of occupational therapy itself demonstrates a failure to measure the impact of interventions (see Chapter 2), a trend that has adversely affected the status of the profession in contrast to more scientifically based disciplines such as medicine (Creek 1997). One response in recent years has been an attempt to find more reliable descriptors for qualitative research while pushing forward the idea that evidence-based practice should not only include qualitative analyses but give them equal weight to those that rely on standardised assessments and numerical scores. Many research papers and journal articles will now employ both methods.

In other ways, phenomenology also had a positive and healthy effect on service provision and has produced new challenges. The focus on the person's own viewpoint led to a much greater emphasis on quality and increasing pressure on service providers to consult with actual and potential users. Marginalised groups who had previously lacked the confidence to assert their own positions began now to do so, while rejecting the definitions, seen as limited and demeaning, imposed on them by politicians, professionals and others in authority. Examples of such developments are the radical Independent Living Movement initiated by physically disabled people themselves, and the emergence of the Social Model of Disability (Box 9.1) with its emphasis on the environmental barriers that are argued to be infinitely more disabling than the impairment itself. We might also draw attention to the various pressure groups from within the minority ethnic communities who have called for culturally appropriate services and training of healthcare

---

Box 9.1 The Social Model of Disability (from Craddock 1996, Finkelstein 1993, Oliver 1999)

The Social Model of Disability was developed from 'The Fundamental Principles of Disability' Union of the Physically Impaired Against Segregation (1976) and asserts that:

- Impairment means the medical or health problem.
- Disability is imposed on top of impairment.
- The term 'people with disabilities' implies that impairments are disabling *per se*.
- The term 'disabled people' implies that people are disabled by other factors, namely environmental, sociopolitical and economic barriers, and by negative attitudes within organisations and society at large which prevent equal opportunities.
- It follows that, once the barrier is removed, for example, by the provision of a hearing aid, spectacles, appropriate access and facilities, and positive attitudes, the person is no longer 'disabled', though he will still have an impairment.
- There is a spectrum between being disabled and non-disabled. The unacceptable term 'able-bodied' implies biological superiority.
- The rehabilitation model places responsibility for change predominantly within the individual.
- The medical model asserts its authority taking the locus of control away from the disabled person.
- Responsibility for change lies within society as a whole and legislation is required to redress imbalances in civil rights for disabled people.
- Disabled people do not necessarily need professional counselling, though they need to be listened to and heard, as do we all. Emotional responses to life events are normal.

---

professionals in self-examination and cultural awareness. We shall be touching on a number of these issues in later sections.

THE HUMANISTIC APPROACH IN PRACTICE

Occupational therapists work in a variety of social and institutional settings across all sectors – statutory, voluntary, private and charitable. We meet people from different walks of life and from other cultures, people who at different stages of their lives are experiencing a wide range of impairments and personal and social difficulties. Some, though by no means all, will have experienced a period of acute care in hospital.

The sick role

When a person is first admitted to hospital, he is likely to lose a degree of autonomy. In the event of an emergency, or a seriously incapacitating illness involving acute admission, decisions may of necessity be taken for him. This should not have to mean that his adult self has been discounted. In practice, however, it often does. Indeed, the expectations of those who are treating him may be that he will quickly adapt to the 'sick role', acquiescing in aspects of the ward regimen and doing whatever he is required with little regard to individual preferences or habits. These expectations are rarely questioned by the 'patient' and if they are he might well be labelled 'difficult'. But it is only in the acute phase of the illness that the person should be expected to accept the sick role, which should, therefore, be seen as strictly time-limited. Once the medical crisis is over and recovery progresses, so the person will hopefully resume responsibility for himself.

Rehabilitation: the person-centred approach

It is at this stage, when the period of rehabilitation and adjustment to residual impairment begins, that the occupational therapist comes into her own, as she treats and supports the individual through the recovery phase of his injury or disabling condition. Her aim will be to restore to the person the autonomy taken from him during the acute phase of his illness, and to do this in a way that addresses the whole person and not just the impairment (Box 9.2).

Client-centred occupational therapy is a partnership between the client and the therapist that *empowers* the client to engage in functional performance and fulfil his or her occupational roles in a variety of environments. The client participates actively in negotiating goals which are given priority and are at the centre of assessment, intervention and evaluation.

Throughout the process the therapist listens to and respects the client's values, adapts the interventions to meet the client's needs and enables the client to make informed decisions.

(Sumsion 2000 p308; author's italics)

Box 9.2 What constitutes good practice along humanistic lines?

- Try to empathise with the person's situation.
- Be receptive and responsive to his story.
- Listen to how he describes his impairment and what it means from his standpoint.
- Try to facilitate looking at different options.
- Try to facilitate solutions that the person has identified for himself, if these are realistic and there are resources to achieve them.
- Be honest in providing relevant information to enable the person to make sound decisions.
- Negotiate and agree the plan for intervention.
- Consider the needs and views of involved family members and carers.

Mattingly and Fleming (1994) describe the person-centred approach in practice as a question of motivating the individual, so that activities have meaning, and tapping into concerns and values deep enough to secure his commitment. They state that 'No matter what the technical expertise or theoretical orientation of the therapist, effective collaboration requires treating the disability as more than a biomechanical matter that can be separated from the experience of the patient'. Box 9.3 gives scenarios where the person-centred approach worked well.

The two-track approach

In some circumstances, for example when dealing with physical injuries that require specific treatment techniques, we may wonder if it would be more realistic to focus exclusively on the objective aspects of treatment. However, the point at issue is not the validity of the phenomenological principle but how 'weakly' or 'strongly' it is applied. Mattingly and Fleming (1994), as we have seen, advocated 'blurring' the phenomenological and biomedical frames, while acknowledging that in some clinical situations, or at certain stages of an ongoing intervention, the biomedical approach would predominate. The case studies in Box 9.4 show the biomedical approach in action. It will be noted, however, that even here something of the person's life context remains present in the therapist's mind, enabling her to share her ideas on treatment with the person or to redirect the therapy along more productive lines.

Box 9.3 Case studies (summarised from Mattingly & Fleming 1994, Sumsion 1997)

A woman in her mid-50s has rheumatoid arthritis. As the therapist takes time to talk with her and to listen, she learns that this woman is concerned about her appearance, her make-up and hair, and her future ability to entertain and go out to dinner again with her husband and friends. Her children and grandchildren are extremely important to her and she doesn't want them to feel embarrassment seeing her in bed or in a wheelchair. Having understood this woman's perspective, the therapist is able to suggest working on energy conservation, allowing herself rest periods, working on transfers to sitting on the couch, and strengthening her arms so that she might hold her grandchildren. Thus they are able to work collaboratively and optimistically together.

An artist cares deeply about her work and is highly motivated to work on strengthening exercises following a hand injury. Dough sculpting fulfils not only the biomechanical goals set to improve range and strength of movement but also accords with her interests.

John is a young Yugoslavian man who has lived in England since the age of ten. He is now in the later stages of AIDS and is nearing the end of his life. It is important to John that he leaves his personal and financial affairs in good order. Although estranged from his family of origin, he has a 'family' of his own consisting of eight of his close friends. The therapist takes account not only of his personal and physical needs in a constricted but cherished home environment but also of his sociocultural, economic, legal and family–political contexts in order to view his case in a holistic light. In dealing with a very complex situation she finds it necessary to examine her own cultural underpinnings in order to be aware of the potential for personal biases.

In the first two examples, a reading of Mattingly and Fleming's original text makes it clear that the therapist is working with a minimum of information about the person. As both men are keen to recover their full physical functioning, they need no other 'meaningful activity' than the one in which they are engaged. The biomedical treatment itself fulfils the requirement to provide activity that is relevant to the person's life and experience. However, in both cases, the therapist is also responding to what she has picked up about the person's background 'along the way'. She also relates to him as an adult who is entitled to an explanation and with whom she can share knowledge. Thus, while carrying out a straightforward medically based intervention, she builds up trust and

---

Box 9.4 Case studies (summarised from Mattingly & Fleming 1994)

An occupational therapist is working with a man with a spinal cord injury and is instructing him in the use of a deltoid aid to facilitate active exercise of his left arm. As she shares her knowledge with him, so he is able to consider the potential of the use of the aid to strengthen his body.

A hand therapist is using a goniometer to measure the range of movement in a man's injured hand. As treatment is often painful and tedious, she explains that the measurements are taken partly for her own records and also to enable him to see his own improvement. Between treatments, she has had some conversation with the man about the effect of the injury on his life situation but although this leads to improved interaction it does not impact in any other way on the treatment.

Both the above are working class men in their twenties. Regaining strength carries meaning for them in terms of self-image and in terms of what they may subsequently make of their lives. They are therefore already highly motivated.

A therapist is treating a man following his second stroke. He frames his problems in religious and existential terms: 'I wish God could do a miracle on me. I can't use my arm as I should'. His is the language of despair. Her response is to reframe the problem in biomedical terms. She praises his efforts so far and explains that the problems are associated with his neglect of his left side. Thus she is directing his way of thinking so that they can work more optimistically together to improve his condition.

Box 9.5 Case study (summarised from Mattingly & Fleming 1994)

Doris was referred to occupational therapy following repair of her right flexor pollicis longus tendon. She reported that the injury was sustained slicing potatoes. Treatment involved a dorsal hand–thumb blocking splint with intermittent dynamic Kleinert traction. Despite consistent therapy attendance and seeming compliance there was declining functional status. An eventual diagnosis of reflex sympathetic dystrophy was made.

Doris's problem at first appeared to be a physical injury requiring straightforward treatment techniques. However, as treatment progressed with limited improvement, the therapist began to adopt a phenomenological approach and discovered that Doris's husband was an apparent drug abuser and that the injury was sustained as Doris resisted a knife attack. Whilst both surgeon and therapist continued to struggle with the lack of function in Doris's hand, and made efforts to help her resolve some of the background issues, they felt that had an accurate medical history been taken earlier, both hand function and the treatment approach would have been different. As it was, doing too little too late prevented maximal healing. Had the real cause of injury been understood at the outset, greater improvement in regaining hand function would have been possible. Whilst the therapist's biomechanical knowledge and skills were essential, they were not sufficient on their own.

---

mutual respect. The interactive approach will increase commitment and hopefully lead to improved outcomes.

In the third example, the therapist ignores the literal meaning of the man's exclamation and addresses herself to its underlying meaning, that is to say, the man's sense of despair. There is no indication that she knows anything of the man's 'story' and her relationship with him at this level is basically intuitive. In the meantime, she 'gets on with the job'. Her explanation encourages and reassures him and brings his ideas and feelings into line with the direction of treatment. The biomedical approach provides the more optimistic view.

Although, in all three examples, it seemed sensible and realistic to focus on the injury, a too narrowly biomedical approach is not without risks. Mattingly and Fleming (1994) provide a case study (Box 9.5) of Doris, a 38-year-old married woman, whose physical dysfunction

might have been treated differently, with improved *physical* healing, if her story had been properly investigated.

Constraints in practice

Heavy workloads and pressures to facilitate safe and speedy discharge from hospital often preclude our getting to know people's anxieties, preferences and ideas in any meaningful way. In many clinical settings, occupational therapists 'may find themselves focusing on self-care activities in order to meet team goals or comply with service constraints to the neglect of other client-identified activities' (Lane 2000). Sometimes, programmes of care are time-limited in order to demonstrate cost and operational efficiencies. In such circumstances, we may tend to be prescriptive in our treatments, ensuring, for example, that assistive equipment is identified and supplied rather than discussing and negotiating options – even though subsequently the equipment may remain unused because we 'won't listen to the person who's going to use it'

(Abbott 1999). Our expressions of so-called 'empathy' may be little more than a form of cajoling, a way of managing the individual and securing his conformity and compliance. And are we not sometimes likely to apply the notion of independence in a dogmatic and unthinking way as an ability to perform activities of daily living, on the assumption that such activity will automatically fulfil the person's lower order needs, enabling him to begin to reclimb his own hierarchy? Not that all practice in activities of daily living is inappropriate; indeed, being able to attend to personal needs is highly likely to increase self-esteem. Rather, the aim is to question at what juncture a judgement should be made, and by whom, regarding continued adherence to a programme that focuses on basic deficiency needs to the exclusion of one that would address being needs.

While we acknowledge that obstacles to good practice do exist within services, and at times can lead to frustration and cynicism, they are not always insurmountable. Lane (2000) points out that where early discharge hospital-at-home schemes are well planned and effective, they offer a more person-centred form of care, with greater opportunities for rehabilitation, than hospital-based services. As we saw earlier, it is possible with real empathy and commitment to develop and maintain a sense of the person even within the constraints of a time-limited, medically orientated intervention. Many of the constraints imposed by services can be overcome with ingenuity, practical imagination and the drive and desire to change things.

If we are to adopt a truly person-centred approach, we will need constantly to re-evaluate our practices. The alternative is that we ourselves may become 'part of the problem'. The continued fulfilment of needs within the person's hierarchy will then be threatened not only by the impact of the impairment but by the attitudes we hold as professional staff. Indeed, it may be that we should now be thinking in terms of a person-*driven* rather than a person-*centred* approach to therapy. This would further shift the balance of power in favour of the individual, who would thereby have greater 'ownership' of his defined goals and a greater commitment to achieving them.

CULTURAL AWARENESS

The Report of the Stephen Lawrence Inquiry (MacPherson 1999) found institutional racism, defined as 'the collective failure of an organization to provide an appropriate and professional service to people because of their colour, culture or ethnic origin', to be deeply embedded in the Metropolitan Police Service. The Report concluded: 'It is incumbent upon every institution to examine their policies and the outcome of their policies and practices to guard against disadvantaging any section of our communities'.

So influential has been the Report that, since its publication, no public body or profession has been able to disregard its findings or consider itself exempt from the suspicion or charge of cultural and racial bias. Nevertheless, progress in addressing these issues has continued to be slow, perhaps not surprisingly as what is involved is a huge cultural shift. As always, there are clear gaps between philosophy and practice. Is our own profession any exception? The Code of Ethics and Professional Conduct for Occupational Therapists (College of Occupational Therapists 2000) requires us 'to be sensitive to cultural and lifestyle diversity and to provide services which reflect and value these' [sic], yet studies have revealed that 'occupational therapists often view the clinical encounter from their own cultural, social and economic perspectives' (Howarth & Jones 1999).

An example of institutional racism within mainstream health and social services might be the lack of provision for language interpreting, with children and often cleaners brought in to translate when serious matters of health are under discussion. This may not only be upsetting for the child but is a clear breach of confidentiality – and yet no-one seems to notice (Parekh 2000).

The term used by sociologists to describe the tendency to view other ethnic groups from the standpoint of one's own culture is 'ethnocentrism'. In the United Kingdom, ethnocentrism has deep roots, going back two or three hundred years to the beginnings of the British Empire. At school, until quite recently, pupils were taught history from the standpoint of 'British interests', never from the perspective of the people whose lands we were occupying. It is a way of thinking that is no longer acceptable in a culturally plural and multiethnic society, yet it continues to be employed, often unconsciously, at the level of everyday professional practice. Ethnocentrism is the very opposite of empathy, which could be defined as the attempt to take in and accept a person's perceptions and feelings as if they were one's own (though without losing one's own boundaries). As such, it stands well outside the phenomenological project.

Empathy is the key to cultural competence. It is simply not possible to be aware of all the social norms, attitudes, customs and beliefs of all the minority groups in our society, although a knowledge of some of the leading differences would certainly be a help. It is possible to be *curious* about other cultures, *appreciative* of other ways of seeing and doing, *understanding* of the pressures and changes affecting minority ethnic communities and *skilled* in the way we ask questions and select activities. Only when we have acquired these competencies can we begin to deliver individualised care that is culturally appropriate. Interventions that take account of the person's cultural experience 'are generally more meaningful, relevant and intrinsically motivating and therefore have greater therapeutic value' (Dillard et al 1992, cited in Fair & Barnitt 1999). Fair and Barnitt go further. In an article with the eye-catching title, 'Making a Cup of Tea as Part of a Culturally Sensitive Service', they assert:

Where culture is not considered by therapists, this may have a significant effect on the appropriateness and outcomes of intervention. There is little benefit gained from the client attempting to make a cup of tea or indeed perform any other functional activity by adopting a method that has little meaning for him or her. The activity will cease to have purpose for the individual and not be therapeutic, potentially making the intervention futile. Therapists must be open to adapting practice to meet the needs of individuals, whichever cultural background they originate from.
(Fair & Barnitt 1999 p204)

Making tea is one fairly minor example of an everyday activity that may need to be looked at afresh by the therapist who aspires to be culturally competent. Other examples, with similarly practi-

cal consequences, are not hard to find. Orthodox Jews use two sinks to separate milk and meat products, a factor that may influence the advice we give on kitchen planning. If finger eating is the norm, then adapted table cutlery may become irrelevant. Religious rituals could preclude home visits at certain times or on particular days. A recent study of the self-care needs of Hindu elders suggests that many individuals in this group may not value independence in the accepted occupational therapy sense of being able to wash, dress and perform other functions unaided – it was expected that family members would help (Gibbs & Barnitt 1999). Box 9.6, extracted from Meghani-Wise (1996), gives examples of different cultural

---

Box 9.6 Cultural behaviours (from Meghani-Wise 1996)

Sikhs (Punjabi)
- do not cut or shave hair (kesha)
- wear a turban
- wear kachha (knee length shorts), which they do not remove in one go, but put one leg in the new pair first
- wear a kangha (semi-circular comb)
- carry a kirpin (dagger)
- wear a kara (bangle)
- do not remove these five Ks
- other personal care customs similar to Muslims

Hindus
- personal care customs similar to Muslims
- jewellery has religious significance and may denote marital status of women
- menstruating women may not cook or have access to areas where prayers are being held

Muslims
- wash hands and mouth before eating
- wash cooking utensils in running water
- wash and bathe in running water; may use a shower or prefer a bowl or bucket
- wash genitals after using the lavatory using the left hand
- may wear jewellery of religious significance

Jews
- do not use razors for shaving
- wear side-locks and keep the head covered
- women cover their head in public
- for prayers men wear a prayer shawl
- men wear a fringed undergarment, only removed for bathing
- pray before and after meals
- wash hands before meals
- use two sinks or bowls to separate meat and milk products

and religious behaviours that will impact upon the occupational therapy intervention. Bear in mind that these relate to orthodox or devout members of each faith. There are widespread variations in religious practice between individuals and groups within faiths and we must be careful not to foist the characteristics of any one religious or cultural community on all of its members.

One of the most pervasive forms of ethnocentrism, arguably shading into racism, is the stereotypical assumption that people belong to homogeneous and enduring communities that are somehow immune to the pressures and changes affecting the rest of society. It is often assumed, for example, that Asian people have extended families who will care for their elders and those family members with disabilities. But this can no longer be taken for granted. With increasing educational opportunities for the younger generation, the adoption of more Western attitudes towards career advancement and the modification of gender role expectations, Asian families may find themselves living geographically apart. A report prepared for the Joseph Rowntree Foundation on the problems facing minority ethnic families caring for a severely disabled child concluded:

Despite stereotypes suggesting the existence of extended supportive families among minority ethnic groups, there was little evidence to support this assertion … Indian and Black African/Caribbean families reported least support from their extended family, with levels of support lower than that [sic] found among the survey of white families. Mothers from all ethnic groups … reported lower levels of support from their partners than white mothers had reported.

(Chamba et al 1999 Ref 539 htm)

A survey of Hindu–Gujerati married couples from the Asian community in Leicester found that although 88% of couples began their lives in extended families, by the time of the survey 63% lived in nuclear-type households (Goodwin et al 1997). None the less, the presupposition of a wider network of family care than is available within the white community has been used by service providers to justify the status quo and save on costs, to the disadvantage of many minority ethnic groups (Patel 1993).

Box 9.7   Guidelines for culturally aware good practice

- Do not make assumptions based on your own cultural values and norms.
- Do not presume, having read about other cultures, that all norms necessarily apply to the individual.
- If in doubt, check it out.
- If language is a barrier, seek help from *adult* relatives or request an interpreter; observe usual boundaries of confidentiality.
- Be prepared to discuss family arrangements and how the impairment affects them.
- Be prepared to ask questions such as:
  - how do you usually do this? Show me your way.
  - is this kitchen equipment similar to yours?
  - do you need any other ingredients?
  - are there any dietary restrictions I need to know?
  - is this a convenient time for me to visit?
- Ensure that assessment paperwork is culturally appropriate

Diversity is a feature not only of the whole of our society but of the communities that make up our society and the generational experiences and family structures within those communities. While it is necessary to have a basic map of the similarities and differences between different ethnic groups, we must beware of seeing any social or cultural formation as static or frozen in time. Otherwise, for all our efforts, we shall end up merely reinforcing cultural stereotypes, neglecting to address the whole person and failing those who are most often at greatest disadvantage (Box 9.7).

LIFESPAN DEVELOPMENT

As we have seen, the therapist working within a humanistic framework relates to the person as far more than a diagnostic category; she considers his impairment in the context of his life-story as a whole. Lifespan theory brings our attention to the type of background issues that the therapist will need to consider as she prepares her treatment programme. Whilst it cannot direct her towards specific interventions, as there is obviously too wide a range, it can help her to identify the broad areas of concern at different stages of life.

In this section, we will consider the lifespan in relation to the three stages of childhood, adolescence and adulthood.

CHILDHOOD

The dependent new-born baby, reared by nurturing parents, learns to trust. As he grows in confidence so he becomes increasingly aware of his own individuality. He relates to a wider circle, perhaps in this society, joining playgroup before starting formal school. Inevitably, conflicts arise as he oversteps safety boundaries, house and social rules, or simply exhausts his parents. Persistent heavy-handed criticism or curbing of his experimentation may lead to rebellion as he asserts his will, or conversely to self-doubt, which sows the seeds of low self-esteem. Imaginative play is important for the development of skills. As a child crawls through a play tunnel, climbs a frame or bounces a ball, he develops not only motor skills but also linguistic and social skills as he takes turns and learns to share. By middle childhood, he begins to develop initiative, defined by Erikson (1980) as a 'truly free sense of enterprise', controlled by a growing conscience, which at this stage is based on internalised distinctions of right and wrong set by significant people in his life. Adults in authority must strike a balance between rightful control, protection and risk taking.

The occupational therapist working with disabled children needs to be able to consider how she may help the parents to encourage their child to develop his full potential. Initially, they will be distressed when their child is born with or acquires some form of impairment, and they will need to be helped to grieve for the loss of expected normality. As parents begin to make the necessary psychological adjustments, so the therapist will suggest ways of improving the child's abilities and thus begin to establish a basis for continued hope for a meaningful quality of life. Bear in mind here that chronic disease in childhood is a vast area. Some diseases are progressive, leading to eventual death, and in these cases a key purpose of therapy is to make a short

life as meaningful and fulfilled as possible. In other cases, the disease process burns itself out or otherwise comes to an end, leaving the child with residual impairments.

As the child becomes conscious of the differences between himself and his peers, so his frustrated outbursts may attract inappropriate discipline. Parents may well experience frustration when he cannot perform the expected ordinary skills of his peers and, whatever delight they may take in his improvements, there will be times when his continued dependency, which has a much longer time span than that of his siblings, will create stress. The therapist should not underestimate this emotional strain and should discuss with parents how and when the teaching of therapy-related skills will be incorporated into everyday routines. Most children, with the exception of those whose central nervous system disorders impair cognition and emotional and behavioural functioning, are of normal intelligence range and should be encouraged to develop in accordance with usual educational practice, though it is likely that absence from school for hospital care and therapy will impact upon their academic progress (Johnson 1994).

A study by Missiuna and Pollock (2000) found that treatment objectives are often prescribed by parents, therapists and teacher *for* the child rather than *with* him. Interestingly, although there was a high level of agreement between parent and child about specific goals, there was far less agreement regarding priorities, parents being more eager that the child pursue academic tasks such as printing and drawing than the self-care and leisure activities preferred by the children. The study highlighted the need to discuss and negotiate options with the children themselves.

Experimentation and exploration are likely to be inhibited by motor dysfunction, so imagination is required to think of alternative ways of encouraging play. A study by Howard (1996) highlighted some of the barriers to different play environments. None of the disabled children in her study belonged to Cubs or Brownies, raising interesting questions regarding factors such as parental overprotection, the child himself not wanting to be the odd one out, difficult access to meeting places and a possible reluctance on the part of leaders to include these children. Many disabled children, she found, played predominantly in their own gardens; non-disabled children could venture further afield. Opportunities similar though not necessarily identical to those available to the non-disabled child need to be found with the therapist acting as facilitator. How she tackles this will depend on the neighbourhood and what is locally available 'but social clubs, self-help groups, equipment, mobility aids and support groups for parents are all possibilities towards the ultimate goal of enhancing the child's independence and preparing him or her for a fully participative adulthood' (Howard 1996 p573). Howard concluded that the occupational therapist is uniquely positioned to assist in this process.

ADOLESCENCE

Adolescence begins with the physical changes of puberty, progresses with the growth and strengthening of sexual and personal identity, and ends at around the age of 18 with the commencement of higher education or paid employment and the ability to live independently. During adolescence, peer groups become key references for experimentation with new roles and identities, as traditional ideas and values are questioned. Healthy conflict with parental authority during this sometimes turbulent period allows for increasing separation of identity from the family. Difficulties in proceeding through this stage may result in identity confusion and uncertainty of roles.

There will be many adolescents who sustain transient physical injuries, for example, fractures resulting from football, skateboarding, climbing and other activities. Their treatment will be essentially biomedical and the encounter with the occupational therapist of too short a duration for all phenomenological issues to be fully addressed; nor do they necessarily need to be.

The therapist can also reasonably expect that personal and sexual matters, the move towards independent living and career choices will be guided by family, friends and those within the educational system. It is far more likely that the occupational therapist will adopt a comprehensive approach with adolescents whose childhood disorders require continued intervention and with those who have experienced trauma or acquired disorders necessitating longer-term treatment.

The work role, or preparation for it, is for most of us a strong identifier, holding out the prospect not only of monetary reward, which facilitates independence, but also influencing and determining social status. In the context of high unemployment rates, many young people, finding their skills unmarketable, have difficulty forming a work identity. If this creates difficulties for the non-disabled adolescent, it falls even harder on the adolescent who is permanently disabled. As disability rights groups assert their needs more vociferously and as equal opportunities policies are better enforced, so we become increasingly aware of the problems facing disabled people in their search for this aspect of role identity.

The extent to which occupational therapists are or should be involved in sexuality issues is a matter of ongoing debate in our professional journals, as is the relevance of sexual orientation to our practice (Couldrick 1999, Northcott & Chard 2000, Williamson 2000). It cannot be within the remit of this chapter to explore these issues in any depth. However, it is relevant to say that disabled adolescents are no different from anyone else in the sexual feelings they experience and wish to express. They have the same need to establish and confirm their sexual identity, and for those who are lesbian, gay or bisexual this may pose particular problems. Jenny Morris makes an interesting comment on the prejudiced assumptions of non-disabled people with regard to the sexual orientation of those who are disabled. 'Disabled people could not possibly be lesbians or gay, and … if we are this is because we cannot achieve a "normal" heterosexual relationship rather than it being an expression of our sexuality' (Morris 1993).

ADULTHOOD

The idea of the biological clock ticking relentlessly from birth to death is one with which we are all familiar. The concept of a 'social clock', which fits into this biological order, has presumed a traditional Western, economically successful climate. In adulthood, the social clock was seen to cover the sequence from stable work role, with the expectation of promotion (often within the same company or profession), marriage and childrearing, retirement and ageing to one's own death. In our society today, many of the assumptions underlying this notion, particularly those relating to early and middle adulthood, are being questioned.

Young couples may choose to cohabit rather than marry; the timing of pregnancy may be deferred as both partners pursue careers; some choose not to have children at all; single parenthood has become more common; divorce may mean reconstituted families. With increasing pressure from gay rights activists, society is being asked to accept alternative lifestyles, with some children being reared within a lesbian or male homosexual household. Employment prospects have become more uncertain with changes in political and economic structure. Many people no longer think in terms of a lifelong career but rather of the need to develop skills to be able to make several career moves during their working lives. Others find themselves facing redundancy, short periods of unemployment or even long-term unemployment, when changes in traditional family roles may have to be made. Finally, concepts of old age are having to change as retired people, who deep down hoped that family would care for them, find themselves living geographically apart from their offspring and, as they become frailer, more reliant upon neighbours and sometimes statutory services, for assistance. Whilst the idea of the social clock may remain true for many, for others it has become an outdated exposition of society's expectations of life pattern.

Early adulthood

Early adulthood is a period of rapid personal development. Becoming an adult involves taking responsibility and building new structures in three key areas: career, friendship networks and intimate relationships. In each of these areas, the disabled young person is faced with additional barriers that make this period of life particularly challenging. The disabled university applicant, for example, must find out which universities offer the best help regarding accessibility to campus, library, canteen, lecture theatre and seminar rooms. Are there computers with appropriate software, a special needs adviser and an accommodations officer who will help him find suitably accessible digs?

Adolescent peer groups have largely broken up by this stage and new groups are formed, which will provide support and a sounding-board as the young adult person makes choices and takes decisions that will shape his future life. Where does the young disabled adult, with the same desires as everyone else, find similar opportunities to form new peer groups and develop his perspectives on the future? If we consider where young people meet and form relationships – parties, gatherings in other people's houses or flats, dance clubs, pubs, restaurants, work venues – the difficulties immediately become apparent. The major problems are obviously those related to access and transport. The disabled young person will need well-developed social communication, self-awareness and appropriate assertiveness skills to ensure that he is not left out.

It is common around this time to seek out a partner with a view to establishing a long-term personal or sexual relationship. Erikson saw this need to share one's life as central to adjustment on a spectrum of intimacy and isolation. Intimacy in its fullest sense involves self-disclosure, vulnerability and closeness to another person without paradoxically losing one's own sense of self. For many disabled people, some of the most painful barriers to intimacy are created by other people's perceptions. Jenny Morris (1993) reveals, from her research interviews, a number of commonly held assumptions that non-disabled people hold about disabled people:

- 'We are asexual or at best sexually inadequate.'
- 'If we are not married or in a long-term relationship it is because no one wants us and

not through our personal choice to remain single or live alone.'

- 'Any able-bodied person who married us must have done so for … suspicious motives and never through love.'
- 'If we have a partner who is also disabled we chose each other for no other reason and not for any other qualities we might possess. When we choose "our own kind" in this way the able-bodied world feels relieved, until of course we wish to have children; then we're seen as irresponsible.'

Such undermining messages, says Morris, 'become part of our way of thinking about ourselves and/or our thinking about other disabled people. This is the internalization of *their* values about *our* lives' (Morris 1993).

Middle adulthood

During the middle period of life, which begins in the early thirties, the main area of productivity is employment, with careers reaching their peak in terms of responsibility. Nevertheless, at this time too, many people reappraise their own values, to balance employment-related achievement with family needs and goals. Knowledge, attitudes and values are passed to the next generation, a process which Erikson terms 'generativity'. This takes place at a formal level within society's institutions and at a personal level in bringing up one's own children and/or contributing to the wellbeing of others. Voluntary roles such as scout leader, youth-group organiser, school governor, magistrate, committee member, church warden and charity worker are examples. Many disabled people today are active in voluntary and community organisations, as staff, committee members, advocates and advisers. Where people fail in their efforts to be generative, they often feel 'a pervading sense of stagnation and personal impoverishment' (Erikson 1980).

Disabled parents face particular difficulties, depending on their specific impairment. Disabled mothers may need specialist care during pregnancy and childbirth. Lifting and carrying a small child may require adaptive equipment not always readily available and therapists may need to be imaginative in helping to design appropriate devices to suit individual parents' ability levels, taking into account energy conservation principles to prevent undue strain and fatigue. Remember, too, that young children run off in play and need retrieving so some disabled parents may need assistance in this respect. Most parents want to be involved in their children's educational and recreational activities. Given the diverse nature of these, coping with the logistics of taking an active role is demanding. Travelling with children is tiring at the best of times. Difficult access to transport systems and/or the high cost of private car ownership (family-sized and suitably adapted) present disabled parents with problems unimagined by many of us.

In our society, paid employment covers a span of around 40 years somewhere between the ages of 16 and 65. These years provide not only income for present expenditure but opportunities for financial investments, including pension schemes, to generate income for the retirement years. This is an important point because unemployed people, who include many disabled people, are financially doubly disadvantaged because they cannot build up adequate pension contributions in addition to those provided by the state benefit.

Recent research on disabled people and employment funded by the Joseph Rowntree Foundation looked at training and preparation for jobs, the application process, maintaining oneself in work and becoming disabled when already in work. The findings indicated that current initiatives often overemphasise preparation and that disabled people were sceptical about training schemes that did not lead to real sustainable jobs with wages at the market rate. Supported employment was found to be a key factor in helping them to maintain the position yet was not readily available. Even when a job was successfully maintained there was often a 'glass ceiling' in promotion terms (Barnes et al 1998).

Major projects that do employ disabled people are most often impairment-specific. The more successful projects were those that moved away from this model and recruited their employees on the basis of common problems shared by a number of groups, such as disabled people, older people and women returners. It was pointed out that changes in the mainstream labour market offered both challenges and opportunities. New technology could be a powerful tool for disabled people, yet there are barriers to its use. Major funders place little emphasis on technology and, where it is available, training is often inappropriate and inadequate. Other developments, such as part-time work, teleworking and self-employed contracts, have the benefits of more flexible hours and could be offered to disabled people, along with the simple, everyday adaptations to the physical environment that are now mandatory (Barnes et al 1998).

If productivity is as central to our professional thinking as we claim, then we are required to keep ourselves up-to-date with current social research in this area and to question and re-evaluate our own practices in work rehabilitation. For some, this knowledge may prompt us to aspire to more influential posts within the statutory sector, or to consider career moves outside it to help initiate more innovative and workable schemes.

Late adulthood

Late adulthood is a time of particular reflection, when the person finally comes to terms with failures and limitations, appraises his successes and sees his life within the context of the meaningful whole. Successful progression through the earlier stages of the life cycle will lead to a fuller integration of the personality, whilst failure to make necessary psychological adjustments leads to a sense of despair, of not having grown inwardly, and may be manifest in criticism, intolerance and disgust towards others (Erikson 1980). Wisdom, not of course restricted to the older adult, may crystallise at this stage.

There is considerable negative stereotyping of elderly people in our society: 'we fill the gaps in our knowledge with dated clichés and misleading prejudices' (Berger 1997). In reality, older adults tend to behave and cope in much the same

ways as they have always done. Many enjoy and contribute to the welfare of grandchildren, and to efforts to benefit the wider society by giving time and valuable expertise to voluntary projects. This is a time for aesthetic enjoyment, when there is leisure for new interests such as gardening, photography, poetry and the arts. These days, many older adults continue to enjoy good health and an active life (including the sexual) well into their seventies, and sometimes beyond, though it is commonly a time when one partner dies with the need for adjustment to this major loss by the surviving partner.

The quality of life in older adulthood depends upon the continuation of friendships, involvement in community activities such as church and social groups and upon financial circumstances which will vary according to early investment opportunities. A point worth noting is that people who migrated to this country as adults may face 'additional poverty, and therefore health risks, as they age. For the pension system depends on lifelong contributions' (Parekh 2000).

Even with failing health, many people continue living in their own homes with various kinds of supportive input, available privately or through statutory services. Some elderly people are cared for by family, although with an ageing population their offspring may be in the retirement years themselves when their elderly parent requires increased assistance. For those who can no longer be maintained in their own or their relatives' homes, the usual next option is residential care, which will be state funded only when personal assets have been reduced to a statutory minimum.

Occupational therapists have considerable input into services for the elderly. Links between these services are of varying quality and can sometimes be confusing. In many areas there is minimum collaboration between 'physical' and 'mental health' teams. As Rigney (2000) points out, 'the divisions are started by hospitals. If you break your leg, you go to a physical hospital and are served by a physical disabilities team on discharge. If you have an episode of depression [you are] discharged to the care of a mental health team'. Whilst she accepts that the particular setting may be a constraint on the therapist who wants to work in a holistic way, she nevertheless urges us to draw on our wide range of skills to identify unmet needs and refer the person on appropriately.

LIFE EVENTS AND RESPONSE TO CHANGE

Throughout life we experience pleasures and disappointments. Some are highly significant, having tremendous impact upon us and requiring time for adjustment. How we cope with them is complex. Various models are available to help the therapist structure and understand this process. These 'models of transition' are devices for analysing an actual experience in a dynamic way, and though they may operate slightly differently for positive and negative experiences, the underlying pattern is similar.

Change and loss may be grouped into different categories. With a short-term transient loss, such as a fractured femur sustained by a healthy active young man, fairly speedy adjustment is expected. Some losses are long-term and enduring. The person diagnosed with multiple sclerosis must adjust not only to the present situation but also to future impairments as they arise. A stroke has different effects on different people; whilst for one person adjustment to residual

upper limb dysfunction may be manageable, for a musician it would be devastating.

The present section focuses on two models of transition, the first developed by Hopson (1981), the second by Moos and Schaefer (1984, 1986). It is important to note that they both refer to the normal ways in which we all respond to life crises. Table 9.1 gives examples of both positive and negative life events.

Hopson's model of transition (1981) proposes a series of stages to be worked through as the person adjusts to change (Table 9.2).

Moos and Schaefer's model of transition (1984, 1986) examines adjustment to life events in terms of adaptive tasks and coping skills necessary to manage the transition or resolve the crisis successfully (Table 9.3). Their work also developed to look specifically at coping with the life crisis of physical disability and the adaptive tasks were enlarged upon (Table 9.4).

Now let us relate these two models to practice. In some settings we will meet the person very soon after he has been admitted to hospital, when both he and his relatives will be in shock. As they react with sorrow, it will be difficult for them to absorb all the information offered. Notwithstanding the self-protective need to deny and avoid painful reality, a growing understanding of the impact of the diagnosis will gradually dawn as they analyse and consider the practical issues. In attempting to relate to healthcare professionals, particularly in an open ward setting, they may present a 'stiff upper lip' but sensitivity

Table 9.1 Life events

Examples of positive desired events		Examples of negative undesired events	
Anticipated	Unanticipated	Anticipated	Unanticipated

Offer of a university place
Getting married
Starting a new job
Receipt of expected
    inheritance
	Falling in love
	Winning a large
	    sum of money
		Death of self or of a loved
		    one following long-term
		    terminal illness
			Routine medical check
			    reveals cancer
			Self or close relative
			    involved in accident
			New-born baby has
			    impairment
			Sudden onset of
			    illness. Coping with
			    demands of disability
			Untimely death of a
			    loved one

Table 9.2 Hopson's model of transition as a person adjusts to change (adapted from Hopson 1981)

Stage	Feelings
Immobilisation	Sense of unreality Shocked disbelief
Reaction	Sharp mood swing: joy to elation; disappointment and sorrow to despair
Minimisation	Overwhelming emotions difficult to live with Intensity of reaction brought under control with more realistic appraisal Elation leads to wider sense of wellbeing or despair is tempered with thoughts that the situation is less dire than imagined
Self-doubt	Ability to cope doubted Accompanying anxieties about future performance Energy levels fluctuate
Letting go	A watershed requiring courage. Placing former lifestyle into different perspective in order to move forward
Testing	Exploring new options that accord with life stage Possibilities and limitations become apparent Hopes raised and dashed Mood changes accompany successes and failures Self-esteem begins to rise
Search for meaning	Striving to gain deeper understanding of meaning of experience, so that lessons may be learned Values and attitudes challenged New insights gained
Integration	The transition process is said to be complete when the life event has been integrated into an overall map of experience and feelings about it are within the context of the whole. That particular life event now shares boundaries with other life experiences and no longer dominates. It is not as though the event had never happened, nor is it that effects will not be felt way into the future; rather it is that the person is now ready to cope with the rest of life, whatever that may bring

Table 9.3 Moos and Schaefer: model of transition – adjustment to life events (summarised from Moos & Schaefer 1984, 1888)

Adaptive tasks

Understanding the significance and confronting the reality of the event	With some events, these aspects are distinct, because a period elapses between one event and the next, e.g. pregnancy to childbirth. With other events, e.g. trauma, illness and disability, the person and family are confronted with aspects of the reality from the outset and realising the significance is ongoing Confronting reality requires action
Maintaining relationships	Within the context of family, work and friendship networks Require energy to sustain
Maintaining a balanced emotional life	Tendency to focus entirely on the event becomes emotionally draining Need to manage extremes of feelings to balance inner life
Preserving self-concept	There may be an identity crisis with a need to preserve one's sense of self

Coping skills

Cognitive: appraisal-focused	Allow logical analysis of and reflection upon the situation, and judgements to be made regarding viable options
Behavioural: problem-focused	Behaviours are observable actions, allowing practical tackling of the situation, such as seeking information and support, and identifying options
Affective: emotion-focused	Enable appropriate expression and containment of emotion in different situations. Sensitivity allows others to do the same Maintaining hope and reaching a stage of acceptance

Table 9.4 Moos and Schaefer: the crisis of physical illness – adaptive tasks (summarised from Moos & Schaefer 1984, 1888)

Illness related	Dealing with pain, incapacitation and symptoms Dealing with hospital environment and treatment procedures Developing and maintaining relationships with healthcare staff
General	Preserving emotional balance by managing upsetting feelings associated with illness Preserving self-concept by revising self-image with changes in physical appearance and by maintaining competence by defining limits of independence and readjusting goals Sustaining relationships with family and friends, keeping communication open and to find emotional and practical support Preparing for uncertain future

on our part, in more private surroundings, may facilitate the expression of deeper fears.

As rehabilitation begins, the therapist's person-centred skills are particularly suited to helping the individual to work through the stages of letting go and exploring new options while encouraging him to have faith in himself and in his own abilities. We must be optimistic if we are to encourage people to progress, but also realistic in our expectations, recognising how difficult it may be for some people to move on. The therapist must be prepared to be the target of negative feelings, sometimes involving anger and verbal abuse. In these cases, our own feelings of frustration are better handled within the context of the team, rather than being projected back onto the person.

As Hopson's model indicates, for many people the next stage is characterised by a search for meaning and a deeper understanding of the experience. A major life event may challenge the person's customary values and attitudes, triggering a transition in which what really matters to the individual is brought into focus. Real friends come forward; unimagined insights and compassion may be gained. For some people, losses and gains balance; for others the scales remain tipped. If disablement provokes a reappraisal of priorities and enables the person to value those things previously taken for granted, then in a sense there has been inner growth. Some people seem able to transcend the most traumatic of life events. The case of Florence (Box 9.8) demonstrates real courage and determination in rebuilding a new life.

Diseases such as some forms of cancer, motor neurone disease and HIV/AIDS carry a poor prognosis. Not only must the person adjust to impairments as they present, during which time the above models may be serviceable but, as the disease progresses towards death, so must he come to terms with the finality of his own life. This process too involves a series of stages, for which the authoritative model is that provided by Elisabeth Kubler-Ross (1970). The five stages identified by Kubler-Ross are presented in Table 9.5. Her work addresses a number of themes: how to examine our own fears of death, how to share the knowledge of terminal illness with the person and how to reach beyond the ostensible meaning of a communication to its underlying meaning which may be hidden. The reader is also referred to Colin Murray Parkes (1998), who addresses the issue of bereavement from the perspective of immediate family and friends.

Box 9.8 Case study (summarised from Aadalen & Stroebel-Kahn 1981)

Happily married and pregnant, Florence, a professional woman whose life was 'rich and fulfilling', sustained a C5–6 quadriplegia in a road traffic accident. Her story tells of how she came to terms with her many losses, 'my marriage as it existed before the accident, our baby, my hands, my legs and feet, my singing voice', later the loss of her sister, which 'released the floodgate', and her divorce, the most stressful adjustment of all, when her husband 'was finally able to acknowledge that there was no way he could live with me and have his needs met … We both feel rotten'.

Others planned her rehabilitation and she was saddened that no-one invited her involvement. She resented being talked *about* 'treated like a piece of wood'. Provision of assistive devices emphasised the permanence of her disability. As recovery progressed she began to derive pleasure from 'sights, sounds and smells' on outings with her husband, though going home proved traumatic. Quadriplegic in her own home and in profound depression 'my feelings were raw. I tried to gain some control over my sense of utter helplessness … I'd bite out at the people closest to me … Jumping the gun on caretakers was one of the ways I was still denying my reality'.

Later 'I discovered I had developed increased risk-taking skills … you see that you can tackle most anything by breaking it down in bits and pieces of challenge'. Although intellectually able to work out her losses, emotionally this proved more difficult. Establishing 'appropriate criteria for worthiness' for herself was demanding in a society that values productivity so highly.

Following her divorce, she began to take charge of her life. As time went on, she made firm friendships and, with a live-in caretaker, began life in her own apartment. 'Visualising and planning for the future, in terms of [my] professional involvement and self-actualisation are ongoing processes', she tells us.

CONCLUSION

There is nothing new in the idea that therapy should address the needs of the whole person. In the late eighteenth century, the pioneers of Moral Treatment in France and England (see Chapter 1) proclaimed respect for the individual and recognised the value of enabling people to engage in activity suited to their particular interests, personalities and gifts. They did this, of course, from the standpoint of their own ideological, cultural and religious presuppositions, an observation that led to the criticism that, however apparently

Table 9.5 Stages of dying (adapted from Kubler-Ross 1997)

Denial and isolation	'No, it can't be true' is a temporary defence mechanism, replaced by partial acceptance and partial denial
Anger	Rage, resentment and anger often displaced on to professional staff, family and God. The person needs attention, tolerance and time to express his feelings so they can be understood rather than judged. Some anger may be connected with no longer being in control so decision making within the boundaries of necessary treatment regimens should be encouraged
Bargaining	Often a hidden stage, when the person bargains with God for extra time although he knows this to be illogical
Depression	Two types of depression identified: • depression concerned with practicalities, such as future provision for family, or making final will, is best relieved by helping the person to deal with these • depression concerned with loss of everything, life itself is best handled with quiet empathy, warmth and touch
Acceptance	A final coming to terms with the inevitability of death, a stage almost devoid of feelings

'holistic', the system was at root a 'gigantic moral imprisonment' (Foucault 1967). What is new and transforming about the phenomenological approach is that it offers at least a partial escape from this 'imprisonment', finding the locus of control within the person. It is transforming in the demand it makes on the therapist to relinquish some of her power – 'doing with' rather than 'doing to' – and sharing her professional knowledge in a spirit of genuine partnership. Indeed, this approach requires a different kind of therapist, one who is 'integrated, transparently real in the relationship', able to accept the client as a separate individual, and 'sensitively empathic' in seeing the world through his eyes (Rogers 1967). With the emergence of new perspectives on disability and cultural difference, it is likely that person-centred therapy will continue to be an essential focus of education and training in occupational therapy.

REFERENCES

Aadalen SP, Stroebel-Kahn F 1981 Coping with quadriplegia. In: Moos RH, Schaefer JA (eds) 1984 Coping with physical illness: new perspectives. Plenum, New York, ch 13, pp 173–188

Abbott S 1999 Planning and implementation of care: the patient's role. British Journal of Therapy and Rehabilitation 6(8):398–401

Barnes H, Thornton P, Campbell SM 1998 Disabled people and employment: A review of research and development work. Policy Press, Partridge Green

Berger KS 1997 The developing person through the lifespan, 4th edn. Worth, New York

Chamba R, Ahmad W, Hirst M et al 1999 On the edge: minority ethnic families caring for a severely disabled child. Policy Press, Partridge Green *www.jrf.org.uk/knowledge/findings/social* care/539htm

College of Occupational Therapists 2000 Code of ethics and professional conduct for occupational therapists. College of Occupational Therapists, London

Couldrick L 1999 Sexual issues within occupational therapy. Part 2. Implications for education and practice. British Journal of Occupational Therapy 62(1):26–30

Craddock J 1996 Responses of the occupational therapy profession to the perspective of the disability movement, Part 1. British Journal of Occupational Therapy 59(1):17–22

Creek J 1997 The truth is no longer out there. British Journal of Occupational Therapy 60(2):50–52

Dillard M, Andonian L, Flores O et al 1992 Culturally competent occupational therapy in a diversely populated mental health setting. In: Fair A, Barnitt R 1999 Making a cup of tea as part of a culturally sensitive service. British Journal of Occupational Therapy 62(5):199–205

Erikson EH 1980 Identity and the life cycle. WW Norton, New York

Finkelstein V 1993 Disability: a social challenge or an administrative responsibility? In: Swain J, Finkelstein V, French S, Oliver M (eds) Disabling barriers – enabling environments. Open University, Sage, London, section 1.4, 34–43

Finlay L 1999 Applying phenomenology in research: problems, principles and practice. British Journal of Occupational Therapy 62(7):299–306

Foucault M 1967 Madness and civilization. Tavistock, London

Gibbs KE, Barnitt R 1999 Occupational therapy and the self-care needs of Hindu elders. British Journal of Occupational Therapy 62(3):100–106

Goodwin R, Cramer D, Sinhal H, Adatia K 1997 Social support and marital wellbeing in an Asian community. YPS for Joseph Rowntree Foundation, York

Hopson B 1981 Response to papers by Schlossberg, Brammer, Abrego. Counselling Psychologist 9:36–39

Howard L 1996 A comparison of leisure-time activities between able-bodied children and children with physical disabilities. British Journal of Occupational Therapy 59(12):570–574

Howarth A, Jones D 1999 Transcultural occupational therapy in the United Kingdom: concepts and research. British Journal of Occupational Therapy 62(10):451–458

Johnson SB 1994 Chronic illness in children. In: Penny G, Bennett P, Herbert M (eds) Health psychology: a lifespan perspective. Harwood Academic, Reading, section 1, 31–50

Kubler-Ross E 1997 On death and dying. Routledge, London

Lane L 2000 Client-centred practice: is it compatible with early discharge hospital-at-home policies? British Journal of Occupational Therapy 63(7):310–315

MacPherson Sir W. The Stephen Lawrence Inquiry: STO1999. Report of an Inquiry by Sir William MacPherson of Cluny, advised by Tom Cook, The Right Reverend Dr John Sentamu, Dr Richard Stone. Presented to Parliament by the Secretary of State for the Home Department by Command of Her Majesty

Maslow AH 1970 Motivation and personality, 2nd edn. Harper & Row, New York

Mattingly C, Fleming MH 1994 Clinical reasoning: forms of inquiry in a therapeutic practice. FA Davis, Philadelphia, PA

Meghani-Wise Z 1996 Why this interest in minority ethnic groups? British Journal of Occupational Therapy 59(10):485–489

Missiuna C, Pollock N 2000 Perceived efficacy and goal setting in young children. Canadian Journal of Occupational Therapy 67(2):101–109

Moos RH, Schaefer JA 1984 Coping with physical illness: new perspectives. Plenum, New York

Moos RH, Schaefer JA 1986 Coping with life crises: an integrated approach. Plenum, New York

Morris J 1993 Prejudice. In: Swain J, Finkelstein V, French S, Oliver M (eds) Disabling barriers – enabling environments. Open University, Sage, London, Section 2.5, 101–106

Northcott R, Chard G 2000 Sexual aspects of rehabilitation: the client's perspective. British Journal of Occupational Therapy 63(9):412–418

Oliver M 1999 The disability movement and the professions. British Journal of Therapy and Rehabilitation 6(8):377–379

Parekh 2000 Report of the Commission on the Future of Multi-Ethnic Britain, established by The Runnymede Trust. Profile Books, London

Patel N 1993 Health margins: black elders' care – models, policies and prospects. In: Ahmed WIU (ed) Race and health in contemporary Britain. Open University, Buckingham, ch 7

Rigney C 2000 Physical or mental health: should we divide? British Journal of Occupational Therapy 63(4):177–178

Rogers CR 1967 On becoming a person. Constable, London

Sumsion T 1997 Environmental challenges and opportunities of client-centred practice. British Journal of Occupational Therapy 60(2):53–56

Sumsion T 2000 A revised occupational therapy definition of client-centred practice. British Journal of Occupational Therapy 63(7):308–309

Williamson P 2000 Football and tin cans: a model of identity formation based on sexual orientation expressed through engagement in occupations. British Journal of Occupational Therapy 63(9):432–439

FURTHER READING

Atkinson RL, Atkinson RC, Smith EE et al 2000 Hilgard's introduction to psychology, 13th edn. Harcourt Brace, London

Berry JW, Poorting YH, Segall MH, Dasen PR 1992 Cross-cultural psychology: research and applications. Cambridge University Press, Cambridge

Cole A, McIntosh B, Whittaker A 2000 We want our voices heard: developing new lifestyles with disabled people. Policy Press, Partridge Green

Levinson DJ 1978 The seasons of a man's life. Ballantine, New York

Levinson DJ 1997 The seasons of a woman's life. Ballantine, New York

Murray Parkes C 1998 Bereavement: studies of grief in adult life. Penguin, London

Sugarman L 1995 Lifespan development: concepts, theories and interventions. Routledge, London

10

Life skills

Marg Foster

INTRODUCTION

Life skills or skills for living are a major area of occupational therapy practice with almost all client groups. It is a vast area with many different facets, which are impossible to cover in detail in one chapter. Whole books have been written on particular aspects of living and the skills for managing them in different settings. Practitioners and people with particular areas of dysfunction can refer to a wealth of texts on the assessment and management of life skills from both professional and personal perspectives.

This chapter therefore aims to present an overview of life skills. It will identify some of the requirements for success in individual areas of function and illustrate ways in which the individual and the therapist may work together to address problem areas. Specific techniques, items of equipment and individual organisation are offered only as illustrative examples; the references given at the end of the chapter will provide the reader with more detailed information in specific areas.

This chapter begins by defining what is meant by 'life skills' and describes their classification, addressing basic transferable skills that apply across most areas and dividing the activities into three overlapping categories: self-maintenance, role duties and leisure. The general development of life skills is discussed, together with the potential implications for an individual of any disruption in his ability to perform everyday tasks. Following this, the possible strategies employed by the occupational therapist in working with the individual, and those closely involved with his care when helping to address and overcome the difficulties, is outlined.

The chapter then discusses basic skills that are transferable to many areas of living – mobility and manipulative hand skills, communication and cognitive and processing skills. Following this, each of the three categories of life skills is covered in turn, describing the types of functional ability each may demand, the types of assessment appropriate to each area and ways in which the therapist and others may help the individual to optimise performance and meet his own occupational performance priorities. The discussion of self-maintenance activities includes sections on the importance of sexuality and image, as well as the day-to-day occupations of feeding, toileting, dressing and undressing, personal cleansing and grooming.

The section on role duties examines the implications for managing a number of different roles. The discussion commences with the examination of the responsibilities and skills associated with the homemaking role. The is followed by discussion on the role of the carer, with particular attention to those who provide support for individuals with particular problems associated with disability. Examples of assistance available to them from both statutory and non-statutory provision is given. The special needs of carers who are themselves managing their own disability, child carers and the needs of parents of children with a disability are outlined. Following this, the worker role is considered. The discussion explores the value of work in maintaining the individual's self-esteem and the occupational therapist's role in assessing an individual's skills and attributes and preparing for resettlement in a former job or exploring alternative options. In addition, some of the various forms of support for employees with disabilities and trainee opportunities are outlined. Finally, two roles related to the worker role – those of the student and the volunteer – are briefly considered.

The final section of the chapter examines the importance of leisure pursuits in helping individuals with a disability to achieve a healthy balance of interests and activities, especially when the worker role can no longer be fulfilled. Leisure pursuits provide an avenue for socialisation, relaxation and mental stimulation, and can provide an individual identity. As such, they constitute a vital component of habilitation and rehabilitation. Options for leisure activities are described, along with ways in which the therapist can support the individual in gaining confidence to return to previous hobbies or take up new interests and to make contacts beyond the family circle.

Throughout the chapter, much of the therapist's involvement reflects a problem-solving, compensatory approach, and ways by which the individual can compensate for loss of function predominate. It must be stressed, however, that the therapist's approach must be determined by the particular problems and needs of the individual and his carers, and that intervention must, above all, reflect the aspirations and priorities of her client. Other therapeutic approaches may be used in particular situations to improve performance in order to overcome dysfunctional areas rather than compensate for their loss or limitation.

WHAT ARE LIFE SKILLS?

Life skills are the abilities individuals acquire and develop in order to perform everyday tasks successfully. They vary from person to person and change throughout the lifespan. Evolving roles and responsibilities influence an individual's balance of occupation, his perception of the relative importance of various occupations and the very nature of the occupations in which he is engaged (Fig. 10.1). Factors such as culture and the individual's social setting also influence the importance of particular skills and attributes. The emphasis given to particular skills in the occupational therapist's intervention should be based on the individual's own priorities, taking into account his desires and aspirations and the demands placed upon him by his various roles.

The acquisition or recovery of a life skill depends not only on the level of its complexity in

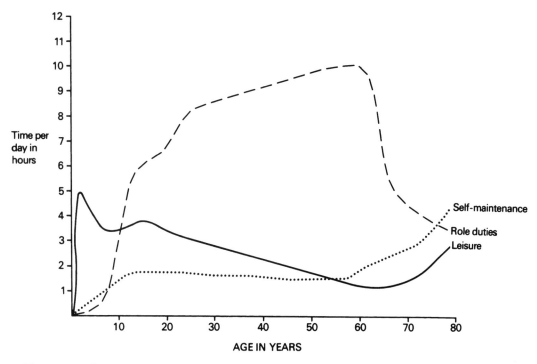

Fig. 10.1 Life skills map for a 77-year-old widow living alone who maintained the roles of housewife, parent and part-time employee until 60 years and nursed her disabled husband until his death when she was 63 years.

relation to the individual's dysfunction but also upon the person's motivation, drive and accustomed lifestyle and roles. Someone who has never had to perform an activity before may have different needs from someone who is relearning a previously familiar activity. The therapist needs to understand the importance and relevance of individual occupations in supporting people's roles in their particular family, culture and environment. Illness, dysfunction or other disruption to a person's routine pattern will disrupt roles previously accepted as normal. Individuals' priorities will vary; for some people independence in self-maintenance activities will be the prime concern. Others may prefer to accept ongoing assistance with self-care tasks in order to conserve energy for other pursuits. For others, the acquisition of skills that will allow them to return to paid employment will be the prime objective.

The occupational therapist will also need to consider the nature of the skills to be addressed. She will need to analyse each skill in terms of its physical, sensory, cognitive, perceptual and social components, and consider to what degree these components may be transferable from one area of living to another. Her primary concern will be with how the individual's skills interrelate in the performance of an activity. Therefore, while she may make frequent use of the specialised measurements taken by other professionals in order to locate specific areas of function and limitation, her particular contribution will lie in her ability to take a comprehensive view of the interrelationship of these skills in the performance of functional tasks and the individual's perceived relative importance of the tasks in the wider context of his life pattern.

CATEGORISATION OF ACTIVITIES

Texts and practitioners have grouped life skills into various different categories, such as 'domestic activities', 'activities of daily living' (ADL) and 'work activities'. Such categories, although useful, often overlap. Money-handling skills, for example, may be considered in any of the three categories. Whilst bearing this fluidity of categorisation in mind, for ease of analysis this chapter has considered basic transferable skills that apply to many aspects of living, followed by the skills necessary for activities organised under the three main headings of: personal self-maintenance, role duties and leisure (Fig. 10.2), but recognises that these categories are not exclusive:

- Basic transferable skills relate to those overarching attributes that can be utilised in many aspects of daily living and include mobility and manipulative hand skills, communication and cognitive and processing skills.
- Self-maintenance skills are those related to addressing the daily personal care needs of feeding, toileting, dressing, personal hygiene and grooming.
- Role duties are those duties that are demanded by the individual's roles and that are not (primarily) related to self-maintenance or leisure. These may include the domestic duties of the homemaker, the academic duties of the student, the work duties of the employer/employee and the duties of the carer.
- Leisure includes those tasks in which the individual participates in order to socialise, relax or pursue interests and hobbies.

Again, the skills included in each of the above categories will vary from one context to another. A lucrative hobby, for instance, may be classified as a work or as a leisure pursuit. Eating a meal may be a matter of self-maintenance but a business lunch may be seen as a role duty and dinner with family or friends as a leisure activity. Moreover, role duties may be perceived differently from one culture to another. A more extensive exploration of such difficulties in classification may be found in Cynkin and Robinson (1990).

However problematic, the categorisation of activities can provide the therapist with a starting point for assessment and helps to ensure that the full range of an individual's occupations and activities is given consideration. It is instructive to ascertain not only the individual's level of

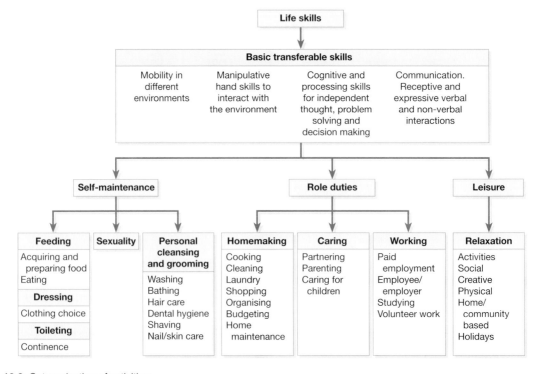

Fig. 10.2 Categorisation of activities.

performance of a given activity but also how he perceives and categorises that activity, as this will provide some insight into his attitudes and priorities. In a study of time use by adults with spinal cord injuries, Yerxa and Locker (1990) identified differences in the perception and classification of activities between the study group, a parallel non-disabled group and occupational therapists. Their study suggests that the increased value accorded to some activities by the group of people with spinal cord injury may be linked to the loss of the work role and reflect the desire to find alternative occupational competency.

In conclusion, although the therapist will need some kind of structure through which she can isolate and assess the various occupations that constitute life skills, she should not apply any categorisation too rigidly but should take time to identify the significance that each activity has for the individual concerned.

DEVELOPMENT OF LIFE SKILLS

Basic transferable skills begin to develop early in life and the range of occupations in which they are used expands with development and life experiences. Skills in self-maintenance are acquired gradually throughout childhood. They improve with practice and many are finally taken for granted. Consider the process of getting up each morning and preparing to go to work or school. On waking, one automatically stretches, climbs out of bed and walks to the bathroom or toilet. One washes, dresses and prepares breakfast, all without much thought. But imagine the thinking and preparation required for people who rely on a wheelchair or prosthesis for mobility; are only able to use one hand; have difficulty with balance, reach or coordination; or whose memory and concentration is limited. These simple tasks, which are taken for granted by the able-bodied person, take on vastly different proportions for many people with significant impairment.

Advice regarding ways of overcoming temporary dysfunction in certain aspects of living may be all that is required for people whose impairment is short term. New learning, relearning or modification of techniques may be necessary for the person with long-term problems and this may entail considerable practice to reach a meaningful level of competence. The therapist who facilitates such learning must be able to analyse the tasks and adapt their performance to individual wishes, needs and capabilities.

The ultimate success of intervention lies in the person's willingness to maintain an often strenuous programme of practice. Use of residual attributes, together with an exercise regimen to strengthen weakened muscles and improve coordination and agility, demands commitment. Periods of frustration, anxiety and depression may affect an individual's motivation and drive. In many situations, much will depend upon the encouragement and support that the individual receives. It is important that realistic goals are set. The number and nature of the activities that a person chooses to manage independently will depend upon his level of ability, his own wishes and standards and those of his family or carers, and the resources available to him.

Intervention should be based on the priorities determined by the individual in consultation with the therapist. A good rapport between the therapist and the client is important in enabling both parties to express and explore the available options openly. If work is a high priority, it may be pointless to strive for complete independence in the morning self-maintenance routine if this leaves the individual too fatigued to meet the demands of his job. In such a case it may be preferable for the individual to be 'interdependent' and accept help or assistance with some tasks. Similarly, for the person living alone, eating breakfast in night clothes may be more acceptable than getting dressed in day clothes only to become too fatigued to prepare breakfast. An individual who diverts his energy to independence only in the self-maintenance activities that are important to him may be better able to fulfil his role duties and to enjoy leisure pursuits than the person who is totally independent in self care. The desire for full independence should be weighed against the balance between physical, psychological and social aspects of living.

Skills in role duties develop through education and practice, as experiences change in line with chronological age and life events (Box 10.1). The schoolchild learns about role expectations in the classroom and playground environment but he can be prepared for some of these demands and experiences before entering school. Similarly, skills learned in the school environment regarding socialisation, adherence to rules, structure and organisation, as well as many of the performance skills related to mobility, communication, reasoning and prioritisation, prepare the child for adult role duties. Where adequate resources are available to enable the disabled child to integrate practically and socially, experience of the normal education system will give him the opportunity to prepare for the rigorous demands of adult living. Additional postschool training schemes may continue this development after formal schooling is completed.

Individuals whose activities as employee or homemaker have been interrupted by illness or disability may need support in regaining the skills and confidence to resume their former role. Similarly, those whose disability has had a significant impact upon performance in their usual role may need help to make the necessary readjustments. Practice in domestic skills in the home or other suitable supported environment may prepare the homemaker to return to their customary role. Activities that stimulate the working situation may be used to assess skills or build levels of confidence for return to employment. Further education or additional training schemes may also support return to employment.

A child learns leisure activities naturally through play. As he develops, his interests expand in accordance with the opportunities available. Such developments often form the basis of lifelong leisure interests. A person who enjoys music at school is likely to pursue it in later life, either actively as a participant or passively as a listener, and the child who is keen on active games or sports may have similar interests in adulthood. Those who enjoy precision hobbies or individual activities such as model building, reading or sewing are more likely to pursue individual rather than team leisure pursuits. For this reason, early introduction to play experiences

Box 10.1 Development stages and associated roles: a summary	
Developmental stage	**Associated roles**
1. Infant	Total dependence – player, learner
	Family member role commences
2. Small child (pre-school)	Family member role increases
	Player role expands – experimentation with roles observed in others
	Friend role commences
3. Child (junior school age)	Increase in roles and experimentation
	Schoolchild
	Family member role continues to increase
	Friend role increasingly important
	Begins to perceive certain roles
4. Adolescent	Student
	Family member role subject to change over time
	Role experimentation – adulthood
	Friend role important – both sexes
	Worker – assumes equal important with friend role
	Player – greater diversity
5. Adult	Partner, parent, homemaker
	Worker/breadwinner
	Leisure and friendship roles
	Social, organisational, cultural roles
6. Older person	Role continuity/gains – family friends, work (paid or unpaid), leisure, education
	Role loss: bereavement, retirement, moving house.

and purposeful activities is vital for the disabled child to provide the foundations for valued leisure pursuits in adult life. Frequently, such opportunities are denied because of the limitations imposed by the impairment or because the demands of daily care leave little time or support for play. Family support and introduction to community resources for leisure activities are of great importance for the disabled child's future development.

Dysfunction gained in adult life may lead a person to devise new ways of pursuing favourite activities or to take up new interests altogether. The therapist should encourage the person's involvement in leisure activities by providing information regarding the resources and opportunities available in the local community for both disabled and able bodied participants.

THE ROLE OF THE OCCUPATIONAL THERAPIST

Habilitation or rehabilitation in life skills in many instances involves the individual together with his family or carers, as well as the medical, para-medical, employment and community services personnel. Success will depend upon the ability of team members to work together, understanding and supporting each other's roles, on the motivation and drive of the individual and on the resources available.

The role of the occupational therapist will vary in accordance with her client's circumstances and needs. As well as providing direct intervention and treatment, she may act as a facilitator, planner, educator, resource person, adviser or liaison officer. She should know and understand the roles of her colleagues in the medical, educational and employment fields, be familiar with community provision for support in self-maintenance and domestic tasks and be aware of local facilities and support for leisure pursuits. She should also be conversant with legislative provision and the financial support available for individuals and their carers. She should appreciate the unique importance of independence in specific skills for each individual and should also be sensitive to the demands of caring that have been placed on the individual and those close to him.

The therapist's intervention usually begins with a thorough assessment of the person's strengths, weaknesses, needs and wishes. In working with individuals to identify areas of difficulty and select goals for intervention, she must also be able to analyse daily tasks and recognise the specific skills and attributes necessary for their successful performance. In almost all cases, her intervention will be based on a collaborative problem-solving approach. However, she will need to be conversant with specific interventions to overcome particular difficulties and improve function. Biomechanical, neurodevelopmental, cognitive or behavioural techniques might all be used to overcome specific impairments and thereby promote independence in life skills. However, for many people with permanent dysfunction, a compensatory rehabilitative approach may be more appropriate. This will involve the modification of techniques and the development of strategies to compensate for functional limitation.

BASIC TRANSFERABLE SKILLS

Basic transferable skills can be utilised to a greater or lesser extent in many areas of activity. They underpin the successes and limitations in performance of other specific activities and are an essential component of most occupations. Current policies in education and training link closely to the development of such skills in many aspects of living and build on their use in many areas of activity. For the purpose of this chapter, these skills include mobility, manipulative hand skills, communication and cognitive and processing skills.

MOBILITY

Some form of mobility is an essential component of independence in almost all areas of self-maintenance and for most role duties and leisure activities. However, this requirement has changed considerably with the advancement of technology. The development of computer systems, including Internet and e-mail communications, have reduced the need to travel to the supermarket, work or other locations. Groceries, advice on health issues, holidays and a vast range of other services can be requested over the Internet and the ability to work from home or communicate with friends at considerable distances is now possible via the computer. The advancement of voice-activated controls and communication systems overcomes the need to manipulate specific items of equipment. However, many people do not have access to such opportunities, or prefer not to use them. The ability to control specific limb movements, to transfer from place to place and to interface with equipment and the environment remain important requirements to success in the wide range of tasks in the daily occupations for these people.

The occupational therapist should assess the person's mobility skills in relation to his environment and discuss whether he is likely to be able to improve his physical condition or whether it will be necessary to use a compensatory rehabilitative approach to facilitate independent function. The ability to negotiate stairs, for example, may be gained through specific treatment to improve balance, muscle strength and range of lower limb movement. This will usually have greater urgency for the person who is living in a two storey house than for someone who is living in a bungalow. Where some impairment is likely to be permanent, consideration should be given to alternative means of managing steps and stairs through seated rising from step to step, adapting the existing home through the provision of a stair raise or lift, or the addition of extra downstairs facilities. In some instances, consideration may be given to choosing a more suitable place to live and this decision should take account of other factors, such as external environmental support and financial implications.

Additionally, the occupational therapist should consider the person's lifestyle requirements with regards to outdoor mobility – the garden, the neighbourhood, at the shops, on the way to work or school, in performing leisure pursuits. Chapter 7 considers the issues regarding mobility in greater depth and should be read in conjunction with the present discussion.

MANIPULATIVE HAND SKILLS

Manipulative hand skills are basic components of independence in most life activities. These manipulative skills may be used in verbal or written communication (to handle the telephone, papers or books, or to use the computer keyboard) in mobility (to manage keys, locks, door handles or use push-button entry systems) or in maintaining a comfortable environment through the manipulation of heating controls, lighting or window mechanisms. Dexterity skills are used when operating taps, setting controls on an alarm clock, using the television or the microwave, opening letters or flushing the toilet. All or any of these skills may be crucial to safety, comfort and independence in life skills and are increasingly important in the use of much modern technological equipment. The wider use of remote controls for electrical equipment, whilst reducing the need for gross mobility, has increased the demands for fine manipulative skills when using unadapted control mechanisms. Modification of such controls can overcome this need but this requires specialist equipment and provision, which is not readily available through regular high street suppliers.

Detailed assessment of manipulative skills, dexterity, grip strength, sensation and coordination, together with analysis of needs and of existing equipment and environmental controls, may be necessary to determine levels of function and dysfunction. Some problems may be overcome by adopting alternative methods when performing activities, for example, using the elbow to depress the toilet flush. Modifications to tools and controls may be necessary to overcome specific difficulties. An immense number of variations are available, ranging from simple alterations to knobs, switches or handles to facilitate grip to sophisticated electronic devices to operate a range of environmental equipment such as door locks, heating controls and the computer. Careful assessment and practice with a number of different options, through services such as those offered by many Disabilities Living Centres, will enable the individual to make the most appropriate choice for short- and long-term needs.

COMMUNICATION

Communication may be defined as the 'passing of information, ideas and attitudes from person to person' (Williams 1968). Communication is an extremely important life skill. We need to move, to eat and to toilet in order to survive, but we also need to communicate to gain assistance with any of these activities. The baby or young child laughs or cries to express feelings, the adult modifies and refines communication skills according to his environment and personal wishes and requirements, and the elderly rely on communication to maintain contact with others in the face of many losses.

Whatever our age, our success in communicating with others determines a large measure of our quality of life.

What is communication?

The range of methods of communication is vast. Communication may be direct or indirect: it may be face-to-face or via an intermediary in verbal, written or expressive form, or through the use of technical appliances. Messages may be conveyed by a smile or frown across a room, or by fax or e-mail transmission across thousands of miles. Whatever its form, communication consists of the same creative and receptive processes: a message or idea is initiated, formulated and presented, to be received, decoded and understood. This process becomes circular as messages are transmitted and responses given (Fig. 10.3).

Problems may occur at any of these stages. Some difficulties will be directly attributable to impairment, others to factors related to learning, culture or social context. The interpretation of messages is not always straightforward. A smile, for example, may be a sign of friendship or welcome or a signal of ridicule or disrespect. The receiver's interpretation may depend upon his previous contact with the sender, on the formality or otherwise of the situation, or on his self-esteem or self-image. Communication problems related to impairment may occur in both the receptive and expressive domains; these are discussed below.

Receptive problems

These are usually related to sensory or perceptual impairments but may also reflect a limitation in cognitive or intellectual capability resulting from, for example, head injury or some forms of cerebral palsy. Receptive problems may also be the result of lack of experience, orientation or cultural understanding.

Sensory impairments affecting communication are predominantly those associated with limited hearing or vision. Visuoperceptual problems and receptive dysphasia affect interpretation of signals or messages. Limited cognition may impede learning and understanding of the verbal and written language as well as the interpretation of non-verbal communications.

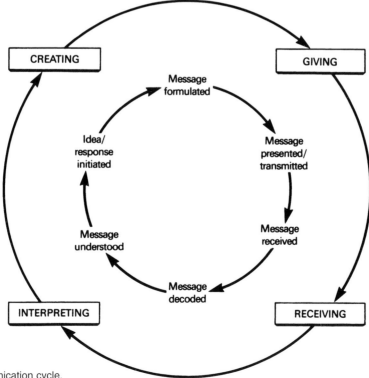

Fig. 10.3 The communication cycle.

Hearing difficulties may be limited to particular sounds or there may be total hearing loss. There are a number of ways of overcoming hearing difficulties, depending on the nature and severity of the hearing loss. A hearing aid or voice amplifier, for example, can improve reception of sounds for those with limited hearing, whilst various forms of assistance may compensate for total absence of hearing. These may include flashing lights on doorbells or alarms, or a vibrator pad placed under the pillow to act as an alarm clock. In all cases, instruction in the use and maintenance of such equipment must be given. Alternative means of communication, such as sign languages or lip reading, require considerable education and practice and are frequently acquired most successfully by those who developed their hearing impairment early in life. The Royal National Institute for the Deaf, speech and language therapists, audiologists, social workers for the hearing impaired and electronic equipment suppliers may provide assessment of needs and specialist support.

Some visual impairments may be overcome through the use of optical aids such as magnifiers or large print books. Where these are not adequate, more specialist means of communication such as Braille texts, sensory maps, taped books or voice recorders may be of assistance. The Royal National Institute for the Blind and social workers for the visually impaired are the experts in this field.

Perceptual difficulties should be identified by the occupational therapist through specific perceptual assessments. Once the problems have been identified, the occupational therapist's role is to explain the deficit to the individual and to help him to practise techniques to overcome particular difficulties. Where perceptual problems are severe and impede a specific means of communication (for example, visual difficulties in shape recognition may prohibit reading), alternative ways of receiving information, such as taped messages, may be necessary.

Problems with reception or understanding may be due purely to linguistic or cultural barriers. In a multicultural society in which people do not share the same language or cultural background, there may be difficulties in translation of messages, differences in understanding due to dialect, culture or lack of familiarity with technical jargon. Therapists should be aware of language or dialect difficulties and every effort should be made to facilitate interpretation by spoken or written means. Professionals tend to use jargon; this should be avoided when discussing issues with the disabled person or his carers because, besides limiting understanding, it further accentuates any perceived disadvantaged role. Where the client and the professional do not share the same language, a recognised professional interpreter should be employed, who understands the culture and language of the client and the professional's role and who is independent of the client's immediate or extended family.

Expressive problems

A number of expressive problems occur as the direct result of impairment. These problems may be with verbal or non-verbal expression or with the practical management of communication equipment.

Verbal expressive problems may be the result of damage to the speech centres in the brain resulting in difficulties in formulating and remembering speech. Problems may also occur due to damage to the mechanisms for articulating speech, for example, the muscles of the mouth, the tongue, the larynx or the trachea. This can occur with neurological disorders such as multiple sclerosis, cerebral palsy or motor neuron disease or may be the result of surgery (for example, laryngectomy). The occupational therapist should liaise with the speech and language therapist to identify the specific problem and the most appropriate ways of overcoming it. Rehabilitation may include practice in speech sound or words in conjunction with visual stimuli, the introduction of equipment, letter or word boards, through which the individual can indicate a request or response, or instruction in the use of more sophisticated means of communication such as voice synthesisers or electronic communicators.

Non-verbal expression may be limited by impairments that affect the control of muscles of the face or upper limbs. Limited mobility of the facial muscles, such as that which occurs with

Parkinson's disease, affects the ability to show responses or emotions facially. Where hypermobility of the facial muscles occurs, as in some people with athetoid cerebral palsy, the control of facial muscles is difficult. Speech may also be impaired in both of the above situations, further adding to the communication difficulties. The listener, or receiver, should be attentive to the response and check they have heard correctly through feedback to the sender. (In this, the sender should, where possible, employ an alternative method of communication, for example, head nodding, pointing or a written response to the receiver's checking feedback.)

Uncontrolled movements of the upper limbs also hinder non-verbal communication. A hand or arm may be used to point, gesticulate, initiate contact by beckoning or emphasise a fact. A sudden spasm of an upper limb may be misinterpreted as an invitation or a rejection. With the permission of the individual it may be beneficial for the therapist to explain such problems to close relatives and carers and to encourage them to verify the meaning of the person's non-verbal cues with him, thus ensuring better understanding.

Written communication may be affected by limitations in hand function or by visual impairment. For handwriting, various modifications may be made to pens or pencils to assist with grasp or control. For those who are not able to write, alternative means of communication by word, such as computers or electronic communicators, may be used. For people who are able to manage some hand function, modified keyboards may be used. Where hand function is not adequate to manage a keyboard, alternative means of operation may be necessary, such as voice activation or the use of other bodily movements. The use of a simple tape recorder to transmit the spoken rather than the written word may be more appropriate in some situations for people whose visual impairment inhibits the use of a keyboard.

Impairments in hand function may also affect the use of other pieces of communication equipment such as the telephone. A number of modifications are available, including those provided by British Telecom, to reduce the need for fine dexterity or motor control in operating telecommunications equipment.

Communication problems may also occur because of difficulties with language, or as the result of limited mobility or social experience. Development of linguistic and social skills are part of normal life experience and maturity and these difficulties may affect anyone, but they may present an additional handicap for people coping with other impairments.

People with mobility problems often have difficulty keeping in touch, even with other members of the family in different rooms in the house. Simple intercom systems may facilitate room-to-room communication. Where there is a need to make contact outside the home, either for work, pleasure or in cases of emergency, a mobile phone or alarm system may be used to alert neighbours, friends or colleagues. A large number of systems are available and careful choice should be made, bearing in mind the needs of all parties involved. The use of computer technology has advanced opportunities to maintain communication with a wider, more varied range of receivers through the use of Internet and e-mail facilities.

Limited social experiences can impede the development of communication skills. This may lead to anxiety in particular social situations because of uncertainty regarding the most appropriate type of behaviour. In some instances, inappropriate behaviour may lead to embarrassment and further handicap the individual. Appropriate advice and support should be provided to enable an individual to develop skills and confidence in social communication in a secure environment. Following this, opportunities should be made for him gradually to integrate into a number of social settings, with support as necessary.

COGNITIVE AND PROCESSING SKILLS

The ability to be independent extends beyond physical capabilities for performing tasks to include the cognitive and intellectual skills necessary for problem solving and decision making.

It is impossible to predict or rehearse all of the situations that person may have to cope with in the community, at home, at work or in a recreational setting. A piece of essential equipment may break down, a helper may fail to arrive, an unexpected social, educational or business opportunity may arise. It is therefore equally important to recognise the importance of cognitive skills in conjunction with physical attributes and to facilitate the development of independent processing skills that will enable each individual to deal with situations as objectively, positively and autonomously as possible.

The development of processing skills may involve re-education and/or readdressing of priorities to take account of changed needs for the person who has had previous life experience. Where disability has occurred early in life, opportunity to practise processing skills may have been limited; such skills may have to be learned and developed from a theoretical base rather than from previous experiences.

Processing skills enable individuals to interpret information and make the most appropriate response in a given situation. They involve the receptive skills to take in and absorb information; knowledge; understanding; analytical and discriminatory skills to interpret facts; imaginative, judgemental and evaluative skills to consider possible implications and outcomes of particular decisions; expressive skills to deliver the response; and practical skills to pursue the chosen solution. Processing skills may be developed gradually; the person may progress from simple choices, such as which items of clothing to wear, to more complex decision making in such areas as budgeting or home maintenance. In each case, the basic facts should be identified and the pros and cons of the available options explored. The individual should then decide upon the option he prefers, provided that all the possibilities have been addressed and no major negative factors or health and safety hazards have been overlooked. The person's choice may not be in line with the therapist or others but, if all the information regarding possible risks, expenditure, and implications for significant others have been discussed, the individual's decision should be respected. This should be accompanied by clear recording of the process by which the decision was made and, if the outcome turns out not to be as the person anticipated, these records

can be used to analyse the possible reasons why this has occurred.

The therapist's objective is to enable the individual to perform such actions practically and independently in his own environment. This may also include working with the individual to develop skills for rationalisation of information, prioritisation of facts and possible implications, and assertiveness to support his decisions, or to manage anxiety regarding the possible outcomes. However, where there are major difficulties with thought processes, such as those that may occur following a stroke or head injury, or where experience is limited and important decisions are involved, it may be safer for learning to occur through theoretical exercises, before practical action is attempted. Problem-solving exercises using case studies or audiovisual materials, specific games involving choice and decision making, individual guidance and group discussions may be used to promote learning. The therapist may take a guiding or facilitating role in such activities, depending on the needs and skills of the individual or the group.

SPECIFIC SELF-MAINTENANCE ACTIVITIES

FEEDING

The consumption of nourishment is the most basic voluntary activity for sustaining life. While those who are unconscious or severely ill may be fed by artificial means through tubes or drips, the usual way of taking nourishment is through taking meals, which involves eating and drinking. Katz et al's (1963) hierarchical scale of independent function recognised the consumption of nourishment as the first activity to be gained (and often the last to be lost) following impairment. Problems with eating or drinking may be related to difficulties with the acquisition and problems with mouth control, chewing and swallowing, loss of taste and motivation to eat or with preparation of food, the availability of appropriate food in relation to culture, diet or personal preferences.

Acquiring and preparing food

The general level of an individual's mobility, the proximity and accessibility of shops and the availability of transport all affect food acquisition. Large supermarkets with wide aisles and suitable parking close to the entrance enable the ambulant person or wheelchair user to take an active part in shopping, although the height of shelves and depth of freezer cabinets may make total independence difficult. Some ambulant people cope well in this environment, using the shopping trolley as a substitute walking aid, but may find the hustle and bustle of a busy supermarket daunting and prefer to use a small local shop where personal service compensates for difficulties in reaching and handling food.

For those who are unable to use supermarkets or small shops themselves, home delivery may be arranged by written or telephone ordering or by Internet shopping services. Alternatively, a member of the family, neighbour, friend or carer may be able to shop from a prepared list. It is important for every individual to retain some control over the purchase of food, through nominating some or all of the items to be purchased. Home delivery services of fresh or frozen foods are available for people with special needs but these vary in different locations.

Preparation of food involves a wide range of skills, dependent upon the type of meal being prepared, the ingredients necessary and the available equipment. Successful practice in the preparation of simple meals may help to build confidence to try more ambitious menus. Frozen, partly prepared or preprepared meals reduce the demands of the task, as do food processors and microwaves. In each situation, attention to safety is of paramount importance. Many everyday labour-saving items designed for all users may help overcome a particular impairment. Kitchen layout and equipment design should be assessed; modifications may be suggested to improve manoeuvrability for the wheelchair user or to increase accessibility for someone with limited reach or poor manipulative skills. Impairments of motor control, reduced bilaterality or limited vision may also pose problems with the use of some kitchen equipment but, with ingenuity, minor modifications and opportunities to try different options, many problems can be safely overcome.

The environment and feeding activity

When considering feeding difficulties, accessibility of the family dining area, the choice of tableware and furniture and the positioning of the individual in relation to the food must all be addressed.

The suitability of tables and chairs should be evaluated. It is necessary to consider whether feeding will be better achieved sitting at the table on a dining chair, in a wheelchair or other chair. A chair with arms will provide more support than one without for those who have difficulty with balance and stability. A slightly higher table and chair may be necessary to accommodate stiff lower limbs. A wheelchair user needs clearance under the table apron; domestic armrests on the wheelchair will facilitate closer positioning at the table. The table must be sufficiently stable to withstand any inadvertent knocks from the chair. When sitting at the dining table is not possible, a cantilever table or tray attached to a chair or wheelchair will enable the individual to dine in the same room with family or others. If this is not possible, meals may be taken in bed with the provision of a stable over bed table of a suitable height.

A winged headrest on the wheelchair may assist the person who has limited control of head and neck movements when feeding but, if tremors or spasms are severe, independent feeding may not be feasible. Where weakness of the upper arm or forearm is the primary cause of difficulty, the use of ultralight cutlery and arm supports or stabilisers may assist. The technique of pivoting the forearm of the feeding arm on the clenched fist of the other hand, resting on the table, will facilitate greater forearm mobility without upper arm movement.

Finger feeding is much easier than using cutlery but is contrary to etiquette in many Western cultures. However, in many Eastern cultures finger feeding is the norm and should be respected. Any specialist equipment used for feeding should be as similar as possible to that used by the general public; unusual specialist equipment that draws attention to the individual's problems should be avoided as far as possible.

Western cutlery is held like a small tool, with the handle pressed into the palm and stabilised by thumb pressure against the middle finger. It is stabilised and guided from above by the index finger, and additional downward pressure for picking up or cutting food is exerted by flexion of the wrist joint. If any of these abilities is limited or absent, as in median nerve lesion, rheumatoid arthritis or tetraplegia, efficiency is considerably reduced. Alternative methods of holding cutlery, such as clip-on or padded handles, or small orthoses to position the fingers in the grip position or stabilise the wrist may assist. A large range of modified cutlery is available and the opportunity to try different modifications will enable individuals to make informed choices on suitability and ease of use.

People who are only able to use one hand often become very dextrous when using an upturned fork or a spoon but may need assistance when cutting food. A number of modified 'knives' are available with a blade that operates through a rolling or rocking action, similar to those of pizza cutters. The user must be made aware of the potential danger of cutting the side of the lips or mouth when using these to take food into the mouth for eating. Many people with strong Islamic beliefs may prefer to be fed rather than use the 'unclean' hand for one-handed feeding.

For people with a limited range of movement or restricted reach in the upper limbs, angled or lengthened cutlery may provide a suitable solution. This must be adjusted to meet individual needs. Swivel cutlery is also available for people with limited wrist or elbow movement or slight difficulties with motor control.

Suitable crockery may enable individuals to become independent and retain dignity when eating. Some manufacturers make deep rimmed plates to match their range of crockery but many of these are expensive and quite heavy. Their weight, while providing some stability when eating, may make them unsuitable for those who are weak, living alone and have to do their own washing up. Some specialist-designed crockery includes dishes that incorporate a shaped rim to assist when pushing food onto the spoon or fork. Plate guards fitted to dinner or breakfast plates may be used in the same way but these are more obtrusive.

The type of food may affect the success of independent feeding. Such foods as tough meat, spaghetti, peas or meringues cause difficulties for everyone and the person with an impairment is no exception. Foods that require slicing or cutting may also pose problems. While a person should not be restricted to a diet of minced meat, mashed potato and yoghurt, particularly difficult foods may be best avoided, particularly when eating out.

Spillage difficulties when drinking may be overcome in some instances by only partly filling the cup, mug or glass, and by using a lightweight beaker, flexistraws or a small piece of narrow plastic tubing clipped to the side of the mug or glass. Bottle carriers of the type used by cyclists can be attached to the side of the chair and fitted with a longer drinking tube. For people who have severe problems with motor control, non-spill beakers may be used. Insulated beakers prevent cooling of hot drinks if drinking is slow and afford protection to the hands for people with heat sensitivity problems. Modern thermal containers with lever-operated dispensers enable hot drinks to be available throughout the day for people who are unable to manage a conventional kettle or pan safely.

Crockery may be stabilised with a PVC-coated cloth or mat or a varnished cork table mat. These are easy to clean, pleasant to look at and do not draw attention to the person's problems. Other forms of specialist stabilising material with rubberised or pimple non-slip surfaces are also available in sheeting or mat form. Even a damp cloth will serve to reduce plate slippage on a flat surface. For people with severe coordination problems, a rimmed tray with a non-slip surface may be necessary.

Difficulties with mouth control, chewing and swallowing

Children may readily accept bright towelling or plastic bibs to protect clothes during meals.

However, these are very demeaning for most adults. A fabric napkin tucked into the neck of a shirt or blouse will absorb drips in a less obvious manner. A plastic-backed fabric bib to match the person's clothing is less obvious than one made from white towelling.

Choice and presentation of food may obviate some of the difficulties when eating. Severe temperomandibular joint involvement in rheumatoid arthritis, facial burns or oral cancer may cause pain and difficulty in opening the mouth. For these people, food cut into small pieces, which require little or no chewing, will be easier to manage.

Eating can be very difficult for people with oral spasticity. Spasms may occur when anything touches the teeth or gums, so food may be better managed by sucking from a fork or spoon with the lips. To overcome tongue thrust, food may be placed to the side or back of the tongue to minimise food loss, but the texture of the food should be smooth to reduce risk of choking.

People who have difficulty controlling head movements because of primitive reflex patterns, such as the asymmetrical tonic neck reflex, should eat or be fed from a central forward position to overcome the abnormal movement pattern. Under no circumstances should the head be tipped back to retain food in the mouth, as this adds to difficulties with swallowing and may cause choking. Problems affecting the fitting of dentures, such as those resulting from a cerebrovascular accident that has affected the facial muscles, should be addressed as a matter of urgency to enable adequate nourishment to be retained.

Obviously, the choice of food consistency and texture is important for many people. Foods may be minced, shredded or liquidised but when a number of different foods are treated this way in the same meal they should be prepared individually to retain their separate colours and flavours. Small regular snacks may be easier and quicker to prepare, eat and digest. A diet that is nutritious and appealing to an individual is more likely to encourage those who are less motivated to eat. It should include adequate fibre, vitamins, protein and carbohydrate and be appropriate to the person's cultural, religious and dietary needs. Difficulties with mouth control may be discussed with the speech and language therapist and the dietician will give advice on dietary needs and specialist foods.

In conclusion, feeding is a complex task vital to human survival. Emphasis has been placed on the essential tasks necessary to obtain adequate nourishment. These should be given priority but it should also be remembered that eating is frequently a social or cultural activity with accepted norms of behaviour. Inability to perform such behaviours may cause anxiety or embarrassment, for the individual, relatives and carers. The individual may become reluctant to join others at meal times or to eat away from home. The therapist has an important contribution to make in helping to identify the precise nature of the problems, which may be as diverse as an inability to respond to a waiter's questions or a loss of inhibitions in drinking or chewing food, and discussing ways in which problems may be alleviated or overcome.

TOILETING

Toileting is a very personal area of life skills and is the activity in which most people wish to regain or maintain independence. For people with severe impairment it is one of the most difficult areas of self-maintenance, and one that is crucial to retaining dignity and remaining independent in one's own home. Problems in toileting may be divided into those caused by difficulties in coping with the environment and manipulating clothing and those that are due to medical conditions that cause continence problems. Frequently, the two aspects are interlinked – the person with problems resulting in urgency may be incontinent because of difficulties with mobility that prevent him from reaching the toilet in time. It should be remembered that there are many different habits concerning toileting in various cultures and religions, particularly Islam; where appropriate these should be identified and respected.

Environmental problems

The toilet is usually the smallest and most inaccessible room in the home. New building regulations will improve the availability of ground floor toilet facilities in new properties but the size of these may still be limited and many people live in older properties with only one toilet upstairs. Even when the toilet is separate from the bathroom, there is not always adequate or suitable space for manoeuvring within the toilet. Access to the toilet may be hindered by steps and structural alterations are often necessary for the wheelchair user. When the toilet and bathroom are separate but adjacent, the removal of the dividing wall to integrate the two rooms may provide more space for manoeuvring. Access may be improved in some instances by widening the doorway, providing a gentle ramp or shallow step and handrails. Installation of a sliding door, or rehanging the existing door to open the opposite way may add space and facilitate better mobility.

The position of the toilet within the room is also important. Wheelchair users usually find a sideways transfer is easier if the toilet pedestal is set further forward from the wall than is usual, and require considerable space to the side of the toilet to facilitate the transfer. The majority of ambulant people with walking problems prefer a pedestal seat that is higher than usual, to facilitate ease of rising. A variety of raised toilet seats are available in different heights; some clip to the toilet bowl and others incorporate handrails in their design. The type of seat may make a difference to comfort and stability; a horseshoe-shaped seat may make peroneal cleansing easier but may be less stable for some users. Ideally, there should be a basin close enough to the toilet to avoid additional movement and exertion when handwashing.

The positioning and size of handrails is a matter of individual need and preference. Horizontal and vertical rails usually offer more assistance than those that are inclined. However, some people find inclined rails of great assistance when rising from the toilet because they support the forearm as well as providing a firm handgrip. A matt finish, either ridged or rubberised, is safer than a chrome finish, which may be slippery when wet, and a rail 3.75–5.00 cm in diameter is more serviceable than a slimmer one. Useful sources of reference include texts such as 'Designing for the Disabled' (Goldsmith 1984), 'Cracking Housing Problems, A Practical Guide to Problem Solving for Disabled People, Occupational Therapists and Carers' (Walbrook Housing Association (1992), 'The Good Loo Design Guide' (Centre on Environment for the Handicapped 1988) and 'Housing Options for Disabled People' written by members of the College of Occupational Therapists Specialist Section on Housing (Bull 1998).

Transfers

Transfer techniques to and from the toilet provide problems for many people, particularly for those people who are wheelchair users. Some people may be able to stand up, take one or two steps, turn and sit down. The continued use of such skills should be encouraged, as this will enable the individual to be more independent in toileting, both at home and elsewhere.

For people who are totally dependent on the wheelchair, consideration of the modes of transfer should be an integral part of the initial wheelchair selection process. If the individual is unable to manage a direct sideways transfer, a portable sliding board may enable him to transfer independently using the mobility and strength in his upper limbs, shoulder girdle and trunk. Detachable wheelchair armrests, chassis design that permits a close approach to the toilet pan, and occasionally a folding or removable backrest, may all facilitate independent transfers by different means. Some individuals, most commonly those who have double above-knee amputations, prefer to transfer forwards onto the toilet and function sitting back to front, facing the cistern.

Sanichairs are available for people who cannot transfer from the wheelchair to the toilet. These can either be propelled by the occupant or wheeled by a helper and positioned over the toilet pedestal (Disabled Living Foundation 1999).

Management of clothing

Undressing, cleansing, washing and dressing must all be considered as part of toileting activity, as well as the use of the toilet equipment. Undertaking these activities in the confined space of the toilet adds to the difficulty for many people. Alterations to clothing, particularly underwear, and discussion of alternative techniques, may enable some people to regain or retain independence. If the person is no longer able to stand and balance, he may be taught to slide forward on the toilet seat and wipe himself from the back, or slide back on the seat and cleanse with his legs apart. Various designs of tongs and paper holders may be used to assist people with limited reach or poor manual dexterity. For the person with a severe level of impairment the use of a bidet, or electrically operated toilet such as the Clos-o-mat or Medic-loo, which dispense warm washing water followed by warm air, may solve cleansing difficulties.

Menstruation can result in discomfort, embarrassment and occasionally depression. Periods may be painful, with heavy loss of blood, and the individual may seek medical advice to suppress or regulate menstruation. Discussion and advice on the merits of different forms of protection, such as self-adhesive pads that adhere to the inside of pants, may assist individuals, particularly younger women, in finding the most suitable and easily managed personal solution. The need for peroneal hygiene to prevent odour and secondary skin problems should be emphasised. Assessment in toileting skill should consider the individual's need to use a conventional toilet. Some individuals may find that using a bottle, commode or chemical toilet is preferable to making major alterations to the home or expending the energy necessary for them to use an ordinary toilet. Assessment should include both day- and night-time needs. For night-time it may be necessary to make arrangements different from those used during the day, taking account of relatives and helpers' needs. Carers who are heavily committed to supporting the person during the day benefit from an uninterrupted night's sleep if they are to continue this role. Urinals, commodes and chemical toilets may provide safe convenient alternatives for night-time toileting. Whatever method is suggested and followed, safety for both carers and users is of paramount importance.

Continence problems

Incontinence is symptomatic of a number of conditions and may be a major contributory factor in admissions to care. Some elderly people, those with neurological disorders such as multiple sclerosis and some individuals with cognitive or emotional disorders may require assistance with continence problems. An understanding approach is necessary for all involved, for incontinence of urine and/or faeces causes the individual acute embarrassment, misery and discomfort. A number of ways of overcoming difficulties can be devised by discussing the problem with the individual and through consultation with nurses, continence advisers and carers. If a regimen has already been formulated, all necessary personnel involved should be aware of the requirements and adhere to them.

Training in a particular regimen is important, whether the individual is wearing an appliance that needs emptying at regular intervals or requires access to toilet facilities at certain times of the day. Urgency or frequency of micturition is a problem that is often made worse by worry, so people need help and reassurance in timing visits to the toilet. This is a very individual matter. Some people may need to empty the bladder every hour through manual expression, while others may need to visit the toilet following meals and at a regular time between meals. Curtailing fluid intake throughout the day is not usually advised because of secondary problems resulting from dehydration but some people may be advised to restrict fluid intake in the latter part of the day to reduce the risk of nocturnal incontinence. Medical advice should be sought in this regard.

A variety of appliances is available for coping with urinary incontinence. Men are often able to manage problems more readily because their anatomy enables them to wear condom-sheath-style appliances unobtrusively. Most women prefer to wear some form of absorbent one-way pad inside protective pants. Several types of pad are available with different absorbency factors, and may be worn with a range of pants that can be pulled up in the usual way or which have drop-front panels or side openings. Faecal continence may be managed through dietary means but if this is not adequate medical advice regarding the use of purgatives or suppositories may be necessary. In some instances, manual evacuation may be the only option.

Clothing for the lower half of the body should be kept to a comfortable minimum and be made from easy-care fabrics that are not likely to cause secondary friction or sweating problems. Wide openings and concealed zips in trousers facilitate dressing and undressing. Separate upper and lower garments are usually easier to manage and a short upper garment is less likely to be soiled than a longer one. Skin care and odour control are equally important for comfort and self-respect. Regular hygiene and careful skin care, together with the use of products to disguise odour, promotes confidence and reduces the risk of skin breakdown.

Psychological stress may affect urinary habits and control. Discussion of problems, reassurance or specialist counselling regarding the predisposing emotional difficulties and anxieties may help to relieve the stress. Confusion, disorientation or loss of memory following neurological damage or deterioration, or factors related to certain drug use, may affect continence. Careful identification of the predisposing factors, together with the development of a regular toileting regimen, may help to alleviate some of the difficulties.

When using a compensatory approach to overcome toileting problems, modifications to the home environment or the provision of sizeable items of equipment should be considered only if absolutely essential, since their value will be limited to facilitating ability within a specific location. Modifications to clothing or toileting techniques, the introduction of a timing regimen, or the provision of small transportable items of equipment or advice may be more helpful overall, as they may be applied in a number of different settings.

The therapist should be able to advise the individual and his carers on the range of help available locally and the advantages of particular equipment and techniques. Detailed information may be obtained from such sources as the Hamilton Index, the Disabled Living Foundation Information Service and the Directory for Disabled People. Independent Living Centres, situated in a number of cities throughout the country, provide assessment opportunities and advice on a broad range of services and equipment, and may provide a retail or referral facility in some cases. Texts such as 'How to get Equipment for Disability' (Mandelstam 1992) and the Disability Rights Handbook, which is updated regularly, provide guidance on the process of accessing services or equipment. In addition, information on local services may be obtained through the local community nursing service and the local social services department.

DRESSING AND UNDRESSING

Everyone expresses their personality to some degree through their choice of clothing. Anyone may draw attention to himself by virtue of his dress. Clothing may enhance a strong feature or exaggerate or disguise a deformity, dependent upon the wishes of the individual. Careful selection or adaptation of clothing may help conceal deformities and to compensate for difficulties with dressing activities.

The ability to dress and undress and to make one's appearance presentable and pleasing to oneself and others requires balance and coordination, joint mobility to facilitate reach, dexterity and muscle strength, insight into the task to be undertaken, sensation and a degree of spatial awareness.

Basic principles

Despite dressing not being an essential task to survival, everyone should be encouraged to change into day clothes rather than to spend the day in night clothes and slippers. This is primarily to boost morale and initiate the psychological move to a 'normal dress' code away from the 'sick role'. However, full independence in dressing should not be pursued rigidly if such activity is likely to fatigue the person unduly. Practical assessment of undressing and dressing abilities should be undertaken and the expectations of rehabilitation should be realistic. Practical assessment will identify those areas in which the individual is independent and those that require practice, exploration of alternative techniques or assistance from others. Specific requirements of cultural dress and potential difficulties between gender and generations should be respected by therapists when carrying out dressing practice.

Undressing is easier than dressing. It is less tiring and should be practised before dressing is pursued. It is usually carried out in the evening, which is comparatively relaxed, and when there is no rush to meet a daytime deadline. This may contribute to success, but cumulative fatigue from the activities of the day may counteract this.

Whenever possible, garments on the upper half of the body should be removed first, followed by those on the lower half and, finally, the shoes. Footwear is usually the last to be removed. This is because if there is a need to stand, it is much safer wearing shoes than only socks or stockings. However, when wearing tight trousers, shoes may need to be removed before the trousers are taken off.

When undressing, it is beneficial to think ahead in preparation for dressing the following day. Clothes to be worn again should be left with the right side out and in the order in which they will be put on.

Dressing will occur in the bedroom for most people. Clothing should be stored to hand and both the bed and a bedside chair may be used for dressing. The chair should be firm and stable, with arms if balance is a problem. The seat should be of a suitable height to enable the feet to be placed flat on the floor when seated. A good level of balance is required to reach up and pull clothes over the head, to lean forward and twist the trunk when dressing the lower half of the body and to reach back fastenings. Sitting or lying on the bed may be easier for dressing for some people whose general mobility and balance is affected.

The room should be warm, comfortable, well lit and as private as possible, remembering that some degree of privacy may have to be compromised in the interests of safety. When planning techniques for dressing and undressing, consideration should be given not only to the person's level of ability but also to his choice and style of dress and to any habitual techniques that have been successfully retained. It is usual to respect any gender habits, such as recognised differences between men's and women's techniques, when removing jumpers, sweaters or other upper half garments. Men tend to grasp the upper back of the garment and pull it over the head, whilst women will more frequently pull it up over the arms and head from the waistband. Such strong automatic techniques may be retained despite perceptual problems or confusion. Special garments, adaptations or equipment to assist dressing should only be used as the last resort, when alternative manual techniques have been fully explored and found to be inadequate.

Careful consideration should be given to the sequence and timing of dressing. Pants and trousers may be put on whilst sitting on the bed before transferring to a wheelchair. Prostheses and shoes should be put on before the person stands. As far as possible, the dressing schedule should fit into the daily family routine, particularly if help is required. Similarly, the therapist should carry out dressing practice at the time that would be 'normal' for the individual, as this will give a realistic picture of the person's capability level at the relevant time of day and will facilitate normalisation for individuals who are confused or disorientated. Ample time should be allowed for dressing practice but the person should not be permitted to become cold or too fatigued. Consideration should be given to the person's pain level, stiffness, slowness and weakness, and help offered as appropriate. This help may only be required temporarily, as specific difficulties may be overcome with practice.

Dressing practice should be carried out by first dressing the upper half of the body, followed by the lower half. The therapist should ensure the person is safely supported on the bed or chair, observe and discuss particular difficulties, and provide advice and assistance when necessary. Particular methods of dressing or undressing must be safe and suited to the individual's practical needs; those that have been worked out by the individual himself, in discussion with the therapist, are most likely to be continued.

Choice of clothing

Clothing that is currently available in high street shops provides the greatest range of choice. It is almost always possible to find readymade clothes that meet individual taste, are suitable according to age and capabilities and that conceal deformities, appliances or wasted muscles. Each person's needs, circumstances and limitations should be considered in the choice of garments. Particular attention should be paid to comfort, as some people have to spend many hours in the same position. Any specially made clothing should be skilfully designed to disguise the problem and should be produced in contemporary materials, styles and colours.

Shopping for clothes is often difficult and frustrating. Many people find the larger stores are more accessible, have larger fitting rooms and offer wider choice. If shopping locally is not possible, reputable mail order firms may provide a solution, as clothes can be tried on at home and returned if unsuitable.

Ideally, garments should be simple and loose fitting, with a minimum of fastenings and with ample openings and gussets. Elasticised waists, cuffs and shoulder straps are easy to manage if they are not too tight. In cool conditions, many people with limited mobility need warmer clothing than those who are able to maintain body temperature through physical activity. Dressing and undressing is easier if fabrics are chosen for their warmth, rather than wearing many layers of clothing to retain heat.

PERSONAL CLEANSING AND GROOMING

Personal cleansing comprises the activities involved in washing all or part of the body. Grooming includes such activities as hair care, dental hygiene, nail care and make-up. Some of these activities are essential to the maintenance of good hygiene and prevention of infection but personal cleansing and grooming also affect general wellbeing, morale and confidence in social settings.

Habits vary considerably from person to person. Some people wash the whole body daily while others wash only certain parts daily and bathe the whole body at less frequent intervals. Hair care and methods of washing may be determined by religious practices and cultural norms, or by familial habits.

Washing and bathing are areas of self care where most people have a desire to be independent for reasons of privacy and dignity, whereas grooming activities are generally less private in nature.

Washing

Most people are able to wash their hands and face, provided they have access to hot water, soap, a flannel and a towel. Such items as tap turners, flannel mittens, soap holders or liquid soap dispensers may make manipulative tasks easier. If the bathroom handbasin is inaccessible it may be possible to use a bowl of water on a stable over-bed table.

The whole body may be washed in a bath, under a shower, or by means of a 'strip' wash or, for those who are unable to attend the bathroom, a 'bed-bath' may suffice.

Bathing is a difficult task for many people who have physical impairments. Considerable strength, agility and balance (including the ability to stand on one leg) are required to step in and out of the bath safely in the conventional manner. The provision of suitably placed fixtures and equipment, such as rails, boards, seats, non-slip mats, stools and bath hoists, may make the task easier and safer (Disabled Living Foundation 1999).

It should be remembered that sitting on a seat above or high in the water can be cold if the room is not heated adequately. Immersion in warm, deeper water can be soothing and relaxing for painful muscles and joints.

Taps and other fittings should be of a design and in a position that facilitates their use. Inset soap dishes, taps and wash basins should not be used for extra support when stepping in or out of the bath, or pulling up from a sitting position, as they are usually not sufficiently stable to take extra weight. Lever taps or tap turners may be of assistance when an individual has difficulty operating conventional taps. Suitably positioned bath bars, trays and shelves will enable accoutrements such as soaps or gels, sponges and brushes to be within easy reach.

Where upper limb dysfunction limits reach to all parts of the body, extended handles on sponges, brushes or loofahs may be of assistance. Trick methods, such as using one foot to rub soap onto the other, may be helpful if one leg has limited mobility.

A well-designed and positioned shower provides a more suitable and safer method of washing for many people. Showering may be easier to manage, more hygienic and more economical than bathing but it can be uncomfortable if the room is cold. Individual capabilities and preferences should be considered before a shower installation is recommended. Shower sprays attached to taps may be easy to manage but suitably designed, thermostatically controlled showers are generally safer for everyone to use.

The position of the shower rose is important; those which are fixed overhead are often unsuitable for a person who is likely to have difficulty balancing in either a sitting or standing position, when bombarded with water over the face and head. The shower rose should be at chest height, and should be moveable to permit all-over washing from a seated position.

The choice of shower tray is also important. Ambulant users may be able to step over a lipped shower tray but a fixed handrail may assist them in this process. A shower tray flush with the floor level with a sloping drainage facility will facilitate the use of a wheeled shower chair when moving in and out of the cubicle.

Shower stools or chairs should have well maintained rubber ferrules to prevent the seat slipping or damaging the shower tray. Some cubicles have built-in seats and others have seats attached to the wall. These should be positioned at a suitable height and depth to meet the individual's needs when transferring and sitting comfortably. Some seats are hinged so they can be raised back against the wall when not required.

If it is not possible to install a separate shower cubicle, a shower spray attached to the bath taps may suffice. Care must be taken to control the temperature of the water. Sitting on a bath seat, it is possible to use the shower to wash, with or without the bath being filled with water.

Drying the body requires grip and coordination to grasp and control the towel, range of movement to reach the extremities and muscle strength to apply sufficient pressure to dry the skin.

A warm room with a radiator or towel rail to warm the towel or bathrobe is most useful. Wrapping in a warm robe or large bath sheet enables drying with the minimum of effort. A length of towel with handles or tape loops at each end reduces the need for good grip and reach and facilitates drying of the back and legs. Thick, soft, towelling mittens may also be of assistance when grip and dexterity are impaired.

Safety is of paramount importance when washing. Heat, condensation and steam make surfaces slippery and may cause dizziness or fatigue. They may impair vision for those dependent on glasses. Bathroom floors should have a non-slip surface and any unnecessary mats or clutter should be removed. Care should be taken particularly when making transfers and, if appropriate, the bathroom door should not be locked and a bath should be taken only when assistance is available in the house in case of emergency. If bathing is required for health reasons, the community nursing service may provide assistance for those who live alone or whose relatives are unable to help.

Some people prefer to have a strip wash seated or standing at the handbasin for reasons of safety or because of difficulties with transfers to the bath or shower. Problems when reaching the lower extremities can be overcome with a long-handled sponge or brush. The room should be warm, as this method of washing can be very cold.

Washing the body is also an important ritual in some religions. Every effort should be made to ensure that cultural norms are understood and the wishes of the individual and his family, particularly regarding privacy and techniques, are respected.

Hair care

If it is not possible to wash hair independently at the handbasin, it may be possible to wash it when bathing by using the shower attachment. In many areas there are mobile home hair-dressing services for people who prefer these, or those who are unable to attend a hair salon. If a person is confined to bed, a hair rinsing tray may be used.

Hair washing, drying and styling is a difficult task. Short, simple, minimum-care styles that do not require regular pinning, setting or plaiting are easiest to manage independently. A more complicated style may be managed with the cooperation of a willing carer, if the individual is not able to cope alone.

Dental hygiene

This is important for everyone but is particularly difficult for people who have problems affecting their mouth or upper limb muscle control. A regular mouthwash may help to maintain oral hygiene. Toothbrush handles may be enlarged to overcome weak grip. Handles may be lengthened and/or angled to assist people with impaired upper limb mobility to reach the mouth. An electrically operated toothbrush may be essential for maintaining oral hygiene independently when hand function is impaired. Cleansing using proprietary materials and/or regular brushing is also particularly important in maintaining oral hygiene with dentures.

Shaving

While women may be able to use a depilatory cream to remove underarm, facial or leg hair, this method is not usually acceptable for removing men's facial hair. Wet shaving with a hand razor is a hazardous business that can be performed satisfactorily only with a steady hand; a battery-operated or electric razor is safer. Elastic or leather hand straps may be used if holding the razor is difficult and a holding bracket angled at the required height can be used when grip and arm control are severely limited.

Shaving may be particularly problematical where there has been facial disfigurement, particularly following severe facial burns. The skin may be sensitive and uneven, and growing a beard may not be a suitable solution as many hair follicles may have been destroyed, resulting in uneven growth. Specialist medical guidance on products that can be used in conjunction with the skin condition is advised.

Nail care

Good care of finger- and toenails is essential for hygiene and appearance and the care of toenails is closely linked with mobility. Nail files and clippers may be attached to small boards to assist stability and grip when cutting finger nails. Toenails often present insurmountable problems and it is advisable to obtain help from the family, the community nursing service or chiropodist, particularly if the feet and toenails require professional attention, for example, for people with poor circulation or diabetes.

When cleaning the fingernails, a curved-handled nail brush that clips around the hand reduces the need for good grip. Suction pads that attach the nail brush to the side of the handbasin may be helpful for people who are only able to use one hand.

Make-up and skin care

A person who has had previous experience of skin care and the use of cosmetics may find continuing the same regimen difficult or impossible due to physical dysfunction. Alternatively, changes in the condition of the skin may necessitate a change in skin care.

Provision of adequate lighting and easily managed containers for beauty preparations may ease the problem when hand function is limited. A suitably placed mirror (which may have a magnifying facility if vision is limited) may be of assistance. Extended handles for powder pads, make-up brushes or lipsticks will enable a person with limited reach to apply make-up.

Where skin damage has occurred, discussion with a trained beauty therapist on types of cosmetic products and their application is advisable. Some baby products or non-allergenic skin preparations can be recommended. Camouflage make-up may be used to boost confidence for people who are particularly conscious of facial or hand disfigurement. After many types of skin damage, particular care should be taken in bright sunlight, as the skin may be more sensitive than prior to the injury.

Personal cleansing and grooming are essential parts of everyone's daily routine. It is important to encourage everyone to take a pride in their appearance, for the sake of identity, morale and hygiene, and in order to maintain social acceptability with carers, friends and workmates.

SEXUALITY

Human sexuality has been defined as a:

… complete attribute of every person, involving deep needs for identity, relationships, love and immortality. It is more than biological, gender, physiological processes, or modes of behaviour; it involves one's self concept and self esteem. Sexuality includes masculine and feminine self image, expression of emotional states of being, and communication of feelings for others, and encompasses everything that an individual is, thinks, feels and does during the entire lifespan. Sexual behaviour, more than any other behaviour, is intimately related to emotional and social well being.

(Kusczynski 1980)

Physical dysfunction and societal attitudes may affect people's sexuality in terms of how they present themselves – personal appearance, dress, interpersonal verbal and non-verbal communication, confidence and social interactions (Parker 1998). Individual experiences and the reactions of others may develop or constrain sexuality. Social opportunity may help to develop sexual awareness and sexual identity. Where impairment has affected personality and psychological processes, appropriate behaviours and presentation skills may need to be relearned.

Learning to express sexuality or develop appropriate social behaviours may be part of life skills training in occupational therapy. Hair care, personal adornment, make-up, dress and personal hygiene are part of personal care activities but all are also means of expressing sexuality.

Communication and interpersonal skills training may include learning appropriate social skills and behaviours. Opportunities to practise and develop these skills and express personal identity in a secure, supportive learning environment will assist the individual when approaching new social situations. Physical dysfunction may significantly affect an individual's abilities in presentation and intimate sexual relationships. Diminution of sensation may limit the pleasure of a caressing touch and difficulties with muscle control may impair physical contacts and non-verbal presentation and expression. Pain and fatigue may curtail activity levels in general and

pain or mobility problems may impede close intimacy. Difficulties with continence of urine or faeces, or the emotional sensitivity of disfigurement or deformity, may cause avoidance of intimate relationships because of the fear of 'exposure' or rejection.

Some individuals' or couples' problems may be addressed through discussion of difficulties and concerns with an informed, supportive professional, who can explore attitudes and emotions and give guidance regarding interventions and alternative strategies. Different methods of coping may include the use of drugs to control tension, spasticity or pain, alternative positions for sexual intercourse and the use of sex aids or alternative techniques to achieve sexual satisfaction. Only therapists who are knowledgeable about sexual problems and interventions, skilled in counselling, aware of their own attitudes and feelings, and comfortable discussing sexuality and intimate sexual relationships, should be involved in this form of therapy. However, all therapists should be sensitive to the possible difficulties and should have knowledge of experts to whom the individual or couple may wish to be referred. These may include specialists from Relate, representatives from the Association to Aid the Sexual and Personal Relationships of People with a Disability (SPOD), specialists from individual disability organisations, sex counsellors or therapists.

Many people are acutely embarrassed when discussing such intimate issues with others and may prefer to read appropriate literature privately. Specific texts and leaflets that address difficulties related to individual diagnoses may give further in-depth guidance for particular problems. Many such advisory leaflets, or references for other sources of guidance, may be obtained from SPOD.

Difficulties with manipulation or hand control may make some methods of contraception difficult. Fears regarding pregnancy (for example, how to cope with childbirth and parenthood or anxieties regarding inherited impairments) may restrict intimate relationships. Additionally, some clinical treatments, particularly drugs, may affect libido, potency or the effectiveness of oral contraception. Guidance on methods of contraception, management of drugs or, in the case of anxieties regarding heredity, genetic guidance or counselling, may resolve or clarify problems.

Sexual relationships may also be affected by changes resulting from physical caring. The lover or partner who is fatigued by the caring tasks may not wish to pursue sexual relationships and carers' views of partners or lovers may be changed by the intimate nursing duties they perform. Specialist guidance and counselling for both parties may help to explore and address the issues involved and identify ways of improving or managing the situation.

ROLE DUTIES

Throughout life we all adopt a number of different roles, for example, as child, friend, employee, partner, carer. Each role imposes a range of duties and tasks to be fulfilled successfully, either by our own standards or in line with the expectations of others. Most people have a number of different roles at one time and may need to consider the demands of each and to prioritise activities to retain a healthy balance in life. While the skills and attributes necessary to fulfil each role often overlap, some roles demand very specific skills (Fig. 10.4).

Individual role demands vary considerably, depending on the person and his relationships with others in the fulfilment of the role. In some situations, duties may be carried out entirely by one person, who may adopt an almost servile compliance to the demands and wishes of others. In other relationships the same roles may be perceived as shared partnerships, each person contributing equally to the completion of tasks.

Individual perceptions of roles influence priorities. Some people value the role of the homemaker above that of the worker and gain satisfaction and pleasure from the achievements and freedom it holds, while others regret the restrictions on career opportunities imposed by the homemaking role. Limited abilities, as well as environmental and societal constraints, frequently restrict the range of roles readily available to the person with severe dysfunction; in such cases considerable effort, ingenuity and support are required to maintain old roles and build new ones.

The following discussion considers the roles of homemaking, caring and working in their broadest sense. Caring includes the parenting role; the role of the worker includes that of the student, employer and volunteer.

HOMEMAKING

Skills for homemaking include planning, organising and budgeting; shopping; preparing, cooking and serving meals; laundry, sewing and mending; and basic home maintenance. Obviously there will be considerable differences in the demands of this role depending on the occupants of the home. A person living alone may need to be independent in all activities because of the lack of help available but will only have himself to look after. The homemaker who is responsible for a number of people will require many additional organisational and negotiation skills to maintain a home environment physically and emotionally suited to the needs and wishes of all the occupants. This will vary, depending on the other occupants and their roles in the homemaking process. Sharing responsibilities for the planning and execution of activities may ease the burden of homemaking for each individual, whereas responsibility for young children, disabled or elderly relatives or members of the family who take no part in domestic tasks will add to the demands placed on the homemaker. Many homemakers also have a worker role and must manage the essential demands of employment alongside their domestic tasks.

Assessment and training or retraining of the disabled homemaker is an area in which the occupational therapist can make an important contribution. Assessment should include details of the type, design and organisation of the person's home, of how many there are in the family, of what help is available from the family and/or other agencies and of whether the appro-

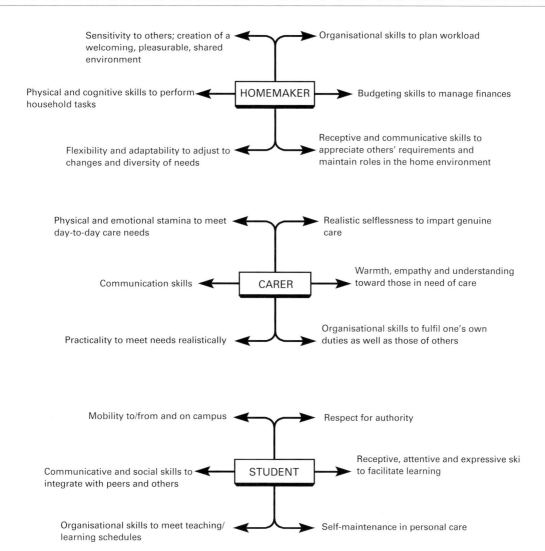

Fig. 10.4 Some aspects of role duties.

priate reorganisation of any of these will make the person more independent or the homemaking role less demanding. When selecting specific areas for intervention the therapist should take account of the person's level of disability, his personal wishes and priorities and other roles he is pursuing.

Intervention must be realistic and practical. The therapist can assist the person who has been in hospital for some time to regain confidence and re-establish a routine. She may help in organising tasks so that each family member has his own duties, for example bed-making,

cleaning his own bedroom, shopping, or preparing vegetables for a meal. For the disabled person, training in specific areas may be necessary, such as balancing on a kitchen stool, safe mobility in the home, optimum working positions or lifting techniques. The therapist can help the person to build up physical stamina and to improve physical and organisational skills, and can recommend appropriate and safe labour-saving techniques.

If the disabled person is not able to perform homemaking tasks, other avenues should be explored. Trombley (1994) states that the 'severely disabled homemaker may be an effective home manager, directing the efforts of other family members or paid household help. She can manage the finances and oversee the shopping'. Trombley states that the experienced householder may manage this with little training but the 'inexperienced homemaker may need practice in hypothetical financial management and in directing others effectively by words alone'. Others may prefer to retain a more active role in home management through modification of methods or techniques or changes to equipment or the domestic environment, only accepting manual assistance in a small number of activities. Whichever role is pursued, careful planning is important to ensure that the workload is evenly distributed and needs are met appropriately.

Forward planning of the week's activities and organisation of tasks, labour and equipment are essential prerequisites to successful completion of activities. Where the person is an active participant, it is important to plan the day so that necessary tasks can be completed comfortably, allowing for rest periods and leisure time with family members or friends.

A compensatory approach may be used where previous methods are no longer possible. New techniques may be tried and the most appropriate ones adopted. Practice in these new techniques will be necessary in most cases. Reorganisation of the home layout to minimise difficulties and facilitate mobility, modification to storage, selection of major items of equipment such as cookers, cleaners and washing machines, and the provision of suitably sited power sources and small items of specialist domestic equipment may all assist the disabled person in many household tasks.

When tasks cannot be completed independently or with the assistance of family members, other sources of help may be sought. Local authority homecare provision varies from area to area in the duties the carers are permitted to carry out. Some may provide assistance only with shopping, food preparation, cooking and serving meals, while others will do laundry and cleaning. The local Meals on Wheels service can meet the needs of the disabled person who has difficulty shopping and

preparing food, but this is not usually available every day of the week. Various voluntary organisations in many localities also provide assistance with domestic tasks in the person's home. Specific individual requirements for the disabled person and his family may be financed in some instances by the Social Fund, a community care grant or the Family Fund. In many areas, local privately organised services exist to help with domestic care. These may be engaged through the use of benefits such as the Independent Living Fund and the Disability Living Allowance, details of which can be found in the Disability Rights Handbook, which is updated regularly. The therapist should be aware of local facilities and services and should advise the disabled person and his family on how to make applications and gain the most benefit from such services.

CARING

In many instances, the occupational therapist is involved in assessing the disabled person for community living. This may be with a view to an individual's return to the community following hospitalisation. It may also be undertaken to find the most appropriate environment in which the home-based disabled person can continue in community living. It is therefore vitally important that the therapist be conversant with the needs, demands and resources for successful community care for both the disabled person and his carers.

Emphasis is often placed on the needs of the disabled person in the assumption that a partner or member of the family will take an active part in his care. Such assumptions infringe upon the rights as individuals of those concerned. Open, informed discussions should take place to identify the resources and options available; each person's wishes should be considered before decisions are made regarding future care. In many situations the outcome may have to be a compromise by both parties in light of the limitations of available resources. However, where compromise decisions are made they should be considered as sensitively and positively as possible to limit any feelings of anger and bitterness that may mar personal relationships between the carer and the disabled person. Information should be provided on services and personnel available to cope with unexpected pressures or crises in caring and, where possible, regular appraisal or reviews to monitor the situation and any changes in needs should be carried out.

The carer

Care may include help with any aspect of life skills. It may be given in the form of advice, guidance and stimulation to support the disabled person in learning how to safely perform a given activity himself, or it may extend to practical assistance to compensate for the person's inability to do the task independently. Each of these forms of care has its own particular strains. The former requires genuine respect and unflagging patience in promoting the person's achievement according to his own wishes and without the imposition of the carer's own standards. The latter type of care may be physically demanding, for example, in terms of lifting and moving the disabled person, and may impose impossible or unrealistic physical strain on the carer. In both cases, care is time-consuming, either in terms of the total number of hours devoted to the care of an individual or by virtue of an ongoing commitment to a daily or weekly schedule.

The Disabled Persons Services, Consultation and Representation Act 1986 extended the provision of the Chronically Sick and Disabled Persons Act 1970. Section 8 of the 1986 Act recognised the rights of carers to request an assessment of needs for the disabled person for whom they are caring that takes account of their ability to continue to provide care. For the purposes of the Act, carers are those who provide a substantial amount of care without remuneration on a regular basis for a disabled person who is living at home. The NHS and Community Care Act 1990 introduced the principle of care management, in which a designated care manager is responsible for assessing and monitoring an individual's needs and the use of support services.

The Carer's (Recognition and Services) Act 1995 linked the rights of carers to the regulations regarding assessment and care management stated in 1990 NHS and Community Care Act. The 1995 Act clarified the rights of carers to assessment and consideration of needs, and particularly recognised the situations of young carers, consistent with the needs of children as stated in the 1989 Children's Act.

Many carers are themselves elderly or disabled and the burden of caring for a loved one who is also disabled, over and above managing their own problems, can cause considerable physical, mental, social and financial strain. Successful caring requires a partnership in which each party recognises and respects the wishes and needs of the other. This should be viewed not just in terms of the demands each places on the other when they are together, but should also be considered in terms of the need for personal space, privacy and periods of freedom from the patient or carer role. Much will depend, therefore, on provision of and access to resources for support to permit respite periods to occur on a regular basis, without feelings of guilt or bitterness and without any sacrifice of safety.

Where the carer has a close relationship with the disabled person, changes in this relationship precipitated by disability may place heavy demands on both partners in their emotional and/or sexual interactions. Sensitive discussion of each other's feelings and needs may enable each partner to come to terms with his own and the other person's wishes and roles, and to find ways of modifying and continuing the close relationship.

Caring also includes childcare and parenting. The stresses of looking after a disabled child may affect the entire family physically, emotionally, financially and socially. In addition to the pressures on parents, those imposed upon siblings must be considered. Siblings may feel jealous of the attention given to their disabled brother or sister, angry at the limitations imposed on the family or burdened by their extra duties toward the disabled child. These feelings should be shared and discussed and the family should be encouraged and supported in finding ways to achieve an acceptable balance of attention and activity for all its members.

Where a parent, particularly the mother, is disabled, practical difficulties may arise in caring for the children, especially when they are very young. Specialist equipment and practical assistance with caring duties may enable the disabled person to fulfil the parenting role safely. Where possible, such assistance should be home based; this will enable the children to develop in their own environment and permit the parent to retain maximum contact with them. Day nurseries should be considered only when homecare is not possible, or where it seems to be necessary for the social development of the older child, as early separation of the child from the parent may affect emotional bonding. As children grow older they should be encouraged to take responsibility for their own personal care but should not be over-burdened with unrealistic domestic duties over and above those normally expected of children their age. Recent research has focused on the situation of children who care, and their needs, particularly in relation to the requirements of the Children's Act 1995. The findings of the research are published in 'Children Who Care – Inside the World of Young Carers' (Aldridge & Becker 1993) and 'My Child, My Carer – the Parent's Perspective' (Aldridge & Becker 1994).

On a more positive note, it should be emphasised that caring can be a pleasure. It can provide friendship and companionship for both parties. Maintenance of abilities and small achievements can be a source of pleasure and pride to the disabled person and to the carer, adding to a fuller appreciation of life and living.

Needs for caring

The support required by carers in order to successfully fulfil their role includes:

- Information about the services available, how to make an application, how decisions are made and how to make an appeal against unfavourable or unsuitable decisions. This information should be given in easily understood terms in the languages of the local community.

- Separate assessment of needs for the disabled person and the carer. Both parties are entitled to this service and the legitimate interests of both parties should be considered equally.
- Consultation: this should occur at all levels *before* care plans are formulated. This should extend beyond the disabled person and the carer to include appropriate external agencies, for example, voluntary organisations, social services or housing agencies, before decisions are made for future care.
- Practical help, which may include assistance with self-maintenance or domestic activities, mobility, employment or home adaptations. Practical help may also include financial provision in the form of benefits, or emotional support through counselling, befriending or self-help groups.
- Relief from care for both parties. Both short and long spells of relief should be considered, ranging from the occasional social or shopping trip to holiday periods. The type of relief should be compatible with each person's needs. However short the relief may be, a regular, predictable service is usually valued most.

Sources of information

The various sources of information about the help available for disabled people and their carers include:

- the National Council for Voluntary Organisations, which provides a directory of voluntary agencies and their roles
- DIAL UK, Disability Alliance and the Citizens' Advice Bureau, all of which provide information on rights and services
- the Equal Opportunities Commission
- the Department of Social Security and the appropriate acts of Parliament, which provide information on statutory provision
- the Association of Carers and the Association of Crossroads Care Attendant Schemes, which consider specific care provision
- many other agencies that provide information and assistance for specific groups of disabled people and their carers.

WORKING

Work may be defined as the purposeful application of effort. Work and work patterns have changed considerably over the twentieth century. Whereas many people used to spend long hours in heavy manual labour, employment in less physically demanding tasks and more flexible, shorter working periods are now becoming the norm. Advances in technology have enabled tasks to be completed by push-button control, which in some instances has led to a need for fewer employees to meet production demands and higher levels of unemployment.

Gains from working

Independence

Work may provide the means to be self-sufficient. Many people work to earn sufficient income to sustain independence in daily living for themselves and their dependants. It is important to consider that those in low-paid employment may not benefit financially from work. Equally, statutory benefits do not usually provide sufficient funding for holidays, outings or other luxuries.

Additionally, many illnesses carry added expense – special dietary requirements, extra heating and transportation costs and expenses for personal care and home cleaning can add to the strain for those on a low income.

Self-esteem/status

It is interesting to note that social class may be determined by occupation (Box 10.2). Some jobs have a status image attached to them that affects the ways in which the individual is perceived by

---

Box 10.2 Work and social class (Registrar General, Somerset House, National Records Office)

Category	Occupation
Social class I	Professional occupations
Social class II	Intermediate occupations
Social class III (N)	Skilled occupations: non-manual
Social class III (M)	Skilled occupations: manual
Social class IV	Partly skilled occupations
Social class V	Unskilled occupations

---

society. The work people do may determine the type of house in which they live, the area in which they live, the people they meet, the items they can afford to buy and, in some instances, the opinions they hold.

Work carries with it a sense of purpose and worth, a role in life, and a responsibility to or for others. Many people who cannot work feel a 'burden on society'. Some lose their self-respect and feel they cannot contribute to the society in which they live. Some still think of themselves as living on charity when receiving benefits or other services to which they are entitled and for this reason (as well as others) they may not apply for the help available to them.

Group membership

Humans are naturally gregarious animals and the need to be part of a group and to have a defined role in society is a constant pull. People can gain support and social contact from those with whom they work. For many people, the primary focus of work is not financial gain but the benefits of meeting others, getting out of the house and being a useful member of society or part of a social and employment circle.

Structure

Everyone enjoys the freedom to do what they want to do, when they want to do it, for a limited period, but for many people this freedom may lose its attraction after a time, as they lapse into apathy because of a lack of variety or purpose to the day. Work, on the other hand, can provide structure to the day, week, month and year. It may determine the individual's allocation of time, type of dress and social behaviours. In so doing it may add to their appreciation of non-work time – in the evening, at weekends, or during holidays – because of the change and freedom it brings.

The role of the occupational therapist

In some instances, assessment for work may be part of an individual's comprehensive programme of treatment; thus the occupational therapist will be familiar with the person's skills and limitations. In other instances, the individual will be referred to the therapist specifically for work assessment or work preparation, and thus may have had no previous contact with her. In either case, both parties should be clear of the purpose of assessment or work preparation, and be able to discuss anxieties, difficulties and options openly.

Further information regarding the role of the occupational therapist with work assessment can be found in Chapter 6.

The demands of the worker

To sustain employment, the worker must be able to meet the demands of the job adequately. These may be many and varied, depending upon the type of employment and the work situation.

Physically, employment demands extra effort and, in some cases, a sustained level of strenuous physical activity throughout the working day. In addition to fulfilling the demands of the actual work tasks, considerable effort may be required by the disabled person in order to travel to and from work. Some work, such as computing or fine assembly tasks, demands a high degree of coordination and dexterity. Some people may find these demands too great if such skills are unpractised or if illness has resulted in significant dysfunction.

Psychologically, any work demands a degree of concentration and adherence to routine. Certain rules and regulations must be followed – acceptable dress, language, social habits, time-keeping and personal hygiene must be displayed. Skills of communication and organisation are required to perform adequately in many situations. Social skills necessary to relate appropriately to employers and workmates, and independence in all activities of self-maintenance, enhance the possibility of successful work resettlement. Awareness of current trends and societal opinions may assist the individual to gain acceptance by workmates in both work and social contexts.

Skills in budgeting, in adjusting personal life around the work routine, or in using public transport, work canteens or specialist equipment may be necessary for successful integration into the workforce.

Work assessment

The work assessment should aim to ascertain whether the person will be able to return to his former occupation or, where this is not considered feasible, to discover his ability to undertake a new job, and the training it may demand. The activities performed in a work assessment may vary, depending on the nature of the employment and the level of dysfunction. Certain skills will be required to greater or lesser extent, depending on the nature of the job. For example, it may be necessary to note the ability of a clerk to sit for long periods, use a typewriter or computer, and write legibly. Lifting, climbing and carrying skills may need in-depth assessment for a bricklayer. However, according to Jacobs (1991) skills will fall into four main groups:

1. Work behaviours (sometimes known as 'pre-vocational readiness' skills (Jacobs 1991). These include ADL, intellectual and social skills such as personal grooming, social conduct, interpersonal skills, self-control, punctuality and time management, attention span, ability to follow instructions, ability to start and finish an activity, problem-solving, independent coping skills and adherence to regulations.
2. Aptitudes and abilities. Jacobs (1991) says that these include 'intelligence; verbal, numerical and spatial ability; form perception; clerical perception; motor coordination; finger dexterity; manual dexterity; eye-hand-foot coordination; and colour discrimination'.
3. Work skills and attainments. These are the skills that the person has previously achieved: through formal employment, in daily living, and through previous academic and practical education.
4. Physical capabilities. These include gross motor skills, such as bending, kneeling, crouching, walking, climbing, lifting, carrying, pushing and pulling, strength and

stamina; upper limb skills such as feeling, reaching, handling, grasping, holding and manipulating; and sensory skills such as smelling, hearing and seeing.

When assessing a person's ability to return to work the therapist should ensure that she is conversant with the skills demanded by the job; this will entail making an ergonomic job analysis. This can usually be done by asking the person himself what the job involves but, where this is not possible, the therapist should ensure she receives accurate information by contacting the person's employer or another reliable source.

Additionally, through questioning, observation of non-verbal behaviours, exploration of previous work patterns and discussion of future options, the therapist should aim to identify the person's motivation and attitude to work, and his priorities for future employment. These may also give insight into the realism the person has regarding his attributes and skills, and the situation of the labour market.

Work preparation

The intervention to prepare the person for work will vary, depending on the nature and type of work, the level of dysfunction, the setting of the intervention and the resources available. The therapist should aim to develop work skills and tolerances, guide the individual in developing realistic aspirations and refer him to appropriate sources for further assistance. This may include any or all of the following:

● Teaching coping strategies in self-maintenance activities. Where personal independence is limited, the therapist aims to minimise dysfunction by suitable means. If the person is severely impaired and needs to attend a work assessment or training centre, it will be necessary for him to have adequate skills or support for coping with self-maintenance before embarking on such a scheme.
● Teaching or improving basic skills. Where confidence or abilities are limited the therapist will be concerned with improving the person's

level of function. This may include practising using public transport, handling money or developing appropriate social skills. Driving a car may require specialist assessment and practice, which may be available through a disabled driving centre or a driving school such as the British School of Motoring.
● Improving psychological and communication skills. If concentration, perception or other mental processes have been affected, the therapist may devise activities to improve these skills. Similarly, if verbal or written communication is impaired, advice and support from the speech and language therapist and practice with various forms of written communication may develop skills and confidences.
● Improving physical ability. As part of the overall intervention process the occupational therapist will be aiming to help the person to regain or optimise physical function when this has been impaired or is limited. The interventions may include activities to improve range of movement, muscle strength, dexterity, coordination and balance. Liaison with the physiotherapist may be advantageous in some instances to coordinate activities to improve specific functions.
● Building or improving work tolerance and work behaviours. Following illness or a long period away from work, many people have difficulty regaining the work habit or sufficient stamina to cope with a full day's work. Impairments, either congenital or acquired, may further affect work tolerances and behaviours. In such situations, the occupational therapist can begin to build up the person's work tolerance through his performance of tasks similar to those required by the job in a simulated workstation. Time periods and output demands should be gradually increased to equate, as far as practicable, to the real work situation. Effort and concentration may be improved through changes in the demands of the activity in terms of muscle strength or complexity of the task. It may also be necessary, when designing the workstation, to consider developing tolerances for specific environmental conditions, for example, heat, cold, noise, dust, heights, outdoor work or fixed bench

work, where these will form part of the real job. The person may need practice to acquire the confidence to work unsupervised, or to attain the necessary levels of stamina and work behaviour suitable for open employment.

● Improving intellectual skills. Assessment enables the therapist to identify the person's level of intellectual performance. Deficits may be the result of injury and impairment, or may have occurred through lack of opportunity to develop specific skills. Standardised assessment or specific tests may be carried out by the therapist, or in conjunction with the psychologist. Following the results of the test, the therapist may provide specific activities to meet or overcome particular areas of deficit, or make recommendations for referral to an appropriate educational agency.

It is often difficult for the therapist to simulate the demands imposed by a full day's work in industry or commerce but, where work behaviours and tolerances are limited, improvement in this area can be initiated while the person is regularly attending the hospital or rehabilitation centre. Practice in simulated work tasks builds up skills and confidences before returning to open employment or making an application for alternative training. Employment regulations and health and safety legislation have restricted opportunities to practise work-related tasks in other areas of the hospital or community, but the employment services work training and Job Introduction Schemes provide opportunities to further work preparation.

Advances in technology, in the form of computers, faxes and electronic links to employers, enable people who have difficulties with mobility, self-maintenance activities or verbal communication to work from a home base. In this situation the psychological demands for concentration and adherence to routine are particularly important to maintain the work pattern in the domestic environment. In the past, home-based employment has frequently been in poorly paid assembly or packing tasks, but advances in information technology have raised job status and the level of remuneration for some people who work from a home base.

Following comprehensive work assessment and/or work preparation, the occupational therapist may recommend return to previous employment. Where this is not possible, the therapist should complete a report for the Disability Employment Advisor (DEA) to assist with advising the individual on the employment opportunities available through the Employment Services. The therapist may also be required to present a report to the consultant, general practitioner or other personnel concerned with the person's future or with his compensation claim.

Giving information and guidance

Frequently, people whose employment prospects are doubtful have little idea of the type of help available to them either for building up fitness for return to work or for retraining for alternative employment. It is often a source of great concern to the person that his future employment prospects seem poor. The occupational therapist should be able to supply accurate and appropriate information on the sources of help available (Fig. 10.5) and on what benefits the person may receive. The therapist may be a member of the team that assesses the person's capabilities and makes direct referral to the Disability Employment Advisor or other appropriate agency.

Ordinary further education courses provide pathways for some disabled people to gain experience and qualifications at an academic and social level, which may enhance employment opportunities.

The resettlement clinic

Some hospitals or specialist rehabilitation centres hold a regular resettlement clinic to determine the future work prospects of individuals undergoing treatment. Such clinics are usually run by the doctor in charge of the unit or the consultant responsible for rehabilitation services. They are usually attended by the occupational therapist, physiotherapist, social worker, a senior nurse attached to the unit (where appropriate) and the Disability Employment Advisor. Occasionally, the psychologist or the person's relatives may also

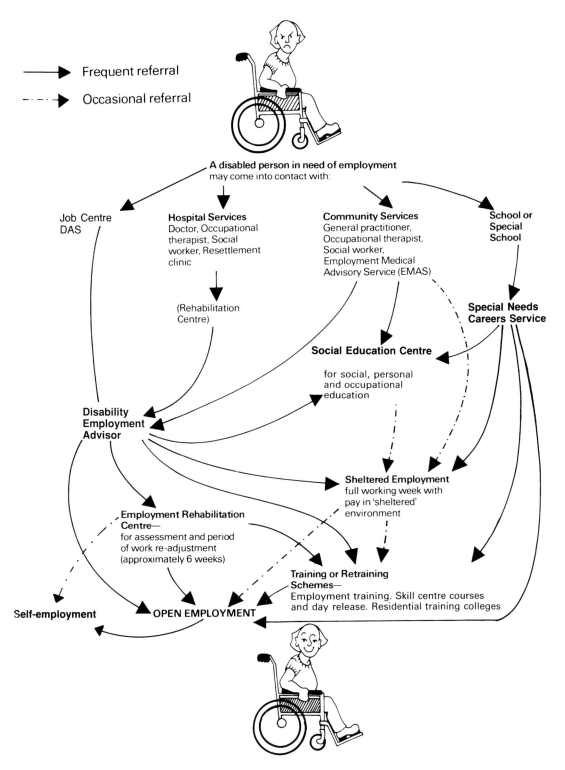

Fig. 10.5 Services available to help the disabled person with employment.

attend. The person's case is presented, his progress charted and his future prospects and options discussed. Where further intensive medical treatment is considered advisable, he may be referred to a medical rehabilitation centre. Alternatively, it may be considered that he has reached his maximum potential and that referral to employment training or support services would be more suitable.

Medical rehabilitation centres

These provide an intensive programme of rehabilitation following serious illness or injury. Individuals may be referred to such centres following initial assessment and treatment in hospital. Such centres have the facilities to build up a higher degree of physical fitness and work tolerance than is possible in most hospital departments. Treatment is provided under medical supervision by a team comprising physiotherapists (who may conduct hydrotherapy and gymnasium work), occupational therapists, speech therapists and social workers. The centres offer a non-hospital atmosphere. Some centres are residential on a weekday basis; residents are encouraged to be personally independent and make their own arrangements for transportation and entertainment during their stay.

Sources of assistance for the disabled worker

The Disablement Advisory Service (DAS)

This is part of the Employment Service Agency and is usually based at the Employment Service area office or Job Centre. The Disability Advisory Service exists to assist both employers and people who are already in employment or are seeking work. It can provide advice on developing and implementing a sound company policy on the employment of people with disabilities, as outlined in their 'Guide to employment for disabled people' (Greater London Association for Disabled People 1997). Specific advice may be given regarding the recruitment, career development and retention of workers with disabilities. A number of special schemes exist to overcome particular difficul-

ties. These include the Job Introduction Scheme, the Special Aids to Employment Scheme, the Adaptations to Premises and Equipment Scheme, the Personal Reader Service for the visually impaired and the Working at Home with Technology Scheme.

The Placing, Assessment and Counselling Team (PACT)

These teams, based in Job Centres and consisting of Disability Employment Advisors and occupational psychologists, aim to provide coordinated services to help people with disability into employment, to promote the value of people with disabilities to employers and to help employers recruit and retain people with disabilities.

They provide advice and guidance regarding employment opportunities, counselling and assessment for work, contact with organisations providing work preparation and training, practical help for employment, work placements and continued support for employers and disabled employees.

Training and work preparation programmes usually extend for a period of six weeks in an environment as similar as possible to the 'real' work situation. Here the person is closely monitored and supported to help establish or re-establish a work routine. Alternatively, the PACT team may advise on educational opportunities in specialist colleges or in mainstream educational establishments with adequate student support.

Practical help may involve the provision of equipment to minimise the effects of the impairment when working, funding for adapting work premises or help with costs for funding a support worker for a person with a severe impairment or for additional expenses incurred by the disabled person when travelling to work.

Work placement aims to place the worker in the most appropriate work environment. This may be in open employment with the necessary support, or may be in sheltered or supported employment, with organisations such as Remploy, Scope or the Shaw Trust. The Disability Employment Advisor acts as a source of information for both the employer and prospective employee. The Job Introduction Scheme

(Disability Rights Handbook) and the New Deal Scheme provide financial incentives to employers to provide a trial period in a particular job for prospective disabled employees.

The Disability Employment Advisor also acts as an advocate for employment of people with disabilities by working with people with disabilities and employers 'to help more employers employ more disabled people more effectively'. The use of the Disability Symbol promotes this. The commitments of employers using the disability symbol are to:

- interview all applicants with a disability who meet the minimum criteria for a job vacancy and to consider them on their abilities
- ask disabled employees, at least once every year, what can be done to ensure they can use and develop their abilities at work
- make every effort, when employees become disabled, to make sure they stay in employment
- take action to ensure that key employees develop the necessary awareness of disability to make the commitments work
- revise the commitments each year by reviewing what has been achieved, planning ways to improve these achievements, and informing all employees of progress and future plans.

Disability Employment Advisors may provide practical information about ways of putting the commitments into practice, where to access expert guidance if an employee becomes disabled and advice on ways of developing disability awareness. They may also aim to give a speedy response to help recruit someone with a disability where a suitable vacancy exists, and provide advice and individual help to access specialist support to facilitate successful employment of a person with a disability.

Employment Rehabilitation Centres (ERCs)

These centres provide opportunities for people who have not been employed for some time following illness or injury and who need a chance to adapt themselves gradually to normal working conditions. The ERCs also assess people's employment capabilities. Courses vary according to individual needs and the facilities offered aim to simulate working conditions and a realistic work atmosphere.

During the stay at the centre, individuals are paid a tax-free maintenance allowance at a higher rate than basic unemployment and sickness benefit. Each person's programme is discussed regularly and reviewed at a case conference.

Employment training

A number of employment training schemes are available for the disabled person on a residential or daily basis. Residential colleges provide training courses for disabled people in a range of commercial and vocational skills. Trainees receive an allowance while on the course. Applications should be made through the local Disability Employment Advisor. Local employment training initiatives vary from area to area and information is available through the Disability Employment Advisor at local employment training or skill centres. Some further education establishments provide day release courses and other employment training courses suitable for disabled people.

Training for work schemes

These are run by the Learning Skills Councils (LSCs) and provide a broad range of training and job development initiatives. The schemes focus on those unemployed and disabled people seeking work who are in receipt of invalidity benefit or severe disability allowance. More information on the range of provision can be obtained from local LSCs.

Sheltered Work and Sheltered Placement Schemes

In the past, when a disabled person was unable to work in open employment, sheltered provision was established under the Disabled Person's (Employment) Act 1944. Originally predominantly based in sheltered workshops, this has been extended to include Sheltered Placement Schemes. These schemes enable people with disabilities who are able to perform a particular job, but at a slower rate than a non-disabled employee, to be employed and paid the going wage for the job. The employer then claims a subsidy from the Employment Service for lost production.

The Disability Discrimination Act 1995 has strengthened the position of disabled people with regard to employment by making it unlawful to discriminate against actual or potential employees based on their disability in a range of employment areas.

Social education centre

For those who are unable to cope with either open or sheltered employment, social education centres run by the local authority offer social and occupational education. As well as simple work tasks performed in a realistic work atmosphere (again, usually under contract to local firms), these centres provide education in life skills such as self-maintenance, homemaking and social interaction. Trainees receive standard state benefits while attending the centre and a small remuneration for the work they produce. Some people may progress to further courses after a period at the centre.

Other initiatives

A variety of local community programmes are available to help the less disabled person who has not worked for some time to regain confidence. These differ from region to region and rely largely on local initiatives.

Some specialist training courses are offered for people with particular impairments; for example, training schemes for visually impaired people are offered by the Royal National Institute for the Blind.

The Rehabilitation Engineering Movement Advisory Panels (REMAP) will also design and provide special items of equipment to assist the disabled person to overcome a particular problem at work.

Self-employment

Able-bodied and disabled people alike may wish to become self-employed, using their skills in a creative or consultative capacity. Starting one's own business can seem very attractive but there are many factors to consider before embarking on such a venture. Realistic, reliable advice regarding available resources and potential pitfalls is of vital importance. Consideration should be given to the viability of the skill or product in question and to financing the venture in terms of materials, premises, marketing and production costs. The physical, psychological and social demands of such a project should be assessed realistically in light of the person's impairment, and the stress that self-employment is likely to cause to the individual and his carers should be considered. The Disability Employment Advisor may be able to advise the disabled person regarding the opportunities and schemes available to him, and advice from banking and business agencies will be invaluable.

The disabled employer

Many people are able to maintain their role as employers despite substantial levels of physical disability. Much will depend on the type of work involved. Cognitive and communication skills are usually the disabled employer's most important personal assets. Modern technology and good support staff have enabled people with limited mobility and very restricted physical skills to continue in the managerial role, using their knowledge and experience to organise and negotiate effectively, and retaining their pride, dignity and the respect of employees and customers.

The Employment Service Agency may provide advice concerning specialist equipment or other resources available to the disabled employer.

THE STUDENT

Studying is included here under the work role because many of the skills necessary for successful schooling are similar to those needed in employment. Both roles require adherence to the rules or regime of the establishment, social skills to communicate with those in authority and with one's peers, practical skills to meet the demands of set tasks and mobility skills to travel to, from and within the school or campus.

The occupational therapist's role is also similar in both situations. She may be involved in assessing and developing skills in relation to the demands of the role, reporting to others about individual needs and providing advice, guidance and liaison between the individual and the establishment to facilitate successful integration.

The 1981 Education Act encouraged increased placement of children with special needs in mainstream schools. This was further supported in the Education Act 1993, which also extended the rights of children and parents to involvement in the consultation and decision-making process. The occupational therapist may be involved in detailed assessment of the child's abilities for the Statement of Special Educational Needs. Areas evaluated may include independence in personal care tasks, fine and gross motor skills and perceptual, cognitive and social skills. The Statement aims to ensure that the necessary provision is available for the child at school. The therapist may be involved in the development of these skills in readiness for school and she may also be required to provide advice to parents and teachers. This may include recommendations on site modifications, handling techniques and special equipment to promote mobility or facilitate teaching and learning.

For the older student, the therapist may assist with the assessment and development of skills for future study, employment and community living.

Many adult and elderly disabled people who are unemployed or retired may consider study as a means of purposefully filling the day without the direct objective of attaining gainful employment.

THE VOLUNTEER

Some disabled people who are not in paid employment use their knowledge and skills in a voluntary capacity to assist others. The range of voluntary activities is extensive and provides assistance to all age groups. People who have skilled knowledge and experience in managerial activities may be valued members of voluntary groups, while others who have particular physical skills or communicative abilities may be able to use these in teaching or assisting others. Personal experience of problems often promotes greater understanding of the difficulties others may be facing. Some people with disabilities become active members of disability organisations or pressure groups which aim to improve recognition and facilities for disabled people in general.

Many people who do not wish to join the paid workforce find that their volunteer 'work' provides structure, satisfaction, pride in their abilities and recognition. In some instances, volunteer work has led to paid work in open employment or to educational or managerial roles in charitable organisations.

In conclusion, purposeful occupation – whether as homemaker, carer, worker, employer, student or volunteer – is a vital component of the disabled person's quality of life. Many disabled people are able to fulfil some if not all of the duties associated with their roles, and the occupational therapist may assist them in recognising, maximising and utilising their skills and in identifying techniques, equipment and resources that will help them to overcome particular areas of difficulty.

LEISURE

Leisure-time pursuits are an important part of any person's daily life. These may include hobbies, sports, exercise, entertainment, holidays, relaxation and play. For the disabled or elderly person who is not able to work, leisure plays an even more important part in living. Leisure activities and involvement in local organisations are a substitute for work and provide opportunities for participation in creative activities and for maintaining or increasing social contacts. They may introduce the person to broader areas of interest and compensate him for the lack of status associated with unemployment.

Initially, leisure activities may help the more severely impaired or elderly person to adjust to a new lifestyle, but later these activities may become more than a time-filler. They may encourage the individual to strive for more knowledge and skills than he had time for previously.

Individual needs differ considerably, depending on the temperament, personality, interests and level of intelligence of the person, as well as on the impairments he may have. The therapist must be aware of such factors before she can guide the person towards fulfilling his needs. She needs to take into account previous interests, for these may still be pursued to advantage by some people; however, for others who have a significant level of impairment, returning to previous activities may cause frustration and accentuate functional losses. Much will depend on the person's desires and the facilities and resources available locally to meet his requirements.

EXPLORING LEISURE OPTIONS

The most important task is to identify what the disabled person would like to gain from leisure pursuits. For some people, socialisation may be the prime objective, while others may see creativity as the most important aspect. Socialisation may involve active participation with others in a social setting or group; alternatively, the individual may be a passive receiver in a social environment such as the cinema, theatre or at a football match. The range of possible creative activities is immense. Some people may wish to join others in classes or groups, while others may prefer to be creative in their home environment if the facilities and materials are available. Others may wish to expand their education and knowledge through adult classes or independent learning methods.

Leisure pursuits may be explored individually, giving an opportunity for the development of relationships away from the carer or family. Such wishes should be clearly identified and discussed to avoid any feelings of rejection on the part of the family or carers. Alternatively, the disabled person and the family may wish to identify activities that all members can participate in together. This may be particularly important for holidays.

Issues such as travel, transport, cost of materials or activities and any special equipment should be explored. Some financial assistance may be available either through reduced attendance fees or through grants or loans from charitable organisations such as the British Sports Association for the Disabled or the Royal National Institute for the Blind. Jay (1984) suggests that many disabled people do not partici-

pate in the wide range of leisure opportunities available to them because of:

- lack of confidence in their ability to participate, which reduces motivation to explore options
- lack of knowledge of how or where to find information about leisure activities.

Confidence

Some people do not wish to join activities specifically for disabled people. They would prefer to participate in activities with people who are not disabled but are concerned about others' attitudes to them and whether they will be able to participate equally. Unfortunately, many may have suffered rejection or overprotection by their non-disabled peers because of their impairment.

The therapist can help such individuals to discuss their anxieties and to explore societal attitudes and can provide opportunities for assertiveness training and confidence building. Where he lacks confidence in his practical abilities to pursue the activity, the disabled person may be able to explore the activity in a day centre before joining a local group or club. Many centres provide a wide range of social and leisure activities with help and guidance from centre staff or peers. Books and reference texts may be obtained from the local library to assist learning.

If communication skills are impaired they may be improved through regular practice in communication techniques in a safe environment in one-to-one and group activities. Social skills training may occur in discussion groups, role play, video exercises and organised excursions. Cognitive skills may be developed through reality orientation, problem-solving games and simple quizzes or through activities or exercises that involve following verbal or written instructions.

A one-to-one introduction may assist both the organisers and the disabled person to share concerns and discuss any special arrangements that may ease anxieties about participation in a club, class or group. In some instances, a relative or carer may be able to accompany the disabled person; this may reassure him, particularly on the first visit. However, if he is happy with his choice of activity he may not wish the relative or carer to continue attending, as this may impede his social integration. It is possible in some instances for the occupational therapist to fulfil this introductory role.

Sources of information

Nationally, information may be obtained from a number of sources. Many charities provide information on the range of activities available to their members. Additionally, the Disabled Living Foundation information leaflets, the Equipment for the Disabled booklets 'Gardening' and the 'Directory of Sports and Leisure for the Disabled' (Disability Information Trust 1997), as well as many other leaflets and books, provide a wide range of information on organisations and equipment specifically for disabled people. On a local basis, information can usually be obtained from the Citizens' Advice Bureau, leisure or education services departments of the local council and from the social services department. Access information and details of facilities available in particular areas can be obtained from city information and access guides, and organisations such as the National Trust provide their own information booklets.

Information about travel can be obtained from the Department of Environment 'Door to Door' booklet, RADAR publications on holidays and travel, and from RAC and AA publications and the 'Directory for Disabled People'. A number of holiday organisations have details of access and mobility facilities in holiday accommodation in resorts in Britain and abroad. Some organisations provide holidays specifically for disabled people and their families.

The range of leisure options

The range of leisure options available to a disabled individual may include:

- practical pastimes such as model-making, gardening, photography, cookery and needlework
- intellectual pursuits, including further or higher education, adult education classes, study and appreciation of music, art, literature, computing and many other areas of interest that may be used for intellectual stimulation or pleasurable appreciation

- active participation in sports or games, ranging from card or board games to more active pursuits such as archery, swimming, riding or skiing
- specific interest collections such as stamps, coins, books, records and many other collectable items
- interests requiring little or no active participation, such as theatre, cinema, television and radio, music or spectator sports
- social clubs which organise particular social activities or outings, either specifically for disabled people or as a broader facility for all.

In conclusion, many opportunities are available for the disabled person to pursue leisure activities at home or in the community. The occupational therapist may introduce leisure interests through therapeutic social activities or may provide information on where to obtain details of services or equipment. She may stimulate the disabled person to explore old skills or interests or encourage him to consider new leisure pursuits. For those who are not able to obtain paid employment, leisure activities provide structure to the day and enhance self-esteem.

Satisfaction, pleasure or achievement in recreational activities can add quality to the day or week and promote a sense of purpose and wellbeing for the disabled person, and may ease some of the emotional burden on relatives and carers.

CONCLUSION

This chapter has attempted to outline the life skills necessary for successful community living. Of necessity, the coverage of each particular area has been superficial. The chapter has addressed the main aspects of self-maintenance, role duties and leisure but the reader will need to explore particular areas in more detail to meet the specific needs for a given individual. Section 4 of this book identifies some of the problems resulting from specific diagnoses but other texts, which provide detailed information on equipment, techniques or particular life skills, should be explored.

Many of the techniques used by the occupational therapist in helping the disabled individual to develop life skills are based on the rehabilitative approach and thus explore ways of compensating for loss of function. However, these techniques should not be used in isolation, as many problems may be minimised or overcome by the use of other therapeutic approaches to enhance physical, intellectual or social performance, and thereby improve function.

Realistic consideration of the individual's personal wishes in the context of his present physical, social, psychological and environmental situation is the crucial factor in devising a strategy that will meet his needs and those of his relatives and carers in developing life skills.

REFERENCES

Aldridge J, Becker S 1993 Children who care – inside the world of young carers. Loughborough University/Billingham Press, UK

Aldridge J, Becker S 1994 My child, my carer – the parent's perspective. Loughborough University/Billingham Press, UK

British Telecom 1997 A guide for people who are older or disabled. BT plc

Bull R (ed) 1998 Housing options for disabled people. Jessica Kingsley, London

Carer's (Recognition and Services) Act (1995). HMSO, London

Centre on Environment for the Handicapped 1988 Good Loo Design Guide. Centre on Environment for the Handicapped, London

Children's Act (1989). HMSO, London

Children's Act (1995). HMSO, London

Chronically Sick and Disabled Persons Act (1970). HMSO, London

Cooper E 1999 Sexuality and disability; a guide for everyday practice. Radcliffe Medical Press, Abingdon, Oxfordshire

Cynkin S, Robinson AM 1990 Occupational therapy and activities health: towards health through activities. Little Brown, Boston, MA

Disability Alliance and Educational Research Association. Disability Right Handbook (updated regularly). Anderson Fraser, London.

Disability Discrimination Act (1995). HMSO, London

Disability Information Trust 1997 Equipment for disabled – gardening; and Directory of Sports and Leisure for the disabled. Disability Information Trust, Oxford

Disabled Living Foundation 1999 Hamilton Index. Disabled Living Foundation, London

Disabled Persons (Employment) Act (1994). HMSO, London

Disabled Persons Services, Consultation and Representation Act (1986). HMSO, London

Education Act (1981). HMSO, London

Education Act (1993). HMSO, London

Goldsmith S 1984 Designing for the disabled, 4th edn. Royal Institute of British Architects, London

Greater London Association for Disabled People 1997 Guide to employment for disabled people. GLAD, London

HMSO 1990 National Health Service and Community Care Act. HMSO, London

Jacobs K 1991 Occupational therapy – work related programs and assessments, 2nd edn. Little Brown, Boston, MA

Katz S, Ford AB, Moskowitz RW, Jackson B, Jaffe MW 1963 Studies of illness in the aged. The index of ADL; a standardised measure of biological and psychosocial function. Journal of American Medical Association 185(12):914–919

Kuczynski JH 1980 Nursing and medical students sexual attitudes and knowledge. Journal of Obstetric, Gynecological and Neonatal Nursing Nov–Dec:339–342

Mandelstam M 1992 How to get equipment for disability. Jessica Kingsley, London

Parker R 1998 Culture, society and sexuality. UCL Press, London

Trombly CA 1994 Occupational therapy for physical dysfunction, 4th edn. Williams & Wilkins, Baltimore, MD

Walbrook Housing Association 1992 Cracking housing problems. A practical guide to problem solving for disabled people, occupational therapists and carers. Walbrook Housing Association, Derby

Williams R 1968 Communication. Penguin, London

Yerxa EJ, Locker SB 1990 Quality of time use by adults with spinal cord injuries. American Journal of Occupational Therapy 44(4):318–326

FURTHER READING

Darnborough A, Kinrade D 1999 Directory for disabled people. A handbook for everyone involved with disability. RADAR/Prentice Hall Europe, Hertfordshire.

Jay P 1984 Coping with disability. Disabled Living Foundation, London.

Mandelstam D 1986 Incontinence and its management. Croom Helm, London.

USEFUL CONTACT

Association to Aid the Sexual and Personal Relationships of people with a Disability (SPOD) 286 Camden Road, London. Tel: 020 7607 8851.

Practice

SECTION CONTENTS

11

Cerebral palsy

Gillian Brown

INTRODUCTION

Cerebral palsy (CP) is most commonly defined as a disorder of posture and movement that is non-progressive in nature (Bax 1964). This definition may serve to confuse rather than explain and therefore requires some clarification. In medical terms, it describes the underlying disorder associated with a variety of cerebral palsy syndromes and the primary cerebral pathology. Functionally, it is the expression of 'cerebral palsy' in the individual child and the consequences for development throughout the lifecycle stages that is most significant. The expression of cerebral palsy may change, or even disappear, throughout early childhood (Davis 1997).

For children presenting with motor difficulties arising from cerebral palsy, there are often other concerns about occupational performance and limitations in performance components. There may also be impairment in other systems of the body, including visual perceptual difficulties and hearing difficulties. Concerns about nutrition and growth with associated feeding problems are common. There may also be cognitive difficulties presenting as global or specific learning disabilities. A child with cerebral palsy is more likely than other children to have a fit or convulsion during his life. The stage at which this can happen, and the subsequent incidence of convulsions or fits, will vary from one child to another. Orthopaedic consequences of postural asymmetry and imbalances of muscular action are frequently seen.

Reviews of clinical classifications of cerebral palsy are based upon the extremities affected and the type of tonal dysfunction exhibited, together with the involuntary movement properties. Davis (1997), for example, classifies cerebral palsy in this way. Children with cerebral palsy will have very individual patterns of movement. This means that no two children are really alike in the combination and extent of their difficulties. The cerebral palsy can present as spasticity, athetosis or ataxia. The presentation of these movement patterns relates to the area of brain that has been damaged, namely the motor cortex, the basal ganglia and the cerebellum, respectively. Single features such as spasticity or ataxia alone are rarely seen. Hypotonia or floppiness may be present and considered as being a presentation of cerebral palsy where muscle disorders have been excluded. Hypotonia may be seen in association with ataxia. Other terms used to describe the 'clinical' signs of cerebral palsy include spastic cerebral palsy (diplegia, hemiplegia and quadriplegia), dyskinetic (athetoid and dystonic) ataxia and mixed. The terms quadriplegia (total body involvement), diplegia (lower limbs usually with some upper limb involvement) or hemiplegia (one side) indicate the extent of involvement. The description of the presentation of cerebral palsy as seen in an individual child helps the therapist to understand how the child's performance may be affected.

THE DEVELOPING CHILD

While a child may have problems with movement identified at any time during the first years of life, the picture will be an evolving one. How the picture evolves depends upon the severity and the extent of these problems, with these becoming more evident as the child's nervous system matures. The altered motor function seen in the young child continues to evolve as the nervous system matures and new motor skills emerge. A changing clinical picture is seen, giving the impression of a progressive rather than a static disorder. The literature suggests that definitive diagnosis is rarely made before 6 months. Davis (1997) reports that delayed motor milestone development is the most consistent presenting feature. The complexity and extent of the difficulties may not be fully realised until the child is 2–3 years old, and sometimes later.

Functionally, problems can occur right across the performance areas and performance components. For example, a child with spasticity, having increased tone affecting their lower limbs, will have difficulty with gaining independent walking, may be unsteady and need to use walking aids. There are also likely to be associated difficulties with the control of the upper limbs as fluency of movement and production of fine control is restricted. A child with ataxia or 'uncoordinated' movement will find play and activity easier in standing and find achieving a stable sitting posture much more demanding. He may overshoot his reach when trying to pick up a toy and his speech articulation may be affected. His movement will be very deliberate and he will find it difficult to vary his speed of movement, as this can exacerbate the ataxia. A child with athetosis, where involuntary movement masks the production of voluntary movement, will find it difficult to achieve a stable working position unaided or without using compensatory techniques such as adopting flexed postures. Excitement and interest in an activity can make the involuntary movement so marked that it is very difficult for the child to be still and this can severely restrict the child's participation in an activity. Eating can be a particular problem as coordinating head control and hand movement can be very demanding.

As the child gets older, parents will often report changes that reflect deterioration in performance areas. The child may remain dependent on adult care and practical physical help to achieve everyday tasks such as dressing, in contrast to his peers who do not have cerebral palsy.

CONSEQUENCES OF DELAYED DEVELOPMENT

The individual child with physical and usually other difficulties is at risk of restricted opportunities to explore his environment. A child's play, seen as an occupation, is vital if he is to develop independence and autonomy. Play is more than a means of providing developmentally appropriate learning tasks. For a child spending so much time in an adult-directed environment, there is sometimes little opportunity for him to develop intrinsic interest in an activity, to be playful or to develop pretend play. There may also be differences in the way that a child with cerebral palsy learns because of the presence of cognitive difficulties and the way that activities and play experiences are offered must be considered. For example, a child who is struggling to concentrate will find a box full of toys too distracting. Initially, a limited selection of tasks might be offered. Equally, the child may be at risk of having difficulties with relating to his peers as a result of being more or less dependent on his parent(s) and other adult carers.

In addition, receptive and expressive language difficulties and difficulties with articulation will impact on a child's capacity to communicate needs and wishes. Where there are marked difficulties augmentative communication may be an option to support occupational performance.

As the child reaches nursery age, a planned transition to a nursery school will ensure the child is well supported at the appropriate times during the school day. Everyone involved will be informed about the level of support required by the child to facilitate full participation in all activities. Cross-agency collaboration and working in partnership with the child's family in line with the Special Educational Needs Code of Practice is required. Effective sharing of information and partnership will continue to be important as the family makes choices about their child's moves onto primary school and then secondary school.

For some children, a decision may be made that a child's special educational needs can be best met in a school offering a developmental or modified curriculum. Sometimes this placement will be on a shared time basis with another local school offering elements of the curriculum for part of the week.

Families will have to face the added demands of caring for a child with lifelong, complex healthcare needs. Each family will react to these demands in unique ways and will evolve their own ways of coping. This will be in the context of their own extended families, the reactions of their local community and society in general. The family may elect to access support from networks within statutory services, specialist services, the voluntary sector and also parental networks and self-help groups. The pattern of accessible support services will vary from one geographical area to another and may require the family to travel considerable distances.

RESTRICTIONS FROM THE ENVIRONMENT

The physical home environment can be restrictive in providing opportunities for developing independence in terms of activities of daily living and in accessing family activity. It is particularly important to enable the child to develop his role within the family and to participate in everyday family life. Achieving this in the home environment places great demands on a family as there are many costs, not least financial ones. Often, there is a need to accept a referral onto the local authority social services department at an early stage in a child's life. This may happen before a greater understanding of the longer-term consequences has been reached. This event can be particularly distressing. The family will also need to be able to negotiate their way through the processes of accessing such help. The whole process of defining the need for facilities to meet the special needs of the child places an emphasis on the reality of the situation for the child and for the family. It can polarise their reactions around their sense of loss.

An accessible environment is equally important at the stage of transition to preschool and then school facilities.

OBTAINING A DIAGNOSIS

There is much debate about the need for early confirmation that a child's difficulties can be explained by a diagnosis. Where this is cerebral palsy, it signifies that this child and his family will need access to services, to provide intervention and support throughout the lifecycle. For the family, the stage of diagnosis may help to make sense of the child's difficulties and be a starting place for their own learning about their child's individual needs.

It is important for the occupational therapist to develop an understanding of the context or place of contact from the family's perspective. Depending on the local patterns of service delivery, the occupational therapist's contact could begin soon after the family has been given a diagnosis and has begun to learn about ways of explaining the child's difficulties. At first, the occupational therapist may be seen as someone who will give more bad news as the necessity of contact with the family confirms the extent of their child's difficulties. Later, after this stage, contact may be associated with the delivery of practical solutions, where delays in processing and accessing practical help may result in reactions of frustration and anger. Parents report that their ability to parent their child is often compromised (Brown 1996) and effective, timely intervention by an occupational therapist can result in a very positive outcome.

PROGNOSIS

With the complexity of the nature of cerebral palsy, there are few clear indicators about the prognosis for an individual child. Generally, most children live to adulthood, although life expectancy is often shorter than normal. With ongoing support there can be significant functional gains across all performance areas. It is useful to consider a wide range of outcomes. At one extreme, there is the recognition of a child's capacity to be able to influence and direct his own care, even when requiring direct practical help for some or all activities during the day. By contrast, there is the provision of a lightweight thumb post orthosis to improve a child's pencil grip.

Overall, occupational therapy intervention will include the following:

- developing the child's skills in the context of his family
- having an impact on the child's environment, both at home and at school
- contributing to the special needs procedures (Special Educational Needs Code of Practice 1996)
- parental education
- providing advice and consultation for the extended multidisciplinary team.

THE INTERVENTION TEAM

Local service provisions for obstetrics and maternity care and for neonatal, primary, secondary and tertiary care will influence the nature of the services that can be accessible for a family with a child presenting with cerebral palsy. In the UK, local authority health, education and social services departments are required to make a cohesive and coordinated response to a child and his family's needs.

For infants, young children and school-age children, medical care will be provided by an acute service paediatrician at local, secondary or tertiary level or by a local community paediatrician, where they exist. Sometimes, a child may be followed-up by a neonatal team and then referred on to local or specialist services.

Primary healthcare teams, with general practitioners and health visitors, may contribute to the identification of concerns about motor difficulties through their screening and health surveillance roles.

At secondary and tertiary levels of care, multidisciplinary teams, sometimes known as Child Development Teams or Services for Children with Special Needs, may be available for assessment and diagnosis and, in some cases, may offer continuing care intervention and support. At stages throughout the child's life, other specialists may be involved. These include paediatric neurologists, orthopaedic surgeons and paediatric surgeons for surgical provision of, for example, a gastrostomy for a child facing complex feeding and nutrition problems.

Condition-specific agencies within the voluntary sector, such as SCOPE, provide information services, assessment services and specialist schools together with support services, which may include advocacy services. Interdisciplinary and cross-agency collaboration is central to the philosophy underpinning effective service delivery. For each discipline, it is essential to be well-informed about the roles and responsibilities of other service providers. Occupational therapy input for a child must reflect this. Graham and Maze (1997) discuss collaboration between an occupational therapist, a physiotherapist and a class teacher in a school setting. Hickling (2000) addresses the provision of a therapy service in an inclusive school setting, using a transdisciplinary approach.

Multidisciplinary and interdisciplinary working requires that the occupational therapist identify the key operational links that should be established. The services making up the intervention team will have evolved over time in local situations.

The roles and responsibilities that individual services may undertake that interact and overlap with the main domains of concern for the occupational therapist are indicated in Figure 11.1.

LIAISON

It is vital that close liaison is maintained with all the other professionals involved with the child. An open working relationship must be achieved with the family if specific interventions offered by the occupational therapist are to be successful and benefit the child. This is important whether the occupational therapist works as part of an extended team on one site or is operationally separate from other people supporting the child and the family. Decisions about timing of intervention will be based on an understanding of the family and child's current situation, gained by appraising information obtained both directly and indirectly.

FAMILY AND PARENTAL ROLES

It is essential to recognise the family structure in relation to the network of services providing intervention. Parents or other family members hold the parental responsibility and provide the day-to-day care of the child, in the context of the individual family. The roles undertaken will vary over time and exist on a continuum of degrees of participation (Brown et al 1997). The occupational therapist will need to be aware of the family's need to change roles and adjust the extent of the input they wish to contribute. Where a child's care is provided outside their own family (and parental responsibility is held by a local authority under 'looked after' arrangements), it is important to establish the interagency arrangements for the provision of care and intervention.

THE CONTEXT OF OCCUPATIONAL THERAPY

Referral to occupational therapy can come from a variety of sources influenced by local management arrangements and patterns of referral. Occupational therapy services for children are usually provided within health or social services but posts within voluntary agencies or schools also exist.

The setting within which the therapist works will influence the role(s) and functions she undertakes. The range can include contributing to the early evaluation and diagnostic stages, making an assessment of the child's developmental status, specific interventions to address problems with performance components and performance areas and referral to other occupational therapists in the other agencies. Contact between an occupational therapy service and a family could be at the early stages only, at intervals or on a regular basis over a short- or long-term period throughout the stages of childhood and into adolescence, before the child is referred onto available adult services. More detail of key tasks is given on page 330.

Multidisciplinary/interdisciplinary intervention matrix from occupational therapist's perspective (Brown 2000)	Occupational performance areas								Performance components			
	Physical health/medical issues	Self care	Communication	Mobility	Education	Play	Environment	Support for the family	Sensorimotor	Neuromuscular skeletal	Cognitive	Psychosocial
Range of services												
Occupational therapist							6					
Physiotherapist		1								7		
Speech and language therapist										8		9
Dietician		2										
Health visitor		3										
Community paediatric nurse		4										
Paediatrician		R										
Clinical psychologist		5										
Educational psychologist												
Classroom teacher												
Class support workers												
Special educational needs officer												
Vision services												
Audiology services												
Wheelchair services												
Social worker												

1 Handling young child

2 Nutrition

3 Weaning and management

4 Augmentative feeding

5 Management

6 Including equipment and/or technique solutions/home modification

7 Motor skills and postural control

8 Oral motor control

9 Parent–child interaction

R Referral on for videofluoroscopy

Fig. 11.1 Multidisciplinary/interdisciplinary intervention matrix from the occupational therapist's perspective.

THEORETICAL FOUNDATIONS FOR INTERVENTION

UNDERPINNING FRAMEWORKS AND CONCEPTS

Hinojosa and Kramer (1993) point out that theoretical material organised around a diagnosis may provide insight into a child's disabilities but does not address the occupational therapist's primary concern with functional capacities.

In the context of a child with cerebral palsy, an appreciation of normal development should underpin occupational therapy intervention. Contradictions and differences appear in the appreciation of the nature of development but it is generally understood that there is a recognisable sequential pattern in all developmental theories (Case Smith et al 1996).

Best practice when working with children also requires the therapist to adopt a family-centred approach. The family forms a crucial part of the child's performance context. Where a child himself may be too young, not ready or not able to understand complex questions, specific observation during everyday tasks and information from the family members may complete the evolving picture of the child's situation.

THE MODEL OF HUMAN OCCUPATION

To anchor occupational therapy practice with children firmly within the core beliefs of the profession, the Model of Human Occupation is used to provide a way of gaining information and guiding the intervention process (Kielhofner & Forsyth 1997). Application of the model allows the therapist to use a theoretical framework as a guide to gather and interpret information collected and to guide intervention. Questions generated from the theoretical perspective of the model will prompt information gathering.

Table 11.1 shows a planned review, taking place during half-term and involving both Christopher and his mother. It gives an example of how the Model of Human Occupation can be used to guide data collection and how other assessment tools can help to enhance this information as required.

The collation of information will be guided by the therapist's understanding of the:

- expectations for occupational performance of a child of this age
- child's physical and sociocultural environment.

Occupational therapists need to be aware of the influence of rehabilitation models on their practice when working with children who cannot be said to have lost skills. The focus will be on the therapist's recognition of the impact of an impairment, restriction in participation and the environmental factors on the occupational performance of the child. This will be underpinned by an understanding of the nature of cerebral palsy and the associated restrictions on the performance areas and performance components throughout the lifecycle.

FRAMES OF REFERENCE

Hinojosa and Kramer (1993) present a range of theoretical frameworks for the occupational therapist to consider when working with a child with cerebral palsy. They advocate that a frame of reference 'offers an outline of fundamental theoretical concepts relative to particular areas of function' (Hinojosa & Kramer 1993). Frames of reference guide the therapist's practice in the assessment of functional capacities and support the conceptualising and initialising of intervention. Each frame of reference identifies the areas of functioning the framework is concerned with on a function–dysfunction continuum. It helps the therapist determine what is functional and what is not functional or dysfunctional and the range of accepted abilities and human performance represented on this scale (Hinojosa et al 1996).

The occupational therapist may consider drawing on a number of frames of reference at different times throughout the child's life and into adulthood. From experience, the following have been found to be the most appropriate:

- developmental

Table 11.1 Using the Model of Human Occupation to identify issues and guide intervention during a planned review of Christopher, aged 8 years, who had right hemiplegia

Subsystem	Areas of concern identified by parent and/or child	Further evaluation required	Options for intervention to be negotiated with mother
Performance			
Age appropriate skills in self care	Cutting food, helping to prepare snacks, eating from yoghurt pot Relies on left hand use	Identify ways of observing these tasks/making detailed task analysis What has worked/not worked so far?	Use of compensatory strategies through adaptive/assistive equipment, e.g. cutting board, clamps, yoghurt pot sits in small bowl or cup to stop tipping
Communication	Writing more than his name	Extent of use of computer – skills Targets set by school Current handwriting performance	Set realistic goals for use of mechanical handwriting, e.g. to write name and address, and use of computer to record work for more than short 'insert' answers on worksheets
Process skills	Maths – has difficulty moving onto mental arithmetic	Consult with class teacher, educational psychologist Investigate numeracy/dyscalcula	Suggest joint task analysis and target-setting session with school, mother, educational psychologist, occupational therapist
Perceptual motor skills	Resists looking at detail in charts, pictures, worksheets	Detailed assessment of perceptual motor skills using standardised tools	Graded introduction of detail based on findings of assessment Provide problem-solving strategies and when to ask for help
Habituation			
Roles	Acts the clown	Other coping strategies	Introduce other strategies Look at feedback for other roles
Habits	Sleeping	Consult with paediatrician/psychologist	Management strategies at home, preparation for bedtime, sleeping arrangements
	Copes poorly with change	Consult with psychologist and school	Routines, timing of explanations about what is to happen
Volition			
Personal causation	'I can't do it'	Consult with school about strategies to gain participation Observation in play	Clear achievable targets Positive feedback Try to set own goals
	Has difficulty sharing	Observation in school, reports from school	Structured play sessions in pairs and then groups
Values	Following some rules at home but lacks self-discipline, gets too excited	Consult with paediatrician/psychologist Look at self-image at home versus school	Support for mother Reinforce positive aspects of behaviour Provide feedback on less acceptable behaviour
Interests	Football cards, videos sometimes to exclusion of other interests	Other potential areas of interest	Extend range of activity in play and participation in household management
Play	Does not play with peers when friends come to visit. Will accept playing one-to-one with mother	Play assessments Information from school/other environments	Maintain contact with peers Look at 'buddy' strategies, structuring play sessions, choice of activities

- compensatory
- biomechanical.

Developmental

As the child grows and develops, a frame of reference that is based on the assumption that the enhancement of skills will need to occur in a sequence, related closely to the stages of normal development, will help address issues of delayed achievement of developmental milestones. Within this frame of reference a variety of approaches may be considered and these will depend on the needs of the child, the philosophy of the service and the knowledge, skills and attitude of the therapist.

Compensatory

This frame of reference acknowledges the child's need for occupational performance and reflects that, in the presence of persistent dysfunction, performance may be achieved only where compensatory methods are used to overcome functional difficulties. For the child with cerebral palsy, compensatory and/or adaptive approaches are often essential to facilitate the undertaking of occupational performance needs.

Biomechanical

The principles of this approach underpin aspects of intervention aimed at increasing the child's mobility and physical competence. It is primarily used to guide thinking in relation to postural management, positioning and the adaptation and supply of mobility equipment.

APPROACHES

Within the developmental frame of reference

Intervention with children with cerebral palsy in the United Kingdom has been influenced by two main schools of thought. These are 'The Bobath Concept', otherwise known as Neurodevelopmental Therapy, and 'Conductive Education' (Brown 1999). Therapists also incorporate the principles of sensory integration into their practice, particularly elements such as sensory diet (Blanche & Botticelli 1995).

The Bobath concept

This is an evolving concept in the United Kingdom. It originated with Karl and Bertha Bobath and considers normal motor development, sensory motor feedback mechanisms, components of movement and sequences in motor development (Mayston 1992). It offers an understanding of the movement continuum for the child with cerebral palsy, the variety in presentation of cerebral palsy with the recognised associated difficulties seen in different children and the effect on the child's development. The concept provides specific intervention techniques.

Conductive education

Originally developed in Hungary, conductive education is practised in a variety of settings in the United Kingdom. As a holistic system of education (Brown 1999) it encourages a child with cerebral palsy to take an active part in his own learning. Five key themes, or pillars, form a framework that guides this system. These are the daily routine, the task series, the use of rhythm, the group and the conductor. It can be considered as an option for early intervention in preparing a child for later inclusive schooling.

Occupational therapists need to understand the main assumptions and thinking underpinning these approaches and how this knowledge interacts with their core occupational therapy practice and beliefs around occupational performance. Recommendations for handling and facilitation techniques need to be linked meaningfully to aims set for a performance area task.

Other approaches

Other non-occupational therapy approaches, which may be accessed by a family for their child with cerebral palsy, include cranial osteopathy, patterning and hyperbaric oxygen therapy. These three forms of intervention are accessible via private or voluntary sector agencies. Currently, undergraduate programmes include little education in any specific intervention approaches for cerebral palsy and further postgraduate study will be necessary.

Levitt (1995) and Finnie (1997) provide detailed information about direct intervention and management for a child with cerebral palsy and how to work in partnership with a child's parents. These texts represent contemporary best practice.

EFFICACY STUDIES

There is unfortunately little reported research about the effectiveness of intervention with children with cerebral palsy. With the studies reported so far, there is a general dissatisfaction with the methodologies used, including the size of the studies and the interpretation of the results of single case study designs. Sadsad (1998) gives a small scale meta-analysis of the efficacy of neuro-developmental treatment, listing ten studies over the period 1990–97.

Hinojosa (1990) investigates mothers' perceptions of occupational therapy (and physiotherapy) intervention. These studies do not focus directly on outcomes in terms of change in individual children. The findings do give indicators about what the parents did and what they did not find helpful. Davis (1997) states that 'it is generally accepted that early intervention will improve outcome by facilitating normal development and by preventing further deleterious effects'. Whether this improvement arises as a result of direct intervention with the child or as a result of creating appropriate learning opportunities for the child through parental education and support, the fact that it happens continues to challenge practitioners to evaluate their interventions.

Stewart and Nyerlin-Beale (1999) investigate whether occupational therapy made a difference to children with cerebral palsy. A specialist paediatric occupational therapist in a social services department undertook the intervention. They conclude that there had been a change in the independence levels of most of the children following intervention and that this change had been facilitated by the occupational therapy intervention.

Pimm (1996), a psychologist, takes a psychosocial viewpoint in his evaluation of mothers and fathers caring for a child or adult with cerebral palsy. His findings suggest that while parents of children with cerebral palsy faced the same pressures as other families, there are unique sets of problems that place additional burdens not only for a parent but other family members too.

There is an ongoing debate about amounts of 'treatment' and anecdotal evidence only that 'more must be best'. Natural parental anxiety and motivation to do the best for their child, and scant contradictory evidence, possibly fuel this. This must pose many questions about what 'treatment' or interventions are effective, when to treat or intervene, how to intervene and with what intended outcomes and for whom? These are important questions, demanding that occupational therapists develop methodologies to explore these issues in the light of clinical governance. This is essential if the profession is to be able to contribute to the future development of clinical guidelines by the National Institute for Clinical Excellence for practice within the field of cerebral palsy (see Chapter 8).

PRINCIPLES UNDERLYING INTERVENTION

An occupational therapist can draw on a repertoire of treatment options from a range of theoretical perspectives (Table 11.2).

Working in partnership with the family of the child must be central to the way that any intervention is offered. A detailed understanding of the way in which an individual family functions will underpin attempts to individualise intervention. A number of frameworks is available to assist the occupational therapist in 'adopting a whole family approach' (Dale 1996). It is important to be aware of the constraints that impact on the intervention that can be offered and to have

Table 11.2 Theoretical concepts underpinning occupational therapy intervention with the child who has cerebral palsy

Theoretical concept	Reference for description of application to practice	Performance areas or components	Function/dysfunction continuum
Model of human occupation	Peganoff O'Brien (1993)	Psychological component – social and self-management	Occupational behaviour – play–work continuum
Activities of daily living	Shepherd et al (1996)	Performance areas	Activities of daily living
Neurodevelopmental frame of reference (Bobath concept)	Blanche & Hallway (1998) Rast (1999)	Performance areas, gross and fine motor skills, quality of movement	Activities of daily living, motor development, sensorimotor development
Biomechanical frame of reference	Colangelo (1993)	Postural control	Physical and physiological influences on motor development
Psychosocial frame of reference	Olson (1993)	Psychosocial skills	Temperament, attachment, interactive skills' play, environmental interaction
Coping frame of reference	Williamson et al (1993)	Self-management	Stress, coping, adaptation
Developmental theories	Hinojosa et al (1996)	Sensorimotor, cognitive, psychosocial and all performance areas	Stage-specific expected norms of development
Sensory integration	Blanche & Botticelli (1995)	Sensorimotor components	Sensory, perceptual processing, neuromuscular skeletal, motor
Visual perception	Todd (1993)	Perceptual processing	Visual attention, memory, visual discrimination

an understanding of the effect of your intervention with the family, as much as the effect a family can have on you as a professional. Dale (1996) advocates adopting 'a negotiating model' where the parent/family members' viewpoints and the professionals' viewpoints are brought together and explored as options for evaluation leading onto a plan for action. In this way, the occupational therapy intervention can be family-centred while keeping a focus on the child's individual needs and welfare. This will enable the therapist to respond to a family's hopes and wishes for their child while establishing a working relationship that can enable the therapist's professional perspective to be explained and aims of intervention incorporated into the child's daily programme in a meaningful way.

The suggested aims set by the occupational therapist are those that often emerge when working collaboratively with a family. For each family the priorities will be those reflecting the family's hopes and wishes, such that the goals are family- or person-driven, and not therapist-driven. Perhaps a family would elect to work on elements of dressing skills first, rather than on developing assisted feeding skills, even though a therapist may consider dressing skills to be less important than feeding skills at the time.

Where in a child's day an occupational therapist has contact will influence the choice of activities undertaken, the approach adopted and whether it is on a direct, indirect or on a consultation level. The work setting and the context of the referral may also influence the role and functions that the occupational therapist is expected to have. Resource issues and agreed patterns of service delivery may also influence such decisions. However, if it is clear that many other people are involved, the occupational therapist will be required to provide information about their viewpoints on the child's needs and how to meet these in an accessible and meaningful way.

Box 11.1 Overall aims of occupational therapy intervention for the child with cerebral palsy: most frequently identified in discussion between the child, the family and the therapist (adapted from Case Smith et al 1996)

- Improve performance components, e.g. improve accuracy when reaching for a toy.
- Enhance performance of functional activities (performance areas), e.g. eating a wafer biscuit independently.
- Modify the performance context, e.g. provide box or stool to use during dressing.
- Support the overall motor programme through complementing therapy aims using the appropriate selection of equipment solutions, e.g. apply active seating principles to selection of toilet seat and transfer/facilitation techniques.
- Minimise restriction on participation and social role function.
- Increase self-esteem and self-actualisation.
- Promote positive interactions and relationships.

The occupational therapy aims need to be presented in such a way that the essence can be incorporated into the management of the child's day and embraced by all involved (Box 11.1).

THE OCCUPATIONAL THERAPY PROCESS

The process involves a sequence of activities with the child, the child's caregivers and others within the child's environment. The process begins from the point of receiving a referral and involves data collection and interpreting information followed by planning and implementing intervention.

SCREENING AND EVALUATION

This may include a decision as to the suitability for occupational therapy intervention and extend as far as using interview, observations or standardised assessment to determine the child's needs, before embarking upon a comprehensive programme of further evaluation and intervention. At this stage the therapist will select a model that reflects the key issues in the referral. This will guide the selection of evaluation tools and decide which occupational performance areas or components will be the focus of intervention. At this stage, the therapist collects essential information about the child and, where appropriate, the child's environment. Current information on the child's health, visual and audiological status will inform the occupational therapy assessment.

Being faced with the challenge of carrying out an evaluation of a child's occupational performance is a daunting experience. Preparation for the process in terms of determining the goals of the evaluation, establishing effective data collection and understanding the concerns and questions posed by the family and other professionals is essential. In this way, the therapist can remain 'open to new ways of understanding the child' (Stewart 1996), actively making decisions about which assessment methods and measures to select and make a sound analysis of the results and formulate recommendations. Six key principles underpin an effective evaluation process (Box 11.2).

In some settings, this evaluation stage and the previous screening stage may be operationally combined, depending on the timing of each stage in relation to the time from referral to first contact or waiting times for intervention post-initial assessment. The occupational therapist's core beliefs about occupational performance will underpin this evaluation process.

Box 11.2 Six key principles underpinning effective evaluation (adapted from Stewart (1996) and Case Smith (1997))

1. *The evaluation process is an ongoing, dynamic process, beginning with the initial referral, continuing through all stages of intervention and ending in discharge.*
2. Evaluation should include methods and measures that are ecologically and culturally valid, and appropriate for the child's age and function.
3. The assessment tools selected will match the evaluation purpose.
4. The child's views will be known where possible.
5. The views and priorities of the child's primary carer must be central to the evaluation process.
6. The outcome should be an in-depth understanding of the child's functional abilities in performance components and performance areas.

Daily living skills, play and school activities are generally the primary focus of occupational therapy. Coster (1998) advocates an occupation-centred assessment of children. The occupational performance of the child will be viewed within the context of his natural environment, including its sociocultural and physical characteristics. This ecological evaluation is likely to include the following: play-based assessment and observation; observation of behaviour and performance of functional tasks; interviews with parents, other carers, and teacher; inventories or scales and standardised tests. Through the use of a combination of these methods, a comprehensive evaluation will be achieved. Richardson (1996) gives a clear analysis of the pros and cons of using standardised testing and comments on tests such as the Gross Motor Function Measure (Russell et al 1989) and the Pediatric Evaluation of Disability Inventory (PEDI; Haley 1997), which have been developed specifically for use with children with physical disabilities. Knox and Usen (2000) undertake a clinical review of the PEDI used with children with cerebral palsy.

The occupational therapist will consider the relationship between the chosen frame of reference and the approaches, techniques and activities used. Stewart (1996) lists examples of evaluations categorised by performance areas, components and context. Case Smith (1997) gives an overview of assessment used in paediatric occupational therapy in the United States and in the same year Chu and Hong (1997) reported on a review of assessments used in the United Kingdom. The only one identified as being developed specifically for use with children with cerebral palsy is the Milani–Comparetti Motor Development Screening Test, which is not readily available in the United Kingdom. A more accessible and useful tool for providing qualitative information about movement is the Toddler and Infant Motor Evaluation (1994). This evaluation gives information that can inform goal setting as well as recording change in gross and fine motor skills. Chu and Hong (1997) suggest that the Test of Visual Perceptual Skills may be useful in the assessment of children with cerebral palsy and problems with motor coordination but, in the absence of validity studies, its usefulness has yet to be determined. For examples of assessment tools available for use with children with cerebral palsy, see Table 11.3.

These assessment tools assist the occupational therapist by extending the understanding of why and how a child is having difficulties in the identified performance areas. Priorities for evaluation are identified in collaboration with the family and the child himself where possible. Evaluation will lead to identifying the immediate and long-term goals of intervention.

INTERVENTION PLANNING

Following evaluation, an appropriate frame of reference provides a theory base to guide the therapist's thinking. Following the interpretation, the results of evaluation appropriate goals are identified. These goals will be developed and intervention plans established in the context of the child's life and that of their family and in the other environments in which they are required to function. The occupational therapy process, with its focus on occupational performance, enables the therapist to become involved in the central activities of the child's life (Case Smith 1996).

PRACTICE ARENAS

It is important to recognise that each child functions in a unique set of environments. Additionally, work settings influence the occupational therapist's selection of theoretical base, activities and method of service delivery. There are strong arguments for evaluating a child's needs based on assessments undertaken across the variety of environments in which the child is asked to function. Unfortunately, resource constraints are likely to impinge upon the occupational therapist's capacity to achieve a truly comprehensive assessment. Strategies will be required to address this. Data can be collected by other members of the multidisciplinary team and shared between disciplines. Decisions in favour of individual or group intervention and on home- or centre-based treatment sessions will be informed by local circumstances. The occupational therapist will see a child in any of the

Table 11.3 Range of relevant assessment tools available for use with children who have cerebral palsy

Name of measure	Author(s)	Performance component/area	Age range
Bayley Scales of Infant Development (2nd edn)	Bayley (1993)	Developmental, comprehensive, evaluation	1 month to 42 months
Schedule of Growing Skills	Bellman et al (1996)	Screening test	Birth to 5 years
Denver Developmental Screening Test	Frankenberg et al (1990)	Screening tool	1 month to 5 years
Beery Developmental Test of Visual Motor Integration (3rd revision)	Beery & Buktenica (1989)	Sensorimotor	2 years 9 months to 19 years 8 months
Test of Visual Perceptual Skills (TVPS)	Gardener (1988)	Sensory	4 years to 12 years 11 months
Motor – free Visual Perception Test (MVPT-R)	Colarusso & Hammill (1995)	Sensory	4 years to 11 years 6 months
Erdhardt Developmental Prehension Assessment	Erdhardt (1994)	Motor	Birth to 6 years
Erdhardt Developmental Visual Assessment	Erdhardt (1990)	Sensory	Birth to 6 years
Toddler and Infant Motor Evaluation (TIME)	Miller & Roid (1994)	Neuromuscular	Birth to 42 months
Milani–Comparetti Motor Development Screening Test	Milani–Comparetti & Gidoni (1967)	Motor	Birth to 2 years
Pediatric Evaluation of Disability Inventory	Haley et al (1997)	Occupational performance	6 months to 7 years
School Function Assessment	Coster et al (1998)	Occupational performance	3 years to 11 years

environments in which he spends part of his day in order to fully understand his occupational performance in all settings. This will include home, preschool setting/school setting, specialist centre or local clinic, acute hospital on an inpatient or outpatient basis.

FREQUENTLY IDENTIFIED AREAS REQUIRING INTERVENTION

An assessment of a child with cerebral palsy often results in numerous areas of concern in a child's functional performance, ranging from dressing and mobility, feeding and toileting to educational activities and functional communication. The common underlying problems may be explained by the presence of deficits in performance components. This would include postural control, muscle tone and coordination. There will also be deficits in cognitive and psychosocial compo-

nents, such as attention span and problem solving, together with self-expression. Difficulties with the way that a child responds emotionally and behaviourally to any given situation may also need addressing.

The performance context formed by the child's age and the environment also affect function, and intervention should therefore address concerns both in component areas and in the context. The family is a key element in the environmental aspects of the performance context, providing an environment in which the child learns and which changes in influence during the lifecycle. The child's psychosocial skills and behavioural responses to demands in life evolve in part in response to the environment created by the family. Family dynamics and the child's temperament can be seen to be closely linked. In early childhood it is misleading to view activities in differentiated categories such as play, learning and self care and rarely does one performance component occur as the only contributor to dysfunction and activities.

The following examples of intervention areas are frequently identified by the child, the family and the therapist as important priorities for intervention (Table 11.4). The examples are listed by age group and aim to guide the goal-setting process (from the developmental and skill acquisition perspective) that will take place in collaboration with the child's family and in consultation with other professionals.

The following section contains a selection of specific examples of interventions frequently identified during such negotiations, giving details of how these performance areas and performance components may be addressed.

PERFORMANCE AREAS

Occupational and task performance requiring assistive technology and equipment

When a child is unable to master the physical or perceptual skills required to perform a task, adaptation may be necessary. Recommendations for equipment will be based on a comprehensive evaluation of the child's capacities and abilities and of the environment in which activity will be undertaken. The parents' and carers' perspectives must be included and considered and results of the evaluation and the development of the recommendations fully discussed with everyone involved. An understanding of the theoretical principles underpinning postural control will support intervention relating to the recommendation and provision of environmental modifications, which includes the identification of equipment solutions to enable the child.

The challenge is to achieve a balance between enabling the child to achieve success and acquire skills, making effective use of the child's activity tolerance, and also providing opportunities to experience developmentally appropriate activities throughout the day. Access to activity and maximum participation in family and school life should incorporate time spent on developing skills but the amount of time and effort expected of the child and family spent on developing skills should not unduly compromise the level of participation in daily activities.

Play

The nature of cerebral palsy restricts play and overall development in two ways. Firstly, where play is a context for learning and practising adaptive responses, a child who has difficulty with interaction risks missing opportunities for this learning. Secondly, a child who has difficulty entering into play has restricted experience of play as a spontaneous, intrinsically motivated, fun activity. Blanche (cited in Parham and Fazio 1997) discusses this viewpoint and emphasises the need to incorporate play into the child's intervention and daily life. The key theme of Blanche's approach is to stress that the therapist is required to enter into play with the child. This premise is central to the way that an occupational therapist may intervene whether directly, through offering play-based sessions, or when making recommendations on ways of incorporating therapy aims into the child's day and into family life. Therefore, the occupational therapist must rise to the challenge of including the essence of play into a child's daily programme. Play is traditionally recognised for its role in the acquisition of functional skills. This has been seen as important, as play serves a function of preparation for adult performance. More recent literature confronts the traditional viewpoint and challenges the occupational therapist to consider the quality of the experience of play as an end itself. Bundy's model of playfulness (1996) offers an observational assessment, the Test of Playfulness (ToP). This guides the evaluation of play rather than performance in play activity. The model of playfulness describes a play–non-play continuum based on an understanding of the individual's perception of control, source of motivation and suspension of reality. Blanche (cited in Parham and Fazio 1997) encourages therapists working within a neurodevelopmental frame of reference to appraise each activity as providing the potential for play and to restore the essence of play into the life of the child with cerebral palsy and in the acquisition of intervention goals. Diamant (2000) gives guidelines for positioning and play, working in partnership with parents to ensure that play and positioning materials are available in the family's environment.

Table 11.4 Examples of frequently identified intervention areas (adapted from Occupational Therapy Practice Guidelines (Colangelo & Gorga 1996) by kind permission of AOTA)

Infant/preschool stage

Performance area	Performance components	Other professional issues	Sample goal	Context	Compensation options
Socialisation	Visual, sensory awareness	Visual acuity and function. Parent–child interaction	Infant will fix and focus on mother's face	Quiet, in bedroom at start of each dressing task	Cushioning to assist positioning so mother can facilitate child's movement
Feeding	Postural control, level of arousal, sensory processing	Nutrition, swallowing and respiration, oral motor skills	Infant will take first stage food from a spoon	At home with mother	Selected infant seat and plastic flat bowl spoon
Dressing	Sensory awareness, sensory processing, postural alignment	Postural management programme, orthotic trunk brace	Infant to pull off sock(s)	While maintaining stable posture	Adult sets up activity with correct size bench and prompts holding onto bench
Play	Sensory awareness, postural control	Object permanence	Infant to explore a toy using both hands	While sitting on floor in quiet room at home	Toy placed on flat tray to stop it rolling away, adult to prompt use of two hands
Educational activity	Fine motor coordination, visual integration, postural control, attention span	Understanding instructions	Child to find and pick out three red pegs	Sitting next to another child in playgroup setting	Correct height chair and table, non-slip mat under flat bowl containing pegs

School-age children

Performance area	Performance components	Other professional issues	Sample goal	Context	Compensation options
Functional mobility	Motor control, social conduct, self-concept	Risk assessment of safety and access	Child will take register to school office	With one-to-one supervision until reaching office	Use of power wheelchair
Toileting	Postural control, fine motor skills	Safety in toilet area and cubicle	Child to reach out and collect piece of toilet paper	After emptying bladder and before standing up	Toilet support frame, repositioned toilet roll holder
Educational activity	Tactile, proprioceptive	Comprehension of task, ability to follow instructions	Child to construct line of coloured blocks to two-colour pattern	Sitting with stability at table in classroom, activity set up by adult	Correct height table and chair, weighted blocks
Functional communication	Fine motor, visuomotor integration, perceptual processing	Other curriculum achievements, knowledge of letter formation	Child will copy under example of name	In classroom, when class asked to put name on work	Selected pencil with grip, non-slip slope surface
Eating	Oral motor skills, fine motor skills, postural control	Swallowing	Child will eat crisps from crisp bag	Packet opened by adult at child's request	Correct size height table and chair or footbox and back pad provided

Family/caregiver education. This is equally as important as achieving child-centred goals. The child's development and management must be supported by extending the parent/carer's knowledge and skills

Bathing/showering	Coping skills, perceptual processing, body scheme, postural control	Moving and handling assessment selection of equipment	Mother will demonstrate positioning and facilitating techniques during transfer to bath seat	Mother will set up bathroom ready for activity	Bath seat at optimum height Positioning techniques
Feeding	Postural control, sensory processing, oral motor control, interpersonal skills	Nutrition, parental stress, safety of swallow	Mother will settle child in an effective position as part of preparing child for feeding	Mother will set up activity and place in home to carry out feeding in relaxed and uninterrupted way	Effective and comfortable position for both mother and child
Activities of daily living – moving and handling	Neuromusculoskeletal, motor, cognition, social, self-management	Moving and handling legislation and its interpretation for individuals in their own home	Mother to plan how to help the child move from place to place, minimising lifting even when child is small	Bathroom/bedroom sequence and layout supports safe moving and handling	Moving and handling equipment solutions in situ, e.g. items ranging from sliding sheet to track hoist with fully supporting sling
Play	Psychosocial, social	Place of play in the family Balance of work – play continuum	Mother to facilitate non-directed play-based activity	Mother to set up play with another child	Effective positioning, selection of appropriate play opportunity

Environmental adaptation

Play, exploration	Sensory processing, postural control, endurance	Use of aid to facilitate walking	Child to explore plants in garden alongside path	Obstacles removed, use of aid prompted by adult	Modified access across door threshold, bag attached to walking aid to collect plants
Bathing/showering	Gross motor coordination, postural control, self-management	Selection of equipment provision of special facilities at home	Child to participate in bathtime activity	Bathtime at home	Modified bathroom bath seat
Productivity – meal preparation	Gross motor, fine motor, cognitive, self-management	Parental expectations Health and safety	Child to assist in preparation of jam sandwich	Standing at worktop in kitchen	Height of worktop, choice of kitchen tools Facilitating techniques to achieve stable standing posture
Community mobility	Motor, cognitive, self-management	Child's developmental stage and independence Health and safety	Child to go to corner shop using powered chair	Buying a paper for parent	Clear access, barriers removed, ramps provided, door/open closure supervised or mechanised

An important extension to this area of work is the way in which the occupational therapist can develop strategies to recognise that play differs from one child to another. Play within the context of the family may also be different from play within the school or playground setting.

Integrating a child with cerebral palsy into family play

Play within the context of the family will be influenced by the family's values, culture and setting. Parents of a child with a disability such as cerebral palsy have the additional responsibilities arising from the particular needs of that child. Hinojosa and Kramer (cited in Parham and Fazio 1997) discuss the role of the occupational therapist in supporting this performance area and comment on the risk that a family might become so child-centred that family activity is dominated by the needs of the child. As a result, the additional time and resources devoted to the child have the impact of restricting recreational opportunities for the family and for individual family members. They go onto explain that enjoyment can be achieved from varying degrees of participation in family activity. The extent of the child's limitations may restrict this participation. The aim can then be to ensure that the child is included to the extent that is possible or, for example, as active spectator or holder and marker of the score board in a team game.

Feeding and eating

Intervention will be based on an understanding of the typical progression through the stages of oral feeding and self-feeding and the likely problems that a child with cerebral palsy may face. Multidisciplinary assessment supported by information about the child's swallowing and respiratory patterns during feeding, gained through medical investigation using videofluoroscopy, will link weaning, feeding behaviours, sensory tolerances, postural control and positions for feeding. The risks associated with feeding, such as aspiration and choking, indicate a methodical and cohesive approach to intervention. The occupational therapist will work collaboratively with local services and consult with specialist tertiary clinics where indicated.

Growth rate and weight gains are often of concern for children with cerebral palsy. This can occur alongside oral motor difficulties affecting the mechanics of feeding. Parents will be striving to ensure that their child is feeding well and gaining weight and this can become their primary focus, taking up much of their day.

For some children, the risks of aspiration and choking are so great, or there is such concern about the child's capacity to gain weight, that a gastrostomy may be indicated. A gastrostomy is a procedure to create a small button in the abdominal wall and specially prepared feeds are passed by tube into the stomach. The feeding is usually carried out overnight once the process has been established. If swallowing is very hazardous and likely to result in aspiration, oral feeding can be avoided by gastrostomy feeding at meal times. Some children may be fed by nasogastric tube for short periods, although it is now generally accepted that this should not continue over extended periods as it interferes with the maturation of swallowing and vomiting reflexes and makes progression to oral feeding even more difficult to achieve.

Strategies to develop self-feeding will be based on effective positioning, motor coordination, hand function and sensory function. Assisted devices are available if the demands of achieving upper limb control create too much stress and compromise activity tolerance and participation. Decisions about aiming for self-feeding, the use of assistive devices or opting for individual adult help will be carefully made so as to ensure safety and effective nutrition.

PERFORMANCE COMPONENTS
Postural management

It is important to be able to recognise the risks of developing deformity for the child with cerebral palsy. Asymmetry in movement and posture and imbalances in muscle tone are likely to result in misalignment or deformity; typically in the foot and ankle, at the hip and knee and at the pelvis and spine. These evolving deformities will be seen in the young child and the rate of change is the indicator for long-term outcomes. Initial aims for the young child will be for postural symmetry in lying, sitting and standing to reduce the opportunities for these deformities to develop. Once a deformity has developed, a coordinated management approach is essential. In some circumstances children can develop dislocation at the hip, which interferes with sitting, is associated with pelvic and spine deformity and can present with pain.

Scrutton (1999) advocates referral onto a tertiary orthopaedic clinic for every child with bilateral cerebral palsy for evaluation of hip dysplasia and the possibility of hip dislocation. The physiotherapist has a key role in contributing to surveillance procedures to highlight the risk of dislocating hips. In partnership, the occupational therapist requires an understanding of the biomechanics of positioning, seating and 24-hour positional management programmes. She should ensure that families have access to advice and monitoring for orthopaedic management and that principles are incorporated into the child's occupational performance throughout his day. A collaborative and integrated management programme is the ultimate aim.

An understanding of the need for postural management on a 24-hour basis has developed gradually since the late 1980s (Box 11.3). The work of the team at Chailey Heritage hospital and school in England has had a significant influence on the management of postural control. Practical application of this developing theoretical base is seen in the design and development of a variety of equipment on the market to greater or lesser extent.

Hand function

When there are problems identified with sensorimotor performance components, hand function will be central to some of the aims for occupational therapy. A child will need to make effective use of hand skills to achieve independence in daily activity. The therapist will need to bring together knowledge about visual perception, sensory function, grasp and release, manipulation and postural control. Hypersensitivity may need to be addressed as acquisition of the early

---

Box 11.3 Principles of postural management (adapted from Pountney et al (2000))

- Management draws on knowledge of biomechanics, muscle and bone adaptation, impact of ability, cognition and musculoskeletal changes, neuroplasticity and motor learning theory and sensory experience.
- Management encompasses the child's position in all activity in sitting, standing and in lying throughout the day, and also during the night.
- Selection of equipment is based upon an understanding of the child's lying, sitting and standing ability.
- Postural management advocates that positioning complements therapy-intervention regimens by continuing correct biomechanical feedback day and night.
- The aim is to promote normal motor development, improve practical ability, reduce deformity and maintain a symmetrical position, and to provide periods of muscle stretch.

---

exploratory play skills is established. Having an understanding of the impact that gross motor difficulties have on hand function for the child with cerebral palsy helps to inform decisions about selecting effective working positions and priorities for developing hand function. For example, a child who finds reaching and grasping for a toy difficult will have restricted opportunities to play independently. A child who can reach but, on reaching, finds his hand remains fisted, will not be able to voluntarily grasp and to hold a toy or a brush. This limits opportunities for a child to use tools. Fritts (1999) discusses the treatment of the hand in the child with cerebral palsy and describes the movement compensations seen.

The use of tools is fundamental to many performance areas. A compensatory and adaptive approach is adopted by Smith and Topping (1996) in the use of a robotic aid to drawing for children with cerebral palsy. A child whose hand remains fisted may not be able to isolate finger movement. This means he has to use gross upper limb movement and the use of more refined switching inputs for toys or for the computer is restricted.

Where demands for hand use compromises overall performance, the use of other parts of the body or other patterns of movement may be used to access switching. A child may be very successful at isolating a head movement, a shoulder movement or a foot movement.

Visual perception

A comprehensive assessment will indicate need for intervention in this area. While performance and specific assessment may indicate need, findings must be seen in the context of the child's comprehension and cognitive skills, so that a developmentally appropriate intervention programme can be developed. Information can also be gained about the presentation of play and learning materials. The impact of any visual impairment must be considered.

ALTERNATIVE INTERVENTIONS

Parents may elect to include alternative interventions in the care of their child. The occupational therapist will need to establish a working relationship where parental choice can be respected and motives behind their selection understood. Such interventions may include complementary therapies such as paediatric osteopathy, non-traditional medical interventions such as hyperbaric oxygen therapy and private practitioners offering a range of interventions. It is advisable to encourage an open and honest attitude to sharing information so that any possible contraindications can be highlighted and areas of potential conflict of advice, techniques or approaches avoided where possible. Where this is achieved, the child will not be overloaded, their wellbeing will be maintained and the parents' need to explore alternative ways of helping their child or seeking resolution of their child's problems can be supported. This scenario will continue to challenge occupational therapists to respond in appropriate professional ways. Being able to discuss the choices available from an informed position rather than responding in a discouraging way will enable the occupational therapist to continue to develop the working relationship with the family members and the child. Vickers (1994) gives a useful overview of the range of complementary interventions and includes advice for consumers on selecting a practitioner. The National Association of Paediatric Occupational Therapists (NAPOT) yearbook gives guidance on selecting private practitioners and can be copied for parents' use.

CONCLUSION

'Cerebral palsy' is a term used to describe a range of conditions that initially present in childhood. There is some debate as to whether all children presenting with motor impairment affecting tone and coordination and associated problems in other systems can be described as having cerebral palsy. The stage of development (for example, before, during or subsequent to birth) at which the damage to the brain that results in

Box 11.4 Case study: Lucy

Lucy was 4 months old when she was referred to occupational therapy by a physiotherapist. She lived with her mother and father in a single unit mobile home. Although still very young, it was clear that Lucy was struggling to gain any postural control. Her interest in people and play resulted in an increase in her muscle tone and associated extensor patterns of movement. Her early referral allowed joint working with the physiotherapist and enabled strategies for handling Lucy and opportunities for play to be introduced in line with normal developmental stages.

Early evaluation was guided by the neurodevelopmental and biomechanical frames of reference whilst being careful to support Lucy's mother in her parenting role.

Over time, it was established that Lucy settled to play when she was helped to achieve a more flexed posture and when she had an opportunity to be an active participant in play activity. Soft seating surfaces, including sitting on a soft rubber spider, helped her to gain trust when being positioned and so enabled her to become tolerant of different working positions. The progression onto seating provided a safe and supportive working and playing position for Lucy, enabling more independence for her and practical help for her mother. Lucy also has visual difficulties and so preparation for movement has been very important. Lucy learnt to work with her mother when changing positions and during activities such as getting undressed or dressed, instead of becoming distressed and resisting. Understanding Lucy's response to positioning and movement informed selection of other equipment items such as a pushchair, a car seat, a toilet seat formed from a stabilised potty and a ladder back chair. This understanding also informed the multidisciplinary team's intervention around feeding.

An early referral to the local authority has resulted in the family being rehoused in an accessible ground-floor flat with a bathroom. This includes a height-adjustable bath and direct access from the bedroom, allowing for future provision of moving and handling equipment.

the child having physical and cognitive difficulties occurs can be the key issue.

Occupational therapists have a crucial role in supporting a family in bringing up their child with cerebral palsy. Knowledge of child development and occupational performance, together with neurodevelopmental, compensatory and biomechanical frames of reference, is required. This is complemented by knowledge of practical solutions to solve the everyday challenges met by the child and the child's family, in the context of the child's own story. A sensitive appreciation of the parent's experience of learning about their child must be central to all contact with a family.

Box 11.5   Case study: Aysha

Aysha and her family became known to the occupational therapy service when she was two. Her family had been living in temporary housing and it was expected that they would be staying in their new home for at least 6 months while permanent housing was arranged. During the first 2 years of Aysha's life, her family had moved so frequently that they had little consistent input from any therapy services. On meeting Aysha it was clear that her reported problems with sitting, walking, eating and sleeping were due to athetoid cerebral palsy with total body involvement. Aysha found it extremely difficult to adopt any stable positions for play or activity. She was unable to initiate changes in posture and spent most of her time lying on the floor, or propped up in the corner of the sofa at home. Her parents reported that she was very difficult to feed and that she would cough a lot during feeding. Collaborative work with the physiotherapist and speech and language therapist identified an approach to establishing more control of movement for Aysha using neurodevelopmental techniques. Her parents were shown ways of handling her and helping her to move. A chair to prompt symmetrical and stable seating provided a good position for play and, importantly, for feeding. The stable position allowed Aysha to hold her head centrally and to bring it forward to receive food, rather than being fed in a reclined position on her mother's lap. This new position reduced the amount of coughing and it was reassuring to see that she was no longer at risk of inhaling food. Future aims will include increasing Aysha's participation in activities of daily living now that she has improved postural control. Further work on feeding will also follow to extend her capacity to take a greater range of food textures and to help her parents understand the importance of good positioning and safe feeding.

Box 11.6   Case study: Julian

Julian, now 13, lives with his mother. He is attending a local mainstream school and finding it increasingly difficult to participate in transfers between standing and sitting. When he was younger he was able to rise to standing from sitting and to return with minimal help. As he has grown taller he has also become stiffer and heavier, and this action has been more and more difficult.

Over the last 4 years, modifications have been made to his home to allow easier access to toilet and bathroom facilities and a stairlift was fitted. This situation was satisfactory but the extra demands on his mother have now led her to decide to opt for rehousing. Julian's mother is the sole carer of a physically dependent young man. Her long-standing back problems are aggravated by the physical demands of having to lift Julian and to facilitate his movement. Practical problem-solving strategies to address the moving and handling difficulties in the home are required but the consequences of Julian's increasing dependency on his mother also need to be addressed. This requires two perspectives to be considered. The provision of moving and handling equipment had to be approached from both a problem-solving and a psychosocial perspective in order to understand Julian's and his mother's reaction to the situation, the effect of changing roles and the need to change their coping strategies. Clearly, if this situation was not fully understood there was a risk that Julian and his mother would reject the provision of equipment. This would place his mother's health and capacity to care for Julian at risk and would also complicate the dynamics of the relationship between Julian and his mother.

At a difficult time of adolescence, when Julian is striving for independence, he is also having to face coping with increasing dependency. There is also the reality that he may not be able to continue to rely on his mother for his care and wellbeing. Julian's mother is very anxious about her own health and emotional needs as they affect her ability to care for her son. She is also concerned about what the future holds.

Provision of moving and handling equipment will at least provide the option of utilising agency carers funded through the local authority. Without the equipment, caring agencies would consider the home situation too high a risk to allow the placement of carers or would restrict the role that they were able to undertake. The decision to accept equipment to allow the use of carers, which would then be available for Julian and his mother to use, may be an acceptable way forward at this stage.

REFERENCES

Bax MCO 1964 Terminology and classification of cerebral palsy. Developmental Medicine and Child Neurology 6:295

Bayley N 1993 Bayley Scales on Infant Development, 2nd edn (BSID-11). The Psychological Corporation, London

Beery K, Buktenica N 1989 Development Test of Visual Motor Integration. NFER–Nelson, Berkshire

Bellman M, Lingham S, Aukett A 1996 Schedule of Growing Skills, 2nd edn. NFER–Nelson, Berkshire

Blanche EI 1997 Doing with – not doing to: play and the child with cerebral palsy. In: Parham DL, Fazio LS (eds) Play in occupational therapy for children. Mosby Year Book, St Louis, MO, ch 13, p 202

Blanche EI, Botticelli T 1995 Combining neuro-developmental treatment and sensory integration principles: an approach to paediatric therapy. Therapy Skill Builders, Tucson, AZ

Blanche EI, Hallway M 1998 Historical perspective: neurodevelopmental treatment in occupational therapy. Developmental Disabilities 21(3), special interest section, quartery, American Occupational Therapy Association, Bethesda, MD

Brown G 1996 The parent's experience of learning about their child. Master's Dissertation, University of East London

Brown H 1999 Conductive education and children with cerebral palsy. British Journal of Therapy and Rehabilitation 6(12):580–584

Brown SM, Humphry R, Taylor E 1997 A model of the nature of family – therapist relationships: implications for education. American Journal of Occupational Therapy 51(7):597–603

Bundy A 1996 Play and playfulness: what to look for. In: Parham DL, Fazio LS (eds) Play in occupational therapy for children. Mosby Year Book, St Louis, MO, ch 4, p 52

Case Smith J 1997 Pediatric assessment. OT Practice 2(4):24–39

Case Smith J 1996 An overview of occupational therapy with children. In: Case Smith J, Allen AS, Pratt PN (eds) Occupational therapy for children 3rd edn. Mosby, St Louis, MO, p10

Chu S, Hong SH 1997 A review of assessments used in paediatric occupational therapy. British Journal of Therapy and Rehabilitation 4(5):228–233

Colangelo CA 1993 Biomechanical frame of reference. In: Hinojosa J, Kramer P (eds) Frames of reference for pediatric occupationals. Williams & Wilkins, Baltimore, MD, ch 8, p 233

Colangelo C, Gorga D 1996 Occupational therapy practice guidelines for cerebral palsy. American Occupational Therapy Association, Bethesda, MD

Colarusso RP, Hammill DD 1995 Motor-Free Visual Perception Test (MVPT-R). Ann Arbor Publishers Ltd, Belford, Northumberland

Coster WJ 1998 Occupation-centered assessment of children. American Journal of Occupational Therapy 52(5):337–344

Coster WJ, Deeney T, Haltiwanger J, Haley SM 1998 The school function assessment: standardised version. Boston University, Boston, MA

Dale N 1996 Working with families of children with special needs – partnership and practice. Routledge, London

Davis DW 1997 Review of cerebral palsy, Part 1. Neonatal Network 16(3):7–12

Diamant R 2000 Partnering with parents: guidelines for positioning and play. OT Practice 5(9):14–18

Erdhardt RP 1990 Development visual dysfunction – models for assessment and management. The Psychological Corporation, London

Erdhardt RP 1994 Erdhardt developmental prehension assessment (EDPA). Revised. The Psychological Corporation, London

Finnie NR 1997 Handling the young child with cerebral palsy at home, 3rd edn. Butterworth-Heinemann, Oxford

Frankenburg W, Dodds J, Archer P, Bresnick B, Maschka P, Edelman N, Shapiro H 1990 Denver Developmental Screening Test. Ladoca Publishing Foundation, Denver

Fritts RDF 1999 Treatment of the hand in the child with cerebral palsy. Developmental Disabilities 22(3), special interest section, quarterly, American Occupational Therapy Association, Bethesda, MD

Gardener MF 1988 Test of Visual–Perceptual Skills (non-motor). Revised. Ann Arbor Publishers Ltd, Belford, Northumberland

Graham J, Maze MK 1997 The evolution of a partnership to meet the special needs of children. British Journal of Occupational Therapy 60(12):521–524

Haley SM, Coster WJ, Ludlow LH, Haltiwanger JT, Andrellos PJ 1997 Pediatric Evaluation of Disability Inventory (PEDI). The Psychological Corporation, London

Hickling A 2000 Education and therapy needs of children with multiple disabilities. British Journal of Therapy and Rehabilitation 7(8):334–338

Hinojosa J 1990 How mothers of preschool children with cerebral palsy perceive occupational and physical therapists and their influence on family life. The Occupational Therapy Journal of Research 10(3):145–161

Hinojosa J, Kramer P 1993 Frames of reference for pediatric occupational therapy. Williams & Wilkins, Baltimore, MD

Hinojosa J, Kramer P 1997 Integrating children with disabilities into family play. In: Parham DL, Fazio LS (eds) Play in occupational therapy for children. Mosby Year Book, St Louis, MO, ch 10, p 159

Hinojosa J, Kramer P, Pratt N 1996 Foundations of practice: developmental principles, theories, and frames of reference. In: Case Smith J, Allen AS, Pratt N (eds) Occupational therapy for children. Mosby, St Louis, MO

Kielhofner G, Forsyth K 1997 The model of human occuption: an overview of current concepts. British Journal of Occupational Therapy 60(3):103–110

Knox V, Usen Y 2000 Clinical review of the pediatric evaluation of disability inventory. British Journal of Occupational Therapy 63(1):29–32

Levitt S 1995 Treatment of cerebral palsy and motor delay, 3rd edn. Blackwell Science, Oxford

Mayston MJ 1992 The Bobath concept – evolution and application. Medicine and Sports Science 36:1–6

Milani-Comparetti A, Gidoni EA 1967 Routine development examination in normal and retarded children. Developmental Medicine and Child Neurology 9:631–638

Miller LJ, Roid GH 1994 The TIME Toddler and Infant Motor Education. The Psychological Corporation, London

National Association of Paediatric Occupational Therapists Yearbook 2000–2001. Information Press, Oxford

Olson L 1993 Psychosocial frame of reference. In: Hinojosa J, Kramer P (eds) Frames of reference for pediatric occupational therapy. Williams & Wilkins, Baltimore, MD

Parham LD, Fazio LS 1997 Play in occupational therapy for children. Mosby, St Louis, MO

Peganoff O'Brien S 1993 Human occupation frame of reference. In: Hinojosa J, Kramer P (eds) Frames of reference for pediatric occupational therapy. Williams & Wilkins, Baltimore, MD, ch 9, p 307

Pimm PL 1996 Some of the implications of caring for a child or adult with cerebral palsy. British Journal of Occupational Therapy 59(7):335–341

Pountney TE, Mulcahy CM, Clarke SM, Green EM 2000 The Chailey approach to postural management. Active Design Limited, Birmingham

Rast M 1999 NDT in continuum: micro to macro levels in therapy. Developmental Disabilities 22(2), special interest section, quarterly, American Occupational Therapy Association, Bethesda, MD

Richardson PK 1996 Use of standardised tests in paediatric practice. In: Case Smith J, Allen AS, Pratt PN (eds) Occupational therapy for children, 3rd edn. Mosby, St Louis, MO

Russell D, Rosenbaum P, Cadman D, Gowland C, Hardy S, Jarvis S 1989 Gross motor function measure: a means to evaluate the effects of physical therapy. Developmental Medicine and Child Neurology 31:341–352

Sadsad C 1998 Research articles pertaining to the efficacy of neurodevelopmental treatment. Developmental Disabilities 21(4):1–2, special interest section, quarterly, American Occupational Therapy Association, Bethesda, MD

Scutton D 1999 A study of children with bilateral cerebral palsy. Journal of the Association of Paediatric Chartered Physiotherapists 90:10–14

Shephard J, Procter SA, Coley IL 1996 In: Case Smith J, Allen AS, Pratt N (eds) Occupational therapy for children. Mosby, St Louis, MO

Smith J, Topping M 1996 The introduction of a robotic aid into a school for physically handicapped children: a case study. British Journal of Occupational Therapy 59(12):565–569

Special Educational Needs Code of Practice 1996 Department of Education and Employment Publication Centre, dfee.gov.uk/sen/code.htm (under revision and out to consultation, 2000–2001)

Stewart KB 1996 Occupational therapy assessment in paediatrics. In: Case Smith J, Allen AS, Pratt N (eds) Occupational therapy for children, Mosby, St Louis, MD

Stewart S, Nyerlin-Beale J 1999 Enhancing independence in children with cerebral palsy. British Journal of Therapy and Rehabilitation 6(12):574–579

Todd VR 1993 Visual perceptual frame of reference: an information processing approach. In: Hinojosa J, Kramer P (eds) Frames of reference for pediatric occupational therapy. Williams & Wilkins, Baltimore, MD, ch 7, p 177

Williamson GG, Szczepanski M, Zeitlin S 1993 Coping frame of reference. In: Hinojosa J, Kramer P (eds) Frames of reference for pediatric occupational therapy. Williams & Wilkins, Baltimore, MD

Vickers A 1994 Health options. Complementary therapies for cerebral palsy and related conditions. Element Books, Shaftesbury, Dorset

USEFUL CONTACTS

The Bobath Centre London: 250 East End Road, East Finchley, London N2 8AU. Tel: 020 8844 3355

Capability Scotland: www.capability-scotland.org.uk

Hemihelp for children with hemiplegia: www.Hemihelp.org.uk

National Association of Paediatric Occupational Therapists: Barton's Cottage, Prestbury Road, Wilmslow, Cheshire SK9 2LL

National Institute for Conductive Education: www.conductive-education.org.uk

SCOPE: www.scope.org.uk

The Family Fund Trust: www.familyfundtrust.org.uk

Muscular dystrophy

Gillian Brown

INTRODUCTION

Muscular dystrophy sits within a range of conditions known as neuromuscular disorders. Common to all these conditions is the progressive weakening and wasting of muscles. One person in 2000 in the United Kingdom will have a neuromuscular disease. This chapter will focus upon the more commonly seen muscular dystrophy and congenital muscular dystrophy.

To fully understand the impact of the conditions known as muscular dystrophy on the child and his family, it is useful to draw upon information about the nature and course of the conditions and the underlying pathology.

DUCHENNE MUSCULAR DYSTROPHY AND BECKER MUSCULAR DYSTROPHY

These are the progressive muscular dystrophies. With first signs in early childhood or early adolescence, these conditions are seen more frequently in boys than girls and can affect several boys in one family. The first physical signs are the progressive muscle weakness affecting the lower limbs and then the upper limbs. The affected muscles show an increase in girth as the muscle fibres are replaced by fibrous tissue (Bakker & van Ommen 1998). Typically, concern is raised by a report of a child being unable to get up from the floor unaided, being unsteady on his feet or sometimes walking on his toes; he is usually unable to run. Physical signs associated with

Duchenne muscular dystrophy usually occur before the age of three (Bakker & van Ommen 1998).

With these physical changes, the child's developmental milestones are interrupted, with the consequence of physical, psychological and social development falling behind. There will be implications as the child enters his school career and effects on the family from the time of diagnosis and onwards through the lifecycle. A family will mourn the loss of the child who appeared normal and now has muscular dystrophy. They will have to adjust their activities around caring for a child with an evolving level of dependence.

By the age of 8–11 years, the child with Duchenne muscular dystrophy will be unable to walk and, by the time he reaches his early teenage years, he will rely on using a wheelchair for mobility. Children with muscular dystrophy may have progressive weakness of the intercostal muscles resulting in respiratory difficulties. One-third of boys with Duchenne muscular dystrophy are found to have an IQ of less than 75. The link between the learning difficulties and the pathology underlying the condition is not understood (Bakker & van Ommen 1998). Unlike the muscle weakness, the learning difficulties are not progressive.

The presentation of the extent and effect of the muscle weakness is variable. For some boys, the Becker form of muscular dystrophy echoes a milder form of Duchenne muscular dystrophy. Some boys' walking mobility will be sustained throughout their lives. Typically, a child with Becker muscular dystrophy can be expected to remain ambulant into adolescence. At around the age of 16 years, the loss of ambulation leads to dependency on a wheelchair for mobility. Those with Becker muscular dystrophy may have involvement of the cardiac muscles and this will require medical intervention. Boys with Duchenne muscular dystrophy do sometimes have cardiac muscle involvement but not the progressive heart failure seen in Becker muscular dystrophy.

Both Duchenne and Becker muscular dystrophy are recessive X-linked genetic disorders. In families known to have muscular dystrophy, the abnormal gene sits on the female sex chromosome, the X chromosome. Being recessive, the normal gene on the second sex chromosome prevents expression of the disease in the females. In contrast, males (who inherit the abnormal gene on their mother's X chromosome) are affected.

LIMB GIRDLE MUSCULAR DYSTROPHY

This is initially noticed as difficulty with walking and running at any time during the first three decades of life, usually from the age of 10 to 15 years. Parents of affected children can often recall subtle difficulties with movement when their child was younger. With limb girdle muscular dystrophy, the symmetrical muscle weakness occurs around the shoulder or pelvic girdles initially, extending later to the lower limbs and then the upper limbs. The most prominent features are limb girdle and trunk weakness (Beckmann & Fardeau 1998). This form of muscular dystrophy has been diagnosed in girls as well as boys.

CONGENITAL MUSCULAR DYSTROPHIES

These are autosomal recessive muscle diseases characterised by very early onset, generalised hypotonia (neonatal or infantile, depending on the type of congenital muscular dystrophy) and muscle weakness with delayed motor milestones. There is likely to be muscle atrophy, early contractures and joint deformities. Respiratory difficulties are also present in some specific forms of congenital muscular dystrophy. Although not a progressive condition like muscular dystrophy, the impact of the hypotonia and muscle weakness on a child's occupational performance and acquisition of skills is significant. Information given in this chapter on the progressive form of muscular dystrophy will guide intervention for a child known to have one of the many forms of congenital muscular dystrophy. Specific information about the nature of each individual child and his condition must support evaluation and intervention for the child.

THE EFFECT OF MUSCULAR DYSTROPHY ON OCCUPATIONAL PERFORMANCE

Functionally, the age of onset and the pattern and extent of muscle weakness will interfere with the expected stages of motor development and the acquisition of skills across the occupational performance areas of self care, productivity (primary schooling) and leisure. Loss of functional mobility through increasing muscle weakness will affect all areas of the child's life and have a subsequent effect on his family. As described above, some dystrophies also present with cognitive difficulties and this also will have an impact on progress. For the family, awareness of limited acquisition of motor skills and the apparent loss of motor skills in the child leads to the reality of the longer-term progressive and deteriorating nature of the condition.

The child will become more dependent upon adults for his physical care and wellbeing. This can lead to frustration for the child, which may manifest in behavioural difficulties. These behavioural difficulties often relate to the coping strategies that the child adopts. A child who is struggling to move around at home may want to insist that he is not left alone or out of direct visual contact with an adult. The child will want to know that he can call on his parents for help. He will be trusting in the care provided by his parent(s) and less accepting of care offered by other potential carers. This places additional demands on the parents.

The child may be frightened of falling over and of being unable to get up again. This fear will affect his motivation to move independently and limit his capacity to make choices about what he wants to do for himself and with other people.

The child's participation in family life, school and community is restricted by the deterioration in physical ability. The environment can severely restrict functional ability.

It is also important to acknowledge the impact on the child's life and his reactions to learning about the changes that he is experiencing. Here each individual child will react in his own ways. One child may respond in a surprisingly passive way, whilst another may express open anger and aggression. At important stages for personal growth and maturation, such as during adolescence, the young person will experience increasing dependence because of the deterioration in physical skills. Expressions of rebellion and frustration during adolescence will be commonplace among their peers. For the young person with muscular dystrophy, as skills are lost and function becomes more limited, this rebellion and frustration will also be connected with these personal circumstances and with others' attempts to offer help and practical assistance. It is important to help the young person and the family to recognise that, while functions may be lost, roles can remain intact. Practical help to assist in the maintenance of valued roles as function and skills diminish is an essential remit of the occupational therapist.

MUSCULAR DYSTROPHY WITHIN THE FAMILY

For some families, diagnosis of one child with Duchenne muscular dystrophy will occur after the birth of second and subsequent siblings, which may mean the possibility of two, three or four children with Duchenne muscular dystrophy in one family. Genetic counselling is now available and early diagnosis of one child allows the family the choice of accessing genetic counselling for subsequent pregnancies. Siblings can elect to investigate if they are carriers of a muscular dystrophy gene and to receive counselling about the risk of having a child with muscular dystrophy. At whatever age diagnosis does occur, a family will need ongoing accessible support from health, social services, education services and voluntary agencies. A national organisation – the Muscular Dystrophy Campaign – has a network of specialist family care officers linked to tertiary centres offering diagnosis and management of muscular dystrophy.

Among the neuromuscular disorders, muscular dystrophy is well recognised. Other forms of dystrophy exist and the nature of each individual child's story should be evaluated carefully to inform understanding of the likely progression and outcome.

PROGNOSIS

Boys with Duchenne muscular dystrophy have a life expectancy of 20–25 years, or longer where respiratory function and cardiac involvement are effectively managed. For limb girdle dystrophies, life expectancy is middle to late adult years, depending on age of onset and progression.

Enormous advances in the understanding of the neuromuscular disorders were made during the 1990s. The application of medical science, especially molecular genetic techniques, has contributed much to medical clinical management of this group of conditions. The evolving genetic techniques have offered preclinical diagnosis, assessment of prognosis, genetic counselling and prenatal diagnosis. The significance of these developments for the families where neuromuscular disorders are identified is yet to be fully understood. A greater understanding of the pathogenesis of the conditions, and developments in gene therapy, will further impact on the interventions available (Emery 1998). For the future, gene therapy may offer hope of treating the muscle pathology.

Families of children with muscular dystrophy can become very resilient and resourceful. They seem to be able to draw on immense personal resources as they strive to provide for their children, while at the same time having to cope with the experience of bringing up a child or more than one child with muscular dystrophy.

REACTIONS TO DIAGNOSIS

In the early days, soon after the confirmation of diagnosis, a family will be seen to react in different ways. Feelings of grief, loss, shock, disbelief and anger will have an effect on family life, on siblings and on family dynamics. Parents often express a need for information about what to expect in the future – for their child with muscular dystrophy and for their family as a whole. Although this may have been outlined by a doctor at the time of giving the diagnosis, parents will work out their own reactions to this and look for more information in their own ways. Some may be able to access the Internet, where an enormous amount of information is available, although often expressed in technical language. Some will take up offers to meet other families in their local area or make links with families through the Muscular Dystrophy Campaign family care officers. A family will also look to their local teams of therapists for this information, as these may be among the most frequently contactable resources for the family.

THE INTERVENTION TEAM

In the United Kingdom, the nature of services providing intervention will vary depending upon the stage of progression of the child's muscular dystrophy. Generally, referral to a specialist neuromuscular team occurs shortly after initial diagnosis to explore the type of condition and to access specialist advice on management. These specialist teams operate from regional or national centres.

Local services may be coordinated by a primary care team through the GP, by a multidisciplinary team at a children's centre in the community or by the local hospital trust. In some areas, a key worker, link worker or case manager scheme may operate. In rural areas, identification may come through the GP when evidence of falls and loss of motor skills in the child is noted. Later in the child's life, the GP may be actively involved in providing and coordinating a support package and will certainly be involved at the later stages of care.

For the family with a child/children with muscular dystrophy, the numbers of professionals they have contact with expands as the child requires more physical help and environmental challenges have to be met.

Multidisciplinary/interdisciplinary intervention matrix for a child with muscular dystrophy from occupational therapist's perspective (Brown 2000)	Performance areas								Performance components			
	Physical health/medical issues	Self care	Communication	Mobility	Education	Play	Environment	Support for the family	Sensorimotor	Neuromuscular skeletal	Cognitive	Psychosocial
Range of services												
Occupational therapist												
Physiotherapist	3.4									5		
Speech and language therapist		1										
Dietician												
Health visitor												
Community paediatric nurse	2.3											
Paediatrician												
Clinical psychologist								6				
Educational psychologist												
Classroom teacher												
Class support workers												
Special educational needs officer												
Wheelchair services												
Social worker												
Family care officer												
Specialist neuromuscular team												
Ambulatory and orthopaedic clinic	7											
Orthotists	8											
Hospice provision												

1 Feeding and swallowing
2 Tissue viability and pressure relief
3 Respiratory function – overnight oxygen
4 Postoperative care
5 Physical activity, muscle strength, management of physical changes and deformity
6 Parent and sibling group
7 Diagnostic services, genetic counselling
8 Scoliosis – monitoring and intervention

Fig. 12.1 The range of professionals that may be involved in the care of a child with muscular dystrophy.

Figure 12.1 indicates the range of professionals that may be involved in the care of a child with muscular dystrophy and his family. It gives suggestions of the areas where interdisciplinary approaches are appropriate. Additional information appears under the names of some of the services likely to be involved.

Wheelchair service. This service will offer assessment and provision of a mobility aid such as a larger pushchair, a transit wheelchair or a self-propelling wheelchair. The service may also make assessments for powered wheelchairs, sometimes leading to the provision of an indoor powered chair initially and/or contribute to assessment and provision of an electrically powered indoor/outdoor chair (EPIOC). Operational policies about provision vary and families will often require support to access funding via voluntary agencies.

Dietician. Some boys with Duchene muscular dystrophy are at risk of being overweight, particularly as they get older, less mobile and less active. Advice to a family about healthy eating for the whole family avoids having to restrict access to sweets and other recognised unhealthy foods for the child with muscular dystrophy.

School staff (including class teacher, special educational needs officer and classroom support assistant). Many children with muscular dystrophy will attend their local primary school. When access to the building is an issue, another primary school may be chosen. For some children, families may elect for a child to attend a special school for some of the primary school years. At the stage of secondary school, creative packages of education can support a pupil through mainstream education. At all stages, close home–school liaison is essential, supported by effective cross-agency and interdisciplinary intervention.

The teaching staff will create learning opportunities, offer modified elements of the school curriculum and support the child's participation in school life.

Family care officers. Provided by the Muscular Dystrophy Campaign to offer support and advice to people affected by neuromuscular conditions, family care officers assist children and adults, as well as their relatives. It is often useful for people to have contact with a family care officer at the time of diagnosis, or soon after, because the implications of the diagnosis can be discussed with a family. A family care officer is the link between the hospital and the home. Although they usually work at a hospital, they make home visits to people in their area. They work closely with consultants and other medical and paramedical staff.

Care manager. This role is frequently fulfilled by a social worker. The care manager is responsible for assessing people's needs for community care and for arranging provision of that care. They can advise on respite care, daycare services in the home and residential care. Social workers will be based in an NHS Trust social work department or in the social services department of the local authority. Some authorities have a specialised Children with Disability Team.

REGIONAL/NATIONAL HOSPICE PROVISION

In some areas, it is possible for families to have links with providers of respite residential care, where a family can stay on site and take advantage of the specialist team of staff available.

Effective cross-agency and interdisciplinary liaison and collaboration can support a family in caring for their child. Anything that limits efficient delivery of available services serves only to complicate life for the family and to add to the stress experienced by that family because it compromises the parents' ability to look after and to care for their child or children.

EVIDENCE-BASED PRACTICE

The Muscular Dystrophy Campaign actively supports medical research into the molecular and cellular level pathology of neuromuscular disease. In contrast, there has been a paucity of research into the efficacy of therapeutic intervention. It is therefore essential that every therapist working within this field conducts intervention in such a way that robust outcome measures and evaluation of their treatment begin to build an acceptable bank of evidence and information around the effectiveness of occupational therapy input. The Muscular Dystrophy Campaign produces literature about current best practice, which is aimed at the families of children with muscular dystrophy. Information is given about the important aspects of management, such as passive movements, as part of managing the physical changes that take place. The literature also explains the kinds of help that families can access, the processes of the local authority for providing disabled facilities and the roles undertaken by the professionals that the family may meet. There is relevant research literature that looks at the impact of intervention on the lives of families and children in the field of cerebral palsy but similar studies are not available in the field of muscular dystrophy. It seems that most information about intervention with children and muscular dystrophy arises from descriptions of practice, for example Tuckett (1998), which gave a schedule of occupational therapy input. With increasing emphasis on the need to demonstrate clinical effectiveness of occupational therapy interventions, it is essential that the impact of the processes for evaluating outcomes is also considered. The process of setting baselines and goals against which change is measured will have a very different meaning for the family and for the child with a progressive deteriorating condition than for the therapist who is setting the targets. This should challenge therapists to look at clinical effectiveness not only as it serves to inform practice but also in how it can provide helpful and meaningful information for the family.

THEORETICAL FOUNDATIONS OF INTERVENTION

Muscular dystrophy affects a child's occupational performance from childhood, into adolescence and into adulthood depending on the age of onset. The story of the child with muscular dystrophy is characterised by the progressive loss of skills during a time of life where the development of skills would be the norm.

Deteriorating performance in self care including functional mobility, productivity (mainly education) and leisure is significant and will benefit from the intervention from an occupational therapist. Loss of skills in these performance areas requires attention, together with the consequences of the inability to acquire skills and the potential loss of roles associated with deterioration in function. Access must be maintained for opportunities to develop and utilise skills during childhood and onwards through the life stages.

ASSESSMENT AND EVALUATION

The Canadian Model of Occupational Performance provides a focus on self care, productivity and leisure. The model acknowledges the capacities of the individual and the influence of the environment, the developmental level and the roles a person occupies on occupational performance. Satisfaction with performance, as well as performance itself, contributes to occupational performance. Attention to underlying skills in the four performance components of physical, mental, spiritual and sociocultural will also be required. This model will guide the therapist in gaining an understanding of the child's specific situation in terms of occupational performance and how the child and his family perceive his situation. This will identify areas of occupational performance that require attention and the significance of these identified areas for the child and for his family.

The Canadian Occupational Performance Measure (COPM) (Law et al 1994) is based on the Canadian Model of Occupational Performance. It is an appropriate subjective measurement tool for use with the family of a child with muscular dystrophy and with an individual child. Consideration of the individual child's ability and readiness to use this kind of measure is essential, based on knowledge of any possible concerns about the child's cognition or language. Law et al (1994) report on the measure being successfully tested on children as young as 7 years of age.

The COPM offers two scores, which represent the person's perceived performance and satisfaction with that performance. It serves as a guide to gather information from the parent(s), the child

Table 12.1 Range of relevant assessment tools available for use with the child with muscular dystrophy

Measurement tool	Author	Age range	Occupational performance area/performance component
COPM	Law et al (1994)	From 7 years	All performance areas
Pediatric Evaluation of Disability Inventory (PEDI)	Haley et al (1992)	6 of months to 7 years	Self care, functional mobility
School Function Assessment	Coster et al (1998)	4 to 11 years (primary)	All in school environment
AMPS	Fisher (1997)	Adolescent to adult	Motor and processing skills
School AMPS	Fisher & Bryze (1997)	School age	Motor and processing skills
Community Dependence Index	Eakin & Baird (1995)	All	10 areas of activities of daily living included in occupational performance

and other people involved in the child's care. Where it is not appropriate to complete the full measure to achieve the scoring it will guide the occupational therapist's approach. Use of a measure such as the COPM maintains an emphasis on the family's key concerns, particularly in the early stages after diagnosis. It can support the therapist's developing understanding of the impact of the condition on the individual family members and assist in negotiating the priority given to addressing specific concerns. Observation of the child's performance and collection of reports from everyone involved in the child's care will also provide key information. This can then be discussed with the family and other professionals involved to support the interpretation of the information gained.

The COPM helps structure and guide the interview process and ensures a focus on the primary concerns of the occupational therapist in the performance areas of self care, productivity (including play and school) and leisure. The measure can also provide information about the efficacy of intervention when it is fully used and administered subsequent to review changes in occupational performance.

During assessment, the focus must be on what the child can and wishes to do and on capitalising his strengths and capabilities. Detailed evaluation of these performance areas can be undertaken using specialist standardised assessment to enrich the information gathered initially. Appropriate tools are listed in Tables 12.1 and 12.2. The

Table 12.2 Range of relevant assessment tools available for use with the family of a child with muscular dystrophy (Stewart & Nyerlin-Beale 2000)

Name of measurement tool	Author
Care Strain Index	Robinson (1983)
Perceived stress scale	Cohen (1983)
The subjective burden scale	Brookes & McKinley (1983)

Assessment of Motor and Process Skills for the school-age child (known as the School AMPS) offers functional, unobtrusive, naturalistic, reliable and valid assessment of the effectiveness of motor and process skills during performance of functional school tasks. After the primary years, tools such as the Assessment of Motor and Process Skills (AMPS) can support evaluation in the home environment. Where indicated, further assessment of specific performance components can also be undertaken, or referred onto other services in consultation with the family. The occupational therapist will need to draw upon other theoretical frameworks to address individual performance components. Figure 12.2 shows the relationship between the therapist's use of COPM and certain appropriate standardised assessments.

FRAMES OF REFERENCE

The concept of occupation for the child includes all activities on the continuum of play to work and is therefore central to the development of the child. Once the areas of concern are identified and an

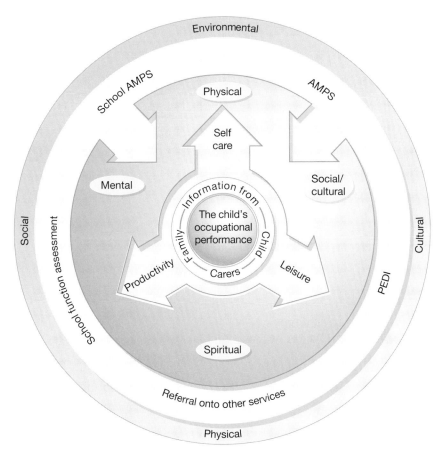

Fig. 12.2 How standardised assessments can augment the information gained following the use of the Canadian Occupational Performance Model.

understanding gained of the priority given to an identified area, attention can be given to finding ways to address the concerns. Occupational therapy will focus primarily on addressing deficits in the performance areas using biomechanical, developmental, compensatory and/or adaptive concepts. Here, appropriate frames of reference will guide intervention (Table 12.3).

The biomechanical frame of reference is helpful when addressing motor components and in understanding the use of orthotic, mobility, postural and orthopaedic-type management strategies. Applying biomechanical principles supports the selection of equipment solutions.

The use of a developmental frame of reference is essential when working on the child's acquisition of skills. Where true developmental acquisi-

tion of skills is not achievable and compensatory and adaptive strategies must be used, a flexible combination of frameworks is required to address motor performance components.

The timing at which a referral to see a child with muscular dystrophy is received will influence the theoretical framework chosen by the occupational therapist, as will the practice context within which the occupational therapist works. For example, an occupational therapist working in a child development team may be asked to see a child who is presenting with language delay and a history of falls in the preschool years. In such a case, taking a developmental approach and helping the family identify specific concerns can assist the family by adding meaning to the need to understand why their son

Table 12.3 Theoretical concepts underpinning occupational therapy intervention that may be used to guide occupational therapy intervention with the child with muscular dystrophy

Theoretical concept	Reference for description of application to practice	Performance component	Function/dysfunction continuum
Model of Occupational Performance	CAOT Guidelines	Focuses on performance areas	Self care, productivity, leisure
Human Occupation frame of reference	Peganoff O'Brien (1993)	Psychological component – social and self-management	Occupational behaviour, play–work continuum
Biomechanical frame of reference	Colangelo (1993)	Postural control	Physical and physiological influences on motor development
Psychosocial frame of reference	Olson (1993)	Psychosocial skills	Temperament, attachment, interactive skills, play, environmental interaction
Coping frame of reference	Williamson et al (1993)	Self-management	Stress, coping, adaptation
Developmental theories	Hinojosa et al (1996)	Sensorimotor, cognitive, psychosocial and all performance areas	Stage-specific expected norms of development

is falling over. It is helpful to illustrate how the contribution of specialist advice can add to the family's understanding of the practical problems being faced by their child. A later referral may require a response to practical problems of access or loss of functional skills in personal care.

It can be helpful to realise the conflicts that can arise between the different theoretical frameworks for the therapist and how parents can struggle with the meaning and relevance of some interventions at different times in the child's life. It is useful to consider how a parent might perceive and respond to a recommendation to use an ankle/foot orthosis, for example. The proposed aim might be to help maintain a foot posture to enable the child to retain the ability to stand with stability and to walk. Parents often question the value of using such orthoses to retain standing and walking, when the child will lose these skills in the future. The therapist will need to explain that, physically and functionally, it is an advantage to maintain the erect postures associated with standing for as long as possible rather than to support only the flexed postures adopted when seated. Another frequent question relates to why a child needs to wear a truck brace to control spinal deformity when the parent does not see the child as having spinal problems. Recommendations for

brace use must be introduced sensitively and discussed thoroughly if the brace is to be incorporated effectively into the child's daily care and family routine. Working within the principles of family-centred practice helps to remind the therapist to be constantly aware of these potential conflicts and the importance of understanding the meaning of any contact or intervention offered from the family's perspective.

Pountney et al (2000 p143) advocates the use of Fleming's three-track reasoning as a process that enables the therapist to apply postural management in the context of the individual child and family (Fig. 12.3). These three tracks of reasoning are procedural, interactive and conditional. Firstly, the procedural track echoes the medical model, problem-solving approach to diagnosis, prognosis and prescription to address functional problems. Here, assessment of the child's lying, sitting and standing abilities gives specific information about options for intervention but does not address the wider issues that can impact on the family. The interactive track helps the therapist to understand the problem when in direct contact with the family, allowing common understandings to develop and extending appreciation of the family's experience and responses. Then, using the information from the procedural and

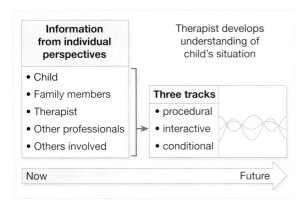

Fig. 12.3 The use of Fleming's three-track reasoning.

interactive tracks, the conditional track brings deeper understandings of the child, now and in the future, and in the context of the child's family. These three tracks are not seen as being sequential but as intertwined and interactive.

USING THEORETICAL KNOWLEDGE TO SUPPORT PARENTAL AND FAMILIAL REACTION TO DIAGNOSIS

In addition to drawing upon theoretical frameworks from the field of occupational therapy, work with families and children requires knowledge of another important area. Occupational therapists need to have a sensitive awareness of the parents' experience of learning about their child and disability (Brown 1996). Literature indicates an emphasis on the field of medicine and initial diagnosis. The parent's reaction to such news, which is sometimes termed the 'concept of adjustment', has been extensively reported by stage theorists such as Kubler-Ross (1969, in Seligman & Darling 1989) who describes the stages of denial, bargaining, anger, depression and acceptance. Dale (1996) cautions that there is some controversy about the idea that parents pass through a series of stages such as those of grief before reaching a point of acceptance or adjustment to their child with a disability. A comprehensive overview of the stages or phases of parents' reactions has been given by Seligman and Darling (1989) around common psychological responses. They describe the initial response of shock and

denial followed by bargaining, sadness, anger, anxiety, adaptation, acceptance or reorganisation.

Featherstone (1980) reports that parents put fear first when they tell their personal stories about their child's disability. It is important to note that not all parents show a 'grief reaction' and that conclusions about a parent's unaccepting or inappropriate behaviour are not made based on their response at any time. Dale (1996) suggests that parents would oscillate between these stages. She stresses that they may accept their child's condition at one period of life but then find it more distressing and more difficult at another period of the lifecycle. Seligman and Darling (1989) highlight that the reactions proposed by the stage theorists may not indeed be experienced sequentially and that they may occur repeatedly. These concepts are particularly useful in helping to develop an understanding of parents' coping strategies, and about how to share information with them. Dale (1996) advises that chronic sorrow and acceptance can coexist as part of a long-term process of parental adjustment. She refers to previous authors' work, such as MacKeith (1973), who also included protectiveness, guilt and embarrassment as examples of parental reactions.

McConachie (1994) reports that research into the impact of a child's disability has changed over time from considering parental reactions as a crisis to recognising their reactions as coping strategies. Each family will respond in their own way and the same event will have different meanings for different families and different members of the same family. However, Dale (1996) highlights the risk that focusing only on coping strategies may mean a family sustaining high levels of stress, which can ultimately lead to burnout.

INTERVENTION

When taking a person-centred approach to intervention it is impossible to know what the child's and/or family's priorities will be. Experience shows, however, that the occupational therapist is likely to be involved in all or some of the areas shown in Tables 12.4 and 12.5. The therapist herself can be guided by the overall aims of intervention, shown in Box 12.1.

For a child with muscular dystrophy it is essential to demonstrate ways in which significant roles can be maintained in the context of diminishing

Table 12.4 Suggestions for intervention strategies for a child with muscular dystrophy

Occupational performance issues	Child wants to, needs to, or is is expected to	Family wants to needs to, or expects the child to	Options for intervention focus/strategies
Self care – personal care	Stand at sink and clean teeth	Be sure risk of falls minimised	Enable access to assistive devices: perching stool adjustable height chair, chunky toothbrush/battery-operated tool Ensure access to correct disability allowances Ensure local authority referral process followed
Self care – functional mobility	Sit down and get up from table and chair	Maintain activity	Correct height chair/powered adjustable height seat
Self care – community management	Get to family car without being carried	Go out in the car	Access to tricycle, or pushchair/wheelchair by referral to wheelchair service
Productivity – paid/unpaid work	Join in sponsored silence	Join peer group activity	Inclusive strategies included in planning event: access/seating
Productivity – household management	Hang up coat on arrival home	Encourage responsibility and independence	Location of coat peg/hanger, timing of activity Provision of information about alternative strategies around dressing
Productivity – play/school	Play with construction set	Play and have fun	Choice of kit, size of tool, working position Advice on goal setting around hand skill acquisition
Productivity – play/school	Join reception class at school	Attend local school	Effective transition planning for school: access, accommodation, equipment, individual help, information on muscular dystrophy
Leisure – quiet recreation	Complete sticker book	Select appropriate activities to support child's independence	Working position, consider size of furniture Location of components
Leisure – active recreation	Go to the park with dad to walk the dog	Include child in family activity	Access to mobility aid, planning outing, distance and tolerance Referral to wheelchair service
Leisure – socialisation	Go to school friend's party	Have peer contact with family of child of same age	Negotiate accessible venue Plan journey and access in advance

Box 12.1 Suggested overall aims of intervention for the occupational therapist working with a child with muscular dystrophy and his family

Overall aims of intervention
- To maintain an optimum level of occupational performance.
- To support the family in the parenting and care of the child.
- To enable the child to undertake everyday activities usually experienced in childhood and throughout life.
- To provide information about compensatory and adaptive strategies to achieve personal care and activities of daily living.
- To ensure supportive and least restrictive environments are available to the child and the family.
- To support transition into the playgroup or preschool, school and further education.
- To ensure access to other services such as the local wheelchair service.
- To liaise with other key operational links.

Table 12.5 Suggestions for intervention strategies for an older child/adolescent with muscular dystrophy

Occupational performance issues	Child wants to, needs to, is expected to	Family wants to, needs to, expects the child to	Options for intervention focus/strategies
Self care – personal care	Wash face, do make-up/shave	Maintain elements of independence	Working position, access to adjustable height sink, minimal effort taps
Self care – functional mobility	Get in/out of bath	Reduce lifting	Facilities to meet changing needs/equipment solutions in place/moving and handling issues addressed
Self care – community management	Use mobility bus to go to cinema	Encourage choice about going out	Skills and knowledge about transport, timetabling, wheelchair proficiency, use of carers, peer buddies
Productivity – paid/unpaid work	Participate in work experience scheme	Support preparation for further education/vocational/work activities	Liaison with school, careers service/transition planning, information about muscular dystrophy
Productivity – household management	Select clothes to wear	Encourage independence and autonomy	Location of clothes, timing of activity
Productivity – play/school	Write spelling list/homework task in book	Support child's learning	Slope top desk Choice of pencil/access to example, location of board in class
Leisure – quiet recreation	Play hand-held electronic game	Find activities child can complete with minimal help	Working position location and mounting of toy
Leisure – active recreation	Watch motor racing	Respond to child's choices of activity	Forward planning, access, facilities, choice of wheelchair, clothing
Leisure – socialisation	Attend youth club with peers	Enjoy peer group contact for their child	Access, transport, respite care arrangement, choice of wheelchair/moving and handling issues addressed

function. Parents can also be supported in identifying these roles for their child. Taking care of a pet, for example, provides opportunities for the child to continue to participate actively on a daily basis. When it is not possible for the child to perform certain tasks such as grooming, feeding or handling, he can continue to own the pet by deciding what food it eats, by asking someone to groom it when he decides this is necessary, by helping to check the pet's health and taking it to see the vet.

It is also important to recognise the need to support the changing role of the parent(s) in orchestrating their child's care and balancing family life and at times electing to accept support from care support workers in the home. Brown et al (1996) describe a model of the nature of family–therapist relationships giving a seven level hierarchy of

family involvement. It serves as a useful guide to the attitudes, knowledge and skills that a clinician requires to operate at each level.

SPECIFIC INTERVENTION STRATEGIES

MANAGEMENT OF CHANGES ARISING FROM PROGRESSION OF MUSCLE WEAKNESS

Weakness affecting mobility

Progressive muscle weakness brings about a loss of skills in walking and then in moving against gravity such as getting up from the floor, standing up from a chair and climbing stairs. Here, the occupational therapist needs to understand the consequences of this change for the child and for the family. Restricted mobility makes it difficult for a child to join in with their peers in boisterous play, making them vulnerable to falls and to being isolated in the playground. This can lead to frustration and opting out. A child's physical dependence brings about practical caring problems for the family. For example, when a child is unable to get out of bed and go to the toilet unaided, it can lead to disturbed nights for the child and the family and require practical issues of continence management to be addressed.

During the early stages of impaired mobility, the use of a tricycle may help bridge the gap for mobility for a child. The introduction of a wheelchair can maintain a child's access to school trips, outings with the local after-school and social groups and being able to join a family outing.

Weakness in upper limbs

Initially, activity against gravity is affected. With progressive weakening of the antigravity and shoulder girdle muscles, the child will need support of the upper limbs to be able to achieve movement. The child will need to place objects and tasks in his lap or on a lower working surface in order to be able to use distal intrinsic hand power and function. Upper limb weakness will have significant impact on the child's capacity to use tools.

Sleep and respiratory problems

Practical problems arise from sleeping disturbances and decline in respiratory function. These need full evaluation by the medical team to ensure that the family and the young person can understand and manage the practical problems they face, and also to reduce anxiety. The use of equipment overnight to assist respiration can reduce dependency on family members/carers and minimise distress.

ENABLING PARTICIPATION
Home and family life

While understanding the importance of maintaining mobility, it is also important to address issues about the child's level of participation in activities with peers and the role that they play. The family will also want to be able to maintain their own contact with social and leisure activities in the community, as well as including the child in everyday family activity such as going to the shops and collecting younger children from school. Recognising the extra demands placed on a family arising from caring for a child with a disability is important if recommendations from therapists are to be incorporated in a child's day and everyday family activity, rather than adding to the demands that the family already has to cope with.

Participation at school

Advice on activity tolerance and energy conservation will be helpful and collaboration regarding curriculum differentiation for the child will also support participation. Here, the learning programme and learning resources are selected individually. Achieving an effective working position, working with a partner and having access to individual classroom support will provide opportunities to accommodate changing muscle power and activity tolerance. For example, using a compensatory/adaptive approach to assist a child who cannot work at a raised painting easel and who finds it difficult to sustain a grasp on a paint brush, can encourage him to choose a more accessible working position and to select alternative tools. An overall goal of producing a piece of work in paint to a given theme can still be achieved in line with the peer group's expected outcome.

Lachina (2000) describes a school-based programme called Project Participate and asserts that 'being there is not enough'. The programme gives a structured approach for an occupational therapist to help school-based staff working with the child ensure the child's maximum participation. This type of programme can be used with the School Function Assessment (see Table 12.1), to make a detailed analysis of the child's performance in the classroom environment allowing specific goals to be set and incorporated into the child's individual education plan.

POSTURAL MANAGEMENT

Spinal curvature (scoliosis) may begin very early in life in young children with muscle weakness, often as early as when the child begins to be supported in the sitting position. This may be a risk for children with congenital myopathies, especially congenital muscular dystrophy. The child will adopt compensatory postures to achieve function. Alternatively, the scoliosis may appear only after walking becomes impossible, for example, in boys who have Duchenne muscular dystrophy. This is usually between the 8th and 12th years. As the boy gets older and less mobile, spending much of the time sitting, the spinal curve tends to increase.

Two important consequences of scoliosis should be recognised. Firstly, as the scoliosis increases, there is progressive tilting of the pelvis (pelvic obliquity). This results in increasing difficulty in sitting, as the weight is no longer distributed evenly between the buttocks. Secondly, scoliosis often results in an alteration of the shape of the chest, eventually restricting the capacity of the lungs and so breathing becomes more difficult (Muscular Dystrophy Campaign 1999). In addition, tissue viability may be at risk in a child or young person who is unable to change position independently. Preventive pressure care and provision of pressure relief equipment in collaboration with nursing services may be indicated.

The child with muscular dystrophy has the disadvantage of being forced by his muscle weakness to assume unusual postures. Stable and symmetrical play and working positions are the aim. Every effort should be made to minimise slouching or leaning habitually to one side when seated, in order to minimise a spinal curvature and its effects. Correct sized furniture (chair height and seat depth with an appropriate height table) to encourage an erect sitting posture is ideal.

Good posture is also important when sitting in a wheelchair, especially as the amount of time spent sitting increases as the child gets older. The arms may need to be used to support the body on the armrests of a chair. Even the position adopted in bed can have an influence, over time, on the development of a spinal curvature. While the spinal posture remains flexible and correctable in early years, there will be fixed deformities later in life.

Orthopaedic management through surgery may be necessary to restore posture and function, particularly around gait, functional mobility and, later, for the management of developing spinal deformity. The occupational therapist will provide support around practical problem solving for the family pre- and postoperatively, including advice on choice of clothes to accommodate plasters or orthoses and the selection of alternative play and leisure activities. Sometimes, forward planning regarding the need for a mobility aid will be required, with appropriate arrangement for access to school site and facilities. The logistics of enabling a child to travel to the school will require collaboration between the family, the school and the provider of school or local authority transport.

OCCUPATIONAL PERFORMANCE

Living with muscular dystrophy produces many challenges but it can be made more manageable by having early access to appropriate facilities and equipment. The overall aim is to gain optimum participation in everyday activity in the home, in school and in the community, in line with the wishes of the child and his family and with normal developmental stages. Maintenance of skills and participation in tasks rather than passive dependence on adult care, will support this aim. Where appropriate facilities can be provided, family functioning can be maintained. Residential placement particularly during the school term may be an option in support of a family continuing to care for their child.

Effective planning and the family's access to support can achieve quality of life for both the child and the family. The pattern of provision does vary across different parts of the United Kingdom and the occupational therapist will need a sound understanding of the availability or limitations of provision.

Self care

As muscle weakness progresses and muscle power declines in the upper limbs, the child's capacity to develop skills or to become independent in self care will be affected. Good positioning, compensatory strategies, including information about easy-to-use styles of clothing, can make a difference. Sportswear trousers made from stretchy soft fabric are easier when dressing than non-stretch, tight-fitting jeans or tailored trousers. Creative choice of fabric and design may be needed to meet particular style needs of the child/adolescent.

As upper power declines further, tasks such as brushing his hair, washing his face and cleaning his teeth become more difficult, such that the child will be dependent on another's help. Support for the upper limbs, through effective positioning to compensate for the lack of anti-gravity power, can enable a child to continue to carry out these tasks, as can the use of items such as an electric toothbrush and a flannel mitten. A change of hairstyle, perhaps to a very short cropped (and maybe coloured) style, as currently favoured by many teenage boys, may eliminate the need to brush his hair – a task frequently not undertaken with enthusiasm by teenage boys at the best of times! A distinctive hairstyle or body piercing may also help a boy express his individuality and provide an area for 'pushing boundaries' where this may not be possible elsewhere. A person-centred approach using joint problem solving encourages active participation and supports autonomy in the maturing child.

When a carer has to undertake care tasks, it is important that the child retains some control and choice over the task. It is important to understand how a child likes to be helped, when that help is required, and to understand how a child feels about having to receive help. Being bathed by an adult at the age of 4 years is a normal and enjoyable part of growing up, for example. However, it is usually neither desirable nor enjoyable for a teenage boy to be seen naked or to be bathed by an adult. Such a situation requires great sensitivity on behalf of the carer if the adolescent is to feel comfortable and in control of a situation. Personal care can be intrusive if not carried out in a sensitive way geared to the individual's needs and wishes. The occupational therapist can support the child in developing skills to communicate their wishes and to exercise autonomy and control over daily situations that they face. Children and young people with muscular dystrophy are often very adept at identifying what help they need and the sorts of practical solutions or equipment they would like to use. The family and the child with muscular dystrophy become expert in identifying the help they need and the occupational therapist can be very effective in supporting this by adopting a person-centred and family-centred way of working.

Productivity

For all children, the activities of the school day and homework should be considered as their productivity. Other individual areas of productivity, for example, pet care or household chores, will require equal attention.

Using learning tools

For the young child, the acquisition of drawing and writing skills is an essential part of the school day. As he progresses through primary school years he will be expected to work more independently, to manage his own time and use frameworks to structure his work.

To enable a child with muscular dystrophy to achieve productivity in these areas, a range of adaptive and compensatory strategies will be required to help with the acquisition of hand skills (Table 12.6).

Computer and assistive technology

Access to computers in schools is increasing and early access to a computer to allow the development of skills is essential for the child with muscular dystrophy. Alternative switching and input devices other than the standard keyboard will be of help, as will the correct set-up and working position for the computer equipment peripherals. Local education resources or exterior agencies

Table 12.6 Adaptive and compensatory strategies required to assist with hand skills required during education

Problem identified	Goal	Possible options
Weak grip	To sustain grip when writing	Thicker pencil, padded pencil
Child unable to copy from whiteboard	Child to copy independently	Individual example located on book rest on desk
Child unable to write more than a phrase on time	Child to be able to record work independently	Use of computer Use of tape recorder and/or scribe
Child unable to hold book	Child to be able to work with book independently	Use of sloped desk top or book rest or document holder
Child unable to copy out list of sums so that answer can be recorded	Child to be able to achieve answer and record answer independently	Use of worksheet with sums already written out leaving space for answer Use of scribe
Child unable to handle apparatus	Child to participate actively in experiment	Child to work with partner Apparatus set up in accessible position Access to individual classroom support

can provide information on different inputs and software to use when distal hand function is maintained but upper limb movement is very restricted. Voice-activated software for access and speed of working where the use of switching is too demanding may be indicated, depending on the child's voice quality and activity tolerance.

Leisure

An understanding of credible, age-appropriate activities undertaken by children and young people will support intervention towards achieving effective occupational performance in the vital area of leisure. This has to be relevant to local geographic and natural communities. Participation in local school and out-of-school social networks and groups may be enhanced by facilitation of mobility and access. When participation in organised social groups becomes increasingly difficult, becoming part of a virtual group through use of the Internet may be an alternative.

ENVIRONMENTAL ADAPTATIONS: THE CHILD'S PERFORMANCE CONTEXT

Home environment

By staying keenly aware of the family's priorities, appropriate solutions to everyday practical prob-

lems can be offered, beginning with the least intrusive ideas such as a chair of an appropriate height to help a child move from sitting to standing. Simple ramps or half steps can also be useful early on and can demonstrate how making changes to the home environment can be helpful. There may be indications for the introduction of more specialised and intrusive equipment, as well as more significant structural changes to a family's home at a later date, and the sensitive use of less intrusive measures in the early stages can help give confidence and aid acceptance of this process. The suggestions offered should be based on the child's and the family's readiness to elect to make changes to their existing ways of coping.

Figure 12.4 provides a framework to guide clinical reasoning and supports the provision of an appropriate home environment for the family with a child with muscular dystrophy.

In the United Kingdom, the Muscular Dystrophy Campaign has published an 'Adaptations Manual' (Harpin 1999) with accompanying fact sheets on equipment solutions. This detailed reference will facilitate discussions with a family regarding adaptations to the home environment. Constraints do exist on local authorities in their capacity to respond to family's needs. Early referral can provide the opportunity for timely intervention to provide appropriate facilities. Early referral also ensures that, where rehousing is indicated, time is allowed for a property to be

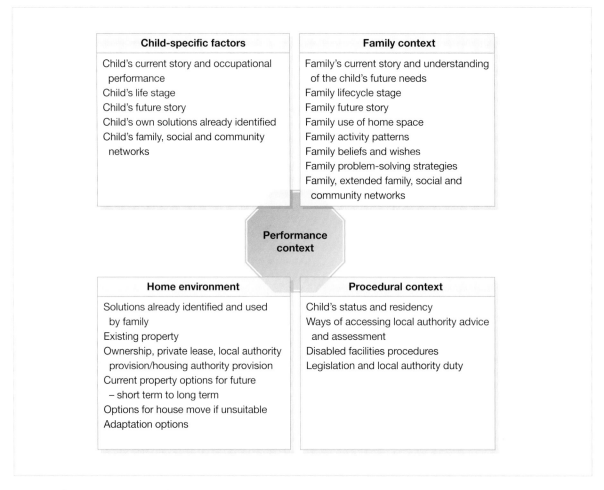

Fig. 12.4 Shaping the child's performance context.

found and modifications put in place, before the family moves home (Box 12.2, Fig. 12.5).

As a child becomes more dependent on others for personal care, a family may make a choice to use care support workers. In the light of moving and handling legislation it is becoming essential that appropriate facilities are in place in the home environment. The absence of suitable equipment may preclude the family from accessing the provision of care support workers in the home, as

---

Box 12.2 Key factors for modification and adaptation of the home environment (adapted from Harpin 1999, with permission)

- Acknowledge progressive nature of disease and evolving disability.
- Accommodate effect of lack of sitting balance and inability to respond to postural change without help.
- Plan with space allowances for use with powerchair.
- Appreciate long-term limitations of the effect of occupational performance deficits.
- Acknowledge upper limb movement compromised by inability to reach hand and raise arms.
- Allow for reduced grip and strength.

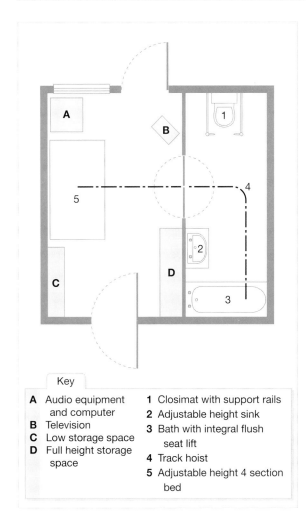

Key

A Audio equipment and computer
B Television
C Low storage space
D Full height storage space

1 Closimat with support rails
2 Adjustable height sink
3 Bath with integral flush seat lift
4 Track hoist
5 Adjustable height 4 section bed

Fig. 12.5 A suitable layout for a bedroom/bathroom facility for a child/adolescent with muscular dystrophy.

well as risking their own health as they care for their child. Ideally, options for provision of equipment need to be available well before the child has significant difficulty with walking and moving about indoors. Where a family has to continue to carry their child, this compromises the health of family members and family functioning is at risk.

School environment

All environments within the school building should be accessible in order to facilitate full

> **Box 12.3** Examples of typical questions that should be asked when assessing the primary school environment of a child with muscular dystrophy
>
> • Where do the child and parent wait to enter the school?
> • How do the other children line up before entering school?
> • Where and how does the child take their coat off and hang it up?
> • Can the child sit on the floor during floor-based activities?
>   – What are the alternatives?
> • Where and how does the child get ready for a PE lesson?
> • Are the toilets accessible, is there room for a carer?
> • How do the other children line up for their lunch?
> • How does the child choose what he wants for lunch?
> • How does the child reach the table with his food tray?
> • How does he manage at break time?

participation in school life. Where this is not possible, creative use of space and school timetabling can change the location of an activity to ensure that it is accessible. Task analysis of the occupations and roles encountered by the child during the school day is helpful to identify and alleviate any potential or real barriers to full access to the school environment and participation in classroom life and the school community. Box 12.3 gives examples of some typical questions that need to be addressed for the child with muscular dystrophy when assessing a primary school environment. For a child at secondary school these questions can be developed in line with the child's stage of maturation and social functioning.

Recommendations for equipment and the need for structural changes in a school building need to be developed in good time to allow for the processes and procedures of the local authority to be followed. It is helpful to identify probable needs when offering advice as part of the Code of Practice to determine Special Educational Need and ways of meeting those needs. Specific information about the child's need for adult help during the school day should be given to support the allocation of classroom support workers.

CONCLUSION

A progressive condition such as muscular dystrophy has immediate and long-term effects on the individual child and his family. The child's occupational performance and family functioning are at risk because of the physical changes taking place and they will all benefit from intervention from an occupational therapist. The family will need to make choices about the kinds of help they want to use and when. For some families, more than one child may be affected and this presents additional very specific challenges for the team of professionals working with them. Accessible services are required that can support a family's changing coping strategies together with allowing the family to elect to use different levels of practical help as the child's needs change and evolve. Close interdisciplinary and cross-agency collaboration is vital if this is to be achieved. The case studies in Boxes 12.4 and 12.5 outline the importance of an occupational therapy input in cases of muscular dystrophy.

Box 12.4   Case study: Tejinder

Background
Tejinder is a 9-year-old boy with Duchenne muscular dystrophy. He has been known to the occupational therapy service since the age of 5 years, when he was diagnosed. His younger brother also has muscular dystrophy. Tejinder and his brother were different from other boys with muscular dystrophy that the therapist had known in that both were very unhappy, angry and probably frightened as opposed to passive and accepting.

Assessment
A person-centred approach using the COPM format, together with an understanding of the nature of the condition and expected developmental stages, guide continuous evaluation and intervention of Tejinder. Monitoring the changes in his occupational performance and physical condition showed that diminishing power and mobility led to priority being placed on self care and productivity areas (school participation) as these have been primarily affected by his diminishing functional mobility.

Functional mobility
Although Tejinder was finding it more difficult to walk and was at risk of falling, he refused to consider using a wheelchair. It was agreed that he would indicate when he was ready to try one. This caused the adults around him much concern but Tejinder's wishes were respected. When Tejinder reported in school that he did want to use a wheelchair, a self-propelling chair was provided as quickly as possible and a referral for assessment for powered mobility was made. He now has an electrically powered indoor outdoor chair (EPIOC) and is independently mobile around the school building and outside with his peers. He also uses the powered chair to go out with his family. Tejinder's progressive weakness meant that he was unable to rise to standing unaided or to sustain standing without support. To facilitate and maintain his occupational performance, and minimise restrictions on his capacity to participate in school activity, moving and handling issues were addressed.

Self care
It had been agreed that Tejinder would have access to a staff toilet at school, which was wheelchair accessible. A compact sit-to-stand-type hoist was recommended following assessment at school in which Tejinder took an active part. When the hoist was demonstrated to Tejinder he became very excited and exclaimed 'That's cool ... I want a go!'. He also agreed to see the hoist at home and is now happy to look at different options for helping himself and his mother. The situation will be monitored as his muscle weakness increases.

Productivity (school participation)
In school, Tejinder resisted most attempts to enable him to participate in learning activities and he would protest loudly and refuse to join in, to the consternation of his class teacher. The teacher had the opportunity to discuss the impact of Tejinder's progressive weakness on his learning, the role he played in class and his choice of coping strategies.

For classroom use, an adjustable height tilting top table has been recommended to allow easy access with the power chair and to encourage a stable and erect sitting posture.

Conclusion
Tejinder appears to be more settled now and he will volunteer to join in discussions about the help that he needs. He perhaps has less fear about the changes that are occurring in his life and is able to accept personal help and the use of practical equipment solutions. Information about changes in Tejinder's situation and indicators about the efficacy of the occupational therapy intervention will be gained using the COPM with Tejinder himself and his family and by collecting and synthesising information from the other agencies involved.

Box 12.5 Case study: Jeremy

Background

Jeremy lives with his parents and younger brother, his dog, cat, two birds and pet rats. He had been known to the occupational therapy service since he was 4 years old, when he was seen as part of a multidisciplinary team assessment arising from concerns about language delay and difficulty with walking. This led to a diagnosis of muscular dystrophy.

Medical situation

Now 15 years old, Jeremy is waiting for an admission date for spinal surgery to control further the deterioration of his trunk posture, pain and consequent increased risks of respiratory and cardiac dysfunction.

Mobility

Jeremy has an electrically powered indoor outdoor wheelchair (EPIOC) with a custom-produced support system that also provides a comfortable seat. This helps him make best use of his physical skills to facilitate occupational performance.

Jeremy's parents use a van-style vehicle so that Jeremy can travel in his chair. It has a ramp and winch to help load the wheelchair while Jeremy sits in it. This has facilitated his access to both school activities and social outings with his family. Having a modified vehicle at his disposal means he can elect to use carers to drive for him instead of having to rely on his parents.

Self care

Jeremy's home has an adapted downstairs bedroom with ensuite bathroom, comprising an Aquanova bath, track hoist and adjustable height sink unit and Closimat toilet. Jeremy also has an adjustable height multiposition bed and pressure sensitive mattress.

Identified priorities

Jeremy is fully aware of the imminent surgery and, while updating the therapist's understanding of his situation, has indicated that his primary needs are related to comfort in bed and use of his wheelchair so that he remains mobile postoperatively. His parents express concerns about the same issues and also their need to be able to care for their son after discharge home. They also want to find ways to offer Jeremy new interests and activities that will be suitable during the weeks following discharge and afterwards.

Assessment and review

The occupational therapist ensured the package of equipment and practical solutions already in situ were working effectively in order to maintain optimum occupational performance across all areas. Current moving and handling issues were also reviewed. Potential changes in Jeremy's physical capacity postoperatively are discussed and practical solutions identified. These comprised an adjustable over-bed table so that Jeremy could continue to access his electronic game (Game Boy) and achieve a good working position for his school work. Other agencies, including the wheelchair service and carer agencies, were informed of the pending admission for surgery.

Conclusion

Keeping the main priorities for Jeremy and his family central to the work undertaken, it was possible to interweave biomechanical information relating to the forthcoming surgery with a sensitive response and proactive support to enable both Jeremy and his family to cope with the ordeal of spinal surgery and life at home afterwards.

REFERENCES

Bakker E, van Ommen GJB 1998 Duchenne and Becker muscular dystrophy. In: Emery AEH (ed) Neuromuscular disorders: clinical and molecular genetics, Wiley, Chichester, ch 3, p60

Beckmann JS, Fardeau M 1998 Limb girdle muscular dystrophy. In: Emery AEH (ed) Neuromuscular disorders: clinical and molecular genetics, Wiley, Chichester, ch 6, p133

Brookes DN, McKinley W 1983 Personality and behavioural change after severe blunt head injury – a relative's view. Journal of Neurology, Neurosurgery and Psychiatry 46:336–344

Brown GJ 1996 The parent's experience of learning about their child. Master's dissertation, University of East London

Brown SM, Humphry R, Taylor E 1996 A model of the nature of family – therapist relationships: implications for education. American Journal of Occupational Therapy 51(7):597–603

Canadian Association of Occupational Therapists 1991 Occupational therapy guidelines for client centred practice. CAOT Publications ACE, Toronto

Cohen S 1983 A global measure of perceived stress. Journal of Health and Social Behaviour 24:385–396

Colangelo CA 1993 Biomechanical frame of reference. In: Hinojosa J, Kramer P (eds) Frames of reference for pediatric occupational therapy. Williams & Wilkins, Baltimore, MD, ch 8, p 233

Coster W, Deeney T, Haltiwanger J, Haley S 1998 School function assessment. The Psychological Corporation, Harcourt Brace & Company: San Antonio, CA

Dale N 1996 Working with families of children with special needs – partnership and practice. Routledge, London

Eakin P, Baird H 1995 The Community Dependency Index. British Journal Of Occupational Therapy 58(1):17–22

Emery AEH 1998 Neuromuscular disorders: clinical and molecular genetics. John Wiley, Chichester

Featherstone H 1980 A difference in the family. Basic Books, New York

Fisher AG 1997 Assessment of motor and process skills, 2nd edn. Three Star Press, Fort Collins, CO

Fisher AG, Bryze K 1997 School AMPS: school version of the Assessment of Motor and Process Skills. Three Star Press, Fort Collins, CO

Haley S, Coster W, Ludlow L, Haltiwanger J, Andrellos P 1992 Pediatric Evaluation of Disability Inventory (PEDI). New England Medical Center Hospitals, Boston, MA

Harpin P 1999 Adaptation manual. Muscular Dystrophy Campaign, London

Hinojosa J, Kramer P, Pratt PN 1996 Foundations of practice: development principles, theories, and frames of reference. In: Case-Smith J, Allen AS, Pratt PN. Occupational therapy for children. Mosby, St Louis, ch 3, pp25–44

Lachina K 2000 All students can participate: including students with disabilities in the classroom. OT Practice March 27:18–25

Law M, Baptiste S, Carswell A, McColl MA, Polatajko H, Pollock N 1994 Canadian Occupational Performance Measure (COPM), 2nd edn. The Canadian Association of Occupational Therapists, Toronto

McConachie H 1994 Implications of a model of stress and coping for services to families of young disabled children. Child Care Health and Development 20:37–46

Muscular Dystrophy Campaign 1999 online available http://www.muscular-dystrophy.org

Olson L 1993 Psychosocial frame of reference. In: Hinojosa J, Kramer P (eds) Frames of reference for pediatric occupational therapy. Williams & Wilkins, Baltimore, MD

Peganoff O'Brien S 1993 Human occupation frame of reference. In: Hinojosa J, Kramer P (eds) Frames of reference for pediatric occupational therapy. Williams & Wilkins, Baltimore, MD, ch 9, p 307

Pountrey TE, Mulealy CM, Clarke SM, Green EM 2000 The charley heritage approach to postural management. Active Design Ltd, Birmingham

Robinson BC 1983 Validation of a caregiver strain index. Journal of Gerontology 38(3):344–348

Seligman M, Darling RB 1989 Ordinary families, special children: a systems approach to childhood disability. The Guildford Press, New York

Stewart S, Nyerlin-Beale J 2000 The impact of community paediatric occupational therapy on children with disabilities and their carers. British Journal of Occupational Therapy 63(8):373–379

Tuckett J 1998 Duchenne muscular dystrophy schedule of occupational therapy input. National Association of Paediatric Occupational Therapists Journal, summer, p14

Williamson GG, Szczepanski M, Zeitlin S 1993 Coping frame of reference. In: Hinojosa J, Kramer P (eds) Frames of reference for pediatric occupational therapy. Williams & Wilkins, Baltimore, MD

USEFUL CONTACTS

Muscular Dystrophy Campaign 7–11 Prescott Place, London SW4 6BS. Tel: 0207 498 0670, www.muscular-dystrophy.org

Advisory Centre for Education www.ace-ed.org.uk
Inclusion website http://inclsion.ngfl.gov.uk

13

Burns

Rosie Gollop

INTRODUCTION

Burn injuries account for approximately 15 000 admissions to hospital and 900 deaths each year. Because of the diversity of ways in which burns can be sustained, all age groups in all sectors of society are at risk. Accidents that result in burns occur within the home, at the workplace, during leisure activities and whilst travelling, and the consequences for the individual are as varied as the causes. The effects of a burn injury upon the individual and his family can be devastating, and successful management and treatment poses many challenges to the occupational therapist, and indeed all members of the burns team.

This chapter will begin by considering the nature of burn injuries, their incidence and their effects on the individual. The role of the many disciplines involved in burns care will be discussed. The theoretical approaches used in the treatment of burn injuries will be outlined, followed by a more detailed explanation of the interventions of the occupational therapist at varying stages of recovery.

Although burn injuries, being mostly unpredictable and acute in nature, can affect anyone, certain gender- and age-related patterns can be defined. In almost all age groups the incidence of burns is greater in males than in females. There is much debate about the reasons for this and a fuller understanding could helpfully inform health promotion campaigns within burn prevention programmes. A simple, and some might argue simplistic, explanation might point towards a tendency for males to engage in more risk-taking behaviour than females, whether at home, work or leisure. However, the many factors, both random and predictable, that combine to result in a burn injury, cannot simply be explained a single theory. What is known is that the majority of burn accidents occur within the home situation and that some, such as scalds in young children, occur almost exclusively within the home. Most fatal burns also occur at home; only 10% of fatal and 18% of non-fatal fire injuries occur in buildings such as factories, hotels, clubs and restaurants. Accidents involving cooking appliances account for 35% of all home fires and 27% of non-fatal and 6% of fatal burns. Smoking-related injuries involving matches, cigarettes, cigars and pipe ash are responsible for an even greater number of casualties; 28% of non-fatal and 39% of fatal injuries. Although the popularity of open fires within homes has declined, burns from gas and electric fires and central heating radiators still account for a significant number of injuries; 13% of non-fatal and 19% of fatal burns (Kemble & Lamb 1987).

Age-related causes of burns follow an identifiable pattern, particularly so in the very young and elderly. Under the age of three, the most common type of burn is the scald injury, frequently occurring in the kitchen or the bathroom. The peak incidence within this age group is between 1 and 2 years, when babies become more mobile and curious, and yet possess a poorly developed sense of danger. The figures in Table 13.1, from one of the United Kingdom's subregional burns units, illustrate the size of the problem.

Table 13.1 Burns and scalds sustained by all age groups

	Total number of burns		Total number of scalds	
	1997	1998	1997	1998
Inpatients	333	288	130	112
Outpatients	305	384	107	218

Within the same unit, the under-5s accounted for approximately 35% of all inpatient admissions in 1997 and 24% in 1998.

Older children sustain burns in a variety of ways, often whilst engaged in unsupervised activities involving, for example, matches, petrol, cooking, plugs and electrical appliances, fireworks and bonfires. House fires, which may involve several members of the same family, frequently involve children of all ages.

From 15 to 60 years of age workplace and road traffic accidents are a major cause of burns, whilst after 60, the effects of ageing, particularly of a decline in mobility and cognition, lead to a significant number of injuries (Dyer & Roberts 1990). Throughout the adult population the abuse of alcohol is a notable factor in the cause of burn injuries. Assaults, injuries involving neglect and self-inflicted injuries constitute a small but important number of burns.

The nature of the burn, and the situation in which it was sustained, is important to the occupational therapist, not only for the information it provides about the individual's background and medical history but also because it may influence the timing and nature of interventions during rehabilitation. This will be examined in more depth later.

The trauma of a burn injury can impact upon the individual's life physically, psychologically and socially. These effects may persist for many months or years after the injury. Noyes et al (1971) have stated that to be severely burned is a devastating experience both physically and emotionally and that the individual may experience extreme psychological reactions that compound physical recovery. The incidence and severity of reactions does not necessarily relate to the severity of the burn, however, but may be connected to other factors such as the individual's own coping mechanisms or their preburn level of activity. For example, a person with a relatively small burn could develop post-traumatic stress disorder that is quite disabling and prevents a return to work.

CLASSIFICATION OF BURNS

The numerous types of burn injury may be classified in the following way:

- Scald – any hot fluid, including hot oil or steam

- Flame – The ignition of clothing from matches or fires, or as a result of explosions
- Flash – the momentary exposure of skin to very high temperatures; often associated with flame burns
- Chemical – includes acids/alkalis in domestic or industrial situations, for example, soda crystals, oven cleaners, cement, industrial cleaning fluids
- Electrical – low voltage, for example, domestic electrical appliances; high voltage, for example, overhead and underground cabling
- Contact – hot metals, for example, oven doors, irons, industrial metals, bitumen. Prolonged contact with extreme cold, for example, frostbite
- Friction – shearing of skin against another surface, usually at high speed, for example, in road traffic accidents
- Inhalation – of smoke or hot gases, often occurring in house fires or explosions
- Radiation – prolonged exposure to sunlight or sunbeds; accidents involving nuclear materials.

DEPTH OF BURN

The depth of injury depends not only on the intensity of the burning agent but also on the time with which it is in contact with the skin. Burn depth is described in Table 13.2.

THE PHYSICAL, PSYCHOLOGICAL AND PSYCHOSOCIAL EFFECTS OF BURNS

The immediate physical effects of a burn injury are not detailed here but can include local and systemic pathologies that, in combination, may be life threatening. Briefly, they include respiratory damage, fluid loss leading to 'burns shock', renal failure, infection, electrolyte imbalance, gastrointestinal ulceration, toxic shock syndrome and burns encephalopathy (Wilson 1997).

The later effects of a burn injury are outlined in Boxes 13.1 and 13.2.

Table 13.2 Depth of burn

Depth of burn	Effect
Superficial	Involves surface epithelium Mildly painful Skin remains intact Heals within a few days
Superficial partial thickness	Involves deeper layers of epidermis or upper layers of dermis Hair follicles, sweat and sebaceous glands spared Painful Heals within 7–10 days
Deep partial thickness	Destruction of epidermis and upper layers of dermis Painful Heals within 3–4 weeks without grafting; cosmesis improved by grafting
Full thickness	Destruction of epidermis and dermis, hair follicles, sweat and sebaceous glands, possibly also of soft tissue and bone Painless Healed by skin grafting

---

Box 13.1 Physical effects of a burn

- Scarring of the skin, and skin fragility
- Contractures of soft tissues and joints
- Amputation of digits, limbs or other body parts
- Visual impairment
- Pain
- Hypersensitivity to extremes of temperature
- Loss of normal body contours
- Impairment of hand function

Box 13.2 Psychological and psychosocial effects of burns

- Denial
- Withdrawal
- Anxiety
- Grief
- Insomnia
- Dependence
- Regression
- Anger/hostility
- Depression
- Isolation
- Alteration of body image
- Guilt

The extent to which an individual experiences psychosocial problems varies enormously. Ward at al (1987) suggested that in burn trauma it is more often the person rather than the injury that determines the emotional prognosis. There is also some evidence to suggest that the incidence of burns is higher in families where there are greater levels of marital disharmony, unemployment, poverty, or a recent history of physical or psychological illness (Cresci 1982, Kolman 1983). The presence or absence of a supportive family can affect recovery significantly, as can the skills of the clinical team.

STAGES OF RECOVERY

The physical and psychosocial difficulties outlined above are not all encountered at the same time; as recovery proceeds the individual passes through a number of stages, each of which brings its own challenges to full rehabilitation. Cresci (1982) and Price (1990) describe the recovery from a burn in three phases: the shock phase, an intermediate/healing phase and a rehabilitative phase. These relate largely to the individual with a major burn, that is, greater than 20% of the total body surface area (TBSA), although individuals with smaller percentage burns may pass through similar stages more quickly.

Shock phase

During this phase, the first 48–72 hours postinjury, the individual is acutely unwell. After an initial period of lucidity, the person may become disorientated or may be sedated or unconscious. Treatment is aimed at supporting the functioning of vital body organs and maintaining fluid and electrolyte balance. If the burn is full thickness it will be initially painless, as nerve endings will have been destroyed. If the individual is conscious he may be anxious, agitated or in denial. There is often little insight into the severity of the burn at this stage and it is not unusual for an individual to talk of the need to return to work within a few days, when in fact they are many months away from such a possibility. Skin grafting procedures are usually started as soon as the person's overall condition is stable; depending on the extent of the injury, grafting may be completed within one or two operating sessions, or may take many weeks. Early debridement (surgical removal of dead skin) and grafting closes the burn wound and minimises the risk of infection. It also reduces the severity of subsequent scarring.

Intermediate/healing phase

During the 2–6 weeks after the end of the shock phase, the individual's overall condition usually stabilises. Wound management continues in the form of dressings or further skin grafting, or both. Investigation of other body systems may take place at this time. For example, a person who was burnt as a result of poorly controlled epilepsy may be investigated by a neurologist in an attempt to prevent a recurrence of the accident. There may have been other injuries sustained at the time of the burn, for example, fractures or a head injury, and management of these may now take precedence.

Rehabilitation usually commences at this stage, although it may be hampered at first by limited mobility, general debilitation and pain. The start of rehabilitation may make the individual more aware of his loss of independence. If the injury is severe there will be a growing awareness of the likely length of the process. There may be feelings of anxiety, outbursts of anger directed towards the care team or feelings of loss, guilt, grief and despair. This can be a difficult time for the individual and a challenging one for those caring for him.

Rehabilitative phase

This frequently extends beyond discharge from hospital and may continue for many months. As independence increases, the individual may need to adapt to a permanently altered status, such as the presence of disfiguring scarring or the loss of a limb. There is also a psychological and social independence to be gained, for it is not unusual for the person to have become quite dependent on the clinical team whilst in hospital. The prospect of returning home and resuming preburn activities can provoke considerable anxiety. There may have been a change of roles within the family structure and a loss of status and authority if a return to work is not possible. If the accident is subject to a police investigation, compensation or insurance claim, this can complicate the rehabilitation process. The late presentation of features such as post-traumatic stress disorder, which can manifest itself long after the physical signs of injury have faded, can catch the individual off guard and cause renewed suffering and anxiety. Even a successful return to work or school does not necessarily mark the end of rehabilitation, for some individuals continue to require surgical interventions, practical advice and emotional support for long periods of time.

Cultural differences

Through all the phases of treatment and recovery, the approach of professionals must be tailored to the needs, beliefs and values of the individual. This is particularly important for individuals and families from ethnic minority groups, whose cultural values may not be widely known or understood by the majority population.

Burn injuries can lead to pigment changes in the skin of people of Asian or African origin. Loss of pigment (hypopigmentation) can occur in areas of partial thickness burn that are not deep enough to require grafting. Sometimes this is a permanent loss, and this often causes a great deal of distress. Cosmetic camouflage can sometimes be very helpful in these instances. People with black skin may also develop increased pigmentation (hyperpigmentation) in grafted areas and this, combined with the fact that black skin tends to develop keloid scarring more readily, is a factor that requires sensitive handling in scar management.

THE INTERVENTION TEAM

Close teamworking is recognised as essential in the management of burn injuries (Leveridge 1991). The complex nature of the individual's needs requires the expertise of many disciplines working towards common goals. Whilst each team member has a specific role to play, there is often some overlap and blurring of boundaries and professionals are likely to vary slightly in the roles adopted within each team. The individual with a burn injury may be treated in a number of environments: accident and emergency depart-

ment, intensive therapy unit, specialised burns unit or general ward. The following description of the roles of team members relates to the disciplines most likely to be involved in a specialised burns unit. The occupational therapist is not included at this stage because it is discussed in detail later in the chapter.

- The **plastic surgeon** usually heads the team and has overall responsibility for the medical and surgical treatment of the burned individual. The surgeon performs primary grafting procedures and secondary contracture release and reconstructive surgery as required. After discharge from inpatient care, the individual's progress is reviewed by the plastic surgeon at regular outpatient clinics.
- The **anaesthetist** is not only responsible for anaesthesia during surgery and major wound care procedures (such as dressings changes) but also coordinates the management of inhalation injuries and advises on pain control.
- The **nurse** provides critical care, wound care and assists in rehabilitation. The role also involves supporting the individual and relatives during the emotional consequences of the injury and coordinating the work of the team during the period of inpatient care.
- The **physiotherapist** has a role in treating the individual with an inhalation burn injury, both by maintaining a clear airway during ventilation and in encouraging coughing and expectoration during recovery. As rehabilitation proceeds, the physiotherapist takes responsibility for range of movement exercises to prevent contracture development, for lower limb mobilising, including stairs assessment and for prescribing gym activities aimed at improving muscle power and tolerance. The roles of the physiotherapist, nurse and occupational therapist may overlap (Bach et al 1984) and it is important that they develop close working relationships with mutually agreed objectives.
- The **dietician** provides nutritional advice and support to the team and the burned individual. Burn injuries impose unique metabolic demands upon the body (Norman 1997) and skilled nutritional management is vital to the healing process.

The dietician assesses the nutritional requirements, plans the dietary regimens and monitors the adequacy of the nutrients provided.

• The **social worker** may have a role to play in addressing the emotional needs of the individual but is also responsible for more practical problem solving, relating to financial and housing difficulties. The social worker often works closely with the occupational therapist in planning a package of support and care for discharge. In situations where abuse or neglect is suspected, both in adults and children, the social worker has a responsibility (statutory in the case of children) to investigate, and to liaise with community agencies, including police and magistrates, as required.

• The **psychologist's** role is in assessing the psychological wellbeing of the individual, and working with him, and frequently the family, to restore psychological wellbeing. The psychologist takes the lead in managing specific problems that threaten to impede recovery, such as sleep disorders, flashbacks, unresolved feelings of guilt and problems associated with altered body image. The psychologist may assess and treat symptoms of post-traumatic stress disorder, working closely with other members of the team. Additionally, some burns teams are fortunate in having the services of a psychologist in providing staff support.

To this list should be added the skills of the hospital teacher, nursery nurse, paediatric community liaison nurse and cosmetic camouflage practitioner (often a trained volunteer with the Red Cross, which has a long history of involvement in this field). When the individual is discharged into the community, the number of professionals involved is likely to increase still further: the general practitioner, district nurse, health visitor, school staff and social services staff may all have a role to play. The diverse nature of the burns intervention team is illustrated in Figure 13.1.

This section would not be complete without acknowledging the importance of the individual's family throughout treatment and rehabilitation. The family can play a crucial role throughout the whole process. In the treatment of children in particular there is much evidence to support the importance of parents participating in care (Campbell et al 1993, Woodward 1968). However, family members have their own needs and con-

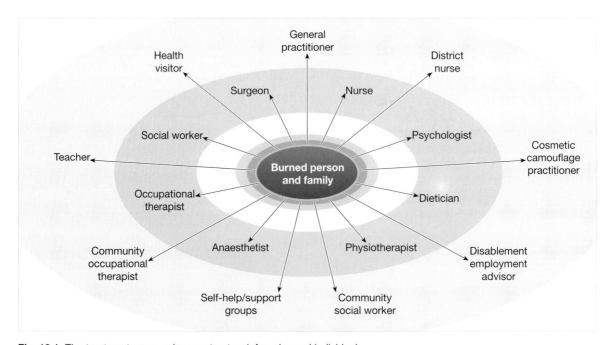

Fig. 13.1 The treatment, care and support network for a burned individual.

cerns and these must be recognised by all team members. The shock of the accident, a sudden role reversal, feelings of guilt and anxiety about the future can all conspire to overwhelm family members in the early days after the injury. Staff should work to build a rapport with families that aims to establish a feeling of support for the burned person and feelings of usefulness and control for the family (Boyle 1997).

THE ROLE OF THE OCCUPATIONAL THERAPIST

THEORETICAL FOUNDATIONS FOR INTERVENTION

The therapist's approach to treatment is essentially humanistic or client-centred. Interventions must be developed in partnership with the individual and often with the family. In the early stages of treatment, a compensatory approach is frequently indicated, with the use of adaptive equipment to aid independence. Such an approach may be used in the long term if there is significant residual impairment or in the prescription of cosmetic camouflage. The use of graded remedial activities to improve strength and tolerance, scar management techniques and the fabrication of orthoses all employ a biomechanical approach to treatment. If the individual is a child, an awareness of the normal stages of development is important, for children may

regress temporarily after sustaining a burn injury and the therapist needs to be able to suggest age-appropriate play activities. A developmental approach is thus required for such circumstances. Finally, a cognitive/behavioural approach is indicated in considering the individual's attitudes to and understanding of their injury, and in helping in the development of coping and problem-solving strategies, encouraging assertive behaviour and in goal setting. A summary of the frames of reference and approaches used in burns treatment is included in Table 13.3.

INTERVENTIONS

Therapists face many challenges in treating individuals with burn injuries. As has been described, burns do not affect a particular sector of society, nor do they follow a predictable pattern of physical or psychological impairment. Treatment may be directed towards a toddler or an octogenarian, and may constitute a single session or a programme spanning several years. The overriding problem may be physical, social or psychological, or a mixture of all three. It is not unusual for different problem areas to assume greater or lesser significance at different times during the treatment period. All of these factors require the therapist to utilise a variety of theoretical frameworks and approaches during treatment. Perhaps the most important is for the approach to be both phenomenological, or client-centred, and interactive. This ensures that the individual's needs

Table 13.3 Frames of reference and interventions

Frame of reference	Phenomenological	Biomechanical	Compensatory	Learning	Developmental
Approach	Humanistic Client-centred	Biomechanical	Rehabilitative	Cognitive/behavioural	Developmental
Techniques	Counselling Person-centred Respecting individuals' hierarchy of needs	Orthoses Pressure therapy Graded remedial programmes	Adapted tools and equipment Alternative activities and techniques Environmental modifications Support from carers	Advice/education Developing coping strategies Problem solving Reasoning Goal setting	Age/stage-appropriate activities

are identified and addressed as effectively as possible and reflects the core purpose of occupational therapy as being 'enabling, empowering and enhancing' (Hagedorn 1995).

The overall aims of occupational therapy interventions in burn management are to:

- maximise function and minimise disability
- promote a return to community and employment
- improve cosmesis
- minimise psychological dysfunction
- educate and inform.

The interventions most commonly used in burns occupational therapy, and the theoretical approaches that guide them, will be examined in some detail. They are:

- prevention of contractures
- functional rehabilitation
- remedial activities, including work assessment
- scar management
- psychological support and treatment
- education.

Prevention of contractures

Soft tissue and joint contractures can occur at any time after a burn injury. Most burns units in the United Kingdom have now adopted a policy of early surgical intervention to heal wounds, so it is less likely that contractures will develop in the early days. As the skin heals, elements within the scar tissue exert a contractual force, restricting range of movement at and around joints and causing functional problems. Contractures initially involve soft tissues only and are correctable but, if left untreated, can involve the mechanism of the joint and become permanent. Certain factors are thought to contribute, these include:

- rapid development of scarring after healing
- reluctance of the person to engage in full range of motion exercises and activities, often because of pain
- inadequate monitoring after discharge; contractures can develop very quickly in immature scar tissue.

Prevention and management of contractures requires the combined approach of the physiotherapist and occupational therapist. The occupational therapist may adopt a biomechanical approach, using custom-made or commercial orthoses to maintain the joint in a corrected position. The use of orthoses in all phases of burn care is well documented and they are used to prevent the adoption of poor postures in the acute phase, to prevent contracture development during healing and to maintain range of movement after contracture release (Bhattacharya et al 1991, Fowler 1987, Leman 1992). If a contracture already exists, an orthosis may need to be applied serially in order to gain a gradual lengthening of fibres. Certain areas of the body are commonly affected:

- first web space of the hand (Fig. 13.2)
- anterior neck (Fig. 13.3)
- axilla
- elbow (Fig. 13.4)
- interphalangeal joints of the little finger
- knee (Fig. 13.5)
- planes of the face (Figs 13.6 and 13.7)
- oral commissures of the mouth (Fig. 13.8).

Orthoses can be particularly difficult for individuals to wear; they may complain of them being hot or restrictive, particularly if worn over pressure garments, and the therapist needs to offer support and encouragement during the period of usage, which may be up to 6 months. Frequent monitoring is required to check fit, skin condition and to make adjustments as necessary. Orthoses are commonly worn at night or

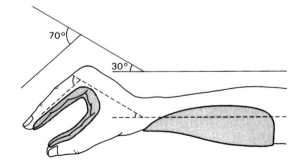

Fig. 13.2 Optimum position for the wrist and hand to prevent contracture.

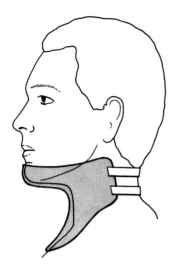

Fig. 13.3 Neck support position.

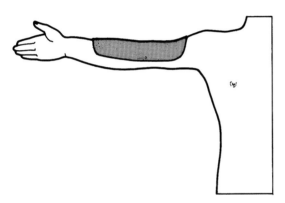

Fig. 13.4 Elbow orthoses. Gutter support.

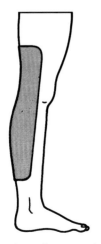

Fig. 13.5 Knee extension gutter support.

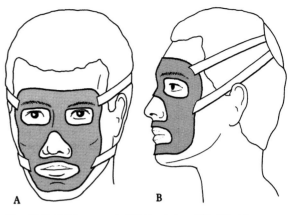

Fig. 13.6 Full face mask. (A) Front view, (B) side view.

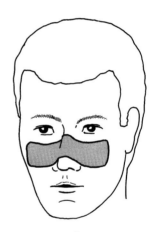

Fig. 13.7 Nose pressure conformer.

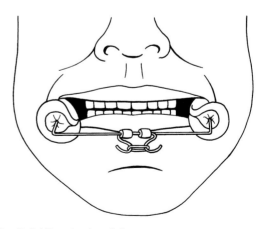

Fig. 13.8 Microstomia splint.

during periods of rest and the person is encouraged to use the affected part functionally at other times.

Functional rehabilitation

This includes activities of personal and domestic daily living and, within the context of burns rehabilitation, may also include wheelchair assessment and home visits. In practice, the burns therapist may find that these activities constitute a relatively small part of case management, as the majority of individuals admitted to the burns unit will have sustained quite small percentage burns that do not seriously impede their ability to self care. However, some circumstances are more likely to require occupational therapy intervention:

- those with major burns, that is, more than 20% of the surface area of the body, or burns affecting the hands in particular
- those whose burns have resulted in surgical amputations
- the very elderly, especially those who live alone
- those with pre-existing medical problems, for example, dementia, multiple sclerosis
- those who have sustained other injuries at the time of the accident, for example, fractures.

There are no standardised ADL assessments specific to burns and therapists must choose an assessment procedure that suits their own needs and fits within the philosophy of their department. The approach for these interventions, which aim to effect the individual's safe discharge from hospital and maximise independence, is both rehabilitative and compensatory. Not everyone will regain full independence and some individuals will return home with a significant degree of disability, whether temporary or permanent. The approach must also be strongly person-centred, with the therapist being sensitive to the potential difficulties of the individual. An example of this might be when undertaking a dressing practice; the person may not yet have wanted or had the opportunity to look in the mirror for the first time after their burn. If the burns are to the face, this is likely to be a difficult occasion, which should not be allowed to happen accidentally. Other points to take into consideration when undertaking functional rehabilitation activities include:

- Individuals with burns to the lower limbs are often unable to tolerate standing for anything more than short periods. Standing still during kitchen assessments, for example, is best avoided, although walking is to be encouraged.
- A routine kitchen or bath assessment may provoke flashbacks and panic attacks; ask how the individual feels about entering an area similar to where the accident occurred.
- A home visit may be a traumatising experience for the same reason; the house may have been fire damaged or returning home may simply prove too strong a reminder of the accident.
- If the individual has a wound infection, any equipment or assistive devices that are loaned by the ward will be subject to infection control procedures. Some infections demand barrier nursing and the therapist should be aware of ward policy in respect of this before beginning any intervention.
- As most burns units are responsible for large geographical and population areas, individuals may be transferred to local hospitals closer to home during the rehabilitative period. Close liaison with other therapists is vital to ensuring the continuation of assessment and treatment.

Remedial activities

As rehabilitation proceeds and the individual is able to leave the ward, attendance at occupational therapy workshops may be appropriate and may continue after discharge from hospital. Children usually perform their own remedial activities through normal play, but occasionally show an initial reluctance to use a hand that has been burned; this rarely persists as a long-term problem. Remedial activities in adults can be used to:

• Promote socialisation and reintegration – the workshop can provide a 'halfway house' between the security of the burns unit and the uncertainties of the outside world. Individuals have the opportunity to 'rehearse' their telling of the injury and gauge other people's reactions; not everyone wishes to elaborate on the circumstances of the injury and this may be their first encounter with people other than supportive family and burns staff.

• Improve biomechanical functioning and encourage normal patterns of movement – emphasis is placed on aspects such as manual dexterity, grip, range of movement at specific joints, the adoption of compensatory postures and overall strength and tolerance.

• Prepare the individual for a return to work – this can be achieved through replicating as far as possible the demands of a working day or of the nature of the tasks required by the work environment. If such replication is beyond the scope of the hospital workshop, the individual may be better served by referral to a specialised rehabilitation centre.

The principles of remedial activities require both biomechanical and phenomenological approaches. The individual may be self-conscious about mixing with other people, concerned about possible damage to newly healed skin or anxious about pain and, for these reasons, the therapist's desire to improve physical function must be tempered by an appreciation of the individual's own concerns.

Further research is required to substantiate the effectiveness of remedial activities in burn rehabilitation. The documentation and analysis of interventions and the use of reliable outcome measures will further the evidence base of occupational therapists' experiences of the utilisation of specific activities and occupations.

Scar management

The development of thickened scarring – known as hypertrophic scarring – is an all too common feature of the rehabilitative phase of treatment. It has the potential to cause much disfigurement, deformity and distress. As its management is often the concern of the occupational therapist, its nature and causes will be described in some detail.

Newly healed skin grafts are initially flat and soft to touch but undergo a rapid change in the first few weeks and months. Typically, they are at their worst 3–6 months after healing. During the active phase of their development the scar tissue is termed immature, and is characterised by being red or purplish in colour, raised and hard, and with a tendency to contract and form into tight bands. Affected individuals frequently complain that the scars are extremely itchy (pruritic). Over the ensuing 6–18 months the scars mature and gradually become paler and softer, although they may remain lumpy to some extent. Factors influencing the development of scarring include age (children and adolescents tend to scar more than adults), race, heredity, location of the burn and type of graft. Much depends on the healing time and on whether or not the burn was grafted; a longer healing time is more likely to lead to a thickened scar.

The mechanism of scar formation is not fully understood but has been the subject of extensive research. In reviewing the literature Scott Ward (1991) describes the process as 'excessive wound repair … typified by overabundant collagen deposition'. The body's response of inflammation leads to increased vascularisation of the wound and a migration of fibroblasts. These fibroblasts synthesise excessive collagen, which is deposited in bundles within the scar tissue. Some of the fibroblasts possess contractile properties and are known as myofibroblasts.

Although the management of hypertrophic burn scarring is often the responsibility of the occupational therapist, working closely with the surgeon, physiotherapists or nursing staff sometimes assume this role. In considering scar management as an occupational therapy intervention it is important to view its effect on the individual as a whole, rather than in a purely biomechanical frame. The presence of scarring, whether or not it affects an area normally exposed, can impact upon social and psychological functioning, as well as on physical functioning. In this respect it is an intervention well suited to the skills and expertise of the occupational therapist. The approaches are therefore not only biomechanical and compensatory, but also phenomenological. Gaining the commitment of the individual is crucial. The therapist can advise, prescribe, inform, counsel and support, but it is the individual who must ultimately decide whether the results achieved by treatment are worth the efforts.

Even the most rigorously followed programme of treatment will not remove scars altogether. Although residual scarring is often minimal and it may be difficult to see where the graft was placed, sometimes the skin remains lumpy, texturally different to adjacent skin, and with altered pigmentation. Black skin that has been grafted often remains hyperpigmented. The textural effect produced by meshed grafts also sometimes persists even when the scar is mature. The therapist, in assessing scar progress, must be sensitive to the individual's feelings regarding cosmesis and offer emotional support and realistic information about the likely outcome of treatment.

In addition to the use of orthoses, described earlier, the treatments available to the therapist in managing hypertrophic scarring are:

- pressure therapy
- massage with emollient creams
- silicone gels
- zinc oxide tape.

Pressure therapy

Pressure has been recognised as having a beneficial effect on maturing scar tissue since the early 1970s, when research by Larson (1971) and others in the United States led to the development of custom-made pressure garments. Pressure therapy remains the mainstay of burn scar management today, in spite of limited research evidence regarding its mechanism. It is thought to effect a realignment of the collagen bundles and may control collagen synthesis by producing a local tissue hypoxia (Johnson 1984).

Early guidelines (Dietch et al 1983) recommended that pressure should be used for any wounds taking more than 14 days to heal, or that has been skin grafted. Pressure exerted by garments should theoretically approximate capillary pressure, that is 25 mmHg (Scott Ward 1991) but a study by Giele et al (1997) in Australia demonstrated that, in practice, pressure garments generate an increase in subdermal pressures of anything between 9 and 90 mmHg, depending on the anatomical site involved.

To be effective, the application of pressure must be continuous, garments only being removed for bathing and massage. Pressure over areas of natural concavity, such as the palm or the clavicular region, can be augmented by the use of inserts or pads made from foam sponge, thermoplastics or elastomers. Care needs to be taken in applying pressure to newly healed grafts, as the scar epithelium is initially quite fragile and the donning or removal of garments can contribute to scar breakdown. In the United Kingdom, made-to-measure pressure garments are available from a number of commercial suppliers, and some occupational therapy departments fabricate their own.

The subject of pressure therapy may be introduced by the therapist or nursing staff while the individual is still in hospital. If there is a self-help or support group, members may visit the ward to share their experiences. If grafting has been extensive, assessment for garments commonly proceeds over several weeks as the various grafted areas heal. For smaller grafts, assessment, measuring and fitting can all be accomplished within a week of healing.

Continued assessment of the fit of garments, the progress of scarring and the individual's feelings about treatment is essential, and monitoring intervals should be discussed at the outset. Children are likely to require more frequent checks because of growth but it is important to remain flexible about follow-up arrangements so that individuals know they can obtain advice and assistance at any time during the treatment. The emphasis throughout is on partnership and easily accessed information. Written information, developed and evaluated with service users, should be offered to supplement verbal information.

People generally tolerate wearing their pressure garments well and very young children appear to view them just as another item of clothing. Users report that they can see the beneficial effects from an early stage and sometimes say that pressure helps to reduce itching. Most complaints arise during periods of hot weather, when use of an electric fan and frequent cool baths are recommended. Occasionally, people are reluctant to leave their garments off when scars are mature, and may need further support in order to do so.

Massage

The sebaceous glands that lubricate normal skin are destroyed in deep partial thickness and full thickness burns. As split skin grafts contain no sebaceous glands, grafted skin is liable to dryness and inelasticity, especially in the early months, and must be rehydrated with topical emollients. There is insufficient research evidence to indicate which type of cream is most effective; in the United Kingdom water-based creams are often prescribed, whereas in other countries lanolin-based preparations are preferred. Creams containing cocoa butter, aloe vera and vitamin E are favoured by some therapists.

Massage is used in conjunction with pressure therapy. As soon as the skin is healed the therapist teaches the individual to massage the scars, gently at first, but with more vigour as the skin gains strength. Creams are applied at least three times a day during the period of scar maturation. Some natural skin lipids are produced by the epidermis and the grafted skin sometimes regains enough lubrication for creams to be left off eventually (Poh-Fitzpatrick 1992).

Silicone gels

Silicone preparations, in the form of gel sheets and oils, are chemically inert materials that have been shown to have beneficial effects on hypertrophic scars. Australian clinicians first described the use of silicone gel in 1982 as an adjunct to pressure therapy, and later research (Ahn et al 1991, Quinn 1987) demonstrated a softening and increased elasticity in scar tissue. The mode of action is still the subject of research but it is thought to be due to hydration, not pressure.

In practice, silicone gels are a relatively inexpensive and simple method of treating healed burn scars. They can be used as an alternative or as an adjunct to pressure therapy, and to line orthoses, as an aid to stretching skin contractures.

Zinc oxide tape

Adhesive zinc oxide tape, applied directly to the healed scar, has been shown to decrease itching and reduce the size of hypertrophic scars, although the body of research evidence in its favour is not great (Soderberg et al 1982). In clinical practice, some individuals find it effective and, for the therapist, it is an inexpensive alternative to silicone for managing small scars.

It is the therapist's responsibility to assess each individual's needs in respect of the most suitable scar treatment. A combination of methods may be chosen, or treatments may change as scars mature. In the absence of firm evidence in favour of one method over another, a full explanation of the practicalities of each can help individuals to be involved with therapists in the decision-making process.

Psychological support and treatment

The extent to which the therapist becomes involved with psychological aspects of recovery depend on personal levels of expertise, the nature of the problem and the roles of other members of the team. Hagedorn (1995) contends that formal counselling is a highly skilled process that occupational therapists should not attempt without appropriate additional qualifications. Informal counselling, however, involves the basic skills that therapists possess and use daily during all types of intervention. A session aimed principally at improving work tolerance, for example, may provide the setting where the individual feels comfortable enough to discuss sleep or relationship problems. The therapist needs to remain alert to cues that indicate that emotional needs require attention. Psychological problems can develop at any stage, and sometimes long after physical scars have healed. It is not unknown for distressing symptoms such as flashbacks and panic attacks to start up to 2 years after the burn injury.

Working principally in a 'physical' setting, the therapist may not feel sufficiently skilled to deal with psychological issues and the recognition of one's own limitations is crucial. All therapists, however, should develop an awareness and understanding of the emotional and psychological difficulties likely to be experienced after burn injuries and should be able to offer support, to listen and to recognise when specialist help is required. For people with visible scarring in particular, returning to situations that will bring them into contact with the general public may be particularly stressful. They may feel accepted by close family members and by the burns team, but the prospect of returning to work, or even of going shopping or engaging in social activities outside the home, can be a source of real anxiety. Relaxation, role play and assertion training are all interventions that may be utilised to good effect in these situations.

Specific, and potentially very disabling, conditions such as post-traumatic stress disorder (PTSD) require a skilled approach (Box 13.3) Clarke (1999) describes therapists' use of purposeful activity, the therapeutic 'use of self' and counselling in the treatment of PTSD, and argues for collaborative practice with other professionals. Regel (1997) describes the use of cognitive behavioural therapies; an approach well suited to team working between occupational therapist and behavioural psychotherapist.

Overall, the therapist should aim to establish a good rapport with both individual and family, to be honest and open about treatment and its limitations, and empathetic and caring in approach. The appreciation of the emotional effects of a burn is a responsibility of the whole team and good team communication and support benefits everyone.

Education

Prior to discharge from hospital, the individual is in daily contact with a range of staff from whom advice and information can be sought. Even after discharge, frequent outpatient appointments are

---

Box 13.3 Case study: John

John was a 54-year-old married man who sustained 32% full thickness burns in a gas explosion. At the time of his accident he was self-employed in the catering trade.

Early occupational therapy interventions centred on establishing a therapeutic relationship with John and his wife and the restoration of personal independence and mobility. As his wounds healed, involvement broadened to include scar management and the prevention of contractures.

During a kitchen assessment John was observed to be showing high levels of anxiety. Although the accident had not occurred in a kitchen, the proximity of gas appliances reminded him of the accident. John was referred to a cognitive behavioural psychotherapist who diagnosed post-traumatic stress disorder. Working with the psychotherapist, the occupational therapist used graded exposure techniques to desensitise John to the anxiety-provoking environment. The triggers for his panic attacks had broadened to include electrical appliances and any naked flames. Several weeks of intensive therapy resulted in John being able to use the electric kettle to make a drink. However, at this point he declined to continue with this part of therapy, finding it too stressful.

John did continue to attend the occupational therapy workshop for activities designed to improve hand function and social reintegration. Although his burn scars were quite visible, this was not a problem for him and did not prevent him from going out.

After many months of treatment it was obvious that John would not be returning to catering. The occupational therapist discussed alternatives and put him in touch with a Disability Employment Advisor. As treatment neared an end John had enrolled on a computer course at his local college and he and his wife were training as counsellors for their local burns self-help group.

---

initially required for wound care, physiotherapy and occupational therapy. However, as attendances reduce, the need for information continues. 'Can I go swimming?' 'Is it safe to go out in the sun?' 'When can I drive again?' these and many other questions are commonly asked, and the therapist may become the primary link between the individual and other team members. This is particularly so if the person is attending regularly for scar management.

Allowing adequate time within treatment sessions for the exchange of information and supplementing with high quality and comprehensive written guidance are important if an individual's need for information is to be met.

MEASURING OUTCOMES

The measurement of outcomes has become important in healthcare as a means by which the efficacy of interventions can be gauged. There are many ways in which outcomes can be measured and in burns, as in many other areas, this is a developing field of interest.

Staley et al (1996), working in the United States, argue that as the improvement of functional ability in burns is a major goal of rehabilitation, levels of functional performance could be a useful predictor of outcome. By identifying appropriate functional outcomes, the rehabilitation process can be improved and therapists can demonstrate that their interventions work. In the United Kingdom, there has been some work by occupational therapists on client-centred goal setting as a method of measuring outcomes (Cook 1995). Goals, which are not condition specific, must be individualised, time related and measurable.

Within the context of scar management, the Burn Scar Index, also known as the Vancouver Scar Scale (Sullivan et al 1990) uses four parameters to document change in scar appearance; pigmentation, vascularity, pliability and height. This has been adapted by others (Baryza & Baryza 1995) to form a simple and practical assessment tool that can be used in clinical research and as an outcome measure.

CONCLUSION

The effects for a person who sustains a burn injury can be shocking and long lasting. Even a small burn can cause significant levels of distress and dysfunction. The aim of occupational therapy is to work in partnership with the individual, family and the therapeutic team to restore function wherever possible and to minimise the physical, psychological and social effects of the injury. Burns is a specialty that is not only challenging but also extremely rewarding for occupational therapists. It provides the unusual opportunity of working with people of all ages, sometimes over many months and years, and of employing a wide range of therapeutic approaches and interventions.

REFERENCES

Ahn ST, Monafo WW, Mustoe TA 1991 Topical silicone gel for the prevention and treatment of hypertrophic scar. Archives of Surgery 126:499–504

Bach J, Draslov B, Jørgenson B 1984 Positioning, splinting and pressure management of the burned hand. Scandinavian Journal of Plastic and Reconstructive Surgery 18:145–147

Baryza MJ, Baryza GA 1995 The Vancouver Scar Scale: an administrative tool and its interrater reliability. Journal of Burn Care and Rehabilitation 16:535–538

Bhattacharya S, Bhatnagar SK, Chandra R 1991 Postburn contracture of the neck – our experience with a new dynamic extension splint. Burns 17:72–74

Boyle S 1997 Social reintegration of the burn patient. In: Bosworth C (ed) Burns trauma management and nursing care. Baillière Tindall, London, ch 11, pp 151–159

Campbell S, Kelly P, Summergill P 1993 Putting the family first. Child Health 1(2):59–60

Clarke C 1999 Treating post-traumatic stress disorder: occupational therapist or counsellor? British Journal of Occupational Therapy 62(3):136–137

Cook S 1995 The merits of individualised outcome measures within routine clinical practice. Outcomes Briefing 6:15–18

Cresci JV 1982 Emotional care of the hospitalised thermally injured. In: Hummel R (ed) Clinical burn therapy. John Wright, Bristol, pp 475–507

Deitch EA, Wheelahan TM, Rose MP et al 1983 Hypertrophic burn scars: analysis of variables. Journal of Trauma 23:895–898

Dyer C, Roberts D 1990 Thermal trauma. Nursing Clinics of North America 25(1):85–117

Fowler D 1987 Australian occupational therapy: current trends and future considerations in burn rehabilitation. Journal of Burn Care and Rehabilitation 8(5):415–417

Giele HP, Liddiard K, Currie K, Wood FM 1997 Direct measurement of cutaneous pressures gained by pressure garments. Burns 23(2):137–141

Hagedorn R 1995 Occupational therapy perspectives and processes. Churchill Livingstone, Edinburgh, p 32

Johnson CL 1984 Physical therapists as scar modifiers. Physical Therapy 64:1381–1387

Kemble JV, Lamb BE 1987 Practical burns management. Hodder & Stoughton, London

Kolman P 1983 The incidence of psychopathology in burned adult patients – a critical review. Journal of Burn Care and Rehabilitation 416:430–436

Larson DL, Abston S, Evans EB, Dobrovsky M, Linares HA 1971 Techniques for decreasing scar formation and contractures in the burned patient. Journal of Trauma 11:807–823

Leman C 1992 Splints and accessories following burn reconstruction. Clinics in Plastic Surgery 19(3):721–730

Leveridge A 1991 Therapy for the burn patient. Chapman & Hall, London

Norman L 1997 Nutritional care in burns patients. In: Bosworth C (ed) Burns trauma management and nursing care. Baillière Tindall, London, ch 9, pp 123–139

Noyes R, Andreason NJC, Hartford CE 1971 The psychological reaction to severe burns. American Journal of Psychosomatic Medicine 11:416–422

Poh-Fitzpatrick M 1992 Skin care of the healed burn patient. Clinics in Plastic Surgery 19(3):745–751

Price B 1990 The burn patient. In: Body image concepts and care. Prentice Hall, Hertfordshire, pp 183–199

Quinn KJ 1987 Silicone gel in scar treatment. Burns 13:S33–S40

Regel S 1997 Burn trauma and post-traumatic stress disorder. In: Bosworth C (ed) Burns trauma management and nursing care. Baillière Tindall, London, ch 14, pp 189–201

Scott Ward R 1991 Pressure therapy for the control of hypertrophic scar formation after burn injury. Journal of Burn Care and Rehabilitation 12(3):257–261

Soderberg T, Hallman G, Barholson L 1982 Treatment of keloida and hypertrophic scars with adhesive zinc tape. Scandinavian Journal of Plastic and Reconstructive Surgery 16:261–266

Staley M, Richard R, Warden GD, Miller SF, Shuster B 1996 Functional outcomes for the patient with burn injuries. Journal of Burn Care and Rehabilitation 17(4):362–368

Sullivan T, Smith J, Kermode J, McIver E, Courtemanche DJ 1990 Rating the burn scar. Journal of Burn Care and Rehabilitation 11:256–260

Ward HW, Moss RL, Darko DF 1987 Prevalence of post burn depression following burn injury. Journal of Burn Care and Rehabilitation 8(4):294–297

Wilson D 1997 Management in the first 48 hours following burn trauma. In: Bosworth C (ed) Burns trauma management and nursing care. Baillière Tindall, London, ch 4, pp 45–63

Woodward J 1968 The burnt child and his family: impact on the family. Proceedings of the Royal Society of Medicine 61:1085–1088

FURTHER READING

Bosworth C (ed) 1997 Burns trauma management and nursing care. Baillière Tindall, London

Bradbury E 1996 Counselling people with disfigurement. The British Psychological Society, Leicester

Leveridge A (ed) 1991 Therapy for the burn patient. Chapman & Hall, London

Partridge J 1990 Changing faces – the challenge of facial disfigurement. Penguin, London

14

Upper limb amputees and limb-deficient children

Vivienne Ibbotson

INTRODUCTION

'Hands play a unique and important role in a person's life; they serve prehensile, proprioceptive and communication purposes' (Lake 1997). The unpredictable loss of one or both hands through trauma, malignancy or vascular disease immediately creates a reduced level of function and a loss of ability automatically to perform everyday tasks. The body is suddenly noticeably incomplete; demonstrative gestures of anger, frustration, caring and comforting are more difficult to perform and during the transitional period there is often a high level of dependency for many small tasks. The impact of the loss on future prospects as the family 'bread winner' is frequently a cause for concern, as financial security will inevitably be of importance. Cultural differences may need to be explored in order to consider the different beliefs and attitudes that will have an impact on the rehabilitation programme.

TRAUMATIC AMPUTATION

Traumatic injuries will involve bone and soft tissue damage and prescription of a prosthesis may be delayed due to oedema, skin grafting or limited range of movement at the residual joints.

Learning new skills should begin immediately to maintain the strength and range of movement in both the affected and residual limbs. Education in prophylactic and preventive healthcare must be initiated to emphasise avoidance of being one handed and promote protection of the residual limb, which will be required to carry out all the manipulative and fine motor tasks in the future. Problems caused by overuse of the remaining arm will seriously jeopardise functional ability.

If the amputation is on the dominant side, occupational therapy intervention must be instrumental in promoting a change in hand dominance. The psychological effect of trauma can often present greater dysfunction than the physical effects. A number of people have poor sleep patterns due to flashbacks, pain or discomfort or because of the amount of stress and anxiety they are suffering.

ELECTIVE AMPUTATION

Amputation surgery for malignancy or vascular disease is considered as a life-saving procedure and treatment for the underlying condition will take immediate precedence to that of prosthetic rehabilitation. Support will be needed during radiotherapy and chemotherapy treatments if these have been prescribed. Occupational therapy intervention will be beneficial in facilitating adaptive behaviour towards this unexpected life event.

The change in circumstances creates a turning point, bringing into question the sense of identity and future role in society. Self-confidence and self-esteem are also affected, bringing about a feeling of failure and incompetence. To face the future, personal change and adaptation are necessary.

Security is challenged with the change in roles within the home and work environment. Leisure pursuits may no longer be possible. As stated by Cracknell (1996), human beings find security in that which they know and it is difficult to look towards a changed lifestyle. On a positive note, the situation can be turned to the individual's advantage, as he may not have previously considered retraining or developing new interests. The significant change in circumstances may open up opportunities never before considered.

It should always be remembered that everyone close to the individual is affected by the amputation and they should always be included in the management of the situation. A realistic approach should be adopted and support and counselling should be offered to the whole family if necessary.

PHANTOM LIMB SENSATION

The majority of upper limb amputees will experience a degree of phantom limb sensation. A few will experience actual pain in either the residual part of the arm or in the amputated (phantom) part of the arm. The duration, severity and form vary considerably and there is currently no acknowledged framework by which these feelings can be explained.

Sensations range from 'pins and needles', itching and cramp to simply feeling that the absent part is still there. Occasionally, particularly if the amputation was due to trauma, the hand can be 'felt' in what seems to be its last position prior to impact. The sensations usually settle to a level that can be tolerated and accepted although it may be necessary for some people to be referred to the chronic pain team, to investigate coping mechanisms to allow the symptoms to be managed.

Fortunately, phantom sensation and phantom pain are now being taken more seriously and extensive research is being carried out both in Europe and the United States.

CONGENITAL LIMB DEFICIENCY

As stated by Marquardt (1983), the birth of a limb-deficient child produces severe shock in the mother, often accompanied by despair and guilt feelings. The initial reaction to the birth is often one of disbelief, sometimes resentment and rejection.

Aetiology

West et al (1995) point out that congenital limb deficiency is a low frequency disability often requiring the services from a number of professions. The aetiology for the majority of congenital abnormalities is unknown and most cases are of sporadic incidence. Research has been carried out extensively and a report by Brown (1996), commissioned by the Department of Health, concluded that further systematic research should be carried out to document what was known about the factors likely to be associated with congenital limb defects.

Advances in ultrasound techniques have enabled earlier detection of limb deficiencies in unborn children. It is crucial at this stage that the professionals involved handle the situation delicately and compassionately and referrals to the correct specialists are appropriately made. This will have a direct impact on how the mother feels throughout the rest of her pregnancy.

Development

The unborn child has no problems at this time but the parents will foresee numerous difficulties ahead and need as much information as they can deal with from this time forwards. It has been known for a mother to think of her daughter's absent left hand and ask where her wedding ring will be worn. A great deal of support and counselling should be offered to help come to terms with the devastating news they have received and prepare them for a happy occasion at the birth. The benefits of ongoing support from the early diagnosis are beginning to be realised through positive feedback from the parents. As the child grows, his physical, psychological and social development will be influenced by the degree of acceptance in the family. The limb absence may attract unwanted attention when in public, particularly if there is a dangling empty sleeve. Parents may themselves be well adjusted within their immediate surroundings but the unwarranted attention they receive from strangers can produce anxiety and stress.

Throughout the first months, the child will have an obvious lack of symmetry and length required for holding and playing with objects in midline. Sitting balance may be affected, as well as crawling. This is more pronounced with higher levels of absence. If balance is affected when walking (this is unlikely with low levels of absence), extra safety measures need to be taken with steps and stairs.

Difficulties can sometimes arise during preschool and early school years, with the introduc-

tion of more and more bimanual activities. Cutting-out, for example, can be accurately achieved without the use of a prosthesis, but the cost is often poor posture and damage to clothing.

Psychologically, children rarely suffer more than any other child within their peer group. Teasing may occur but should be dealt with rationally. It seldom escalates into bullying.

During teenage years, children may feel more self-conscious and begin to think ahead to life after school. Work prospects will be limited but, provided the child and family are realistic in their expectations, rewarding occupations can be entered into. Although opportunities may be improved with the use of a prosthesis, each job of work should be assessed individually and advice given according to the tasks involved.

As with acquired amputation, education concerning adaptive techniques, posture and protection of the residual arm should be explained to parents and teachers. Where it is thought the limb-deficient side would have been the dominant side, assessment of writing and fine motor function will alleviate problems early in the rehabilitation programme.

Multiple limb deficiency

Multiple limb deficiency naturally has greater impact on the child and family. Use of prosthetics should be explored carefully as to the benefits gained compared to learning other compensatory techniques.

Loss of more than one limb will seriously affect the heat regulation of the body. Prosthetics – whilst offering a degree of mobility and/or upper limb function – will most likely be so heavy and cumbersome as to interfere with the already limited independence. The restricted residual body area will be covered by the suspension for upper and lower limb prostheses, dramatically reducing the body area for vital heat regulation. The amount of energy required to use a number of prostheses effectively must be taken into consideration and it may be preferable to encourage use of a wheelchair for much speedier mobility, requiring less energy consumption.

THE INTERVENTION TEAM

ACQUIRED AMPUTATION

On admission to hospital, the consultant will decide on the course of action, primarily involving nursing staff, pain care specialists and the consultant in rehabilitation medicine. It is important to endeavour to make the individual as pain free as possible prior to surgery (Barnes & Ward 2000); this has been shown to have a bearing on the level of postoperative pain. A report by a working party of the Amputee Medical Rehabilitation Society (1992) recommends early involvement of the consultant in rehabilitation medicine, to advise on the preferred level of amputation for optimum prosthetic care. This also applies to individuals undergoing elective surgery (Fig. 14.1).

It is important to provide as much information as possible preoperatively to raise awareness of the rehabilitation process postoperatively. However, as early as 1967, Ley and Spelman looked at studies dealing with memory aspects of information-giving to individuals in hospital and found that only a small proportion of the information was retained after 24 hours.

Postoperatively, the physiotherapist will begin exercising both upper limbs, promoting reduction of oedema and maintaining a full range of movement at all joints. At this stage it is advisable for the nurse and occupational therapist from the Limb Fitting Centre (which may be referred to by a number of titles, for example, Artificial Limb and Appliance Centre (ALAC), Mobility Centre, Disablement Services Centre, depending on its location) to visit the ward, to advise on wound care and early functional activities. Early success in personal care assists in motivating the individual.

Following discharge, the care programme is transferred to the local Limb Fitting Centre; there are approximately 40 of these nationally but not all have facilities and expertise for upper limb prosthetics. The team here is comprised of the consultant in rehabilitation medicine, prosthetist, occupational therapist, nurse and, if indicated, physiotherapist. Advice will be provided on the

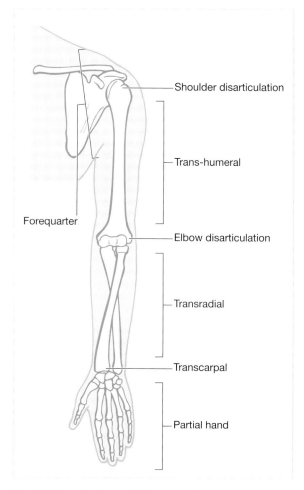

Fig. 14.1 Levels of upper limb amputation.

pros and cons of prosthetic use; nursing and occupational therapy intervention are available whether or not the individual chooses to have a prosthesis, as independent living is of importance to everyone.

Other team members include family and friends, teachers, employers and the clinical psychologist. Contact with a Disability Employment Advisor may be needed if the individual is unable to return to his previous job.

Involvement with support groups is beneficial; someone who has been through a similar experience is the best person to relate closely to the new amputee. Everyone else can only imagine how it must feel (Fig. 14.2).

CONGENITAL LIMB DEFICIENCY

The intervention team here differs slightly from that dealing with acquired amputation. If diagnosed at the scan, the maternity staff should offer the parents maximum support, including early referral to the Limb Fitting Centre. The family, the consultant in rehabilitation medicine and the occupational therapist will discuss the implications and future management together. It is advisable for the family to be put in touch with the national support groups, as well as other families who have been through the same experience. If required, a clinical psychologist can provide counselling.

Following the birth, the team will be joined by the prosthetist who will be responsible for all the prosthetic hardware. Good rapport is essential between all parties, as the family will be visiting the centre for many years. Liaison with the health visitor as well as involvement with playgroups, nursery and mainstream school staff will ensure everyone caring for the child is working towards a common goal (Fig. 14.2).

THEORETICAL FOUNDATIONS FOR INTERVENTION

The role of the occupational therapist is defined in the standards and guidelines document 'Occupational Therapy in the Rehabilitation of Upper Limb Amputees and Limb Deficient Children' produced by the College of Occupational Therapists Clinical Interest Group in Orthotics Prosthetics and Wheelchairs (College of Occupational Therapists 1995).

As always, the occupational therapist's ultimate aim is to rehabilitate the individual to a maximum level of independence and she will, of necessity, adopt various treatment approaches that frequently overlap.

With regard to the physical aspects of the dysfunction, the compensatory approach is implemented throughout. Success will depend considerably on how the individual's psychological and emotional stresses are overcome through the therapist's use of the humanistic approach.

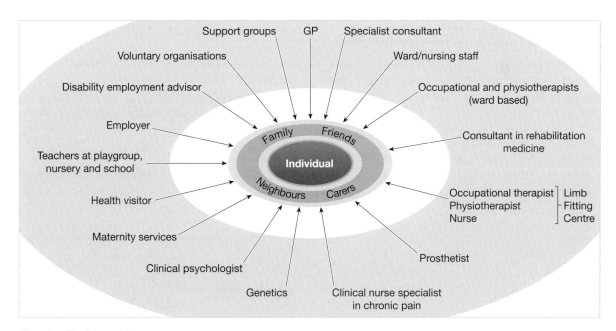

Fig. 14.2 The intervention team.

Exploring the individual's own view of their circumstances before embarking on identifying and prioritising goals establishes the importance of working in partnership. A client-centred approach reflects the humanistic beliefs of the therapist, respecting opinions and helping build confidence and self-esteem by identifying problems and potential solutions with rather than for each person. Although carers' opinions and expectations should be sought, it is the individual's expectations that are of primary concern. Sansom (1997) states that the individual's expectations may in fact widely differ from those of the carers. It is important to empower individuals by allowing involvement in the decisions that affect them, to take control of their changed circumstances.

Attention must be paid to maintaining or improving function in the proximal parts of the amputated limb. Specifically based on physical activity, the biomechanical frame of reference will be used to promote strength and range of movement, as good upper body strength is needed to tolerate and operate an artificial arm.

It cannot be stated too strongly that every person is an individual and should be treated as such. Each set of circumstances is unique. The amputation is only a part of the whole problem to be faced and it is incumbent upon the therapist to take a sensitive and realistic overview of the situation. Although the main focus is on helping the individual to learn how to use a prosthesis functionally, independence remains a priority of those choosing to wear either a cosmetic prosthesis or no prosthesis at all. It is equally important to support, counsel and advise this group of people.

Cultural beliefs may make it difficult or impossible to demonstrate to the individual their ability to reshape their own life, accepting what has happened and taking responsibility to move forward.

When dealing with children, developmental techniques will primarily be used. Individuals with a congenital limb deficiency have particular concerns at each stage of their development and need continuity in care and guidance. Adaptive skills will be employed when teaching how to use a functional prosthesis, using cognitive skills to process the information and solve problems.

Based on the ability to learn, information provided by the therapist will offer the right climate for informed decision making to take place. The range of options available to the individual and his family, together with the implications, will be discussed. Education can be provided by demonstration, observation, and verbal interaction as well as written documentation. It is advisable to provide a wide range of useful information for each recipient.

The number of upper limb amputees and limb-deficient children is very small. Treatment in the acute phase is carried out in the ward setting, where staff rotation and such low frequency disability creates a difficult situation for establishing expertise in this specialist group of patients. Ham (1986) makes reference to educating all staff groups as part of the recommendations possible in the wake of the McColl Report (1986), and Gaine et al (1997) advocate early involvement in the rehabilitation process, as this significantly affects the outcome.

Although a number of upper limb amputations are carried out as an emergency procedure, and therefore involvement of the Limb Centre will begin postoperatively, elective amputation offers an opportunity for considerable preparation, support and counselling. The Amputee Medical Rehabilitation Society (1992) refers to the benefits of early referral for patients with both acquired amputation and congenital limb deficiencies, particularly as the client group is small and resources scattered. Bearing in mind the specialist nature of this client group, it is perhaps understandable that there is a paucity of literature and research available to support interventions. Further research is needed to provide evidence of the value of specific occupational therapy approaches and interventions.

INTERVENTION

ASSESSMENT

Each person has a unique set of circumstances. Age, gender, cultural, family and social background, reason for and age at amputation, site and side of amputation, and hand dominance are all individual.

When dealing with people with acquired amputations, assessment begins by building up background information on the above areas, extended to include:

- secondary factors that may have an impact on the treatment outcome
- relevant past medical history
- functional ability prior to surgery
- previous psychological status.

Assessment of a child with a limb deficiency will differ from the above, as less background information is necessary. Family history and a history of the pregnancy, as well as any medication taken, are usually documented. Although this does not necessarily have a direct bearing on the rehabilitation of the child, it does provide useful information for supporting and counselling the parents.

IDENTIFYING PROBLEMS

For individuals undergoing surgery due to trauma, there may also be many other injuries to consider. It may not be possible to intervene for some time to deal with the limb loss. Healing may be delayed and scar tissue or excessive residual oedema may prevent early prosthetic provision. Although a temporary prosthesis can be fitted, it should be noted that the fit of this device would rapidly change due to the changing shape of the residual part of the arm.

Tolerance to the prosthetic socket can also be affected by hypersensitivity, the presence of neuroma or phantom pain.

Psychological problems may present a higher priority than the physical dysfunction and should be addressed as early as possible. A change of hand dominance may be indicated; depending on the person's lifestyle this could be either a mere irritation or have major implications. Someone who rarely writes (perhaps signing only bank documents or greetings cards) will adapt more quickly than someone who relies on the written word for their livelihood or particular leisure pursuits.

Losing all or part of one or both upper limbs creates difficulties in all aspects of daily living. Assessing the individual's level of independence, identifying problem areas and intervening with an acceptable solution affords early success for the individual. This raises confidence and self-esteem, decreases the level of dependency required immediately postoperatively and improves motivation.

Allowing the individual to take an active part in identifying and prioritising problems, together with assisting in the treatment plan, encourages him to take control of his changed circumstances. Use of the Canadian Occupational Performance Measure provides a valuable tool to focus on client-centred goals and rehabilitation.

The treatment programme should centre on those activities meaningful to the individual and have a preventive and prophylactic approach in order to protect and preserve the remaining parts of the body.

Success of the treatment programme can be affected by a number of external factors. As the Limb Fitting Centre is a regional resource, it may be necessary for the individual or the child and his family to travel long distances. Family circumstances, low income and transport availability all have a bearing on the frequency of treatment sessions. It may even be that the individual is affected by travel sickness and is therefore not well enough on arrival to carry out the remedial activities. If there is a problem attending the Centre, it is advantageous to arrange local therapy input if at all possible. However, this is time-consuming for the Limb Centre therapist as she will need to spend time with the local therapist regarding the prosthetic rehabilitation and monitor the progress from a distance.

Disadvantages of wearing a prosthesis must also be discussed with the individual. Examples of these are as follows:

- Depending on the site, important sensory feedback and sometimes movement can be impeded.
- The prosthesis may be heavy and hot and the straps uncomfortable.
- A skin reaction may arise from the materials used, or an existing skin condition may be

aggravated. This can usually be resolved but it takes time and perseverance to find a satisfactory solution.

- Self-consciousness may be increased, especially in teenage years when many individuals are particularly sensitive concerning appearance and performance.
- Frequent visits to the Centre will be necessary, especially during the growth years of children and the initial stages of rehabilitation of adults.

However, these negative aspects must be balanced against the more positive reasons for gaining expertise with a prosthesis:

- The body image is completed and may reduce unwelcome stares from strangers.
- Whichever side is affected, it will provide a non-dominant assister.
- Bimanual activities can be learned or recommenced.
- Return to work may be accelerated.
- If expertise is gained with a prosthesis, the individual will still be reasonably independent should anything happen to the remaining arm.
- When prescribed for a congenital absence, the child will grow up with an image of himself as being two-handed. Experience will be provided upon which to base an informed decision regarding prosthetic wear during teenage and adult life.

OCCUPATIONAL THERAPY INVOLVEMENT

Acquired amputation

Preoperative

It may be possible for the therapist to be involved preoperatively, particularly if an elective amputation is to be considered. This early introduction allows the relationship with the therapist and the rest of the team to develop. As individuals and their families will be involved with the rehabilitation process for a number of years, it is essential to build up an atmosphere of trust and confidence.

Discussion at this point will centre on how the individual is going to cope postoperatively. Although the therapist and other team members may be more concerned about ensuring the person is as pain free as possible and that his general health and wellbeing can withstand surgery, the individual and the family are usually more concerned about life after surgery. The humanistic and client-centred approaches used by the therapist ensure that these concerns are dealt with early.

It is then possible to explain the advantages of preoperative preparation. Counselling of both the individual and the family may be necessary. If amputation surgery is to be carried out after many years of corrective surgery, there are often unresolved problems surrounding this. Referral to the clinical psychologist may be required to explore these issues, deal with them and prepare to move forward. The amputation needs to be seen as a positive option and not a negative result of failed surgery, as is sometimes felt by the individual.

A great deal of information is available but this does not mean that all of it must be provided. This again reflects the client-centred approach that must always be taken. Armed with written information and presented with photographs, slides, books and video information, as well as having a demonstration of relevant prostheses, becomes overwhelming for an individual who is only just beginning to realise the magnitude of what is about to happen to his body. This early situation must be approached with sensitivity and compassion. It should always be remembered that everyone close to the person is affected by the amputation and should therefore always be included in the management of the situation.

However, individuals and their families are more frequently referred to the occupational therapist after discharge from hospital, when healing has occurred and they are ready for the first prosthesis.

Postoperative

It is not usual to provide a temporary prosthesis or gauntlet, as it is possible to fit a prosthesis as soon as the wound is fully healed. If the dominant hand has been affected, advice is given on activities to promote a change in dominance as soon as possible. The individual will need to develop skill in controlling his new dominant hand, as well as the prosthesis.

All aspects of ADL should be assessed. This is an important area directly related to the individual's independence and one that affords early success and a boost to morale.

Following surgery, a compensatory frame of reference may be used, providing equipment to assist in some areas of independence. Later, provision of a prosthesis will come into this category, as it is with this piece of equipment the individual will work towards becoming 'two handed' again.

Reduction of hypersensitivity and oedema and maintenance of range of movement and muscle strength will be improved using the biomechanical approach, grading the exercises and activities according to individual needs. Advice and education will continue postoperatively, using the learning frame of reference as individuals' attitudes to their circumstances and approach to rehabilitation are explored.

Prosthetic

When attending for the initial appointment at the Limb Fitting Centre, the rehabilitation team will carry out a general assessment and discuss the prosthetic options available (Fig. 14.3). The individual may feel vulnerable, frightened and worried, although he will probably not admit to this until much later when recalling his initial feelings. It is therefore important to establish a relaxed, informative relationship while instilling confidence for future visits to the Centre. Both the prosthetist and therapist provide valuable lines of communication between the individual and doctor, as in many instances there is still an aura of authority surrounding the medical profession that may inhibit a free flow of feelings.

With the provision of a functional prosthesis, adaptive techniques are used to teach operation, control and natural, effective use of the prosthetic terminal device. A terminal device is an implement fitted into the wrist section of the prosthesis. Several (detachable) devices may be provided for use with a body powered prosthesis, as one device alone is not able to carry out even some of the complex, sophisticated movements of the human hand. The devices are many and varied, for specific tasks (Fig. 14.4).

Congenital limb deficiency

It is frequently said that children born with a limb absence have the benefit of never having known what it is like to be two handed and will therefore adapt much better to life with one hand. This does not mean that the child will grow up without any problems.

Preprosthetic

It is essential that children and their families be referred as early as possible to the Limb Centre. A firm relationship with the rehabilitation team built on trust and confidence and promoting a positive attitude can begin. At this time the parents can be supported, counselled and helped in every way possible to come to terms with what they will inevitably feel to be a failure on their part in not producing a perfect child.

The need for parents to be given the opportunity to discuss hopes and fears for the future, even at such an early age, should be recognised. Introduction to other families can be a considerable advantage, as they are in a strong position to understand what the family is going through. Support for families of upper-limb-deficient children is also available through Reach, the association for children with hand or arm deficiency (see Useful Contacts, p393).

Regular contact with the rehabilitation team at the Centre is important, even if a limb is not prescribed for some months, as the family should not be left feeling isolated or uninformed. The need for both upper limbs to be used fully to ensure development occurs as symmetrically as possible, together with helping the child to integrate the prosthesis into play, is emphasised.

The developmental frame of reference will be used consistently as the child grows and needs change, incorporating age-appropriate activities into the treatment programme.

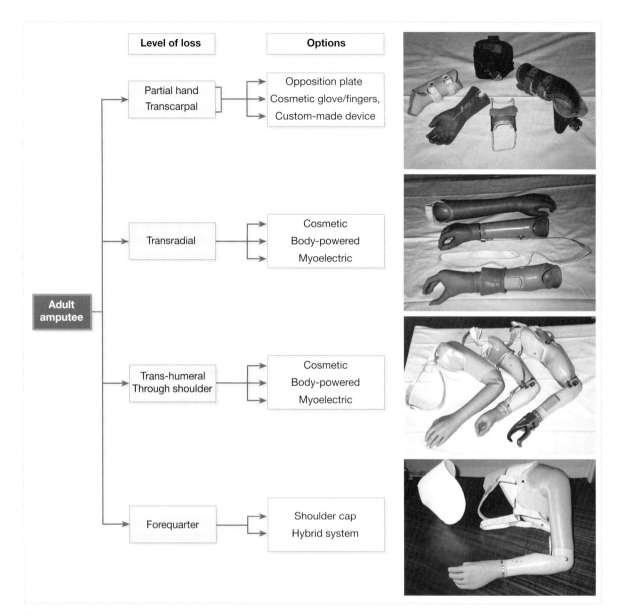

Level of loss	Options
Partial hand Transcarpal	Opposition plate Cosmetic glove/fingers, Custom-made device
Transradial	Cosmetic Body-powered Myoelectric
Trans-humeral Through shoulder	Cosmetic Body-powered Myoelectric
Forequarter	Shoulder cap Hybrid system

Adult amputee

Fig. 14.3 Basic prosthetic options for an adult amputee.

Prosthetic

When the baby is approximately 6 months old, the fitting of the first prosthesis will be prescribed. This is a light, plastic, one-piece socket and fixed hand, fitted on to the baby's arm with an elastic cuff to prevent it slipping off easily. The fitting of this arm immediately completes the baby's body image and will encourage him to be two handed. At this early stage, biomechanical and compensatory approaches will be used to encourage the idea of having another hand to help when playing. Provision of the prosthesis will help reduce stares from strangers when away from home, as the baby will appear two handed. This can provide tremendous psychological support to the parents during this time.

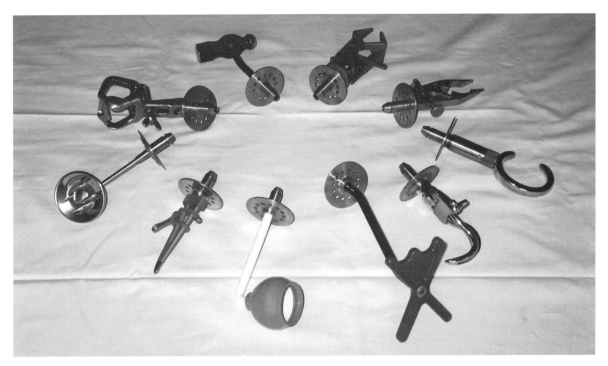

Fig. 14.4 A variety of frequently used terminal devices. Clockwise from centre top: bell pein hammer, universal tool holder, long-nose pliers, Williams 'C' hook, split hook, snooker cue rest, driving appliance, tweezers, potato holder, spade grip.

Introduction of a functional prosthesis is appropriate from the age of approximately 18 months (Fig. 14.5). This may take the form of a body-powered prosthesis or an externally powered prosthesis. The body-powered prosthesis is attached and activated by an arrangement of straps passing across the shoulders and under the opposite armpit. Objects can be picked up and dropped by using shoulder and elbow movement to open and close the terminal device. An externally powered prosthesis can be operated either by means of a pull switch or a single site electrode, offering voluntary opening with automatic spring closing.

It is important to recognise that a child cannot fully operate a prosthesis until he has reached the appropriate stage of 'developmental readiness'. Several training sessions will be arranged to encourage full use of the prosthesis and to show the family how best to supervise activities at home between sessions. Regular appointments are recommended to monitor changes in needs, particularly as the child grows. In all cases, the time required will be greatly affected by motiv-

ation, home circumstances, available transport and travelling distance.

Implementing intervention

The majority of occupational therapy treatment sessions are carried out on a one-to-one basis. Initially, the therapist will concentrate on educating individuals (whether children and their parents or adults) in how the prosthesis is put on and taken off and how the components work, as well as how to keep it clean. Details of the wearing pattern will be provided; it is far more beneficial to wear it for a short time every day than for several hours once a week.

The first step in using the prosthesis begins with learning how to operate the terminal device. How this is done depends on the type of prosthesis prescribed – whether body powered or externally powered (myoelectric prosthesis). From the age of $3\frac{1}{2}$, a myoelectric prosthesis will usually be operated by means of two electrodes, offering voluntary opening and closing.

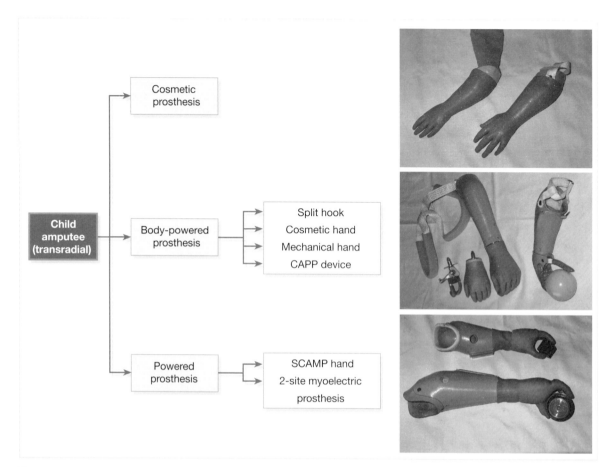

Fig. 14.5 Basic prosthetic options for a child amputee.

Suitability for this system can be assessed by using one of the Otto Bock myotrainers (Fig. 14.6). This piece of equipment greatly assists the decision-making process for the rehabilitation team.

The next stage is to learn how to gain control of the prosthesis, using it effectively and appropriately. The higher the level of loss, the more complex this process becomes. A programme of practise and learning ensues, the length of which varies according to the individual; someone with a high level or double amputation will take considerably longer to achieve independence and prosthetic competence. In all cases, the time required will be greatly affected by motivation, home circumstances, available transport and travelling distance.

Control of the prosthesis is taught by using the terminal device beginning with basic, unilateral activities. As the socket covers the residual part of the arm, sensation is reduced. It is therefore necessary to concentrate more closely on the activity, relying on eyesight and problem-solving skills to position materials and objects suitably.

The tasks should be easy to complete; for example, stacking cubes, to ensure immediate success. As confidence grows, the activities are graded in complexity, incorporating different sizes and weights of objects; working in different planes requires the terminal device to be repositioned. A range of activities, for example, a shapes board – drawing round a template and cutting out – can be timed. This provides a baseline to measure against when retesting. It is necessary to emphasise that you are not undermining anyone's intelligence with such basic activities. Practice using solid objects is prefer-

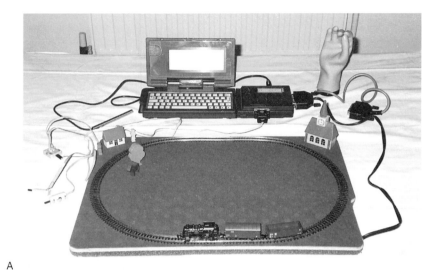

A

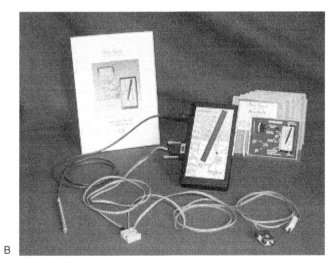

B

Fig. 14.6 (A) Otto Bock Myoelectric Trainer and its successor (B) the Otto Bock Myoboy. This equipment provides invaluable information when assessing for the appropriateness of prescribing a myoelectric prosthesis.

able to damaging valued items of property at home. Ultimately, it should be possible to hold an egg without breaking it, or a tomato whilst slicing it.

Once control has been established, the isolated movements can be combined together into a natural sequence, for example:

- collate and staple several sheets of paper together
- fold neatly to a predetermined size
- put into an envelope

- seal and address the envelope
- open the envelope
- take out and unfold the contents.

The third stage in prosthetic training is to incorporate all the skills learned. A woodwork project requires the drawing-out of a pattern. The design must be cut out, sanded, and so on before assembling and adding the finish. This involves the use of two hands in a natural, effective way. During this time, it may be necessary to demonstrate a number of different terminal appliances. If the dominant right hand has been affected, use of the hammer in the end of the socket may be preferred to using the non-dominant hand, as eye–hand coordination will need to be considered.

A short list of activities for use with children is suggested below:

- cutting out
- threading
- riding a tricycle
- board games
- dressing up
- Play doh
- baking
- Lego®/construction toys
- drawing/stencils
- ball games.

As well as focusing on independence in personal and domestic activities of daily living, hobbies and pastimes should be encouraged. Information and help with activities such as playing a musical instrument may be required to enable full integration with their own peer group.

This is also a very important area for adults. People now have more leisure time at their disposal with many opportunities available. One activity that seems to act as a catalyst is driving. Advice and information can be provided regarding the type of appliances that may be necessary. Referral to a fully accredited Driving Assessment Centre may be required, particularly for individuals with a high level of loss.

During the entire rehabilitation process, liaison will be continuous with many agencies. Regular review appointments at the Centre require ongoing communication with the consultant and prosthetist regarding the achievements of individuals. Feedback is received from the clinical psychologist where appropriate and referrals for physiotherapy intervention are made if joint or muscular problems arise.

Involvement with children requires liaison with the family, health visitor and all pre- and mainstream school staff on a regular basis.

As well as contact with the family and employers, adults may request assistance in contacting agencies involved in further education or to liaise with the Disability Employment Advisor regarding work prospects. Visits to the individual's home, school or workplace are carried out as required, as it is in these settings that the most time is spent (Box 14.1).

Support groups can play an important role in rehabilitating the upper limb amputee. As has been mentioned before, someone who has already been through what the new amputee is going through is best placed for understanding, supporting and advising on how to overcome problems.

Box 14.1 Case study

Mr P. is 24, married, and has a 4-year-old son. He works in a paper mill and suffered a transradial amputation to his dominant right hand when his arm became trapped in a machine.

Referral was 2 days postadmission; Mr P. had full range of movement at all remaining joints, complained of phantom pain and problems with sleeping due to flashbacks. The pain clinic team became involved and his request for counselling noted. General information was provided verbally, supported by written documents for future reference. Basic ADL was assessed and small items of equipment provided. Advice was given regarding changing hand dominance, with emphasis on writing.

Discharge home was within 1 week of admission. Mr P.'s anxiety had increased over this period, with worries regarding his future and financial situation being expressed. Support was provided by the social worker. A home visit took place within 1 week of discharge. Mr P. felt he was coping reasonably well physically but was extremely frustrated with the lack of fine motor skill in his left hand.

Mr P. was fitted early with a prosthesis. Occupational therapy sessions were arranged on a regular basis and a work visit carried out. He currently wears a body-powered, self-suspending laminated socket using a number of terminal appliances for household and DIY activities. He has returned to his place of work after retraining in computer technology and wears an Otto Bock powered Greifer during working hours. He is proficient with both types of prosthesis and needs very few items of equipment to achieve independence. Counselling sessions provided by the clinical psychologist, occupational therapy intervention, attendance at the monthly support group and the support from his family, have all combined to provide a successful outcome.

REFERENCES

Amputee Rehabilitation Society 1992 Amputation rehabilitation. Recommended standards and guidelines. Amputee Medical Rehabilitation Society, London

Barnes MP, Ward AB 2000 Textbook of rehabilitation medicine: Oxford University Press, Oxford

Brown N 1996 Congenital limb reduction defects. HMSO, London

College of Occupational Therapists 1995 Occupational therapy in the rehabilitation of upper limb amputees and limb deficient children. Standards and guidelines. CIGOPW, Manchester (see Useful Contacts)

Cracknell E 1996 Life span development. In: Turner A, Foster M, Johnson SE (eds) Occupational therapy and physical dysfunction. Churchill Livingstone, Edinburgh, ch 3

Gaine et al 1997 Upper limb traumatic amputees. Review of prosthetic use. Journal of Hand Surgery (British and European) 22B(1):73–76

Ham R 1986 Improvements possible in the management of the amputee in line with the McColl Report. Physiotherapy 72(10):520–522

Lake C 1997 Effects of prosthetic training in upper extremity prosthesis use. Journal of Prosthetics and Orthotics 9(1):3–9

Ley P, Spelman M 1967 Communicating with the patient. Staples Press, London

Marquardt EG 1983 A holistic approach to rehabilitation for the limb deficient child. Archives of Physical Medicine and Rehabilitation 64:237–242

McColl Report 1986 Review of artificial limb and appliance centre services, vol 1. DHSS, London

Sansom M 1997 Occupational therapy. In: Goodwill CJ et al (eds) Rehabilitation of the physically disabled adult. Stanley Thomas (Publishers), Cheltenham

West et al 1995 Helping to solve problems with spina bifida: 1. Prescription of the TRS project in organising services for low frequency diagnostic groups and 2. Cognitive deficits often seen in young adults with spina bifida. European Journal of Paediatric Surgery 5 (Suppl 1):12–15

FURTHER READING

For a comprehensive list of books and papers, please refer to the CIGOPW (1999) publication 'Upper Limb Prosthetics Booklist', CIGOPW, Manchester (see Useful Contacts)

USEFUL CONTACTS

Amputee Medical Rehabilitation Society, c/o Royal College of Physicians, 11 St Andrew's Place, Regents Park, London NWI 4LE

Clinical Interest Group in Orthotics, Prosthetics and Wheelchairs (CIGOPW), c/o S. Kennedy, Occupational Therapy Department, Rehabilitation Unit, Withington Hospital, Nell Lane, Manchester M20 2LR
http://homepages.enterprise.net/cigopw

Reach, the association for children with hand or arm deficiency. Mrs Sue Stokes, General Secretary, 25 High Street, Wellingborough, Northants NN8 4JZ

15

Acquired brain injury

Carol Collins   Jackie Dean

INTRODUCTION

Acquired brain injury may be defined as an injury to the brain that has occurred since birth. The term 'acquired brain injury' includes traumatic brain injuries, such as open or closed head injuries, and non-traumatic brain injuries such as those caused by strokes and other vascular accidents, tumours, infectious diseases, hypoxic metabolic disorders and toxic products taken into the body through inhalation or ingestion (Table 15.1). The term does not include brain injuries that are congenital or produced by birth trauma (Medical Rehabilitation Accreditation Commission 1996).

This chapter will focus on brain injury acquired through trauma because this is thought to be the most common cause of brain injury (Kurtzke 1984). Most estimates agree that two to three males sustain traumatic brain injury for every one female and that the peak ages for traumatic brain injury are in the 15–24 years range (Anderson & McLaurin 1980). Prevalence estimates and incidence reports in epidemiological studies vary because of the range of definitions of head injury and methods of data collection. Jennett and MacMillan (1981) cited estimates of incidence of hospitalisation following head injury as between 200 and 300 per 100 000 of the population per annum. The Medical Disabilities Society (1988) estimated that the lowest figure is about 75 000 cases per annum. Tennant (1995) reached a considerably higher figure for the North West of England, which, if extrapolated

Table 15.1 Causes of acquired brain injury

Type of injury	Cause
Trauma	Closed – the skull is not penetrated but the brain is shaken violently within the skull Open – the skull is penetrated, e.g. gunshot wound
Haemorrhage	Around the brain – extradural, subarachnoid and subdural Inside the brain – intracerebral
Metabolic	Due to severely reduced supply of oxygen to the brain (hypoxia) caused by, for example, choking, carbon monoxide poisoning, cardiac arrest or drowning Due to severely reduced supply of glucose which is essential for metabolism to the brain, for example, caused by insulin overdose
Nutritional	Due to lack of essential vitamins, usually in the context of general self-neglect and often associated with alcohol misuse
Infection	Due to viruses such as herpes simplex and HIV Encephalitis due to bacteria Meningitis and brain abscess due to fungi and other infections, usually in people with HIV or immunosuppressant drugs
Toxic	Alcohol Heavy metals such as lead and solvents
Other examples	Thrombosis blocking the blood supply to the brain

nationally, would reach an annual figure of more like 140 000.

Jennett and MacMillan (1981) estimated that approximately 20% of those hospitalised for head injury have sustained a moderate or severe injury. Of the remaining 80% who suffer mild head injuries, many endure ongoing difficulties (Levin et al 1987).

Falls are the leading causes of head trauma, accounting for more than half the injuries incurred by infants, young children and by persons in the 64 and older age range (Goldstein and Levin 1990). Injuries from road traffic accidents account for approximately half of all head injuries in other age groups (Royal College of Surgeons 1999). Assaults from blows to the head or a penetrating weapon account for a further 10%, recreational activities for 10–15% and accidents in the workplace and domestic accidents for 20–30% of injuries (Royal College of Surgeons 1999).

ASSESSING THE SEVERITY OF TRAUMATIC BRAIN INJURY

The severity of traumatic brain injury falls within a continuum ranging from a mild blow with virtually no lasting ill effects to catastrophic injuries in which the person enters a state of waking and sleeping with no evidence of purposeful responses. Those who are said to have suffered a mild brain injury are likely to experience a range of continuing problems known as postconcussional syndrome. Typical characteristics are dizziness, impaired concentration, fatigability, depression and restlessness. After 3 months, 79% still have persistent headaches, 59% have memory problems and 34% are still unemployed. Only 45% of those who have sustained a minor injury will have made a good recovery after 1 year (Royal College of Surgeons 1999).

A number of recognised measures are used to assess the severity of traumatic brain injury (Table 15.2).

The resulting deficits can result from the primary injury and also from the secondary forms of brain damage, possibly due to anoxia or infection following the initial trauma. The extent and severity of the resulting deficits are directly related to the primary and secondary brain damage sustained by the individual.

ASSESSMENT OF RECOVERY

An assessment of the level of cognitive functioning can be made by using a scale developed by

Table 15.2 Assessing the severity of traumatic brain injury

Name of scale	Assessed features	Rationale for use	When required	Evaluation
Glasgow Coma Scale (GCS) (Teasdale & Jennett 1974, 1976)	Eye opening ability (1–4) Motor responsiveness (1–6) Verbal responsiveness (1–5)	Scale developed to assess the neurological state to provide a method of detecting deterioration Used as a diagnostic tool and to predict outcome	Assessment of client who presents as being in a coma Frequently used on admission to Accident and Emergency	A score of 8 or below indicates true coma
Post-traumatic Amnesia (PTA) (Moore & Ruesch 1944)	The time period for continuous day-to-day memory to be restored from the point of injury. This should not be confused with the first remembered event following injury	Used to determine intensity and type of rehabilitation Useful cognitive rehabilitation cannot take place if the individual is in a state of post-traumatic amnesia Used as a diagnostic tool and to predict outcome	Prior to commencing rehabilitation or determining readiness for discharge	<5 min – very mild 5 min–1 hour – mild 1–24 h – moderate 1–7 days – severe 7 days or more – very severe
Period of unconsciousness (Eisenberg 1985)		Used as a diagnostic tool and to predict outcome	When establishing the severity of the injury for diagnostic purposes	15 min or less – minor More than 15 min but less than 6 h – moderate 6 h or more – severe 48 h or more – very severe
Period of retrograde amnesia (Goldberg & Bilder 1986)	Assessment of the period of time between the individual's last memory prior to the injury and the time of the injury	Used as a diagnostic tool and to predict outcome	When establishing the severity of the injury for diagnostic purposes	<30 min – mild

the Rancho Los Amigos Hospital in America (Hagen et al 1979). The scale describes a number of levels of awareness with progressive cognitive functioning and behavioural responses (Box 15.1). It can be used to track improvement, to evaluate

potential, for planning and placement purposes and to measure treatment effects (Lal et al 1988).

Following initial assessment to determine at which level the individual is functioning, treatment is then administered in accordance with the developmental pattern.

Box 15.1 Rancho Los Amigos scale (Hagen et al 1979)

1. No response (coma).
2. Generalised response (inconsistent and non-purposeful).
3. Localised response (specific but inconsistent response to stimuli).
4. Confused – agitated (heightened state of activity with decreased ability to process information).
5. Confused, inappropriate, non-agitated.
6. Confused appropriate.
7. Automatic – appropriate.
8. Purposeful and appropriate.

FUNCTIONAL IMPACT

A traumatic brain injury is sudden and frequently catastrophic. There is no preparation or period of adjustment prior to sustaining injury and permanent disability and therefore individuals and families are not able to develop coping strategies over a period of time before the condition reaches a critical stage.

THE IMPACT ON LIFE STAGE DEVELOPMENT

Sustaining an injury in early adulthood interrupts a highly productive part of life and the impact is therefore far-reaching within a wide range of activities involving friends, family members and colleagues and in all areas of the person's occupational performance. Erickson (1963) believed that young adults are involved in working towards the development of intimacy with others as opposed to isolation from them. This intimacy includes the ability to commit to institutions (e.g. work, college, sports clubs) and partnerships, and the experience of cooperating and sharing with others even when this necessitates sacrifice and compromise. He stated that those who are not able to develop a sense of intimacy live in a world apart, absorbed by himself/herself.

Important decisions in the early adult years include career and lifestyle choices. It is usual for the young adult to leave the parental home and establish a new nuclear family. The young adult usually develops a few meaningful relationships and friends commonly share parallel interests. Interruption in this development will have implications for the development of a future lifestyle.

THE IMPACT ON FUNCTIONAL AREAS

The effects of traumatic brain injury are wide and varied but the majority will result in a complex mix of physical, cognitive, behavioural, emotional and psychosocial difficulties. These will require skilled management to maximise functional performance skills and minimise residual difficulties.

The physical deficits can be a combination of spasticity and hypotonic muscle tone and ataxia. Individuals can become wheelchair dependent or make a good physical recovery up to premorbid levels. Some individuals may suffer chronic fatigue, even though they have no apparent physical deficits. Others may experience problems with sensation; visual, perceptual and spatial disorders; and difficulties with speech, language and memory. Impairments in executive functioning are often the result of damage to the frontal lobes of the brain and include difficulties in planning, initiating and organising activity, making decisions and judgements, and the ability to self-monitor; the individual can also be subject to impulsiveness. A high proportion of the brain-injured population develop post-traumatic epilepsy.

Overall, few traumatic brain injuries result in individual sites of isolated damage. It is common for a brain injury to be more diffuse as a result of axonal shearing caused by the mechanical forces exerted during trauma, thus resulting in the typical complex mix of difficulties. The implications in a client's functional abilities in the areas of self care, productivity and leisure can be far reaching.

It is important to recognise that functional performance is greater than the sum of the individual component parts of a task that, on assessment, the person may appear to have the skills to perform. The person must have sufficient intent, motivation and purpose to successfully, consistently and reliably perform a task.

The long-term implications of the residual deficits can be realised only by the injured person, their family and social contacts, and only over a period of time. Once the life-threatening phase is over family members frequently experience a sense of relief. As the process of rehabilitation progresses, there are likely to be feelings of optimism, hope of recovery and a return to the preaccident lifestyle. A critical stage is the time the person returns to the community, attempting to pick up the threads of their previous lifestyle or coming to terms with the necessity to construct a new life.

A person injured in the very productive part of life could have difficulties in all the spheres engaged in prior to sustaining their injuries, that is, there will be implications for their ability to care for themselves, return to work including driving, implications for partners and families and in social and leisure pursuits.

Initial assessment of those with damage to the frontal lobe areas and who have made a full physical recovery can be overly optimistic and it is only over a period of time that the real implications of functional disability and psychosocial problems emerge. In the United Kingdom, few services are equipped to deal with these difficulties in a planned and cohesive manner. Those with untreated emotional and mood disturbances frequently develop a number of challenging behaviours that can have devastating consequences for the long-term outcome of lifestyle and opportunity. Those who have the most severe emotional and behavioural changes are found to have family members who experience the highest level of burden. This can result in divorce, separation and/or the rupturing of long-term relationships. Partners frequently express negative feelings, saying that they have become more of a minder and carer rather than a friend and lover.

Those with emotional and/or behavioural problems are frequently ostracised by social groups and can be targeted unfairly and even taken advantage of, e.g. physical, sexual or financial abuse.

THE INTERVENTION TEAM

Few specialist services within the statutory system in the United Kingdom can offer dedicated brain injury services with long-term follow-up. The acute care for people with brain injury is generally excellent. Long-term follow-up services, however, after this initial period of treatment and rehabilitation remain fragmented. The independent sector has many dedicated brain injury services, with extracontractual referrals from Health Authorities and Social Services being commonplace. The health and social care professionals, assistants and voluntary workers involved may vary depending on both the stage of recovery and the extent of the permanent injuries sustained.

In the initial stages, hospitalisation is likely, the length of time will depend on the severity of the brain injury. At this time the medical model is more likely to be dominant.

In the early stages of rehabilitation, the interdisciplinary team caring for the injured person will be large. Physiotherapists and occupational therapists, orthotists and suppliers of equipment might well be necessary in the overall treatment and management of physical disability. Outstanding medical issues could require the intervention of physicians, surgeons and skilled nursing care. A dietician might be needed, because some people will be fed via a percutaneous endoscopic gastrostomy site or require carefully balanced nutrition because of their poor ability to take adequate foodstuffs. Speech and language therapy will be required for the assessment of any swallowing disorder and speech and language functioning.

As recovery progresses and medical stability is achieved, more intensive intervention from occupational therapists, physiotherapists, speech and language therapists and neuropsychologists, with their respective assistants, will dominate the rehabilitation. This interdisciplinary team will assist the individual to achieve functional competence commensurate with the level of cognitive recovery. Neuropsychology intervention is vital in the assessment of mood, emotional disturbance, cognitive damage and behavioural difficulties. This will enable the design of treatment programmes for the adequate management of these most important factors.

As the individual progresses into the community, therapeutic intervention continues along with job coaches, social workers, voluntary organisations and day centres providing structure for the brain-injured population. In the United Kingdom, organisations such as Headway and the United Kingdom of Acquired Brain Injury Forum (UKABIF) can provide much support for individuals and families. It is important to note that family members should be considered key members of the team at all stages in the rehabilitation and long-term management of individuals with brain injury. It is often the case that Social Services departments designate their teams for those with physical disability, mental health problems and learning disability and it is generally accepted that the needs of the brain-injured population may require services from all three sectors. As a result of this, a number of local authorities are now developing dedicated brain

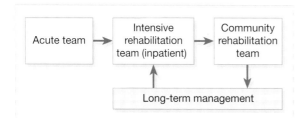

Fig. 15.1 Flow chart demonstrating the feedback loops for rereferral.

injury teams for the long-term support of such individuals.

Rehabilitation is more likely to take place following the achievement of medical stability. However, it is likely that some individuals will require a short period of intensive rehabilitation some years postinjury and a mechanism of rereferral is essential in the long-term management of the residual difficulties (Fig. 15.1).

A key worker or case manager may be responsible for the coordination of an individual's care and community rehabilitation (University of Warwick 1998). This person, who will keep in touch with the individual and the family over a period of time, will monitor progress regularly and help to prevent a build-up of problems. This key worker, who may or may not be an occupational therapist, ensures a safety net through the ability to rerefer if difficulties exist. Additionally, the key worker provides a vital support system for the family, who are themselves key long-term members of the rehabilitation team.

INTERVENTION

THEORETICAL FOUNDATIONS

The complexity and multiplicity of problems experienced by brain-injured people present challenges and demands to the rehabilitation team. The therapist will need to draw from a broad theoretical base and will need to demonstrate sound clinical reasoning skills. Each individual poses different problems and needs and a person-centred approach to intervention is essen-

tial. This must take account of the stage of recovery, level of deficit and the environment in which the person is placed (see Chapter 2).

The occupational therapist is in a significant position through the entire care pathway – from intensive care, through the rehabilitation process and on into the community – to consider the generic picture of the individual and to explore the specific approaches required. The therapist will require a clear knowledge of the component skills associated with the tasks attempted by the person throughout his daily life, and a sound understanding of the impact of the person's disability upon occupational performance. The individual with brain injury may present with a cocktail of physical, behavioural, cognitive, emotional and social problems and the therapist will need to explore the interplay of these deficits and their impact on the individual.

Exploration of the literature reveals expansive study of the deficits following injury but less evidence as a basis for the efficacy of practice relating to the components of occupational performance. There is a paucity of evidence written by occupational therapists and this is clearly a focus for the profession in the future.

ASSESSMENT

Assessment of the brain-injured person is a dynamic process, and it is important that the colateral assessment of other team members is taken into account. It is important that the therapist remains aware of the context in which the assessment takes place and the demands of the environment upon the individual. The occupational therapist provides crucial information to the team with respect to a person's functional ability in relation to their occupational performance needs.

The therapist needs to observe and interact with the individual in a measured and reflective way. Consideration should be given to identifying retained skills and strengths, as well as defining deficits. There is no standard model used by therapists working with this group but the therapist needs to work in a person-centred way during assessment. As the person may not have the cognitive skills to identify realistic personal goals, a framework that can be used on their behalf in a person-centred way, utilising information from the family and from life development theories, and taking account of the impact of cognitive, behavioural and emotional changes, is indicated (see Chapter 2). It is suggested that the model proposed by Reed and Sanderson (1992) – Personal Adaptation through Occupation – would provide the initial generic base required. This model is appropriate because it takes a broad view of the individual within his environment and guides towards clear reasoning of appropriate approaches to intervention and realistic goal definition.

Once an overall picture has been gained, standardised assessments might be used to gain more detailed information in specific areas. Standardised assessments and evaluation tools are becoming increasingly available to the therapist. Commonly used tests include:

- The Chessington Occupational Therapy Neurological Assessment Battery (COTNAB; Tyerman et al 1986).
- A large battery of functionally based assessments through the Thames Valley Test Company as screening measures (e.g. the Rivermead Behavioural Memory Test, the Behavioural Assessment of the Dysexecutive Syndrome (BADS), Hayling and Brixton Test, the Test of Everyday Attention).
- Batteries of tests through the Psychological Test Corporation. Many of the tests available for mental health are usefully applicable to brain injury.
- The Assessment of Motor and Process Skills (AMPS) and the Functional Independence Measure (FIM) are becoming more common, particularly as it is suggested that these provide documentable outcome measures.

As outlined earlier in this section, whilst such assessment is important, it does not replace the unique and irreplaceable role of the therapist in relating inability to everyday function and the individual within his environment. Great care and skill must be used in choosing standardised measures and the validity of predictiveness through isolated test results.

A broad-based assessment, with detailed standardised assessment where appropriate, coupled with knowledge gained about the person as an individual and linked to appropriate life stage theories, will lead to the establishment of person-centred priorities within proposed intervention, and to clear aims and objectives. Having identified the individual's occupational performance needs, the therapist will necessarily draw on a range of frames of reference and approaches at different stages of the person's recovery.

FRAMES OF REFERENCE

In the early stages treatment will focus, for example, on the promotion of recovery, whereas later techniques will become increasingly compensatory. Different rehabilitation services may specialise in particular types of difficulties and may, therefore, focus on a particular frame of reference in response to the needs of those they are treating. Frames of reference and approaches commonly found to be most appropriate are outlined below.

Developmental frame of reference

Neurodevelopmental/neurophysiological approaches

Based upon the normalisation of muscle tone, inhibition of abnormal reflex activity and promotion of normal movement, this approach facilitates normal movement through handling, sensory stimulation or through inhibitory positioning (Bobath 1978).

Sensorimotor approach

Cutaneous stimulation, use of temperature (heat and cold), proprioceptive input and rhythm may be used (Rood 1962) in a controlled way to facilitate normal movement in a goal-directed way.

Sensory integration

This approach is more frequently used with children but techniques are used with brain-injured people in the early stages of recovery, particularly when working at an automatic level with those who have a low level of consciousness. Treatment focuses on promoting normal reflex responses and voluntary movement through provision of controlled sensory stimulation. Stimuli are provided through vestibular, proprioceptive, tactile, visual and auditory channels (Ayres 1972, 1979).

Biomechanical frame of reference

This frame of reference uses the principles of mechanics as they relate to the human body. It focuses on the posture, position, mobility and handing of the person in relation to himself, others, orthoses, equipment and the environment. People with brain injury may also have concomitant injuries, which indicate use of this response.

Learning frame of reference

Behavioural approaches

Behavioural approaches to learning frequently underpin rehabilitation programmes. Cognitive impairments may result in the inability to retain learning or to monitor socially appropriate behaviour. Programmes may focus on the reinforcement of positive or appropriate behaviours, adaptation of the environment and the consideration of antecedents to antisocial behaviours or aggression. Behavioural approaches may be used to habituate skills through modelling and chaining techniques.

Cognitive approaches

Increasingly, strategies based on cognitive approaches to learning are employed. They may be used in the development of strategies to address cognitive deficit and to modify behaviour. It has been known for some time that it is the cognitive and personality problems following brain injury that create the greatest challenges to outcome and to those caring for survivors.

Cognitive behavioural approaches

Cognitive behavioural approaches, whereby individuals link their emotion, behaviour and thought processes, are used as intervention techniques to address cognitive deficits, e.g. perceptual difficulties, memory strategies, problem-solving techniques and also in the management of secondary psychological consequences, such as anxiety, depression, anger management and grief reactions.

Compensatory frame of reference

Many deficits experienced by brain-injured people are not curable through therapy. Function, however, is restorable through the development of strategies and systems appropriate to the individual and which compensate for lost skills.

Some or all of these approaches might be seen in the pathway from acute care to the community. There is no prescription to follow with the brain-injured person. Intervention follows a process dependent upon the impact of injury upon the individual and his environment, and his needs related to his desired occupational performance.

GUIDELINES FOR INTERVENTION

There are a number of factors that may influence recovery and these are early intervention, appropriate rehabilitation, family support and environmental factors and long-term follow-up:

- Therapeutic intervention should commence as early after injury as possible.
- Emphasis should be placed on addressing the impact of the combined sequelae for the individual rather than on each individual deficit.
- It is vital that the rehabilitation team is well coordinated and that its members communicate well. Consistencies of approach and clear communications are vital. Brain-injured people are prone to 'mixed messages' and do not cope well with ambiguity.
- In the early stages of recovery, stimulating the individual towards restored function is an appropriate intervention. Consideration should also be given to the introduction of strategies to deal with cognitive sequelae and of the need to train in specific tasks. Therapy

thus focuses on microdeficits and macrodeficits simultaneously.

- Intervention needs to be based in real life environments using normal activities with the person's occupational needs clearly in focus.
- Throughout treatment planning, emphasis should be placed on the cognitive, emotional and behavioural consequences of brain injury, as well as on physical sequelae.

ACUTE CARE

Occupational therapy in neurointensive care

People in the early stages after acquired brain injury may be nursed on specialised units and/or the intensive therapy unit of the hospital. The occupational therapist will often become involved even before the person is medically stable (Scott & Dow 1995).

To accommodate the fact that the person is unable to participate in planning and decision making at this stage, a person-centred approach to treatment will require the therapist to make decisions on the person's behalf (see Chapter 2). In this, the therapist will be guided by her knowledge of the physical and cognitive sequelae of brain injury and intervention will be planned accordingly. In the latter stages of this phase the therapist will be guided by knowledge of the person from relatives and friends when planning specific intervention.

Aims of treatment

- Establish the level of arousal by systematic observation, controlled stimulation and reference to multidisciplinary assessment.
- Prevent deformity and promote good positioning.
- Promote orientation within the environment.
- Facilitate family involvement in rehabilitation and offer support.

SMART: Sensory Modality Assessment and Rehabilitation Technique.   The SMART was developed over a 10-year period by occupational therapy staff at the Royal Hospital for Neurodisability. It is a standardised assessment tool for people referred with a suggested diagnosis of persistent vegetative state.

The SMART provides a structured sensory programme, which assesses the five senses as well as movement, communication and wakefulness. It has been recognised for some time that as many as 50% of diagnoses of persistent vegetative state may be wrong. This tool is therefore invaluable in assisting therapists to maximise potential for the individual to interact purposefully with his environment. Use of this assessment will ensure that the person receives an accurate assessment of his level of awareness prior to judicial decisions (Gill 1996a,b).

Areas of intervention by the therapist may include measurement of arousal levels and appropriate coma stimulation, consideration of post-traumatic amnesia levels, splinting and positioning, and seating. Avoidance of raised intracranial pressure is a central concern at this stage and changes in position may require medical supervision. Early assessments of cognition and function may be made and person-centred therapeutic goals established by the therapist/family, as already described. Care should be taken at this stage, because recovery is at such a fluid level that baselines are not reliable. The person's condition will fluctuate from day to day, and hour to hour. Assessment at this stage can relate only to the treatment session in hand. A pattern of recovery will evolve gradually and careful monitoring will increase effective planning as the person moves through levels of consciousness. Treatment times should be regular, frequent and graded to the individual's tolerance.

Family education.   At this stage, the role of the occupational therapist is particularly relevant to the family members. At a time when they are exposed to a plethora of incomprehensible and unwelcome clinical information, and are faced with an unresponsive relative connected to complex life-preserving machinery, the relationship with the occupational therapist can be extremely important. Along with other team members, the occupational therapist needs to develop skills in explaining brain injury to the injured person's family. She needs to outline her role in the intervention of the brain-injured person and explain clearly how her intervention will affect the rehabilitation process. Early aggressive therapy has been associated with decreased total length of rehabilitation and higher cognitive levels at discharge (Mackay et al 1992).

Involvement of relatives in the process, directing their stimulation of the injured person, increasing their confidence to interact with the passive recipient and encouraging practical activities, such as collation of familiar personal items, photographs, interest lists, can go a long way towards establishing engagement and assisting the grief process to which the relatives are exposed. Education is important in helping the relatives to understand the process of recovery and to avoid unrealistic expectations.

Returning from coma

As the person emerges from coma he will frequently go through a period of marked agitation, possible aggressive behaviour and confusion. This may include rocking (stereotyped repetitive purposeless movements of the trunk), thrashing, attempting to hit, bite or pinch others, pulling out tubes and catheters, shouting, attempting to get out of the chair/bed or wandering.

The major focus of therapy will be on the performance components of communication, motor control and basic personal care as the building blocks to higher skills. These should be achieved through functional activity. Distraction levels are high and the person will quickly lose interest outside the framework of goal-directed activity at this stage. The therapist will continue to take a leading role in establishment of these goals and a person-centred approach remains essential in defining treatment goals.

Aims of treatment

- Appraisal of levels of orientation.
- Decrease of agitated behaviour by management of the environment.
- Promotion of familiar, meaningful activity and routines.

- Introduction of orientation aids and strategies.

The person might require management by tranquillisers, particularly if he has concomitant injuries such as fractures. Frequently, however, this period of confusion can be addressed through environmental modification and sensitive handling. Tranquillisers can slow recovery and the occupational therapist might be asked to advise regarding behavioural management. Careful risk assessments should be made.

People can become fixed on an idea to explain their environment and situation or a desire to accomplish a particular task. The therapist should focus on engaging the person in meaningful activities within the limits of his capacity. Emphasis is placed on decreasing the agitated behaviour by minimising overstimulation and confusion in the environment. The person is 'stimulus bound', that is, he responds in a stereotypical way to the environment. If uncomfortable or overstimulated then he will respond according to the environmental or physical stimulus with agitated behaviour.

During this stage of recovery, much of the person's behaviour is non-purposeful and his attention span is short. The therapist should promote familiar, simple activities. The more the activities can be associated and approximated to a normal routine, the better. If an activity leads to an increase in agitation, consideration should be given to the levels of stimulation inherent within the task.

The environment should promote as much autonomy as possible within the limits of safety. Management of risk is important. People can engage in bizarre activities (Box 15.2), often as a result of misinterpretation of cues in the environment.

The environment should provide orientation prompts that are in context. Therapists should be careful not to overload the person by providing too much information at once. The therapist should prompt with one instruction at a time and wait for the person to respond or to complete each instruction. The therapist may need to model tasks or initiate activity by guiding the person

---

Box 15.2   Example of reaction to environmental cues

Whilst Sam was waiting for his meal he began trying to eat the pattern off his placemat and drink from his empty glass. This behaviour continued despite efforts from the nursing staff. The therapist deduced that Sam was responding to the cues provided by his place setting. Removal of these environmental antecedents and distraction by engaging Sam in conversation prior to mealtimes quickly eradicated the behaviour.

---

physically. Tasks that are 'overlearned' or that are normally completed at an automatic level are the easiest for the person to carry out; washing, cleaning teeth, dressing, feeding, pouring a drink, lighting a cigarette or loading a CD are all activities that may fall into this category.

Becoming increasingly goal directed

As the person becomes more able to follow instructions and maintain attention, rehabilitation can intensify. The individual will begin automatically to develop independence in areas where he has adequate contextual cues and which are within the limits of his physical disability. He will still require a highly structured, low-stimulus environment to promote this process. Increasing use can now be made of environmental cues and prompts, checklists, orientation aids (clocks, calendars), and the commencement of habitual use of external memory aids. Intervention focuses on sensorimotor difficulties and cognitive skills.

As the person develops increased awareness it is important to involve him in the process of goal setting and the establishment of priorities in intervention at a level that is appropriate. People with brain injury at this level of recovery may not be able to set realistic goals but it is important that they begin to take charge of limited choices to maintain engagement and to promote feelings of autonomy. Using a person-centred framework, such as Maslow's hierarchy of needs (Maslow 1970), physiological needs can be addressed as a base to higher skills and priorities. Basic needs, such as continence, feeding and personal care, are addressed in the first instance, building towards higher skills having re-established a pattern to the daily routine.

Aims of treatment

- Manage the environment to provide controlled stimulation.
- Promote increased independence in appropriate daily living skills through re-establishment of basic routines relevant to the individual at an automatic or prompted level.
- Promote orientation and reduce confusion.
- Encourage the development of normal movement patterns through positioning and physical facilitation.
- Initiate the use of external strategies to ameliorate cognitive difficulties.

POSTACUTE STAGES
General considerations

Currently, the focus of rehabilitation remains on the acute and intermediate stages of recovery. Emphasis continues to be placed on physical dysfunction and, despite our knowledge of the long-term consequences of brain injury, the vast majority of people in the United Kingdom have little access to services in the community, nor do they receive sufficient support or rehabilitation beyond the first few months after their injury.

Domain specificity

Brain-injured individuals have difficulty transferring skills from one environment to another. Rehabilitation environments need to be as close as possible to reality whilst maintaining sufficient consistency and safety for the individual to explore their independence in a controlled, measured way. Teaching memory skills in a department does not mean that the individual will be able to transfer these to everyday life.

Developing routines and structures within the hospital environment is insufficient to meet the demands of everyday life. Ability in the therapy kitchen or on a brief home visit does not in itself indicate reliability of performance on a day-to-day basis.

Errorless learning

People with brain injury learn from success as opposed to trial and error. Procedural learning remains intact and mistakes will often become part of routine or habit. Procedural learning may also be used to re-establish a daily framework or to develop new skills through the use of checklists and proactive prompting (Box 15.3).

Strengths not weaknesses

Throughout this stage, emphasis should be placed on retained strengths as opposed to deficits. It is the retained skills and abilities that provide the compensatory strengths to overcome the challenges faced. Problems and failures consistently confront the brain-injured person. This can lead to a negative spiral of avoidance, poor self-esteem and helplessness. People learn to withdraw from situations that they find difficult or, alternatively, become increasingly chaotic and inappropriate in their behaviour.

Identifying occupational performance needs

Once the individual has a raised level of consciousness and becomes more goal orientated and purposeful, he enters the most active rehabilitation phase. The persisting sequelae of acquired brain injury are varied and individual. Survivors of brain injury are often left with sensorimotor disturbance and cognitive, emotional,

---

Box 15.3 Errorless learning
D, an amnesic person, was involved in a rehabilitation programme involving use of a computer. He had never used a computer before and the therapist noted that he tried to get into the software on screen by randomly pressing keys. After several days, the therapist observed that D consistently followed the same erroneous pattern – he had habitually learned to fail at the task. The therapist proactively introduced a written sequential checklist that D was prompted to follow. After several days the cues were decreased and within a short period the checklist was also abandoned because D had learned how to open the software correctly.

---

behavioural and social problems that require intermittent or intensive therapy for months and years postinjury (Klonoff et al 1986). The interaction with the wider environment, therefore, will demonstrate the impact of the person's disability on occupational performance needs. In the early stages, emphasis tends to be placed upon goals in self care, but with less awareness of issues related to goals surrounding productivity and leisure. It is important that the therapist does not lose sight of these long-term issues when establishing intervention. Intervention is always directed towards the fulfilment of appropriate occupational performance needs.

Physical and cognitive sequelae and their impact on occupational performance

Physical sequelae

The neurological insult of brain injury results in varied problems in the nature and level of recovery (Table 15.3). The current emphasis during inpatient rehabilitation continues to focus upon promotion of motor recovery, often neglecting to address other areas. Sensorimotor deficits may be the result of neurological damage or as a result of concomitant injuries (e.g. fractures, internal damage, burns). Approaches and goals of treatment will vary accordingly. Generally, in promoting recovery, treatment is based on a developmental frame of reference. Approaches to treatment are outlined elsewhere and should be read in conjunction with this chapter (see Chapter 3).

Post-traumatic epilepsy can occur; severity often diminishes over time but it can persist. Continued monitoring by a neurologist usually results in appropriate treatment. The therapist should be aware of any first aid response to a seizure and how to monitor the person during an attack. Awareness should be raised with respect to the potential risks and to side-effects of antiepileptic medication.

Cognitive sequelae

Attention. There are several tests available to the therapist that are useful in the assessment of

Table 15.3 Physical sequelae

Sequelae	Functional difficulty	Effect on occupational performance	Principles of intervention
Changes in muscle tone as a result of damage to motor pathways	Paresis or paralysis	Loss of normal movement patterns leads to difficulty in daily living skills Increased risk factors, loss of role in family and possible wider environment Limitation of leisure and social activities	Inhibition of abnormal movement and posture and facilitatory approach to normal movement Facilitatory handling and modification of environment (Bobath 1978)
Ataxia resulting from reduced proprioceptive input or cerebellar damage	Reduced coordination Lack of smooth movement Balance problems	Loss of coordination and clumsiness leads to difficulty in daily living skills such as feeding, dressing and personal care Reduced balance and/or coordination leads to increased risk of falls Social and leisure activities reduced	Proximal dynamic weight bearing and placing activities Weighting of body parts – this rarely achieves more than a dampening effect Use of compensatory approaches and adaptation of environment to maximise function Prompting to pace activity within limits (Bobath 1978, Balliet et al 1987)
Difficulty in the initiation and termination of movement	Problems of arousal and fatigue Premotor planning difficulties Apraxia Problems terminating movement (motor perseveration)	Difficulty commencing activities and in completing, pacing and sequencing tasks May achieve automatic movements but limit more complex goal directed activity	Hierarchical prompting, written and verbal checklists following task analysis. These may be developed as self-instruction 'Chaining' of tasks by gradually reducing prompts at the start or end Clear definition of start and end points in tasks
Sensory disturbance	Tactile or proprioceptive loss	Poor feedback increases risk of abnormal movement patterns Neglect of limb leads to difficulties in daily living tasks Loss of tactile sensation causes safety issues Cultural environment may expect the use of specific limb for certain activities Social activities limited through diminished function	Use of compensatory approach to encourage use of vision Encourage use of affected limb in bilateral activity Position limb in view (Bobath 1978, Rood 1962)
Special senses: • Visual disturbance Deficits in visual fields Reduced eye movement • Hearing Loss as a result of 8th cranial nerve damage • Smell Damage to front of head associated with cranial nerve damage Often associated with poor outcome as it links with severe injury and frontal lobe damage • Taste Less common but reduced in people with loss of sense of smell	Blurred vision, double vision, scanning problems Deafness, tinnitus Inability to smell noxious substances Loss of sense of taste and appetite General reduction in information from environment	Loss of special senses can impact on daily living skills such as driving and eating Increased risk in internal and external environments Increased risk of isolation and limitation of social activities	Consultations should be available to explore potential for reduction of problem by treatment. This might include prisms, magnifiers or hearing aids Promotion of compensatory strategies to reduce impact on occupational performance, such as scanning strategies, use of head movement, reduction of noise in the environment

attentional difficulties. In particular, the Thames Valley test batteries, Paced Auditory Serial Attention Test (PASAT; Gronwall 1977).

Information can also be obtained by careful and systematic observation in therapy and in functional tasks. The therapist should question the person's ability to sustain activity, how distractible he is, whether he can maintain conversation or divide his attention between two tasks. Activities that a person could previously manage automatically require greater effort and problems with attention can create widespread impact on occupational performance.

There is mixed evidence that remediation techniques are useful (Ponsford & Kinsella 1988, Sohlberg & Mateer 1987) but cognitive demand can be reduced by practice and habituation. Verbal self-instruction can be helpful. In the acquisition of new skills it is usual to rehearse verbally prior to carrying through a task and instruction will often be internalised as the activity becomes increasingly familiar and demand on attention is reduced. Written checklists can be used to perform a similar purpose, enabling the person to maintain engagement in a task, reducing demand on impaired capacity and facilitating return to the activity in hand after losing track.

Perceptual problems. Perception is the process of organising, interpreting, storing and responding to information received from one or more sensory organs (Zolton et al 1986). Perception enables us to make sense of the environment.

Whilst other neurological problems may result in specific perceptual disability, the diffuse nature of acquired brain injury creates additional problems in assessment and treatment. Functional problems are sometimes attributed to a perceptual difficulty when they have been produced through combined effects of cerebral damage. Care should be taken in the analysis of assessment measures to consider the wider perspective and to make a detailed functional analysis through careful structured observation. Specific difficulties are referenced within the framework of treatment for cerebral vascular accident.

In the past, intervention focused on remediation techniques. There is some evidence that in the acute stages of recovery a stimulatory approach to perceptual deficits might be helpful but there is less evidence that skills generalise from one environment or task to another.

Again, compensatory techniques such as structuring the environment, cueing devices within the environment specific to the individual and the task, self-instruction and checklists are useful. Practical, functional approaches are the most effective, as are those that are task orientated. Behavioural learning theories and approaches can be useful in specific task training.

Memory. One of the most common persistent problems following acquired brain injury is memory dysfunction. Problems arise at the levels of attending to information, of processing, of encoding and storing information, and of being able to retrieve information. It is a person's ability to remember things proactively that predominantly affects his ability to manage daily life and is a priority within therapy.

Ongoing deficits can be ameliorated through specific training that is task orientated; by developing internal strategies using mental imagery, rhyming and mnemonics or by the development of external strategies such as diaries, notebooks and planning devices. Demands on a reduced memory function can also be minimised by development of routines and a structured lifestyle (Kapur 1995, Miller 1992, Wilson 1989).

Historically, the practice of remembering has been the most widely used form of memory therapy. There is no evidence to suggest that practising memory games, or exercising the 'memory muscle' is effective. Recognition that this is ineffective has led to the use of internal memory strategies. This might include forming bizarre visual images or verbal rhymes to assist retention and recall. These strategies are employed by mnemonists and are popular within programmes marketed at the general population to 'improve your memory'. Advertising campaigns employ similar strategies to help trigger our recall of specific products.

In reality, these techniques are only of limited functional use and do not replace the use of external aids. With the expansion of modern technology there are increasing numbers of electronic devices available that act as prompts, such as the Neuropager (Wilson 1997). Palm-held computers are complex to use but can benefit people with a high level of retained reasoning skills, insight and the ability to initiate behaviour.

In general, whilst all devices are worth consideration for the individual, it is difficult to replace the versatility, flexibility and personalisation of pen and paper systems. The act of categorising, sorting and writing down information provides a prompt and a level of elaboration that assists the amnesic person in itself.

To be of functional use, systems should be proactive and simple to use. Journals can also be of use to help people to maintain a monitor of thoughts and feelings but it is the development of ways to achieve planned activity that will have the greatest impact on independence. To be of use, such systems should be used at an automatic or habitual level. Ironically, many people with brain injury are reluctant to use such systems, not least because they remind them that they forget. The therapist needs to use behavioural learning theory to reinforce practical use. Staff and family should be encouraged to prompt activity by directing attention to the external aid as opposed to offering a direct prompt. The therapist should be persistent, as these compensatory aids will be the framework for autonomy in the long term.

Language. Specific language problems will be treated by the speech and language therapist but frequently people will present with functional problems that are overlooked. Reading, writing and social language skills need to be assessed in different environmental settings and the occupational therapist can play an important role in facilitating evaluation of the functional impact of language disorder to the individual.

Deficits should be considered when presenting information through verbal or visual prompts. The therapist should also always work towards individual strengths. She may become involved in the recommendation of communication aids. Behavioural problems can arise as a result of frustrated communication and multidisciplinary decisions may need to be made as to the optimum timescale to introduce such aids. Generally, compensatory strategies to language should be used

only when they assist language development or where further recovery is unlikely.

Dysexecutive problems. Problems with executive skills are often associated with frontal lobe damage to the brain. Impairments in these skills, perhaps more than any other, contribute to the failure of the brain-injured population to achieve its potential (Table 15.4). Signs of dysexecutive problems can be subtle and difficult to assess.

It will be noted that these problems are products of mental processing and are rarely seen in isolation. Disorders in executive functioning result in a gradual downward decline in independent activity (Fig. 15.2). This can be reduced by:

- Establishing routines and structure to daily living. The therapist needs to draw on behaviour learning theories to reinforce this process. She must ensure that routines are within a framework of a concrete and predictable environment.
- Developing an infrastructure of external systems and strategies designed to provide the person with the means to structure his own environment.

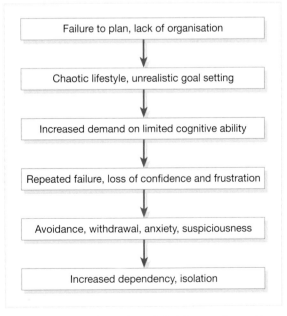

Fig. 15.2 Downward negative spiral of dysexecutive problems.

Table 15.4 Dysexecutive problems

Area of difficulty	Functional deficit	Impact on occupational performance
Organisational skills	The person has difficulty with tasks requiring prioritising, sequencing and timetabling	The person fails to attend appointments, fails to complete daily living skills, avoids activity or becomes chaotic
Realistic goal setting	The person has difficulty identifying personal goals or projecting their desires and needs in to goal-directed behaviour	Person has difficulty evaluating their lifestyle. There is an imbalance of occupational performance components. Person has sense of failure
Motivation (goal-directed behaviour)	As the person has limited realistic goals, they have no direction or reason to initiate activity	Person avoids activity or finds it harder to engage in meaningful activity. Can lead to secondary mental health issues
Decision making and judgemental skills Predictive skills	Person has difficulty identifying problems, generating options and evaluating consequences	Poor life decisions are made. Increased safety risks, increased dependence on others. Increased vulnerability
Impulsivity	Person reacts to internal and external stimuli without evaluation	Increased risk of safety or neglect. Increased vulnerability
Insight and awareness	Person is unaware of, or denies, level of their problem	Person has increased risks associated with safety and vulnerability
Self-monitoring and evaluation	Person has difficulty measuring their ability and does not learn consequentially	Person has problems evaluating their performance during productivity and leisure pursuits. Difficulty in maintaining productivity
Perseveration	Person becomes fixated on an idea or behaviour. Is extremely rigid and has difficulty moving to another task or idea	Person has problems completing daily living skills and in exploring options
Social perception	The person has difficulty 'reading' social situations and empathising with others	Inability to behave appropriately in social situations during productivity and leisure pursuits. May lead to social isolation and secondary mental health issues
Abstract thinking	The person is only able to focus on 'here and now'. Can think only in concrete parameters	Difficulties with generating options for problem solving, empathising with others, evaluation and predictive skills

- Training in well-practised 'emergency' strategies for use when routines fail, or when meeting non-predictable events.
- Over learning of routines and skills within different environments.
- Training in problem-solving techniques that enable the person to turn abstract difficulties into a concrete frame. The therapist helps the person to externalise a behaviour that most of us carry out spontaneously and internally. Whatever sequence of steps is taken, the person must be allowed to identify the problem in concrete terms, to identify alternative options to deal with the problem, to select an option by considering their abilities/potential difficulties, to consider the likely outcome and to evaluate the outcome of his decision.

Behavioural changes. Behaviour and personality changes are commonly associated with acquired brain injury. Sometimes changes can be so severe that they prevent reintegration into the community and meaningful independence. Behaviour problems include physical or verbal aggression, disinhibition, motivation problems and impulsivity. Psychiatric disorders may also follow brain injury. Anxiety and depression are common, obsessive–compulsive symptoms and paranoid ideations are frequent and suicide levels are increased in this population. Psychotic disorders may also occur.

It is arguable whether these changes are as a direct result of brain injury or secondary to cognitive difficulties. Again, symptoms should not be viewed in isolation and premorbid personalities and dynamics should be considered. Problems may be exacerbated by the person's lack of awareness and insight.

Much work in brain injury has centred around the behavioural frame of reference. Simply, behaviour training changes automatic responses by changing reinforcement/consequences for that response (Brooks & McKinlay 1983, Skinner 1953, Wood 1987). Changing the precursors to the behaviour and shaping the environment to maximise success is paramount. Techniques are employed to increase or decrease targeted behaviours. It is important that programmes are designed individually according to the individual's problem behaviours, his current level of awareness and cognition and his occupational performance needs. Target areas and mode of reinforcement should be clearly defined and explained to the person and his family. Whilst appearing initially straightforward, it is important that the therapeutic milieu is supportive of the techniques employed, that staff are trained and able to understand the initial escalation in problem behaviours and that a suitable and consistent reinforcement regimen is available.

Working towards occupational performance goals

The long-term outcome of the rehabilitation process must remain a priority at all stages of intervention. Whilst it is not possible to predict outcome in the acute stages of recovery, the therapist must be careful to establish realistic goals and take care not to reinforce unrealistic or unfeasible long-term options. Sadly, the majority of brain-injured survivors are discharged home as soon as they are considered by medical staff to be mobile and sufficiently orientated to cope outside, on the false premise that they will recover more quickly in a familiar environment. The family may be all too willing to have their relative back home but in fact the problems are only just beginning. It is increasingly acknowledged that availability to continuing services over many years is required if a person is to maximise potential for reintegration and adjustment (University of Warwick 1998).

People are found in community settings at all levels of physical, cognitive and behavioural recovery. The therapist will continue to draw on several frames of reference as outlined throughout this chapter.

At some point, the person will reach a plateau of recovery and here his long-term settlement should be considered. Careful and detailed planning is important and involves establishing the resources required for the individual to maximise his quality of life. The availability, desire and capability of the family to be involved with support should be considered prior to establishing a detailed care plan with appropriate assessment of the risks involved. The establishment of a routine involving, as far as possible, balance of self care, productivity and leisure areas, is essential to enable both the individual and his carers to re-establish a life pattern appropriate to all their needs.

It has already been identified that people with brain injury do not generalise skills well from one environment to another and care should be taken throughout the rehabilitation process that strategies, systems and skills are appropriate to use within the community. Some people remain unsupportable outside a residential environment, or require continued access to a specialised resource. Attention should be made to the quality and appropriateness of the long-term sheltered environment in this case.

Family roles

The impact of the brain injury is dramatic and immediate. Whilst the family are immediately grateful that their relative has returned, they often expect the injured person to return to their former role. Adaptation to changed roles and dynamics within the family are sometimes difficult to accommodate. Counselling may assist some families to resolve this process, whilst readjustment of family roles remains a reality.

Driving

Ability to resume driving is a high priority for most adults and, for adolescents, permission to start learning. This is a highly sensitive area and guidelines remain limited, with the exception of legal restrictions created by epilepsy. Many former drivers can perform driving skills at basic levels but come up against difficulties as operational skills move to a strategic level. The therapist has a legal responsibility to advise the brain-injured person that they should inform DVLA about their accident and the implications of insurance validity.

The therapist needs to have a clear awareness of the limitations and psychological concerns that should be assessed. Driving assessments and lessons from driving schools or referral to specialist centres may be necessary.

Employment

To many people, having meaningful employment is a mark of recovery and independence. The more severe the injury, the less likely is successful return to work. Problems with time keeping, social skills, disruptive or socially inappropriate behaviours and poor monitoring skills all contribute to difficulties in maintaining employment. Supported employment and the use of job coaches can assist in identifying problems and establishing strategies to ameliorate or explain difficulties for employers. The rehabilitation process should explore vocational or prevocational skills.

Employment services can offer help in finding supported employment. Voluntary work placements can assist but, increasingly, the work skills required are comparable with those required for paid employment. Volunteer placements can sometimes be more easily supported or accommodate part-time hours.

College courses can also be useful and it is important for younger survivors to receive adequate education. Most adults access college courses as a step towards a career or for leisure. Brain-injured people have difficulties with new learning and classroom environments, and courses have a limited lifespan. Education should, therefore, be considered an alternative option, providing the course is carefully chosen and the person is adequately supported. The point within the programme that this is introduced is also critical if it is to be successful. For some people, the establishment of alternative productivity roles through responsibilities related to domestic activities such as gardening, pet care or homecare, for example, can act as an alternative to community-based productivity. Routine attendance at a daycare facility can also be viewed in this way.

CONCLUSION

This chapter has provided a brief overview of the multiplicity of difficulties facing people with brain injury and the challenges facing the rehabilitation team. Some of these difficulties and challenges are illustrated in the case study in Box 15.4. They necessitate a broad spectrum of skills, approaches to therapeutic intervention and sound understanding of the impact of disability on occupational performance. It is essential that inexperienced therapists have adequate supervision when working with this group. The occupational therapist plays a key role within the team at all points in the care pathway.

Box 15.4   Case study

Background

Darren, a young man of 19, lived at home with his mother, uncle and younger sister in a council house. He worked as a trainee chef. He enjoyed playing sport and socialised regularly with his friends. Darren suffered from epilepsy, which took the form of tonic–clonic seizures but which was well controlled with medication. This did not affect his work but posed limitations on his future prospects.

Medical history

Darren was admitted to intensive care following a road traffic accident. His Glasgow Coma Scale was 5 on admission. Early intervention involved acute care followed by rehabilitation in a Younger Disabled Unit. Darren was admitted to a specialist brain injury rehabilitation unit 2 years postinjury. His placement was funded by statutory services. On admission:

- **Physical**: Darren was non-weight bearing because of extent of his disability. He had increased muscle tone on his left side with severe contractures of his left upper limb. His right side was ataxic and he had severe dysarthria. His epilepsy remained. Functionally he remained highly dependent on others.
- **Cognitive**: Darren had reduced cognitive ability and poor memory skills. He was able to communicate his needs to a limited extent but was easily cognitively overloaded.
- **Social**: Darren was highly dependent. He had severe behavioural problems and had caused many injuries to staff. This behaviour had led to a breakdown in care arrangements and social isolation. His friends had gradually terminated contact with him.

Assessment

Using Reed and Sanderson's model of Personal Adaptation Through Occupation (1992), together with information from his family and guided by a knowledge of life development theory, the occupational therapist identified the following occupational performance goals on Darren's behalf (see Fig. 2.3) in each performance area:

- **Self care**: Darren will assist with washing his face and hands, cleaning his teeth and taking a shower. He will help to dress himself by helping to control the limb being dressed/undressed and by making guided limited choices over what to wear each day.
  Darren will learn to feed himself.
- **Productivity**: Darren will be facilitated to make choices related to limited options in his choice of activity. He will wipe dirty surfaces after mealtimes and in the rehabilitation kitchen.
- **Leisure**: Darren will be helped to make choices related to limited options in leisure activity. He will participate in organised individual outings in low stimulation environments, on site options initially.

Theoretical framework

A learning frame of reference using a cognitive behavioural approach was most appropriate due to Darren's reduced cognitive abilities. A combination of the developmental frame of reference, using a neurodevelopmental approach (appropriate due to Darren's raised muscle tone) and the compensatory frame of reference (appropriate because of the permanent nature of Darren's physical losses) were used when addressing his physical performance needs.

Intervention

Feeding is given as an example of intervention in one performance area, subdivided into three performance components: physical, cognitive and social:

- **Physical**: Strategies were taught to compensate for ataxia. A 'dinner fix' bowl was used initially. Darren progressed to use of a lip plate and non-slip mat.
  Proximal stability was facilitated in order to increase distal control. A high table was used to stabilise the trunk and functional seating was used to further anchor Darren's pelvis.
- **Cognitive**: Darren's ability to concentrate at mealtimes was facilitated through environmental control. Noise levels were reduced and stimulation kept to a minimum.
- **Social**: To help Darren perform appropriately in a social environment when eating, a programme of graded exposure to more demanding social environments enabled him become more tolerant of social demands.

Outcome measures

- **Physical**: Darren is able to feed himself independently at mealtimes.
- **Cognitive**: Darren is able to exercise more control over his behaviour so that he can begin to make basic choices and tolerate greater levels of stimulation.
- **Social**: Darren can participate in social gatherings at mealtimes.

Conclusion

Although Darren remains highly dependent, his increased level of occupational performance allows him to be cared for in a variety of environments.

REFERENCES

Anderson DW, McLaurin RL (eds) 1980 Report on the national head and spinal cord injury survey. Journal of Neurosurgery 53 (suppl): SO21

Ayres AJ 1972 Sensory integration and learning disorders. Western Psychological Services, Los Angeles, CA

Ayres AJ 1979 Sensory integration and the child. Western Psychological Services, Los Angeles

Balliet R, Harbst KB, Kim D, Stewart RV 1987 Retraining of functional gait through the reduction of upper extremity weightbearing in chronic cerebellar ataxia. International Rehabilitation Medicine 8:148–153

Bobath B 1978 Adult hemiplegia: evaluation and treatment. Heinemann, London

Brooks DN, McKinlay WW 1983 Personality and behavioural change after severe blunt head injury. Journal of Neurology, Neurosurgery and Psychiatry 49:549–553

Eisenberg HM 1985 Outcome after head injury. Part 1: general considerations. In: Becker DP, Povlishshock JT (eds) Central nervous system trauma. Status report. Washington DC: National Institutes of Health. As quoted in Neuropsychological Assessment 1995. Oxford University Press, Oxford

Erickson E 1963 Identity and the life cycle. As quoted in Willard and Spackman's Occupational Therapy, 7th edn, p70. JB Lippincott Company.

Gill H 1996a SMART and persistent vegetative state, Part One. Occupational Therapy News October:12–13

Gill H 1996b SMART and persistent vegetative state, Part Two. Occupational Therapy News November:14–15

Goldberg E, Bilder RM 1986 Neuropsychological perspectives: retrograde amnesia and executive deficits. As quoted in Neuropsychological Assessment 1995. Oxford University Press, Oxford

Goldstein FC, Levin HS 1990 Epidemiology of traumatic brain injury: incidence, clinical characteristics, and risk factors. As quoted in Neuropsychological Assessment 1995. Oxford University Press, Oxford

Gronwall D 1977 Paced auditory serial addition task: A measure of recovery from concussion. Perceptual and Motor Skills 44:367–373

Hagen C, Malkmus D, Durham P, Bowman K 1979 Levels of cognitive functioning. In: Downey CA (ed) Rehabilitation of the head injured adult. Comprehensive physical management. Professional Staff Association of Rancho Los Amigos Hospital. As quoted in Neuropsychological Assessment 1995. Oxford University Press, Oxford

Jennett B, MacMillan R 1981 Epidemiology of head injury. British Medical Journal 282:101–104

Kapur N 1995 Memory aids in the rehabilitation of memory disordered patients. In: Baddeley DA, Wilson BA, Watts FN (eds) Handbook of memory disorders. John Wiley and Sons Ltd, Chichester, pp 532–556

Klonoff PS, Snow WG, Costa LD 1986 Quality of life in patients 2–4 years after closed head injury. Neurosurgery 19:735–743

Kurtzke JF 1984 Neuroepidemiology. Annals of Neurology 16:265–277

Lal S, Merbitz CP, Grip JC 1988 Modification of function in head injured patients with Sinemet. Brain Injury 2:225–233. As quoted in Neuropsychological Assessment 1995. Oxford University Press, Oxford

Levin HS, Mattis S, Ruff RM, Eisenberg HM, Marshall LF, Tabbador K, High EM Jr, Frankowski RF 1987 Neurobehavioral outcome following minor head injury: A three-centre study. Journal of Neurosurgery 66:234–243. As quoted in Ponsford J 1999 Traumatic brain injury: rehabilitation for everyday living. Psychology Press, Hove

Mackay LE, Bernstein BA, Chapman PE, Morgan AS, Milazzo LS 1992 Early intervention in severe head injury: long term benefits of a formalised programme. Archives of Physical Medicine & Rehabilitation 73:635–641

Maslow AH 1970 Motivation and personality, 2nd edn. Harper & Row, New York

Medical Disabilities Society 1988 The management of traumatic brain injury. Royal College of Physicians, London

Medical Rehabilitation Accreditation Commission 1996 Adapted from the 1996 Standards Manual and Interpretive Guidelines for Medical Rehabilitation Accreditation Commission CARF 1996

Miller E 1992 Psychological approaches to the management of memory impairments. British Journal of Psychiatry 160:1–6

Moore BE, Ruesch J 1944 Prolonged disturbances of consciousness following head injury. The New England Journal of Medicine 230:445–452

Ponsford JL, Kinsella G 1988 Evaluation of a remedial program for attentional deficits following closed head injury. Journal of Clinical and Experimental Neuropsychology 10:693–708

Reed K, Sanderson S 1992 Concepts of occupational therapy, 3rd edn. Williams & Wilkins, Baltimore, MD

Rood M 1962 The use of sensory receptors to activate and inhibit motor response, autonomic and somatic. In: Sattely C (ed) Developmental sequence, approaches to treatment of patients with neuromuscular dysfunction. Brown and Co, Dubuque

Royal College of Surgeons 1999 Report of the working party on the management of patients with head injuries. Royal College of Surgeons, London

Scott AD, Dow PW 1995 Traumatic brain injuries. In: Trombly CA (ed) Occupational therapy for physical dysfunction, 4th edn. Williams & Wilkins, Baltimore, MD, pp 705–773

Skinner BF 1953 Science and human behaviour. Free Press, New York

Sohlberg MM, Mateer CA 1987 Effectiveness of an attention training program. Journal of Clinical and Experimental Neuropsychology 9:117–130

Teasdale G, Jennett B 1974 Assessment of coma and impaired consciousness: a practical scale. Lancet 2:81–84

Teasdale G, Jennett B 1976 Assessment and prognosis of coma after head injury. Acta Neurochirurgica 34:45–55

Tennant A 1995 The epidemiology of head injury. In: Chamberlain MA, Neumann V, Tennant A (eds) Traumatic brain injury rehabilitation. Chapman & Hall Medical, London

Tyerman R, Tyerman A, Howard P, Hadfield O 1986 The Chessington Occupational Therapy Neurological Assessment Battery. Nottingham Rehab, Nottingham

University of Warwick 1998 Warwick study – the national traumatic brain injury study. Centre for Health Service Studies, University of Warwick, Coventry

Wilson B 1989 Memory problems after head injury. National Head Injuries Association, Nottingham

Wilson BA, Evans JJ, Emslie H, Malinek V 1997 Evaluation of NeuroPager: a new memory aid. Journal of Neurology, Neurosurgery and Psychiatry 63:113–115

Wood RL 1987 Brain injury rehabilitation: a neurobehavioural approach. Croom Helm, London

Zolton B, Giev E, Freidstat B 1986 Perceptual and cognitive dysfunction in the adult stroke patient, 2nd edn. Slack, New Jersey

FURTHER READING

Baddeley A 1997 Human memory, theory and practice. Psychology Press, Hove

Gronwall D, Wrightson P, Waddell P 1990 Head injury: the facts. Oxford University Press, Oxford

Muir-Giles G, Clark-Wilson J 1993 Brain injury rehabilitation. A neurofunctional approach. Chapman & Hall, London

Ponsford J, Slone S, Snow P 1996 Traumatic brain injury rehabilitation for everyday adaptive living. Psychology Press, Hove

Powell T 1994 Head injury: a practical guide. Winslow Press, Bicester

Williams WH, Evans JJ, Wilson BA 1999 Outcome measures for survivors of acquired brain injury in day and outpatient neurorehabilitation programmes. Neuropsychological Rehabilitation 9(3/4):421–436

Wood RL, Eames PG 1989 Models of brain injury rehabilitation. Croom Helm, London

16

Spinal cord lesions

Sue Cox Martin   Michael Curtin

INTRODUCTION

A spinal cord lesion is commonly the result of damage to the spinal cord following a road traffic or industrial accident, fall, sporting accident (e.g. rugby, diving and horse riding) and/or violence (e.g. shootings or stabbings). In the United Kingdom, approximately 25 000 people have a traumatic spinal cord lesion and there are an estimated 750 to 1000 new cases each year (Glass 1999).

Approximately 15 000 people in the United Kingdom have a non-traumatic spinal cord lesion (Glass 1999). Non-traumatic causes of spinal cord damage include infections (e.g. transverse myelitis, abscess and polyneuritis), tumours, thrombosis in one of the spinal arteries, haemorrhage, demyelinating conditions (e.g. multiple sclerosis), congenital deformities (e.g. spina bifida) and scoliosis.

Whether the cause of the spinal cord lesion is traumatic or non-traumatic the presenting signs and symptoms are similar. The impact for the individual, family, friends and the community in which the person lives is enormous. The effect the impairment has on each person, however, is unique and as a result each person must be considered individually during rehabilitation.

It is well recognised (Grundy & Swain 2001) that admission to a hospital or unit with experience of working with people with spinal cord lesions, as soon after injury as possible, is beneficial both physically and psychologically for life-long follow-up and to avoid complications.

417

TYPES OF SPINAL CORD LESIONS

In general, spinal cord lesions will produce either tetraplegia or paraplegia, depending on the level of damage.

- **Tetraplegia** refers to a lesion in the cervical cord resulting in loss of motor power and sensory input in the lower limbs, trunk and upper limbs with disturbance of bowel, bladder and sexual function. The degree of upper limb involvement will depend on the level of the lesion.
- **Paraplegia** refers to a lesion in the thoracic, lumbar or sacral cord resulting in loss of power and sensory function in the lower limbs and trunk. The upper limbs are not involved but the level of lesion will determine the degree of paralysis and the extent to which bowel, bladder and sexual function are disturbed.

In addition to the level, the spinal cord lesion is referred to as complete or incomplete.

- **Complete** refers to damage that results in total loss of motor power and sensation below the level of the spinal cord lesion.
- **Incomplete** refers to the preservation of some motor power and/or sensation below the spinal cord lesion. Incomplete lesions are categorised according to the area of damage and are referred to as anterior cord syndrome, central cord syndrome, posterior cord syndrome and Brown–Séquard syndrome (Table 16.1).

CLASSIFICATION OF LESIONS

The simplest method of classifying spinal damage is to define the lesion according to the most distal uninvolved spinal cord segment together with the skeletal level (Fig. 16.1). For example, a lesion could be classified as 'tetraplegia, complete or incomplete, below C6 (meaning that C6 is the most distal uninvolved spinal segment), due to dislocation of the C5–6 vertebrae'.

The classification of lesions is described more fully in Ditunno et al (1994) and Glass (1999).

Table 16.1 Categories of incomplete spinal cord lesions

Type of lesion	Features
Anterior cord syndrome	Damage primarily to the anterior spinal tracts, resulting in disruption of pain, temperature and touch sensations, but leaving some pressure and proprioceptive sensation. There may be some recovery in movement
Central cord syndrome	Damage primarily to the central part of the cord, resulting in loss of arm movement with some sparing of leg movement. Bladder and bowel are often partially spared. Sensation is often intact. There may be some recovery beginning in the lower legs and moving upwards
Posterior cord syndrome	Damage primarily to the posterior part of the cord, which may result in poor coordination of movements despite having good muscle power and pain and temperature sensation
Brown–Séquard syndrome	Damage primarily to one side of the cord, resulting in disruption of muscle power on the injured side but intact pain and temperature sensation. The muscle power on the non-injured side of the cord is intact but pain and temperature sensation is disrupted

Apart from paralysis below the level of damage, a spinal cord lesion can result in many other immediate and long-term physiological effects and complications. Bromley (1998) and Grundy and Swain (2001) describe these complications, and their medical and surgical management.

PHILOSOPHY OF SPINAL CORD LESION REHABILITATION

INDEPENDENCE

Rehabilitation is a process of learning to live with one's disability within one's environment (Trieschmann 1988). For people who have a spinal cord lesion, rehabilitation involves a dynamic process that starts at the moment of injury and continues for the remainder of a person's life (Whalley Hammell 1995).

The period of hospitalisation following a spinal cord lesion is the first stage of rehabilitation. The

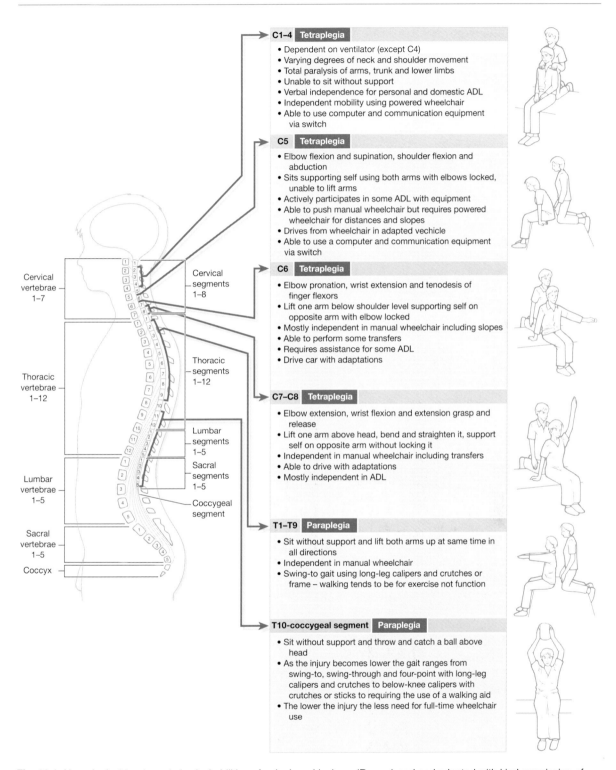

C1–4 Tetraplegia

- Dependent on ventilator (except C4)
- Varying degrees of neck and shoulder movement
- Total paralysis of arms, trunk and lower limbs
- Unable to sit without support
- Verbal independence for personal and domestic ADL
- Independent mobility using powered wheelchair
- Able to use computer and communication equipment via switch

C5 Tetraplegia

- Elbow flexion and supination, shoulder flexion and abduction
- Sits supporting self using both arms with elbows locked, unable to lift arms
- Actively participates in some ADL with equipment
- Able to push manual wheelchair but requires powered wheelchair for distances and slopes
- Drives from wheelchair in adapted vechicle
- Able to use a computer and communication equipment via switch

C6 Tetraplegia

- Elbow pronation, wrist extension and tenodesis of finger flexors
- Lift one arm below shoulder level supporting self on opposite arm with elbow locked
- Mostly independent in manual wheelchair including slopes
- Able to perform some transfers
- Requires assistance for some ADL
- Drive car with adaptations

C7–C8 Tetraplegia

- Elbow extension, wrist flexion and extension grasp and release
- Lift one arm above head, bend and straighten it, support self on opposite arm without locking it
- Independent in manual wheelchair including transfers
- Able to drive with adaptations
- Mostly independent in ADL

T1–T9 Paraplegia

- Sit without support and lift both arms up at same time in all directions
- Independent in manual wheelchair
- Swing-to gait using long-leg calipers and crutches or frame – walking tends to be for exercise not function

T10-coccygeal segment Paraplegia

- Sit without support and throw and catch a ball above head
- As the injury becomes lower the gait ranges from swing-to, swing-through and four-point with long-leg calipers and crutches to below-knee calipers with crutches or sticks to requiring the use of a walking aid
- The lower the injury the less need for full-time wheelchair use

Cervical vertebrae 1–7

Thoracic vertebrae 1–12

Lumbar vertebrae 1–5

Sacral vertebrae 1–5

Coccyx

Cervical segments 1–8

Thoracic segments 1–12

Lumbar segments 1–5

Sacral segments 1–5

Coccygeal segment

Fig. 16.1 Neurological levels and physical abilities of spinal cord lesions. (Reproduced and adapted with kind permission of World Health Organization 1996.)

focus of rehabilitation during this stage is not only on the acquisition of skills to enable a person to get out of bed but also to assist the person in finding the reasons for getting out of bed (Tam 1998, Trieschmann 1988). The aim of rehabilitation is for each person to achieve independence. Whalley Hammell (1995) and Sumsion (1999a) define independence not as a physical state but as an attitude in which an individual takes on responsibility, solves problems and establishes his own goals.

To obtain independence in this sense during rehabilitation, the focus must be on education to enable the person to manage all aspects of his care and to become an expert in understanding and dealing with his body. In this way, he learns to adapt to changes and begins to achieve his desired level of competence and control of his daily life (Spoltore & O'Brien 1995, Tam 1998, Whalley Hammell 1995). For rehabilitation to be considered successful, this must occur despite the person's level of lesion. The therapist can help the person adjust to the fact that, although he may need to face losses in terms of function, he will not necessarily need to lose roles. Independence in occupational performance can mean that the person continues to make decisions, identify goals and plan outcomes while devolving the functional aspects of the tasks involved to someone else.

Although the rehabilitation must include the opportunity to practise self-care tasks such as grooming, bathing/showering, dressing and mobility, these must not be done to the exclusion of a person's many other needs (Pentland et al 1999, Whalley Hammell 1995). It is the resolution of these other needs that will make for a more complete and successful reintegration into the community and will contribute to a person's ability to cope following a spinal cord lesion. These needs include attending to the individual's spiritual, emotional and cognitive dimensions and working with them to obtain their work and leisure, in addition to self-care, goals.

CLIENT-CENTRED APPROACH

The process of encouraging a person to take control is achieved through using a client-centred approach. Sumsion (1999b p56) defines client-centred occupational therapy as:

… a partnership between the therapist and the client. The client's occupational goals are given priority and are at the centre of assessment and treatment. The therapist listens to and respects the client's standards and adapts the intervention to meet the client's needs. The client actively participates in negotiating goals for intervention and is empowered to make decisions through training and education. The therapist and client work together to address the issues presented by a variety of environments to enable the client to fulfil his/her role expectancies.

THEORETICAL FOUNDATIONS UNDERPINNING INTERVENTION

CANADIAN MODEL OF OCCUPATIONAL PERFORMANCE AND SPINAL CORD LESIONS

In using a client-centred approach, occupational therapy intervention may be based on the Canadian Model of Occupational Performance (CMOP; Canadian Association of Occupational Therapy 1997). This model places the person at its centre and emphasises that the occupations he does and the way he does them are a result of the dynamic interaction between him and the environments he inhabits (Fig. 16.2). The model can be used both as an assessment tool, using the Canadian Occupational Performance Model (COPM), and as a guide to intervention. The use of COPM enables the individual and the therapist to explore issues, establish individual priorities and reflect upon the outcomes of intervention.

Spirituality is the primary component of the person. It is considered to give meaning to all the things he does in everyday life. It underpins the reasons for his decisions and choices (Sumsion 1999a) and is essential for his sense of dignity and self-worth (Egan & Delaat 1994). A sense of purpose and meaning to one's life may be disrupted following a spinal cord lesion as a person learns how to live with a (usually) sudden, permanent impairment that profoundly impacts on everything he does as well as on the hopes and plans he holds for the future.

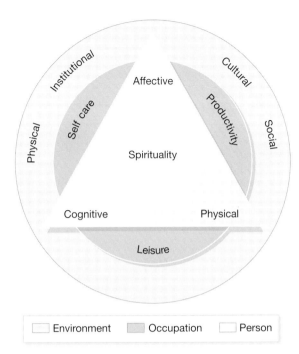

Environment ☐ Occupation ▨ Person ☐

Fig. 16.2 Canadian Model of Occupational Performance. (Reproduced with kind permission from Canadian Association of Occupational Therapists 1997.)

It is a person's spirituality combined with his physical skills (sensory, neuromusculoskeletal and motor components), affect (psychological, emotional, social and self-management components) and cognition (higher brain functions required for thinking) that enable him to perform a multitude of occupations. These occupations can be categorised into the three performance areas of: self care or activities of daily living, work and productivity, and play or leisure (American Occupational Therapy Association 1994, Canadian Association of Occupational Therapy 1997). Following a spinal cord lesion a person usually has paralysis affecting the sensory, neuromusculoskeletal and motor components below the level of injury. The residual physical impairment will alter the way a person performs many of his occupations. Competence in his occupational performance will also be dependent on his affect and the effectiveness of his psychological and emotional coping strategies. In most cases, a person's cognitive abilities are not seriously impaired following a spinal

cord lesion and can be used throughout rehabilitation to enable him to develop relevant problem-solving strategies and to learn to live with his new level of function.

The opportunities and potential to perform occupations is also affected by the environments a person inhabits or is influenced by. The CMOP identifies four environments that can influence occupational performance:

- The **cultural environment** refers to the groups he belongs to, such as an ethnic group or group of people who share similar values. The groups' attitude towards disability will determine how well he can reintegrate into each group following a spinal cord lesion.
- The **physical environment** refers to the man-made and natural surroundings in which he lives. Following a spinal cord injury it is usual that at least some adaptations will need to be made to make this environment accessible.
- The **social environment** refers to the relationship the person has with other people, be it at home, at work or in the community. How these people react and accept the person following a spinal cord lesion will influence his participation in many occupations.
- The fourth environment is **institutional**. This includes the legal, economic and political influences on a person. Following a spinal cord injury factors such as disability benefits, employment rights and community care packages will contribute to the opportunities he has to lead a fulfilling life.

FRAMES OF REFERENCE

Once priorities for intervention have been established, the therapist will decide on the most appropriate frame(s) of reference for use in each area. Given the nature of the effect of a spinal cord lesion, principles of the following frames of reference are likely to prove most effective:

- The **biomechanical** frame of reference will guide the therapist when approaching issues related to physical function, particularly those related to muscular skeletal difficulties.

- The **learning** frame of reference – using an educative approach, the therapist can assist the person to acquire independence by identifying a range of options for problem solving and helping him gain knowledge so that he can make the most appropriate decisions related to the restoration of occupational performance in all areas.
- The **compensatory** frame of reference can be used effectively where skills and functions have been lost permanently. For example, remaining skills may be adapted using new techniques, or 'trick' movements may be required. Roles and/or functions may be adapted to eliminate the need to perform lost functions. Alternatively, these lost skills may be compensated for through the supply of financed environmental modification, services or equipment.

INTERVENTION TEAM

As well as an occupational therapist, an interdisciplinary team of professionals will be working with the spinal injured person throughout his rehabilitation. This interdisciplinary team includes professionals working in the hospital and the community to ensure that the person is reintegrated back into his community as effectively as possible. The team will include physiotherapists, nurses, psychologists, social workers, radiographers, dieticians, podiatrists and doctors. Rehabilitation engineers and speech and language therapists may be involved for people with more complex needs. For rehabilitation to be effective, the team must work with the person, educating him about his lesion and encouraging him to determine and work towards his own goals (Glass 1999). It is important that the team includes the person's family and friends throughout the rehabilitation period to ensure that the programme will be effective.

REHABILITATION FOLLOWING A SPINAL CORD LESION

FOCUSING ON THE PERSON DURING REHABILITATION

The effect of a spinal cord lesion on a person will depend on the level and extent of injury (Grundy & Swain 2001). Other significant factors may include age, gender, cultural background, personality, physical build, religious beliefs, social and educational background, marital status and financial position.

Spirituality

Whatever the situation or circumstances, the personality of a person and his wants, desires, beliefs, likes, dislikes, fears and prejudices do not necessarily change as a result of a spinal cord lesion (Glass 1999). His spirituality, the meaning and purpose to his life, however, may initially be disrupted and he may be confused. One of the tasks during rehabilitation is to encourage the person to find and define a purpose to his life again, to find that inner strength required to lead a fulfilling life (Sumsion 1999a, Whalley Hammell 1995).

There is no one magical approach that will work for everyone, as each person is different (Grant & Lundon 1998). What appears to be important is for the therapist to respect each individual and to portray honest but positive beliefs conveying messages of hope and acceptance (Sumsion 1999a). The occupational therapist needs to listen closely to a person's expressed needs, while working in partnership with him to meet these needs. The therapist will also need to provide him with opportunities to learn about living with a spinal cord lesion to encourage him to think about how he will realistically deal with many of the issues he will face. The concept of independence is closely associated with spirituality. Encouraging the person to achieve his desired level of competence and control of his daily activities will contribute to re-establishing meaning and purpose to his life.

Affect

As each person adjusts to the physiological effects of the spinal cord lesion they will experience a wide variety of emotions (Gatehouse 1995):

- He may not believe what has happened and deny the extent and effect of the lesion.
- As he realises the extent of the injuries and the long-term prognosis, he may experience feelings of depression and hopelessness.
- He may feel anger at what has happened and direct this anger at staff, visitors, other patients or himself.
- As he begins to accept what has happened and starts to think about the effect it is going to have on his life, he may experience feelings of anxiety and vulnerability.
- When he starts to compare his life before to his possible life after the lesion he may feel upset and experience feelings of loss or grief.

The emotional reactions he experiences must be accepted as part of the process he has to go through as he learns to cope with his impairment. Although there is no definitive way of dealing with his reactions, rehabilitation workers need to be honest, informative and encouraging. Listening to him and respecting what he says is important. His emotional reactions are real and opportunities must be provided to allow him to express his feelings. Assisting him to find ways to deal positively with his emotions and to work through them is important for learning to live with a spinal cord lesion (Glass 1999).

To encourage the person to express his emotions the therapist must spend time building up rapport with him, his family and friends soon after admission. This will provide the basis for the trust that will be vital throughout the months of rehabilitation and the process of resettlement in the community.

Immediately following a spinal cord lesion, it is common for a person to spend a period ranging from a few days to weeks on bedrest until the vertebral column, spinal cord and any other injuries are stable enough for sitting. A long period on bedrest may cause him to withdraw and become demotivated so, during this period, it is important that he remains stimulated and is kept aware of what is going on (Glass 1999).

The occupational therapist should encourage him, along with his family and friends, to be involved in planning the day's activities. This may include what to eat, what to watch on television or listen to on the radio, doing crosswords or quizzes, reading or listening to newspapers, magazines or books, or writing to relatives and friends. He should be encouraged to participate as much as possible in some of his self-care occupations, such as eating or brushing his teeth, washing his face and upper body.

His ability to do things and to be involved in what is happening while on bedrest can be facilitated by the use of equipment. Overhead adjustable mirrors and prismatic glasses may enable greater vision whilst in the supine position. For individuals with a tracheotomy it is important to encourage communication either via lip reading or using communication equipment. The standard nurse call system will be suitable for most individuals to contact the ward staff. For people unable to use the standard system, the occupational therapist adapts or replaces the existing switch or controls. This will enable those with cervical lesions to call for assistance and, if combined with environmental control equipment, to operate electrical devices, such as a television, stereo and fan independently.

Cognition

As rehabilitation is primarily about a person learning to live with his impairment, a therapist's responsibility is to educate him about his injury so that he can be fully informed about what has happened and the possible outcomes, so he can make realistic goals. This encourages him to be an active participant throughout the rehabilitation process (Tam 1998). Whalley Hammell (1995 p9) states that:

… people learn best when they are helped to define their own problems, decide on a course of action and evaluate the consequences of their decisions. This learning process will provide the means to solve problems creatively, to address the client's own concerns and to address situations not encountered during the formal rehabilitation programme.

Active participation, rather than being a passive recipient of a programme, is essential for facilitating a person's self-determination and sense of control (Ozer 1988, Pollock 1993, Whalley Hammell 1995). Facilitating the person's active participation should begin soon after admission and continue throughout rehabilitation.

Physical

Occupational therapists, along with other professionals, will work to reduce the effect that a spinal cord lesion has on the physical abilities of the person. This will include the maintenance of joint range of motion and muscle strength, the prevention of contractures and pressure sores and the establishment of a bowel and bladder routine.

Hand and upper limb management

One area that occupational therapists particularly focus on in the early stages is the maintenance of joint range of motion and muscle strength of the hands and the upper limbs of people with tetraplegia. This is because good hand and upper limb function is essential for physical independence in many self-care, work and leisure occupations. Krajnik and Bridle (1992) and Sutton (1993) outline several principles of management of the upper limbs:

- Maintain full range of passive movement in all joints of the upper limb, hand and wrist. Bromley (1998) provides descriptions of how to position and passively range the joints of the upper limb.
- Encourage active movement and use of the upper limb and hands to manage daily occupations.
- Prevent contractures and swelling, particularly if the option of tendon transfer is to be considered at a later stage.
- Maintain the functional position of the hand, supporting the palmar transverse arch, stabilising and supporting the thumb in opposition and abduction and maintaining adequate web space.

- Maintain the usual cosmetic appearance of the hand (to facilitate positive feelings of self-image and self-esteem).

Splinting. Splints are used to position the hands and can generally be divided into four different categories (Curtin 1994):

1. Resting or paddle splints (Fig. 16.3A), which support the whole hand and forearm. They are used to maintain the alignment of the joints and cosmetic appearance of the hand and are suitable for those who have very weak or absent wrist extensors and finger muscles.
2. Wrist extension splints (Fig. 16.3B) support the wrist in extension. They are worn by those who are unable to maintain their wrist position against gravity but who have elbow flexors. They may enable the individual to use his hands to do such activities as push a manual wheelchair, use a keyboard and hold utensils for writing and eating.
3. Short hand splints (Fig. 16.3C) maintain the web space and prevent hyperextension of the metacarpophalangeal joints. Usually the individual will have good wrist extension but an imbalance between the extrinsic and intrinsic finger muscles.
4. Tenodesis splints (Fig. 16.3D) are worn to shorten the long flexor tendons of the fingers to facilitate a firmer tenodesis grip. There is little agreement on how best to facilitate a tenodesis grasp. Several splinting suggestions are shown. For any of these splints to be appropriate the wrist extensors must be strong with only flickers or no active movement of the fingers and thumb. Care must be taken to ensure that the flexor tendons do not overtighten.

Whichever splints are used, the occupational therapist is responsible for monitoring and ensuring their effectiveness.

Tenodesis grip. Individuals who have a complete spinal cord lesion at C6 usually develop the 'trick' tenodesis movement as a result of the natural tightening of the flexor tendons (Krajnik & Bridle 1992, Sutton 1993). This has the potential

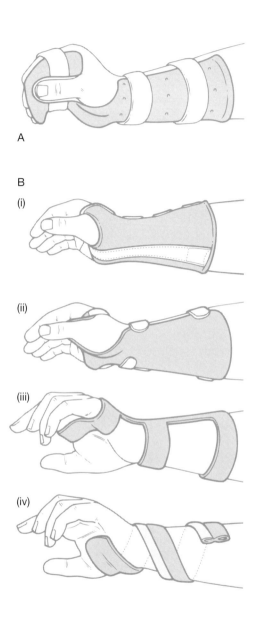

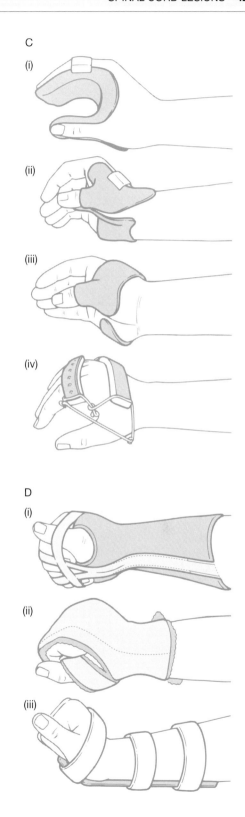

Fig. 16.3 Splinting used to enhance occupational performance. (Reproduced from Curtin 1994 with kind permission of Macmillan Press Ltd.) (A) Resting pan or paddle splints. (B) Wrist extension splints. (i) Futuro-type splint, (ii) long opponens splint, (iii) dorsal cock-up splint, (iv) spiral splint. (C) Short hand splints. (i) short resting pan or paddle splint, (ii) short opponens splint, (iii) thumb post splint, (iv) commercially available MP flexion splint. (D) Tenodesis splints. (i) Taping method, (ii) Heidleberg splint, (iii) volar splint.

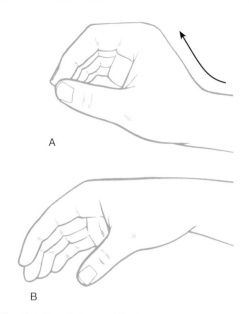

A

B

Fig. 16.4 Tenodesis grip. (A) Wrist extension. (B) Wrist flexion.

to increase a person's physical independence and decrease the reliance on assistive devices. Wrist extension causes the fingers to flex naturally and the thumb to adduct and flex (Fig. 16.4A). Flexion of the wrist causes the fingers to extend at all the joints and the thumb to abduct and extend (Fig. 16.4B).

Although tenodesis occurs naturally, it may need to be facilitated to ensure that the tendons tighten efficiently, particularly the flexor tendons of the thumb. Splinting (see Fig. 16.3D), combined with a passive range of movements, is a means through which this can be achieved.

Upper limb function and high tetraplegia. People who have a complete spinal cord lesion at the neurological level of C4 or above will have no active movement of their upper limbs and hands. Initially, it is important that the joints of the upper limbs and hands are passively ranged to prevent contractures and joint deformities. In conjunction with the passive range of motion of the hand joints, a resting pan splint (see Fig. 16.3A) can also be used to help to maintain the normal curvature and appearance of the hand (Whalley Hammell 1995). The flexibility of the upper limb and hands along with the absence of deformities will make it easier for the carer to wash the upper limbs and trunk and to dress the person.

FOCUSING ON THE PERFORMANCE AREAS DURING REHABILITATION

Self care

Moving into an upright position

Once a person is given the medical clearance to mobilise from bedrest, the physiotherapist, nurse and occupational therapist work closely to enable the progression to sitting in a wheelchair to be as smooth and positive as possible. The individual will require careful psychological preparation as the first time he gets out of bed may be the occasion when he realises the full implication of his lesion. In preparation, a team member will discuss with him what will happen and how this may make him react in order that he can be in control and trust the team. People with lesions in the high thoracic and cervical regions will need to understand that the effects of postural hypotension (i.e. feeling sick and dizzy) are normal reactions of the body. All individuals will need to be aware that their balance and sensation will be affected. Prior to sitting the individual up, the team must:

- ensure that there are no medical complications
- ensure appropriate braces and/or collars are fitted if he is to be sat up beyond 45°
- choose a suitable wheelchair and wheelchair cushion
- choose an appropriate hoist and supportive sling
- be informative and encouraging to maintain and boost his confidence and self-esteem.

Wheelchair and cushion selection

Careful selection of a wheelchair and cushion is essential to ensure that both are supportive and functional. Individuals with paraplegia will most often get up into a standard self-propelling wheelchair, which they are able to propel and manoeuvre straight away. They should be taught that their hips, knees and ankles should be positioned at 90°. Those with tetraplegia will most often get up into a reclining or a tilt-in-space wheelchair, which offers support to compensate for the weak or absent movement of their trunk, upper limbs and neck. They should gradually learn about positioning their hips, trunk, upper limbs and neck in a midline position while sitting in the wheelchair. Chapter 7 includes information about the assessment of a person for a wheelchair. Ham et al (1998) also provide detailed information.

To reduce the risk of developing pressure sores, the individual will require a cushion with good pressure-relieving properties. Additionally, he will use the most appropriate means of relieving his pressure while in a sitting position.

Initially, individuals will use their wheelchairs for short periods. This will be increased slowly each day according to their tolerance and the condition of their skin. It is important that progress is steady and that the individual feels as safe and confident as possible in his new situation in order to enable him to progress his level of performance.

Wheelchair mobility

Once an individual can tolerate sitting in the wheelchair for several hours, he will be encouraged to participate in activities from his wheelchair. Whenever possible, an individual with paraplegia or low tetraplegia should be encouraged to push themselves around as a means of maintaining and building up muscle strength and encouraging balance. Gloves with or without fingers should be worn to protect desensitised areas of the hand and provide extra friction when self-propelling the wheelchair (Fig. 16.5). Individuals with no active wrist movement may require additional support using a wrist extension splint (see Fig. 16.3B). Individuals with little or no active movement in their upper limbs will require a powered chair.

The range of appropriate wheelchairs for people with high tetraplegia, particularly those on a ventilator, is not extensive. For an individual who wants to operate a powered wheelchair, the selection of the most appropriate method to control the wheelchair, including joystick, chin control, head switches, sip-puff control and a combination of scanning and switch devices, requires careful assessment and practice.

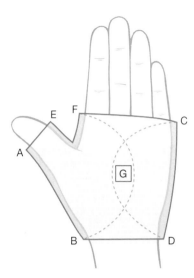

Fig. 16.5 How to make a pushing glove. (1) Draw the person's hand shape with a flat palm and thumb in extension onto tracing paper or greaseproof paper. Mark the metacarpophalangeal heads of the fingers, the IP joint of the thumb and the wrist joint. (2) Allow sufficient space around the hand and thumb and draw the pattern shape as shown. (3) Fold along line AB. Trace the shape of the thumb from A–E–F. From F, draw a semicircle to the wrist at B to form an overlap of the glove on the back of the hand. (4) Fold along line CD. From C, draw a semicircle to the wrist at D to form the overlap on the back of the hand. (5) Open out the paper and cut out the pattern. Try the pattern on the person's hand to ensure that the thumb width is sufficient and that the overlap on the back of the hand is adequate. Modify if necessary. (6) Use the pattern to cut out two gloves in firm leather. (7) Cut out two extra palm pieces of leather to reinforce the palm of the glove and to give traction for pushing the wheelchair. Use leather, suede, rubber or pimple rubber. (8) Sewing. For leather, use a strong thread and a special needle for leather. Try to match the colours of the thread and the Velcro to the leather. (a) Sew the reinforcement onto the palm; (b) sew the Velcro on so that the 'loop' piece overlaps with the 'hook' piece at G; (c) sew around the thumb web apace $\frac{1}{4}$ inch from the edge.

The occupational therapist should be aware of the extensive range of manual and powered wheelchairs. The person must be assessed carefully and guided to select a suitable wheelchair once his balance, strength, comfort, posture and functional ability have achieved the optimum and an anticipation of lifestyle has emerged.

Vehicles

Being mobile within the community is important in terms of accessing work, social and recreational activities (Whalley Hammell 1995). Those who have good power in their upper limbs and good balance will usually be able to drive a car with an automatic or adapted gearbox and standard hand controls. Individuals with weakness in their upper limbs and trunk may require more adaptations. The person will usually require assessment, guidance and practice lessons before being confident.

Some wheelchair users, especially those using powered wheelchairs, may wish to remain in their wheelchairs when travelling in a vehicle. There are many vehicles to choose from and great care is required to match the choice of powered wheelchair with the vehicle to enable access and headroom. The vehicle will require extensive adaptation if the individual is to drive from a powered wheelchair. Mobility Assessment Centres can provide comprehensive information and advice on all aspects of mobility.

Transfers

The range of transfers an individual will achieve will depend on their level of lesion, age, gender, body proportions, physical strength, technique and motivation. It is anticipated that most young people with paraplegia will become independent in wheelchair transfers from bed, car, armchair, toilet, bath and floor. Older people, and those with higher lesions, may be dependent on equipment (e.g. sliding board) or assistance, while others will need to be transferred using a hoist.

There are three basic types of independent transfers from a wheelchair:

1. Legs-down sideways transfers (Fig. 16.6).
2. Legs-up sideways transfer. This is basically the same as the legs-down transfer but the individual lifts his legs onto the surface he is transferring to (e.g. bed or car) before lifting his bottom off the wheelchair cushion.
3. Front-on transfer (Fig. 16.7).

During rehabilitation, transfers to and from varying heights are practised so that techniques can be learned and adapted to meet personal needs and situations. For bed transfers, the bed and the wheelchair should ideally be the same height. All three methods may be used. For arm-chair transfers the wheelchair is positioned at an angle to the armchair and a legs-down transfer used.

Transferring on and off a toilet is much easier if the toilet seat is the same height as the wheelchair seat and cushion. Often, however, the toilet seat will be lower. The toilet seat should be padded to reduce the risk of pressure sores. The method of transfer will depend on the space available but, where possible, the wheelchair should be placed alongside the toilet at a slight angle and a legs-down transfer used.

Transfers in and out of the bath are achieved either over the side or over the end of the bath. The water must always be run and tested before the individual gets into the bath. Hot water should never be added once in the bath. In the event that the individual has difficulty either lifting himself in or out of the bath, a wide range of equipment is available, such as bath boards, bath seats and bath lifts. Equipment should always have a padded seat. There are also bath cushions available to protect the skin from the hard surface of the bath.

Transfers on and off a shower chair will usually take place from the bed and any of the three methods may be used. If a wall mounted, padded shower seat is used a legs-down sideways transfer is used.

The technique used to get in and out of the car will depend on an individual's ability and the type of car. Generally, it is easier to transfer into a three-door car as the doors are wider. A common technique to get into a car is the leg-up transfer, where the individual places his feet into the footwell of the car prior to moving his bottom onto the car seat.

Hoists. Many individuals will require the use of a hoist either short or long term. More details about the use of hoists can be found in Chapter 7.

Communication

The ability to communicate is essential to people who have restricted mobility, as to be independent they have to inform others how and when to assist them (Lipner 1997, Whalley Hammell 1995). Communication is also an essential skill

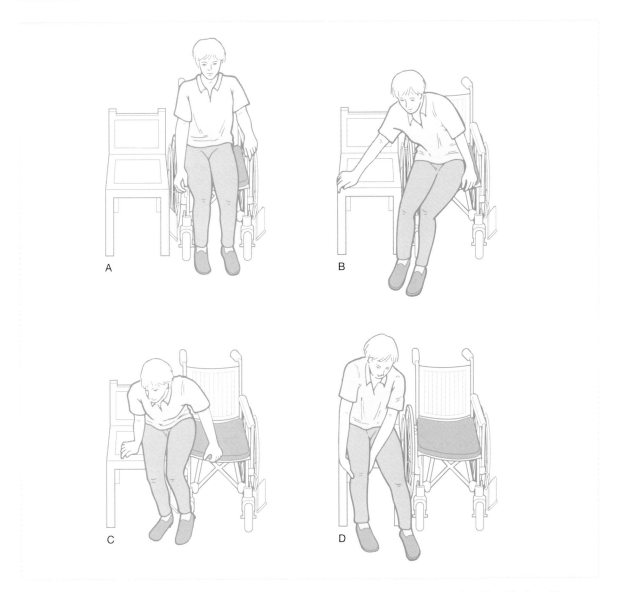

Fig. 16.6 Legs-down transfer. (A) The wheelchair is positioned either beside, or at about 45° to the side of the bed. The footplates are lifted and swung away if necessary and the nearside armrest is removed. (B) The individual lifts himself forwards on the cushion to position his feet flat on the floor. He reaches over with one hand to prepare to lift his bottom off the wheelchair cushion. (C) With one hand on the wheelchair cushion and the other on the surface he is transferring to, he lifts his bottom across, taking care to avoid the rear wheel. (D) He then lifts his legs closer to the surface he has transferred to. The reverse procedure is used to transfer into the wheelchair.

required for many daily occupations, particularly those that involve interacting with other people.

Verbal communication. Using the telephone becomes paramount as a means of communicating with people. A large variety of equipment is available commercially to assist with holding the

handset, to enhance the voice volume or to enable the person to talk hands-free (Stern 1997). For those individuals unable to operate standard equipment, an environmental control system may be beneficial in providing an alternative means of accessing the telephone. These systems

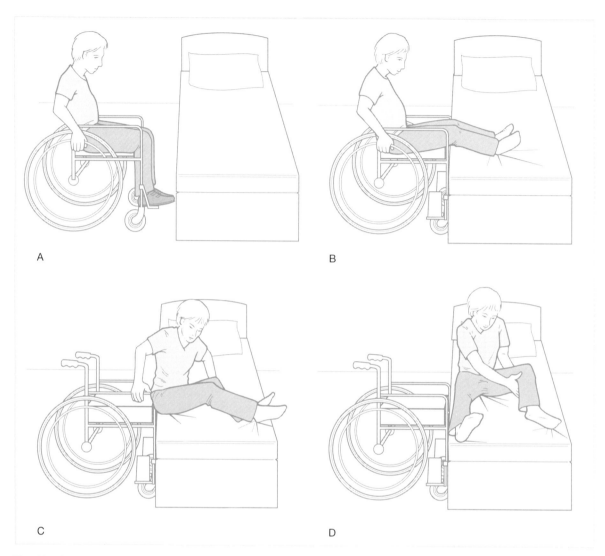

Fig. 16.7 Front-on transfer. This transfer is used only when the environment or the physical abilities of the individual necessitates its use. Sliding sheets are available to assist this type of transfer and to cut down on the sheering forces and friction on the heels. (A) The wheelchair is placed facing the sides of the bed. (B) The person lifts his legs from the footplates onto the bed one at a time. The footplates are then swung away and the wheelchair moved forwards until the front of the wheelchair touches the bed. (C) The person then lifts himself forwards from the wheelchair onto the bed. (D) Once he is on the bed, he lifts his bottom and his legs to make himself comfortable. The procedure is reversed for transfer into the wheelchair.

are accessed via a switch and often have other features, to enable the individual to operate other electrically powered equipment including a television, intercom, computer, lights and radio (Bain 1997).

Written communication. An individual with weak upper limb movement may be able to write using a small adaptive pen holder made from thermoplastic material. An individual with no upper limb movement may be able to use a mouth stick to write. This enables him to achieve a signature or mark as a personal touch on cards, letters and cheques. Using a computer may become a necessity to communicate with friends and for business. Computers with adapted software and hardware enable individuals with little

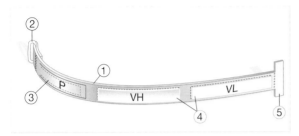

Fig. 16.8 Making a universal cuff. (1) Cut out the strap in leather or webbing to accommodate the individual's hand and the tool to be held. (2) Sew on the plastic loop. (3) The pocket (P) should be the width of the person's palm and is stitched on three sides. (4) Sew on the Velcro 'hooks' (VH) and 'loops' (VL). (5) Sew on an extra tab of material. This end is threaded through the plastic loop to enable the individual to fasten and release the Velcro independently.

or no upper limb movement to word process and the Internet makes it easier to access and send information. Bain and Leger (1997) provide more information on this topic. Current information can be provided by AbilityNet, listed in the Useful Contacts section (p439).

Reading. Whenever possible, individuals are encouraged to use their upper limbs to turn pages of books, newspapers and magazines. A range of alternative methods is possible depending on an individual's ability, including using rubber thumblets, a mouthstick or a universal cuff to hold a rubber-tipped rod (Fig. 16.8) and some commercially available aids. The book or magazine can be placed on a book-stand or table for people who have difficulty holding it. When an individual is unable to use alternative methods, electrically powered page-turners operated via a switch are available commercially. Other options are talking books, having friends or family read to them or accessing reading material via a computer.

Personal care

During bedrest, an individual may become dependent on others for many aspects of care. Some people, due to the level and extent of their injury, will not be able physically to participate in self-care activities. For these people, the goal of intervention is to learn how they would prefer these activities to be done and to become verbally

independent in instructing others how to do these activities for them.

For people who develop the potential for some level of physical independence in their self-care activities, the occupational therapist will begin to facilitate their active participation once their injuries have stabilised and they become more mobile. Initially, adapted methods or adapted tools may be necessary but the need for these should be reassessed as an individual's ability and function improves. Depending upon his abilities, becoming skilled at personal aspects of care can take anything from a few days to several months of practice and perseverance.

The therapist's clinical skills combined with the client's resourcefulness can achieve creative ways of achieving satisfaction with performance in self-care activities (Whalley Hammell 1995).

Eating and drinking. Using commercially available or custom-made adapted cutlery or a universal cuff (see Fig. 16.8) with an ordinary fork or spoon can facilitate eating. When an individual has loss of hand sensation, insulated cups and mugs may be useful initially, particularly for safety. Flexible straws may also be necessary for safe and independent drinking, particularly for those unable to hold and lift a cup.

Personal hygiene. To enable a person with weak grip to hold items such as hairbrush, toothbrush, shaver and make-up applicators, leather or webbing universal cuffs (see Fig. 16.8) can be made in various sizes. Cuffs enable a person who can lift and coordinate their arms and wrists, but who has no finger strength or grip, to perform these tasks. A large range of brushes and combs with various handles are available commercially. Handles using thermoplastic splinting material can be moulded to fit around handles of electric toothbrushes, hairdryers and showerhead when necessary.

Dressing. Once an individual with paraplegia is able to maintain his sitting balance and is free from external bracing, he will be ready to learn to dress and undress on the bed. One possible technique is described in Figure 16.9. In time, he will perfect his own dressing technique. The level of independence achieved in dressing will depend on the level of lesion, age, physical

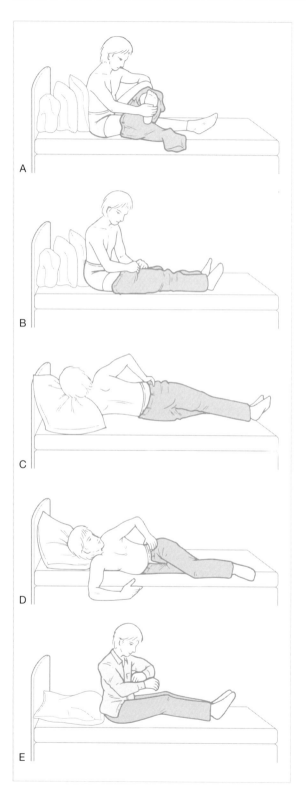

stamina, agility, body shape and motivation. It is not uncommon for people with tetraplegia to choose to have assistance from a carer with dressing and undressing, as they are often unable to dress fast enough or to a self-imposed acceptable standard or because they may find it too tiring.

Sexual issues following a spinal cord lesion

Although an individual with a spinal cord lesion may initially feel inadequate and unsure of his sexuality, it is usual – with time, emotional support and opportunity – for him to learn to feel confident about himself and sexually attractive. For people to feel attractive to others they need to feel good about themselves, have an open mind and a willingness to experiment. A good supportive relationship with a partner will go some way to being mutually satisfying to both. As a rule, however, a person's sexual desires will not alter following a spinal cord lesion. Staff must respect each person's sexual preferences and be open-minded enough to provide appropriate support.

Physically, there will be some changes that will affect sexual function, such as the ability to move around, the ability for men to maintain an erection, the feeling of orgasm and the preparation required prior to intercourse. The changes will

Fig. 16.9 An example of a dressing technique. (A) The person sits up in bed. He lifts and bends one leg at the knee so that the foot rests on the opposite knee or thigh. Socks, which should be seamless, are put on in this position before underwear or trousers. This prevents seams becoming caught in or between the toes. Generally, loose garments are easier to put on than tight ones and it is advisable that all back pockets or studs, which could cause extra pressure, are removed. (B) Underwear and trousers are put over the feet in the same way as the socks and pulled as high up the thighs as possible. (C and D) The individual returns to a supine position and pulls the garments up at the front as far as possible. He then rolls from side to side several times to pull them over his bottom. It is important that all layers of material are smooth. Shoes are put on the same way as the socks, although care needs to be taken that toes remain flat inside the shoe. Generally, shoes should have few seams and be a size larger than usual to accommodate oedema and allow plenty of room for the toes. (E) The person can then choose whether to dress the top half of his body while sitting on the bed or once he has transferred into his wheelchair.

depend on the person's level of injury and whether the damage to the spinal cord is complete or incomplete.

Men's fertility usually decreases after a spinal cord lesion although many will still be able to father children either independently or through medical intervention. Women's menstrual periods may stop for a few months following spinal cord lesion but will eventually return. A woman's fertility is not affected and she is able to become pregnant. This is not recommended within the first 2 years of a traumatic lesion because the vertebral column needs time to become stable and strong and her body needs to adjust to the lesion. Pregnancy will usually be normal. She must, however, be particularly vigilant of pressure relief as she becomes heavier and bigger. She may be unaware of the onset of labour and assistance may be required for the delivery of the baby.

Further information on sexuality following a spinal cord lesion can be found in Gatehouse (1995) and Glass (1999).

Productivity

Home management

Wherever possible, an individual should be given the opportunity to participate in domestic tasks that are appropriate to his roles. This may include making hot drinks; using a microwave, washing machine or vacuum cleaner; and changing a duvet cover. The extent to which an individual performs these tasks will depend upon his functional ability and his motivation. However, it is important that the person experiences activities relevant to his domestic situation to boost confidence and skill and to begin to anticipate and problem-solve issues that might arise. For those planning to return to live at home alone or to live with carer assistance, the ability to perform or direct domestic tasks may become a vital part of a care package. It is important to recognise that living independently may involve the person employing someone to do various tasks for him. In this case the person may need to learn skills relevant to recruiting and employing staff and have access to resources to support this process.

Paid and voluntary employment

Work provides a person with a role, an income, personal satisfaction and an opportunity to socialise (Darnbrough 1995). Returning to employment after a spinal cord lesion is usually a long process and some people wish to become settled at home before considering employment. Some may have an understanding employer, accessible work environment and a suitable job, which may contribute to the individual's motivation to return to work. The advance of computer technology has made a large contribution to the work prospects for people with a spinal cord lesion. The occupational therapist will work with each person to investigate work issues. This may involve investigating alternative employment, further training or education or a change in career. Advice may be required on adaptations to the work environment, equipment or routine to enable the individual to return to his or her former employment, school or college.

A significant barrier to returning to work, other than personal motivation, is access (Whalley Hammell 1995). Access to and around the work environment may not be suitable for an individual using a wheelchair. When investigating work issues, the individual and the occupational therapist should consider factors other than specific work issues. His morning routine of personal hygiene, washing and dressing, whether performed independently or by a carer, may affect the time he is able to start work. Relying on public transport or taxis or the possibility of using his vehicle should be considered. The possibility of flexible working hours or of working part-time or from home may be options, and these require negotiation. For many, the return to work is seen as a major step in the re-establishment of previous roles.

Some individuals may have sufficient income from benefits or compensation and decide not to undertake paid work. For these individuals, voluntary work may fulfil their needs.

Leisure

Occupational therapists assist the individual to identify recreation and leisure interests, skills, opportunities and appropriate activity. It is vital that he has a healthy balance between daily living activities, work and recreation or leisure (Whalley Hammell 1995). This is discussed further in Chapter 2. In some cases, the individual can return to his previous recreation and leisure activities. Some may return to a previous interest but in a different role (e.g. he may become an adjudicator or instructor rather than a participant or play a role on the management committee of a sports club). Some adaptations or changes in techniques may be required but the possibility of returning to these activities should be investigated.

During rehabilitation, the individual may take the opportunity to become involved in a variety of social, sporting, creative and interactive activities. These activities may include going to the pub, shopping, participating in interest groups, such as photography, and trying out various sports, such as wheelchair basketball, rugby, tennis and archery. This will provide him with the opportunity to develop confidence and practice skills to enable him to partake in a variety of activities within the community.

FOCUSING ON THE ENVIRONMENT

Returning home

An occupational therapist should be planning the individual's return home from the day of admission. Due to the complex nature of a spinal cord injury and the long-term planning necessary to reintegrate each person, an early referral to community services is essential.

People live in a variety of different circumstances and, whenever possible, they will usually want to return to their existing home. As soon as it is appropriate, a home visit with community staff is arranged. The aim of the home visit is to establish at an early stage whether return to the property is appropriate for an overnight or weekend stay, and eventually on a permanent basis. If his previous accommodation is not suitable, alternatives will need to be addressed for the acquisition of more suitable property.

An overnight or short-term stay at home may be facilitated through the use of essential environmental adaptations that enable the individual to undertake his acquired level of occupational performance as far as possible. Some of these environmental adaptations may be:

- temporary ramp/s at one entrance
- putting a single bed in a living room or dining room
- using a commode or shower chair for toileting if the toilet is inaccessible
- having a bed bath or washing from a bowl if the bathroom is inaccessible.

The occupational therapist will discuss this arrangement with the family and establish any issues related to overnight stays. Family members and friends should be provided with appropriate training from the team on how to assist their relative whilst he is away from the specialist centre. Once he and his family or friends feel confident, they will be encouraged to spend weekends away from the centre, as this provides opportunities to learn and to boost his self-esteem and motivation. Spending time away may enable him, his family and friends to decide upon what plans they wish to make for long-term resettlement.

If alterations to a property are necessary, obtaining funds to contribute towards the cost of the alterations must be considered. The procedures involved in making alterations to a property require careful thought and planning and can take many months.

As well as the availability of suitable accommodation, organising an appropriate care package tailored to the individual's specific needs involves staff from both the hospital and the community and can take time. In the event of an individual's rehabilitation being completed before long-term accommodation is available, alternative interim accommodation closer to his home should be sought.

SPECIAL CONSIDERATIONS

PEOPLE WITH INCOMPLETE SPINAL CORD LESIONS

People with incomplete spinal cord lesions will show a mixture of problems and, as a result, it may be difficult to be specific about how the lesion will affect their prognosis and function (Edwards 1998). It is unlikely that a person will make a total recovery. As each person is individual, it is best to see what he is having difficulty doing and work through ways to overcome them.

For this group of individuals, consideration should be given to:

- Muscle spasms often commence earlier and are often stronger. It is important to prevent the spasms from causing deformities:
  - frequent re-evaluations are essential to monitor the return of any muscle activity.
  - he must be encouraged to be involved in daily living activities. Long-term goals should be set but should also be flexible as the muscle and sensory return is unpredictable.
- Although the effect of an incomplete spinal cord lesion may not appear to be as severe as a complete lesion, people who have the former often have greater difficulty coping with their impairment. This is mainly due to the uncertainty of their prognosis.

CHILDREN AND ADOLESCENTS WITH SPINAL CORD LESIONS

Many of the rehabilitation goals for children and teenagers who have a spinal cord lesion will be similar to those of adults. There are, however, some issues that are specific to children:

- The child and his family must be involved during the whole rehabilitation programme. The parents or main carer will need to be consulted about their child and kept informed but the child should also be consulted and informed so that he is encouraged to take control of his rehabilitation.

- Rehabilitation must take into account the child's developmental stage and consider how he can achieve the subsequent developmental stages encompassing the attainment of relevant cognitive, social, emotional, as well as motor, skills.
- As the body of a child is still growing and developing it is vulnerable to many deformities following a spinal cord lesion. There is a high risk of scoliosis and lordosis. The vertebral column needs to be stabilised and the child will probably have to wear a body brace and callipers.
- Children should be encouraged not to sit for long periods. Although a wheelchair will be required for taking part in many activities, a child may be provided with a prone trolley, standing device and/or a walker to maintain an erect position, in an effort to maintain the anatomical position of the pelvis and hips (Bergstrom 1998).
- Some children may have difficulty transferring independently, as their arms are shorter in proportion to their trunk compared with adults.
- Any equipment provided or adaptations carried out in the house must take into account that the child will change physically, emotionally and socially, and as such his needs will alter.
- Guidance and advice may be required during the primary school years, secondary school years and the transition stage after school when children enter into their early adult years and begin to consider the option of leaving home.

SPINAL CORD LESIONS IN ELDERLY PEOPLE

Falls are the most common cause of spinal cord injury in the elderly and cervical injuries are the predominate result of this trauma. Several considerations must be taken into account with this client group (Whalley Hammell 1995):

- Many elderly people have other significant medical problems, which may complicate rehabilitation following spinal cord lesion. Elderly people may be more prone to contractures and stiff joints, skin breakdown, decreased endurance and increased fatigue, and perhaps a reduced level of function. Rehabilitation may take longer.

- The use of a wheelchair is advisable, particularly when ambulation is not functional or when stamina is significantly reduced.
- It is possible that an older person's social support systems may be limited or non-existent due to family and friends dying or moving away. This may have implications for the outcome of resettlement.
- As most elderly people will not be in paid employment, the focus of rehabilitation will be on activities of daily living and on leisure, recreation and socialisation.

AGEING WITH A SPINAL CORD LESION

Due to a tremendous improvement in the medical care and the success of rehabilitation over the last few decades, people with spinal cord lesions are surviving into old age. Although a spinal cord lesion is a stable condition, the effects of growing older can have a big impact on the independence of a person (Whalley Hammell 1995). Some possible complications include:

- Decrease in muscle strength will have implications for those people who use a manual wheelchair and who are independent in transferring. The repetitive action of propelling a wheelchair may result in painful and arthritic joints of the upper limb, particularly the shoulder. If this occurs, a person may have to consider other options for propelling a wheelchair (e.g. a powered wheelchair for long distances) and for transferring (e.g. using a transfer board or self-hoisting to ease the strain). For those people who could walk, a wheelchair may be considered for travelling longer distances if they begin to find walking exhausting.
- Increased fatigue may be a result of decreased muscle strength or a compromised cardiorespiratory system. If fatigue becomes significant, energy conservation techniques

may have to be used to ensure the person's independence is maintained.

- Osteoporosis – the loss of bone mass – causes the bone to become very fragile and individuals may be prone to fractures.
- The skin becomes more wrinkled and drier as a result of ageing making it more prone to breakdowns and the person is at a higher risk of developing pressure sores.
- Ageing brings with it changes in bladder and bowel continence and a person with a spinal cord lesion may have to look at other ways to manage these functions as they get older.
- There is also an increased risk of infection due to a less resistant immune system.

The social, financial, psychological and physical issues associated with ageing may have a big impact on people who are growing old with a spinal cord lesion. These issues will need to be considered in the long-term rehabilitation of people with a spinal cord lesion.

PEOPLE WITH VERY HIGH TETRAPLEGIA

This group have no upper limb function, minimal head control and rely on a ventilator or diaphragmatic pacing for respiration. They have a lesion between the C1 and C4 neurological segments. Those with a lesion at C4 are usually able to breathe independently of a ventilator. All aspects of rehabilitation appropriate to people with tetraplegia are relevant to this group who have the added difficulties of limited communication, total physical dependence on others and the immeasurable psychological trauma of being reliant on a ventilator for life.

Occupational therapy input for these people is considerable (Whalley Hammell 1995). The therapist will need to be knowledgeable in the range of appropriate equipment and technology that may benefit the individual and facilitate a satisfactory quality of life (Bain & Leger 1997). This technology will probably include items such as:

- a powered wheelchair, which can be operated independently by the user and which will carry the ventilator

- vehicle conversions, which enable the person to be a passenger while seated in their wheelchair
- software and hardware, which facilitate independent access to a computer
- an environmental control system to control electrical appliances in the home and to call for assistance.

Living at home involves the establishment of personal need plans and care packages to ensure that the person has the relevant level of support. This support is required to ease the physical demands on family relationships. Despite the person being totally physically dependent on others, it is important that he learns to be verbally independent and take control of what is done for him in his environment. He will need to become very familiar with his care routine to be able to advise others on what needs to be done, including turning regimens, hoisting procedure, positioning in the wheelchair, settings on ventilator, suctioning techniques and bowel and bladder management techniques.

CONCLUSION

A spinal cord lesion can be a result of traumatic or non-traumatic damage. It results in complete or incomplete paraplegia or tetraplegia and leads to many immediate and long-term physiological, psychological, social and emotional effects and complications. Rehabilitation for people who have had a spinal cord lesion is not a short-term process, in many ways it is a lifelong process. The initial phase of rehabilitation, however, which commences once the person is admitted to hospital, is essential to enable him to learn how to deal with his needs as well as how to live autonomously. The essence of rehabilitation is to empower the individual with the confidence to have control over his own life and to be able to live the life he wants to live. Occupational therapists play an essential role in assisting and supporting people to meet their own needs (Box 16.1).

Box 16.1   Case study: David

David was a 21-year-old graphic design student on holiday in Majorca with his girlfriend, Paula. He dived into the hotel pool and hit his head on the bottom. He was taken to the local hospital, flown back to the United Kingdom and admitted to a spinal centre. On examination he was found to have a fracture dislocation of C6/7 resulting in a complete tetraplegia at C6.

David was managed conservatively, with his head in skull traction for 8 weeks. X-rays at this time showed that healing was satisfactory. He began to sit up using a profiling bed; a firm neck collar was required for sitting beyond 45°. He was profiled for increasing periods over 2 days and then transferred into a reclining wheelchair with a Jay 2 cushion. To ease the nauseous and dizzy symptoms of postural hypotension he wore antiembolotic stockings and an abdominal binder, and was given a small dose of ephedrine prior to sitting up in the wheelchair.

Initially, he spent 15 minutes in a wheelchair. This was increased daily over the next 2 weeks until he could tolerate 8 hours sitting in a wheelchair and did not experience any problems. He progressed to a non-reclining standard wheelchair and began to attend the physiotherapy and occupational therapy departments.

In physiotherapy, David worked on relearning balance, neck and arm strengthening. In occupational therapy he wished to work on the self-care occupations, eating and teeth cleaning. Independent wheelchair mobility was also encouraged and David was provided with pushing gloves.

Four weeks after initial mobilisation David was able to remove his firm collar. Over the next 6 months he worked on increasing his strength and functional ability so that by the time he was discharged he was able to:

- move independently on the bed
- propel a lightweight wheelchair independently, including managing slopes
- transfer in and out of bed using a sliding board
- transfer in and out of the car with a sliding board and assistance
- undress independently and put himself to bed at night
- wash, shower, clean his teeth and shave independently. He found dressing frustrating and time- and energy-consuming and decided to accept help to enable him to use the time and energy on chosen activities
- make a hot drink and toast independently
- put compact discs onto the stereo
- use communication equipment including a computer keyboard, make a signature using a writing splint and use a telephone.

continued

Box 16.1 *continued*

David went to a specialised centre to be assessed for vehicle adaptations, which would enable him to drive a car. He decided to wait, however, until he had completed his studies before purchasing a car.

David was studying at a university that could cater for students with special needs and he was provided with adapted accommodation. He deferred his course for a year and then resumed his course with the help of a personal assistant.

David was discharged from the spinal centre to his parents' home where he had been able to spend weekends with relatively few alterations. His father made a ramp to the front door, the dining room was converted to a bedroom/sitting room and the ground floor toilet was converted to a shower/toilet. David's parents carried out the work to the house themselves using the offer of help from friends and neighbours.

On completion of his course, David became engaged to his girlfriend Paula and got married 6 months later. They had applied to the local authority for housing and were offered a two-bedroom bungalow by a local housing group. David uses a care package to supplement the help that Paula is able to provide for him as she works at the local school as a cook. David secured employment with a local company in their marketing department. He has a very full social life, enjoys going to concerts and meeting friends. He keeps fit by swimming once a week at the local pool. David and Paula are planning to have a family in the future.

REFERENCES

American Occupational Therapy Association 1994 Uniform terminology for occupational therapy, 3rd edn. American Journal of Occupational Therapy 48(11):1047–1054

Bain B 1997 Environmental control systems. In: Bain B, Leger D (eds) Assistive technology: an interdisciplinary approach. Churchill Livingstone, New York, pp 119–139

Bain B, Leger D 1997 Assistive technology: an interdisciplinary approach. Churchill Livingstone, New York

Bergstrom E 1998 Spinal cord injury in children. In: Bromley I (ed) Tetraplegia and paraplegia: a guide for physiotherapists, 5th edn. Churchill Livingstone, Edinburgh, pp 197–212

Bromley I 1998 Tetraplegia and paraplegia: a guide for physiotherapists, 5th edn. Churchill Livingstone, Edinburgh

Canadian Association of Occupational Therapy 1997 Enabling occupation: an occupational therapy perspective. CAOT Publications ACE, Toronto, Ottawa

Curtin M 1994 Development of a tetraplegic hand assessment and splinting protocol. Paraplegia 32:159–169

Darnbrough A 1995 Work. In: Gatehouse M (ed) Moving forward: the guide to living with spinal cord injury, 1st edn. Spinal Injuries Association, London

Ditunno Jr JF, Young W, Donovan WH, Creasey G 1994 The international standards booklet for neurological and functional classification of spinal cord injury. Paraplegia 32:70–80

Edwards S 1998 The incomplete lesion. In: Bromley I (ed) Tetraplegia and paraplegia: a guide for physiotherapists, 5th edn. Churchill Livingstone, Edinburgh, pp 167–196

Egan M, Delaat MD 1994 Considering spirituality in occupational therapy practice. Canadian Journal of Occupational Therapy 61(2):95–101

Gatehouse M 1995 Feeling. In: Gatehouse M (ed) Moving forward: the guide to living with a spinal cord injury. Spinal Injuries Association, London, pp 8-1–8-11

Glass C 1999 Spinal cord injury: impact and coping. The British Psychological Society, Leicester

Grant DD, Lundon K 1998 The Canadian model of occupational performance applied to females with osteoporosis. Canadian Journal of Occupational Therapy 66(1):3–13

Grundy D, Swain A 2001 ABC of spinal cord injury, 4th edn. British Medical Association Publishing Group, London

Ham R, Aldersea P, Porter D 1998 Wheelchair users and postural seating: a clinical approach. Churchill Livingstone, Edinburgh

Krajnik S, Bridle M 1992 Hand splinting in quadriplegia: current practice. American Journal of Occupational Therapy 46(2):149–156

Lipner H 1997 Augmentative and alternative communication. In Bain B, Leger D (eds) Assistive technology: an interdisciplinary approach. Churchill Livingstone, New York, pp 99–118

Ozer M 1988 The management of persons with spinal cord injury. Demos, New York

Pentland W, Harvey AS, Smith T, Walker J 1999 The impact of spinal cord injury on men's time use. Spinal Cord 37(11):786–792

Pollock N 1993 Client centred assessment. American Journal of Occupational Therapy 47(4):298–301

Spoltore TA, O'Brien AM 1995 Rehabilitation of the spinal cord injured patient. Orthopaedic Nursing 14(3):7–16

Stern L 1997 Telephone communications in the home: a vital link. In Bain B, Leger D (eds) Assistive technology: an interdisciplinary approach. Churchill Livingstone, New York, pp 89–98

Sumsion T 1999a Overview of client-centred practice. In Sumsion T (ed) Client-centred practice in occupational therapy: a guide to implementation. Churchill Livingstone, Edinburgh, pp 1–14

Sumsion T 1999b A study to determine a British occupational therapy definition of client-centred practice. British Journal of Occupational Therapy 62(2):52–58

Sutton S 1993 An overview of the management of the C6 quadriplegic patient's hand: an occupational therapist's perspective. British Journal of Occupational Therapy 56(10):376–380

Tam S 1998 Quality of life: theory and methodology in rehabilitation. International Journal of Rehabilitation Research 21(4):365–374

Trieschmann RB 1988 Spinal cord injuries: psychological, social and vocational management, 2nd edn. Demos, New York

Whalley Hammell K 1995 Spinal cord injury rehabilitation. Chapman & Hall, London

World Health Organization 1996 Promoting independence following a spinal cord injury: a manual for mid-level rehabilitation workers. World Health Organization, Geneva

FURTHER READING

Morris J 1989 Able lives: women's experience of paralysis. The Women's Press, London

Morris J 1993 Independent lives? Community care and disabled people. Macmillan, London

Somers M 1992 Spinal cord injury: functional rehabilitation. Appleton and Lange, Norwalk

USEFUL CONTACTS

AbilityNet Warwick, PO Box 94, Warwick, Warwickshire CV34 5WS. Freephone: 0800 269545. Fax: 01926 407425. Web://www.abilitynet.co.uk

Association to Aid the Sexual and Personal Relationships of People with a Disability (SPOD), 286 Camden Road, London N7 0BJ. Tel: 020 7 607 8851

Back-up, Room 102, The Business Village, Broomhill Road, London SW18 4JQ. Tel: 020 8 875 1805. Fax: 020 8 877 1940

Banstead Mobility Centre, Damson Way, Orchard Hill, Queen Mary's Avenue, Carshalton, Surrey SM5 4NR. Tel: 020 8 770 1151. Fax: 020 8 770 1211

British Sports Association for the Disabled, Mary Glen Haig Suite, Solecast House, 13–27 Brunswick Place, London N1 6DX. Tel: 020 7 490 1919

British Wheelchair Sports Foundation, Guttman Sports Centre, Harvey Road, Stoke Mandeville, Aylesbury, Buckinghamshire HP21 9PP. Tel: 01296 84848. Fax: 01296 24171

Centre for Accessible Environments, 60 Gainsford Street, London SE1 2NY. Tel: 020 7 357 8182

Disability Information Trust, Mary Marlborough Lodge, Nuffield Orthopaedic Centre, Headington, Oxford OX3 7LD. Tel: 01865 227592

Disabled Living Foundation (DLF), 380–384 Harrow Road, London W9 2HU. Tel: 020 7 289 6111. Fax: 020 7 266 2922

Mobility Advice and Vehicle Information Service (MAVIS), Department of Transport, TRRL, Crowthorne, Berks RG11 6AU. Tel: 01344 770456. Fax: 01344 770692

Spinal Injuries Association (SIA), Newpoint House, 76 St James's Lane, London N10 3DF. Tel: 020 8 444 2121. Fax: 020 8 444 3761

17

Upper limb trauma

Theresa Baxter   Helen McKenna

INTRODUCTION

The hand is personal and individual and gives the upper limb its importance and uniqueness. It enables the acquisition of information and the execution of activity that allows the individual to interact with the environment. The hand functions efficiently only if the proximal joints are both stable and mobile, and the combination of the elbow and mobile shoulder unit enables the hand to reach any part of the body with relative ease. The posture and movement of the hand and upper limb convey a wealth of information from skill and beauty to sexuality and power, therefore dysfunction can have wide ranging consequences affecting a myriad of activities, from carrying out a highly technical task to stroking a pet.

Hand and upper limb injuries are very common and can affect a broad spectrum of people in all walks of life. However, they are most common during young adulthood as a characteristic of this period is adaptive behaviour related to engagement with an increasing amount of social, sport and recreational pursuits, which predisposes to injury (Christiansen & Baum 1991). Many of these activities involve competitive or contact sports such as rugby and football, which makes possibility of injury more likely. Also, this is the time when engagement in employment occurs, again opening up the possibility to exposure to injury.

In the majority of cases, the injuries are not related to any degenerative disease process and the nature of the trauma is transient, so the individual will experience only a limited period of dysfunction before returning to their former lifestyle and occupation. However, some individuals may experience severe trauma, which can result in residual and permanent impairment that will necessitate adaptation of their lifestyle. The problems that may occur are many and varied; these may include brachial plexus lesions, which most frequently occur as a result of motorcycle accidents where the rider experiences a traction injury to the brachial plexus due to violent abduction of the neck and shoulder (Dandy 1989), fractures to the humerus and forearm, and injuries to the nerves, tendons and soft tissues of the hand.

Occupational therapists have for many years been involved in the restoration of function and purposeful activity with individuals with upper limb injuries, this being a natural development from the profession's philosophical base and concern with occupational performance (Early 1998, Melvin 1985). An effective therapist needs to have a thorough understanding of upper extremity anatomy, physiology, kinesiology and psychology, as well as an understanding of the process of tissue healing, surgical and disease process and outcomes (Kasch 1989, 1998). In essence, the occupational therapist can only enhance hand and arm rehabilitation by capturing the physical, contextual and psychosocial aspects of functional return (Toth-Fejel et al 1998). Occupational therapists have a vital dual role – they promote the physical rehabilitation of individuals to help them return to their preinjury activities and they provide the valuable psychological support that helps the individual to survive the ordeal of injury, pain and dysfunction and ultimately helps them regain the confidence to try activities and consider alternative ways of performing them when necessary.

This chapter examines the functional impact of upper limb injuries on the individual and the role of the occupational therapist in enabling the individual to resume a meaningful and productive lifestyle. It also explores the psychosocial impact of an upper limb injury to an individual, pain and pain management, and the importance of teamwork in caring for an individual with upper limb injuries. This is followed by consideration of the application of theoretical principles when undertaking assessment and treatment. Then follows the occupational therapy process, starting with data gathering and followed by assessment techniques. The final section of the chapter considers types of intervention and concludes with a case study illustrating factors explored throughout the chapter.

PSYCHOSOCIAL IMPACT OF INJURY

Until recently, the major focus of upper limb surgery and rehabilitation was on perfecting technique, and occupational therapists followed on from surgeons in maintaining a predominantly technical and medical model in their approach to therapy (Bear-Lehman 1983). With advances in splinting materials, assessment packages and technical treatment media, such as the Baltimore Therapeutic Exerciser (BTE), as well as the pressures of the modern health services, therapists have not always taken time to consider the psychological impact of the injury to the individual. In exploring an individual's needs from a purely technical and functional base, a therapist may never find what is important to that individual (Crabtree 1998) and, yet, it is acknowledged that meaning has a considerable impact on the therapeutic process between the individual and the therapist.

Blumenfield and Schoeps (1993) compare the psychological trauma of injury to the hand with injury to the face, stating that 'amputations or deformities to the hand may have as much impact on the person, and consequently, the family, as a deformity of the face'. If the hand is to remain functional, it is difficult to hide the result of disfigurement and deformity. In the early stages of management, the effect of this may be masked by the dressings and the generalised shock of being injured (Jones 1977). However, as the days and weeks pass it may become evident that the individual is becoming increasingly distressed by the appearance of the limb. An individual's reaction to injury is not always proportional to the extent of the physical damage to the hand (Boscheinen-Morrin 1985). The individual may also be experiencing a reactive depression to the event or have developed post-traumatic stress disorder (PTSD) through reliving the traumatic event leading up to the injury and, as a result, there will be a significant impact upon the individual's occupational performance. There may be periods of withdrawal or denial, during which the individual abdicates responsibility for the limb or refuses to accept the severity of the injury.

The psychological effects of upper limb injury can be great, resulting in feelings of anxiety, depression and loss of control and self-esteem. It is essential that the therapist takes time to address these needs, which may ultimately affect the outcome. Fear and anxiety are generally decreased by providing information about the condition and the treatment involved, and it is important that sufficient emphasis is given to this despite the probability of the pressures of a very heavy caseload. Careful ongoing assessment of the individual's psychological make-up and status is recommended. Often, the variation in outcome of injury will depend more on a person's personality and motivation (Chin et al 1999) than any other factor.

An individual's enthusiasm to participate in their rehabilitation programme can be affected by many factors, such as their perspective of the relative importance of their hand both from a practical as well as a body image point of view (Chin et al 1999), the perceived severity of the injury, efficacy of the rehabilitation process and the patient–practitioner relationship. It is recognised that most patients are satisfied by physicians and occupational therapists who are knowledgeable, trustworthy, confident and enthusiastic.

PAIN MANAGEMENT

Pain may also be a major factor in coping with the upper limb trauma. Acute pain is to be expected immediately after injury or surgery. Acute pain is an important warning mechanism and serves a function in guiding the therapist and the individual in preventing further damage to the healing process. Chronic pain, however,

serves no biological purpose but has a considerable impact upon an individual's life, with the person experiencing major difficulties in multiple facets of living (Strong 1996). Upper limb injury may also jeopardise an individual's and family's livelihood, leading to financial and employment difficulties.

OTHER FACTORS

Many other factors may have a considerable effect on an individual's progress through the rehabilitation programme and also on their general compliance to treatment. An individual may be labelled non-compliant or lacking in motivation when there may, in fact, be language or cultural barriers, physical limitations such as poor vision, cognitive impairment or a low level of literacy, which may affect the person's ability to follow verbal or written instructions.

Family and financial commitments may prevent an individual from attending appointments regularly because they may need to work, particularly if they are self-employed, in order to maintain their family or secure their job. The individual may be the main carer in a household with children or ageing relatives and routine clinic appointments may not fit with their lifestyle and occupational roles.

THE TEAM

Teamwork is of paramount importance when treating an individual with upper limb trauma and the most important member of the team is the person themselves. Tubiana (1985) recognised that a person's desire for a good result in upper limb trauma was essential to the success of the rehabilitation programme. It is easy for the therapist to adopt a reductionist approach and to formulate goals and treatment programmes without consulting with the person concerned. However, such programmes are more likely to be ineffective or fail if this first rule is ignored. Consideration of the individual's needs and goals are essential. Issues such as access to therapy, timing of appointments, information giving, clear communication and liaison between professionals ensure a streamlined and comprehensive programme approach is achieved.

Meaning and understanding are very important to the individual and will help to capture attention, lift spirits and prove to be a powerful incentive to deal with the mundane aspects of the rehabilitation process (Crabtree 1998).

The team may consist of physician, surgeon, physiotherapist, nurse, psychologist, social worker, interpreter, orthotist, prosthetist, resettlement team, counsellor, voluntary agencies and employer. However, all these professionals can seem overwhelming and best results will be obtained when the individual feels confident and in control and when the professionals are focused on his agenda and not their own.

Essentials of the team should be coordination and communication concerning protocols and guidelines of care, joint working where appropriate and clear role identity, understanding and appreciation of each other's skills. An example of this may be working with an individual who has a rotator cuff tear. The surgeon may perform a rotator cuff repair, the nurses will provide postoperative care on the ward, the physiotherapist and occupational therapist will work towards helping the individual to regain control of the glenohumeral joint and scapula and to strengthen the rotator cuff. Referrals may be made to a social worker and to the community occupational therapist for a community care package if the person is elderly, and the GP and district nurse will take over the person's medical care on discharge. Collaborative working needs to be the essence of the team and, as can be seen from Figure 17.1, the occupational therapist may be the key person who works alongside the injured person from the early stages of hospital care, through to outpatients and community rehabilitation, and finally into resettlement. Communication and clear reporting will therefore be paramount in the therapist's repertoire of skills.

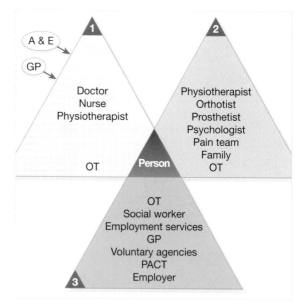

Fig. 17.1 Three distinct stages of team intervention.

THEORETICAL FOUNDATIONS OF INTERVENTION

The ultimate aim of intervention should ideally be to maximise return of function and facilitate a positive adjustment to any residual impairment. This may involve the application of a number of theoretical frames of reference and approaches to achieve goals that are realistic and meaningful to the individual.

The biomedical approach to upper limb rehabilitation has often been seen as the favoured approach of therapists working in busy hand therapy units. Its focus is on the diagnosis and treatment of disease and injury and the traditional biomedical beliefs that a disorder entails a breakdown in the machinery of the body, which can be put right by applying the appropriate scientific and physical remedies (Young & Quinn 1992).

In the late 1970s and early 1980s, the reductionistic influences of medicine continued (Christiansen & Baum 1991) alongside the many advances in surgery, microsurgery and implantation (Callahan 1983). However, therapists working in hand rehabilitation once again returned to their philosophical foundations of being occupation-centred and maximising adaptation to impairments. Although recognising the importance of in-depth knowledge of anatomy, physiology, kinesiology and biomechanics, they also recognised the importance of implementing an occupation-centred approach to their interventions. This is critical to the success and livelihood of individuals in overcoming the limitation to their injury and impairment (Melvin 1985). Therapeutic occupation is one of the profession's oldest traditions and can enrich the process of upper limb rehabilitation by establishing mutually agreed goals of recovery with the individual and adding meaningfulness to the clinical experience.

Therapists working with individuals with upper limb injuries can draw upon a wide range of theories to underpin their practice. They may use a biomechanical frame of reference, with the belief that purposeful activities can be prescribed to remediate the loss of movement, strength and endurance. This can be seen when working with an individual with hand oedema, where the therapist will use the biomechanical frame of reference to underpin her thinking, using her knowledge of anatomy and physiology when determining the degree and type of oedema, the current status of the hand and the intervention process to be adopted (Palmada et al 1998). Linked with this will be the assumption that if these prerequisites are addressed, the individual will automatically regain functional skills. The risk is then of becoming too exercise focused using 'high tech' exercise equipment and remedial activities and not addressing the occupational aspects of therapy. However, there is no guarantee that biomechanical gains, for example, increased range of wrist and shoulder movement, will lead to the functional outcome of an individual being able to self-feed (Dutton 1995). Functional outcomes are important to individuals if they are to return to their former lifestyle and therefore should form the basis of any evaluation process.

A therapist may choose to use a compensatory frame of reference, particularly if involving the individual in a work hardening programme. In this case, it will be essential for the therapist to address the physical, psychosocial and cognitive demands of the person's job and, where possible, look towards identifying standardised evaluation procedures to measure the effectiveness of the intervention and to consider the functional outcomes. Consideration may be given to supplying adapted tools or equipment, modifying the working environment in consultation with the individual and their employers and advising on financial help and benefits.

Working with individuals with upper limb trauma may involve consideration of the learning frame of reference. This educational approach will assist the therapist, working in partnership with the individual, to understand the implications of the injury and will facilitate them in making informed choices about the treatment programme. This may be particularly relevant with individuals with cumulative trauma disorders where the intervention may include an educational programme exploring anatomy of the limb, job modification, joint protection principles and correct use of body mechanics (Lawler et al 1997).

There are occasions when a cognitive behavioural approach may be an essential part of the intervention. Some individuals may present with adjustment disorders, such as stress, as a result of the trauma they have experienced, and may need to practice relaxation techniques. Others may present with factitious disorders or conversion neurosis, where they present with exaggerated symptoms or return repeatedly to the clinic with damaged splints and no clear reason why this damage happened (Barnitt 1996). Close communication with the individual and other team members, as well as clear policies, will help the therapist to deal with such problems.

Identification and recognition of the unique requirements of each individual, and respect for a person's choices and preferences, reflect the application of the humanistic approach. The design of an intervention regimen should be influenced by the lifestyle, interests, experiences and motivation of the individual, as well as the therapeutic requirements of the injury. A humanistic approach to treatment will facilitate collaboration between the therapist and the individual; for example, if the individual expresses an interest in making a cot for his unborn child or a bird table for his garden, and this is appropriate to his treatment needs, then he will be more motivated towards his rehabilitation and become an active participant in his rehabilitation.

Upper limb management does not rely exclusively on one type of approach to intervention. It may incorporate a range of approaches, depending upon the needs of the individual and the source of the injury. For example, an individual who presents with flexor tendon injuries to the hand may have experienced a work-related injury, trapping his hand in a piece of machinery, or the injury may be due to self-mutilation following a suicidal attempt, or due to glass cuts to the palm following a fight in the pub or it may be the result of a domestic accident when carving the Sunday roast. All of these individuals will require a personalised programme of intervention based on a variety of approaches.

The therapist's clinical reasoning supporting the choice of intervention needs to consider the microcomponent of hand function to yield successful functional outcomes, but also requires knowledge of psychosocial, contextual and subjective factors that will influence the individual's ability to cope with the problems of everyday living and to adapt to the limitations that interfere with their role performance (Callahan 1983, Christiansen and Baum 1991, Melvin 1985, Toth-Fejel et al 1998).

As with other aspects of intervention, to be effective when working with upper limb injuries, occupational therapists need to base their decision-making process on the best evidence available (Muir-Gray 1997). Consideration needs to be given to new technology and the latest surgical techniques being used in theatre. In considering the expectations of the individual being treated, it may be useful to carry-out a patient satisfaction questionnaire or to do an audit of non-attendees for therapy to explore how their needs could be met and how treatment could become more client focused. Atroshi et al (1999) recommends the importance of using patient-based health status outcome measures as part of the evaluation of treatment. Atroshi also points out that a significant advantage of using standardised instruments in outcome assessment is the possibility of comparisons across studies, so that regular audit can be carried out to consider the clinical effectiveness of the intervention. It is also important for the therapist to consider the professional expectations related to a particular individual's needs and it is here that reflective practice can be a useful tool for looking back over similar cases in providing a general baseline to the intervention process.

The occupational therapist needs to be aware of the natural process of human development and of the stages of acquisition of hand function. This is particularly important when working with children with upper limb trauma. When working with any age group, choice of intervention (particularly when using activities to promote function) should always be age appropriate, purposeful and meaningful to the person being treated. If the activity has no meaning for the individual then its performance will not be therapeutic (Creek 1996). Activities such as transferring water with a bulb pipette from one container or another, or moving pegs on a board game, will not necessarily have meaning for the person (Golledge 1998) and are at best used as minor or 'warm-up' parts of the intervention process, which will move towards a more purposeful and contextually relevant protocol for the individual. If they are to be used as a major part of the intervention due to the local unit policies or limited resources, then a clear explanation should be given about how these activities are focused on biomechanical gains and how this can be applied to functional and meaningful activity in the person's everyday life. They also need to be graded appropriately and changed regularly as the person progresses and the old adage of 'it's not what you do but the way that you do it' comes into its own when considering remedial games. It is important to try to use activities that can be replicated or utilised in the home so that the person is more motivated towards following through the treatment in the home environment and to the realisation that treatment is not a complex activity that can only be carried out in the department twice a week but has to be part of daily activities.

INTERVENTIONS

DATA GATHERING

Thorough data collection is vital if the therapist is going to develop the most effective intervention protocol with the individual with upper limb trauma. A starting point may be the person's medical records, where information will be given on surgical procedures and future treatment planned. If multidisciplinary notes are kept then there will be entries from other members of the treatment team who are involved. Discussion with members of the team is useful at this stage to ascertain their involvement and future aims. It may also be valuable to consider the X-rays and other test results, as these may have an impact upon the programme of treatment.

Interviewing and history taking is invaluable in planning an intervention programme that will be effective for an individual. It helps to provide a context for understanding the presenting problems and their impact upon the lifestyle of the individual. Demographic data will be collected such as age, hand dominance, other medical conditions, occupation and interests (see Box 17.1), but other useful information gained will be the person's attitude towards the injury, understanding of the condition, motivation and expectations of the outcome of treatment (Boscheinen-Morrin 1985, Christiansen & Baum 1991, Kasch 1998). A study by Chen et al (1998) clearly demonstrated that volition and an internal locus of control had considerable impact on an individual's compliance to treatment. Through the interview process, the therapist can engage an individual in the process by giving him a sense of control over his treatment and reducing the fears that arise from lack of understanding of what is to take place.

Observation of the injured individual is crucial in upper limb rehabilitation and the therapist's observation should start at first contact. Observations can be carried out in two ways: spectator observations, where the therapist discreetly observes the individual's function, or staged observation, which can be with or without

***

Box 17.1 Interview/observation assessment

Medical history

1. **Diagnosis** – type of injury, secondary problems.
2. **Prior/current treatment** – physiotherapy, surgery, drugs.
3. **Presenting symptoms** – oedema, pain, scars, infection, decreased movement.
4. **Relevant medical factors** – diabetes, heart condition, allergies.
5. **Reason for referral** – splinting, work rehabilitation, ADL, mobilisation, etc.

Personal history

1. **Occupation** – type of job, location.
2. **Job analysis** – responsibilities, working positions, functional/cognitive demands.
3. **Social/family background** – children, pets, dependants.
4. **Leisure interests** – hobbies, social activities.

Psychosocial status

1. **Motivation** – eager to participate, uncooperative.
2. **Mental status** – low in mood.

Cognitive status

1. **Level of understanding** – sees need for therapy, able to follow instructions.

Personal goals and expectations

To return to work, to care for family, return to rock climbing, etc.

Functional ability and requirements

Currently unable to use arm and hand for self-care activities.

Other significant factors

Single parent, self-employed.

***

the knowledge of the person, for example, dropping a pen for them to pick up or presenting an appointment card in the midline and seeing how and which hand is used to pick up or hold the item (Stanley & Tribuzi 1992). Insight into the person's psychological attitude to their injury may be gained by watching how the limb is held; it may be hidden from view or swathed in bandages, the individual may look fearful, or arrive with an entourage of people. The arm may be held motionless, suggesting that the person is in pain or has psychologically amputated or disassociated himself from the arm.

ASSESSMENT

Assessment should never be rushed, time given over to an assessment will reap benefits in the treatment process. Only a complete assessment will allow a coherent plan of treatment to be established and highlight the importance of the needs of the individual and the appropriate timings of the intervention (Tubiana 1995). Individuals will gain confidence from feeling that they are receiving clinically effective treatment and the therapist will have a clear baseline from which to measure intervention outcomes. Not all assessment and evaluation techniques are standardised. Some therapists will choose to use standardised tests while others will use tests that have been devised locally, often in conjunction with other members of the team.

Observation will include skin condition, with consideration being given to the colour and status, whether there is oedema or scarring present, and the presence of any deformity of the limb. Physical assessment (Table 17.1) will include measurement of joint movement with a goniometer, oedema with a volumeter or tape measure, dexterity and coordination, strength, pain, temperature and adherence or mobility of the scarring. Many other assessments may include proprioception, touch pressure threshold with monofilaments (Fig. 17.2), two-point discrimination and stereognosis, particularly if the median nerve is involved.

The most important assessment to consider, both from the occupational therapist's point of view and from that of the individual, is functional assessment. Physical evaluation, although useful, does not give the whole picture and although the individual's hand and arm may be considerably impaired according to the measurements, adaptation to the impairment and ability to carry out a variety of activities independently may already have occurred. What the therapist needs to observe is how these are carried out, what compensation techniques are being used and if it is appropriate to continue in this manner. However, the therapist needs to be aware that functional assessments can be highly subjective and the tests too insensitive to measure quality of

Table 17.1 Physical assessment

Areas to consider	Points to consider
Pain	Visual analogue scale, time of day, location, intensity, initiating factors
Oedema	Defuse or localised, brawny or soft, reason for oedema, e.g. infection, poor elevation Volumeter or tape to measure
Range of movement (ROM)	Time of day, who is measuring, analgesia Use of Odstock tracings or goniometers for measuring
Strength	Gross, lateral, tripod and two-point pinch grip Commercially available devices to measure, such as the Jamar dynamometer
Joint stability/stiffness	Check all joints, including elbow and shoulder
Dexterity	Pick-up tests may be used
Scars	Are they raised, mobile, tethered, painful?
Wound/tissue status	Healing or infected?
Sensation	Lack of or hypersensitive?
Temperature	Recognition of hot or cold?
Two-point discrimination	Use weight of the device to control force applied, test both moving and static, test only the fingertips
Touch/deep pressure	Test with monofilaments
Localisation	Most appropriate after nerve repair, usually recorded by mapping

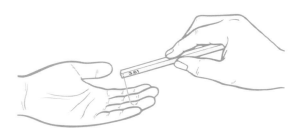

Fig. 17.2 The use of monofilament to assess proprioception.

function rather than the individual's ability to perform a specific task (Tubiana et al 1996). There are a variety of standardised function tests on the market, some of the most common are listed in Table 17.2.

Table 17.2 Standardised tests

Test	What it measures	Comments
Bennett Hand Tool Test	Timed tool manipulation using screwdriver and wrenches	Bilateral normative data
Crawford Small Parts Dexterity Test	Measures dexterity in two parts using tweezers, pins, screws, etc.	Uses familiar tools
Jebsen–Taylor Hand Function Test	Consists of seven subtests that represent various hand activities	Each test is completed with non-dominant and dominant hand. Results compared with normative data
Minnesota Rate of Manipulation Test (MRMT)	Consists of rectangular base using checker-like discs, measures placing, turning, uni- and bilateral function	Time-tested and compared with normative data
Moberg Pick-up Test	Uses an assortment of everyday objects for bilateral activities	Time-tested, no norms established, quick and easy to administer
Nine Hole Peg Test	Object is to place nine pegs in holes in any order to test dexterity	Time-tested, results compared with normative data
O'Conner Test	Fine dexterity manipulation of small pegs on a peg board	Commercially available, quick and easy to use
Purdue Peg Test	Includes five subtests assessing assembly skills	Time-tested, scores measured against normative data based on gender and job types
Sequential Occupational Dexterity Assessment (SODA)	Measures dexterity and allows observation of the performance of self-care-related activities	Originally validated for road accident patients. Quick to administer
Sollermann Test	Measures grip – 20 subtests	Gives good overall measure of function
Valpar Work Samples	Nineteen work samples, which act as a screening tool measuring worker characteristics	Tests can be used individually or in multiple groupings

A functional capacity evaluation should not be a standalone evaluation. Observation, a client self-report and physiological measures will be necessary to give a full accurate picture (King 1998). However, depending on the individual, the environment in which treatment is taking place and resources available, functional assessment may also include a variety of non-standardised tests as well as functional ADL-type activities such as fastening buttons, writing and preparing food.

Oedema

Oedema is a common problem following upper limb trauma and hand surgery. Oedema in the hand results in joint stiffness and can hinder and restrict movement. If left untreated it can lead to fibrosis, pain and an inability to carry out daily activities (Giudice 1990). Oedema is a natural response to trauma and requires speedy and aggressive intervention to prevent permanent disability and stiffness. Oedema may be the result of the individual being overprotective of the limb and it is essential that the therapist ensures that the person understands the importance of early mobilisation to restore function. The therapist can facilitate a variety of treatments with the individual. The most effective is elevation of the limb. This permits gravity to increase the rate of venous and lymphatic flow away from the extremity (Palmada et al 1998). Other intervention strategies include string wrapping or coban wrapping from proximal to distal (Fig. 17.3), followed by retrograde massage (Hunter et al 1995). Other forms of external intermittent and continuous compression may be employed using pressure sleeves, gloves and bandaging.

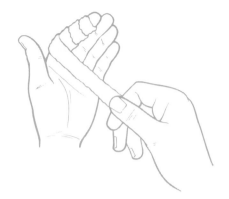

Fig. 17.3 Application of coban wrapping to control oedema.

Introduction to early activity, some of which can be performed in elevation, is essential. Activities need to be carried out within the person's pain tolerance (McEntee 1995) and should follow-on from oedema control strategies. Activities need careful analysis (see Chapter 6) to ensure they are appropriate to the needs of the individual, and may include a range of remedial activities, workshop projects, daily living tasks and use of the Baltimore Therapeutic Exerciser (BTE) and the Microprocessor Controlled Upper Limb Exerciser (MULE). Care should also be taken to mobilise adjacent joints. Splintage may be used to maintain the integrity of the ligaments and to maintain the hand in an optimum position to commence function (Fig. 17.4). An individual home programme would be recommended (Palmada et al 1998) to continue the oedema control in the home environment, to motivate the person and facilitate involvement in the treatment process as an active rather than a passive recipient.

Sensation

Increased or decreased sensibility can greatly compromise an individual's ability to be func-

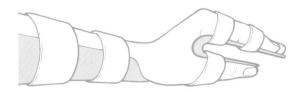

Fig. 17.4 Hand splinting in the POSI position.

tionally independent. Some people with traumatic hand injuries may develop hypersensitivity as a result of amputations, scarring and crush injuries. Complications that may occur include scar formations of regenerating axons, neuromas and adherence of the nerve to its bed (Clark et al 1993). The effects can be extreme, leading to reluctance and, in some cases, complete avoidance of the affected upper limb. The occupational therapist can devise a programme of intervention with the individual that may include massage, percussion, rolling over the affected area with graded textures, vibration and immersion in various particles, for example, rice, beans, polystyrene balls. All these activities are preliminary to functional activity and are graded towards the person's tolerance level. Most people, once guided through the programme, can continue it at home. However, if the problem is particularly severe then a structured functional programme may be necessary. This programme will be graded, taking into consideration the person's lifestyle, occupational and personal requirements. Occasionally, in the early stages of treatment, gel cushioning can be provided to protect the affected area. This will encourage earlier return to active use of the limb. However, the therapist must take care not to allow the person to become dependent on this protection.

Activities that can be carried out include woodwork, wood turning on an electric lathe (which provides vibration), use of the BTE, use of the computer with adapted keys or switches and domestic activities such as baking, which will require immersion in flour and the rolling out of pastry, all of which will help to desensitise the limb.

Cold sensitivity is a common problem following injury. It can be a major disability to those who work outdoors and is reported in up to 85% of individuals who have sustained upper limb injuries (Craigen et al 1999). The therapist will need to educate the person in care of the limb, emphasising the importance of keeping it covered in cold weather.

Lack of adequate sensation can also prevent an individual from using their upper limb effectively. Following peripheral nerve injury or repair, the individual will have difficulty interpreting sensory information and, without sensation, smooth and skilled movement cannot be achieved and the in-built protection system is lost. For those who lack protective sensation, both an educational and compensatory approach will need to be used.

Callahan (1995) advises that the individual should be educated in care of the affected limb and indicates the following points in the care package:

- avoid exposure to excessive heat or cold
- care to be taken in handling sharp objects
- provision of padded handles to avoid low-grade pressure in gripping
- avoidance of prolonged grip
- alternating of activities to rest tissue areas
- regular observation of the skin for signs of stress
- good skin-care regimen.

Goals of treatment will be education of the individual in protection of the limb and the maximising of function in accordance with the person's needs (Clark et al 1993). A home programme will be a significant aspect of the intervention programme. To ensure compliance, the therapist will need to involve the person in the planning and goal setting and facilitate a sense of control and responsibility. Weekly goals may be beneficial along with regular reviews and opportunity to meet others with similar needs (Chen et al 1999).

Pain

It is important to establish an individual's pain levels early in the assessment process to avoid unnecessary pain that may compromise the therapeutic relationship and result in high levels of fear and anxiety. It is necessary to establish whether the pain is constant or intermittent; if there are any aggravating factors; and the nature, location and intensity of the pain. The individual's subjective assessment of pain may provide useful information about his or her general attitude and ability. Visual analogues and pain questionnaires may also be helpful.

It is important to ensure that the pain is well under control during therapy so that the person can gain maximum benefit from the treatment session. If the analgesia is proving to be ineffective then consultation with the consultant or GP is advised. Treatment in a warm and friendly environment can often help the individual to come to terms with the injury. The group setting can provide support and encouragement to individuals. Interventions may include rhythmical purposeful activities within the pain limits, application of heat or ice, massage and, in some cases where pain is persistent, application of transcutaneous electrical nerve stimulation (TENS). This will usually be done in conjunction with the pain management clinic and the physiotherapist. The occupational therapist may also focus on purposeful and meaningful activity engagement, activities of daily living with consideration of adaptive techniques and provision of equipment, relaxation training, coping skills training and stress management (Strong 1996).

ACTIVITIES OF DAILY LIVING (ADL)

It is important for the therapist working with an individual with upper limb injuries to consider daily activity requirements. This should take place as early as possible in the intervention process. Immediately post injury it may be necessary to instruct the person in compensatory techniques or provide equipment. For example, in the case of a person with a flexor tendon repair, it may be appropriate to provide a person with a one-handed knife and fork to prevent frustration and avoid the possibility of the person attempting to use the affected limb inappropriately and thus compromising the surgical repair. It is important that the provision of compensatory devices does not detract from the therapy being provided to restore function. Equipment that is adapted in a way that encourages function and can be graded to address the changing status of the individual can be valuable in restoring function and independence; for example, the use of padded cutlery, which can be decreased in size as grip improves.

ADL questionnaires can be useful screening tools and may provide valuable information to help in prioritising the most essential areas for intervention.

SPLINTING

Splinting is a very useful modality in the rehabilitation of the upper limb and can provide a valuable adjunct to exercise. Splints can be used to support and immobilise healing tissues, hold or stress soft tissues to enable soft tissue extensibility, stabilise mobile joints in order that the corrective exercise force can be directed to the stiff joint or adherent tendon. Dynamic splints can be used to provide a resistive force to increase muscle strength, as well as to apply a corrective stretch to joint contractures and tendon adhesions. The opportunities for creative splinting are many, so long as there is a clear clinical reason for application and the individual understands the requirements and reasoning of the application.

WORK ASSESSMENT AND REHABILITATION

The individual's ability to participate in work and leisure activities should be addressed in the treatment process. Early in the intervention, the therapist should hold a long-term vision with regards to an individual's occupation requirements.

The four main areas for consideration in a work rehabilitation programme are: flexibility, strength, endurance and task simulation. Exercise and remedial activity to increase range of movement is followed by activities to strengthen weakened muscles. Therapeutic putty, grip-strengthening devices, heavy workshop activities and the BTE simulator are frequent techniques utilised to strengthen muscles weakened by injury and to aid in reconditioning those that are used for work-related activities.

When sufficient power returns to enable a person to carry-out work tasks, the emphasis progresses to that of increasing the individual's endurance levels. In the later stages of treatment, job tasks are included to ensure that an individual's capabilities match the specific demands of their work. The BTE is especially helpful at this stage of treatment as it is space-efficient; easily graded in terms of time, resistance and movement; and has the added benefit of providing the person and therapist with feedback on performance and progress.

A job site visit maybe appropriate if the person is to return to paid employment, this will enable the rehabilitation programme to be relevant and to clearly establish the job requirements from both the employer and the individual concerned. Early return to light duties is recommended, if possible, as this will help to maintain work habits and general fitness.

HOME PROGRAMME

In the current economic climate, with ever-increasing financial constraints on therapy services, home rehabilitation programmes are becoming frequently used. A home programme of activity, which is carried out several times a day, 7 days a week, can often be more effective than an intensive, therapist-led session once a week. This also prevents the individual from developing the philosophy that treatment ends when they leave the ward, department or rehabilitation unit (Salter 1987). At the centre of any home programme should be a high level of clear communication, which will take the form of a written home exercise programme, preferably with clear diagrams and personalised to each individual's special requirements. Clear verbal instructions and demonstrations are essential and need to be reinforced at regular intervals. Compliance is necessary if a home programme is to succeed (Chen et al 1999). Therefore, the early sessions should emphasise education. Reviews and upgrades of the programme are essential as compliance levels can be seen to fluctuate throughout treatment. This type of programme is particularly well received by individuals who have to return to work, are caring for others or may have other difficulties in getting to the hospital.

CONCLUSION

When treating individuals with upper limb trauma it is important to see the person as a 'whole' and not as a 'fractured radial head' or 'flexor tendon repair'. The therapist not only needs to turn her attention to the injured limb but should also consider the many physical and psychosocial needs of the individual. The impact of the injury needs to be considered, along with the goals and needs of the person involved (Box 17.2). Surgical and therapeutic intervention in this specialism is evolving rapidly and therapists need to be vigilant about keeping up-to-date with current literature so that they are best placed to offer the most effective and justifiable interventions.

Box 17.2 Case study: Graeme

Graeme is a 42-year-old man who sustained a road traffic accident (RTA) with lacerations to his upper limb. He subsequently developed tetanus, which resulted in autonomic dysfunction, respiratory arrest and renal failure. Whilst on ITU it was noted that he had neuropraxia of the radial nerve of his right arm. Graeme was referred to occupational therapy for assessment and intervention.

Physical examination

A radial nerve palsy, decreased extension of the wrist, metacarpophalangeal joints and thumb. Oedema, stiffness, reduced grip strength and a sensitive, dry, tethered scar.

Personal history

Post Office delivery worker with a partner and two children. Graeme's leisure interests are gardening, betting on the horses and socialising with friends.

Psychosocial status

Motivated, with a good understanding of current physical status.

Personal goals and expectations

To return to full-time employment and look after his partner and children.

Functional abilities

Limited independence in personal activities of daily living (PADL) and domestic activities of daily living (DADL).

Other significant factors

Poor general health due to prolonged stay in hospital, residual effects of infection, resulting in limited tolerance to activity and high levels of fatigue.

Initial intervention

In the acute inpatient phase, Graeme was fitted with a splint to put his hand and wrist in a position of safe immobilisation (POSI) with elevation and retrograde massage. Subsequently, he was fitted with a dynamic splint to encourage range of movement (ROM) and better function. Adapted cutlery was issued to increase independence, and PADL activities commenced and energy conservation advice given.

Intermediate intervention

Following discharge, intermediate intervention took place in outpatients. This commenced with reassessment, job analysis and goal setting.

A light workshop programme was initiated using remedial activities, the Baltimore Therapeutic Exerciser (BTE), scar management and desensitisation.

Further splinting, including a night extension splint, to overcome the contractures at the elbow. A home programme was provided. Group work was encouraged to increase motivation.

Final stage intervention

A heavy workshop programme was developed, where woodworking provided the opportunity to work on fitness and endurance levels as well as grip strength and dexterity of the hand. Further liaison took place with employers who were prepared to offer light duties and reduced working hours.

Discharge saw Graeme returning to full-time employment, enjoying his hobbies and exploring his new found skills in woodworking!

REFERENCES

Atroshi I, Gummersson C, Johnsson R, Sprinchorn A 1999 Symptoms, disability, and quality of life in patients with carpal tunnel syndrome. The Journal of Hand Therapy 24A(2):398–403

Barnitt RE 1996 Factitious disorders in occupational therapy: sad cases or incorrigible rogues? British Journal of Occupational Therapy 59(2):50–55

Bear-Lehman J 1983 Factors affecting return to work after hand injury. The American Journal of Occupational Therapy 37(3):189–194

Blumenfield M, Schoeps MM 1993 Psychological care of the burn and trauma patient. Williams & Wilkins, Baltimore, MD

Boscheinen-Morrin J, Davey V, Conolley WB 1985 The hand – fundamentals of therapy. Butterworth, London

Callahan A 1983 Hand rehabilitation and occupational therapy. The American Journal of Occupational Therapy 37(3):166

Callahan A 1995 Methods of compensation and reeducation for sensory dysfunction. In: Hunter J, Mackin PT,

Callahan A (eds) 1995 Rehabilitation of the hand: surgery and therapy, 4th edn. Mosby, St Louis, MO, vol 1

Chen CY, Neufeld PS, Feely CA, Skinner CS 1998 Factors influencing compliance with home exercise programs among patients with upper extremity impairment. The Journal of Occupational Therapy 53(2):171–179

Chen CY, Neufeld PS, Feely CA, Skinner CS 1999 Factors influencing compliance with home exercise programs among patients with upper extremity impairment. The American Journal of Occupational Therapy 53(2):171–179

Chin KR, Lonner JH, Jupiter BS, Jupiter JB 1999 The surgeon as a hand patient: the clinical and psychological impact of hand and wrist fractures. The Journal of Hand Therapy 24A(1):59–63

Christiansen C, Baum C 1991 Occupational therapy: overcoming human performance deficits. Slack Inc., New Jersey

Clark GL, Shaw-Wilgis EF, Aiello B, Eckhaus D, Eddington LV 1993 Hand rehabilitation – a practical guide. Churchill Livingstone, New York

Crabtree JL 1998 The end of occupational therapy. The American Journal of Occupational Therapy 52(3):205–214

Craigen M, Klienert JM, Crain GM, McCabe SJ 1999 Patient and injury characteristics in the development of cold sensitivity of the hand: A prospective cohort study. The Journal of Hand Therapy 24A(1):8–15

Creek J 1996 Making a cup of tea as an honours degree subject. The British Journal of Occupational Therapy 59(3):128–130

Dandy DJ 1989 Essentials of orthopaedics and trauma. Churchill Livingstone, Edinburgh

Dutton R 1995 Clinical reasoning in physical disabilities. Williams & Wilkins, Baltimore, MD

Early MB 1998 Physical dysfunction practice skills for the occupational therapy assistant. Mosby, St Louis, MO

Golledge J 1998 Distinguishing between occupation, purposeful activity and activity, Part 1, review and explanation. British Journal of Occupational Therapy 61(3):100–104

Guidice ML 1990 Effects of continuous passive motion and elevation on hand oedema. The American Journal of Occupational Therapy 44(3):189–194

Hunter JM, Mackin PT, Callahan A 1995 Rehabilitation of the hand, 4th edn, vol 1. Mosby, St Louis, MO

Jones M 1977 An approach to occupational therapy. Butterworth, London

Kasch MC 1989 Hand rehabilitation. The American Journal of Occupational Therapy 43(3):145–147

Kasch MC 1998 Acute hand injuries. In: Early MB (ed) Physical dysfunction practice skills for the occupational therapy assistant. Mosby, St Louis, MO

King PM 1998 A critical review of functional capacity evaluations. Physical Therapy 78(8):852–866

Lawler AL, James AB, Tomlin G 1997 Educational techniques used in occupational therapy treatment of cumulative trauma disorders of the elbow, wrist and hand. The American Journal of Occupational Therapy 51(2):113–118

Mctree PM 1995 Therapist's management of the stiff hand. In: Hunter J, Mackin PT, Callahan A (eds) Rehabilitation of the hand. Mosby, St Louis, MO

Melvin JL 1985 Roles and functions of occupational therapy in hand rehabilitation. The American Journal of Occupational Therapy 39(12):795–798

Muir-Gray JA 1997 Evidence based healthcare: how to make health policy and management decisions. Churchill Livingstone, Edinburgh

Palmada M, Shah S, O'Hare K 1998 Hand oedema: pathophysiology and treatment. British Journal of Therapy and Rehabilitation 5(11):556–564

Salter M 1987 Hand injuries: a therapeutic approach. Churchill Livingstone, Edinburgh

Stanley B, Tribuzi S 1992 Concepts in hand rehabilitation. FA Davis Company, Philadelphia, PA

Strong J 1996 Chronic pain: the occupational therapist's perspective. Churchill Livingstone, Edinburgh

Toth-Fejel GE, Toth-Fejel GF, Hedricks CA 1998 Occupation-centered practice in hand rehabilitation using the experience sampling method. The American Journal of Occupational Therapy 52(5):381–385

Tubiana R 1985 The hand. WB Saunders Company, Philadelphia, PA, vol 11

Tubiana R, Thomine J, Mackin PT 1996 Examination of the hand and wrist. Martin Dunitz Ltd, London

Young ME, Quinn E 1992 Theories and principles of occupational therapy. Churchill Livingstone, Edinburgh

FURTHER READING

Hunter J, Mackin PT, Callahan A 1995 Rehabilitation of the hand: surgery and therapy, 4th edn. Mosby, St Louis, MO, vol 1

Jacobs K 1991 Occupational therapy – work related programs and assessments, 2nd edn. Little, Brown & Company, Boston, MA

Jebson P, Kasdan M 1998 Hand secrets. Handley & Befus, Philadelphia, PA

Kapandji 1982 The physiology of the joints. Churchill Livingstone, Edinburgh

Lankveld W, Bosch P, Bakker J, Terwindt S, Franssen M, Reil P 1996 Sequential occupational dexterity assessment. The Journal of Hand Therapy 9(1):27–31

Moberg E 1958 Objective methods of determining the functional value of sensibility in the hand. Journal of Bone and Joint Surgery 40B:454

18

HIV/AIDS

Sandie Woods   Camilla Hawkins

INTRODUCTION

According to the Department of Health (1992) 'HIV infection represents perhaps the greatest new public health challenge this [the 20th] century'.

HIV stands for Human Immunodeficiency Virus. The virus was originally isolated in Paris in May 1983 by Luc Montagnier. It belongs to a group of viruses called retroviruses, which prevent the immune system from working properly. Normally, the body can fight off infection but HIV is able to infect key cells (called CD4 cells) that coordinate the immune system's fight against infection. A few CD4 cells are actually destroyed by being infected; others, including CD4 cells that are not themselves infected, no longer work properly (National AIDS Manual (NAM) May 2000).

AIDS stands for Acquired Immune Deficiency Syndrome. It occurs after HIV damage to a person's immune system. A damaged immune system is unable to protect the body against certain specific 'opportunistic' infections and tumours. These are so called because they are caused by organisms that are normally controlled by the immune system but which take the opportunity to cause disease if the immune system has been damaged. Different people with AIDS may experience different clinical problems, depending on which specific opportunistic infection they develop. A term 'syndrome' means that the collection of different signs and symptoms are all part of the same underlying medical condition (NAM May 2000).

The World Health Organization (2000) and UNAIDS (United Nations AIDS organisations) estimated that, by the end of 1999, 33.6 million people would be living with HIV worldwide, 23.3 million of whom would be in sub-Saharan Africa. This was an increase on the 1998 figures of 33.4 million. The end of 1999 recorded 40 372 individuals with HIV in the United Kingdom (Communicable Disease Report January 2000).

Despite greater knowledge and understanding about HIV/AIDS there are over 2000 new HIV infections reported each year in the United Kingdom (Department of Health (DoH), 2000). With the encouraging reduction in death rates but the increasing infection rate, the number of those living with HIV in the United Kingdom is set to double by 2010 (All Party Parliamentary Group on AIDS 1998).

UK trends from the DoH HIV strategy show that the number of children with AIDS remains small, but is increasing. The number of deaths attributed to AIDS is falling but the prevalence of HIV is increasing. The integration of HIV/AIDS and Sexual Health Strategies aims to promote effective joint working (DoH 2000/0306).

There is now a greater understanding of HIV/AIDS. Tests to show the level of the virus in the blood (the viral load) and the number of white blood cells in the blood (the CD4 count) give a much more accurate picture of the disease process and the changes that occur when someone is infected. The viral load and CD4 count help guide decisions about whether and when to start medication. They are also used to identify if the medication is being effective and to consider the risks from opportunistic infections at certain stages in the disease process. Other tests include resistance testing and therapeutic drug monitoring to check adherence, absorption and interactions. All increase knowledge and guide practice.

A wide range of medication is now available. Combinations of drugs are taken (combination therapy) to increase the effectiveness, reduce the risk of resistance and greatly improve the prognosis for those with HIV/AIDS (Anderson & Weatherburn 1998). Highly active antiviral retro-viral therapy (HAART) enables different combinations of drugs to be tried to achieve the best result with the fewest side-effects. Other advances have included improved regimens to reduce the number of tablets taken each day, thus simplifying the procedures around how and when they are taken and thereby improving adherence. Some individuals are unable to continue with combination therapy because of side-effects, resistance to medication or problems with adherence.

It is important to remember that although many advances have been made, the treatments are expensive and in many countries treatment is not affordable or available. There have been moves from several drug companies to cut the cost of medication to the developing countries and decisions about costs should become clearer shortly.

HIV/AIDS may now be considered to be a chronic disease – a slow-moving, long-lasting pandemic with specific HIV-related diseases (Fee & Krieger 1993). There is a continuing need for health education around transmission and prevention of HIV, as well as an ongoing need for research into treatments.

Evidence-based practice has been described as a dynamic process requiring ongoing reflection and change at a number of levels (Lloyd-Smith 1998). It is therefore essential that occupational therapists keep up to date with the best research evidence in this rapidly changing field (Entwistle et al 1996). A number of AIDS websites exist to inform decision making and ensure effective intervention.

EFFECTS OF THE HIV VIRUS ON OCCUPATIONAL PERFORMANCE

The impact of the HIV virus may result in a wide range of changes in performance, including physical, affective and cognitive impairment. These may be due to the effects of the virus, opportunistic infections, tumours and neurological conditions.

PHYSICAL EFFECTS

Symptoms such as fatigue, diarrhoea, fever night sweats and weight loss may occur early in the disease. The individual may experience a rapid change in appearance as a result of weight loss and this will affect body image. Diarrhoea and generalised fatigue may result in the person being unable to care for themselves and they may become dehydrated and in need of medical attention. Conditions affecting the lungs, such as pneumocystis carinii pneumonia (PCP) and tuberculosis (TB) can result in shortness of breath with exertion. Climbing stairs, walking any distance and carrying out daily living skills may become increasingly difficult.

Progressive multifocal leucoencephalopathy (PML), although affecting only around 4% of people with AIDS, can cause a variety of symptoms. Physical manifestations may include loss of balance, weakness on one side of the body and visual and speech disturbance, all of which affect function.

Studies suggest that about one-third of those with symptomatic HIV will experience peripheral neuropathy. This may be due to the direct effect of the virus on the nervous system, as a side-effect of the medication or resulting from drug or alcohol use. The major symptom is pain, which may vary from mild tingling to a burning sensation affecting mainly the feet and less frequently the hands (NAM 2000). This can result in mobility problems and affect safety both within a home environment and in the community.

Cytomegalovirus (CMV) is a member of the herpes family of viruses. It may be present in up to 50% of the adult population but does not present problems with fully functioning immune systems. However, in those with advanced HIV disease it can lead to a number of complications including visual loss, gastrointestinal damage and encephalopathy, all impacting on the individual's lifestyle and wellbeing.

PSYCHOLOGICAL EFFECTS

Many psychological effects may accompany the loss of physical ability. Emotional reactions may be due to the shock of receiving the diagnosis and may be accompanied by distress, anger and fear. Psychiatric symptoms may be a direct effect of the HIV virus on the brain or due to opportunistic infections or tumours. Individuals may have had a past psychiatric history, which would put them at greater risk of developing mental health problems following infection (Dew et al 1990). Substance misuse may also lead to psychological changes (Catalan 1999).

Psychological changes may include depression, anxiety and suicidal ideation. Other conditions such as bipolar disorder and schizophrenic-type symptoms with delusions and hallucinations may be evident in some individuals.

Stress, anxiety and panic attacks may lead to individuals withdrawing from previously enjoyed activities and contact with others. Low mood and fears for the future may result in self-neglect or self-harm, which may include the use of recreational drugs and high intake of alcohol as a coping mechanism.

For parents with HIV there are concerns over the immediate and longer-term care needs of children plus thoughts of what to tell children and when. For parents of infected children there may be feelings of guilt and worry about their children's health. Parents with increasing disability may face psychological distress trying to keep the family together, with members of the family infected or affected by the disease.

COGNITIVE EFFECTS

A proportion of those with HIV will experience a change in cognitive performance, which can be due to a number of causes. These may include the HIV virus directly invading the brain, encephalopathy, PML, toxoplasmosis and Kaposi's sarcoma. The degree of cognitive change will vary from mild to moderate brain impairment (British Brain and Spine Foundation 1998). Results of studies of individuals with HIV who experience brain impairment suggest that between 10 and 16% of infected individuals will suffer cognitive impairment. It is suggested that the number of those with viral activity in the brain may be higher but that the virus may not impact on their normal functioning (AVERT 1998).

The cognitive changes experienced will range from mild impairment with signs of forgetfulness and difficulties with planning and problem solving through to severe dementia resulting in difficulties in attention, concentration, speed of thought and all areas of cognitive functioning. Changes in personality and behaviour may accompany HIV brain impairment and will affect performance and relationships.

SOCIAL EFFECTS

A diagnosis of HIV will have an impact on an individual's social situation. Changes in education, training and employment due to changes in health can mean reduced income and changes may often occur in roles, relationships and opportunities. There may be fears around confidentiality, especially with numerous hospital appointments and medication regimens to follow. There may be changes in lifestyle, with the person no longer being able to continue with work, domestic or leisure pursuits due to ill health or loss of income.

CULTURAL ISSUES

To ensure equal access to services within the UK it is essential to consider cultural needs and differences when carrying out an occupational therapy programme.

When English is not the first language it is important to identify whether an interpreter is required.

If diagnosed HIV positive in the United Kingdom, individuals from countries without access to medication may have to remain in the United Kingdom without the support and care of their extended family. To return home could mean little or no access to combination therapies or treatment for opportunistic infections.

For those living in the United Kingdom as asylum seekers, possibly having faced the death of family members, receiving the news of being HIV positive can create further trauma. Some may be reluctant to receive help from the statutory services because they fear for their immigration status

(Refugee Council 2000). Failure to seek medical treatment may result in increasing isolation and poor health. There may be misunderstanding and fears around the role of hospitals and hospices for those with HIV. Individuals may see them as places to die and education is required to understand the role they have in rehabilitation, respite, long-term and terminal care.

Individuals may have come from a country where treatment may have been from a doctor or nurse and have little concept of an interdisciplinary approach to care. They may be confused by having to work with a number of different people and it is important that explanations are kept simple and that time is given to prevent confusion and enable the person to readjust to a different approach.

It is essential to build a relationship of trust to enable individuals to express fears, concerns, needs and to develop a therapeutic relationship.

SPIRITUALITY

The Canadian Model of Occupational Performance (Law et al 1997) places spirituality at its core (Fig. 18.1). Spiritual needs are seen as an essential requirement for meaningful, holistic, person-centred occupational therapy intervention.

The term 'spirituality' may be interpreted in different ways. It may be defined as the need for meaning in life, especially when faced with the many changes experienced with HIV/AIDS. It can also mean hope to face the difficulties and challenges presented and to cope with the future. Spirituality addresses the need for belief and faith to make sense of the world. Urbanowski and Vargo (1994) describe the expression of spirituality as 'the experience of meaning in everyday life activities'. Egan and Delaat (1997) define spirituality as 'our truest selves, which we attempt to express in all our actions'.

For some people, spiritual or religious issues may be helped by talking to a chaplain. Individuals may seek support by telling others their diagnosis and coping with complex changes in their lives. In the late stages of the disease they may wish to look at issues of death and dying and make arrangements around their death.

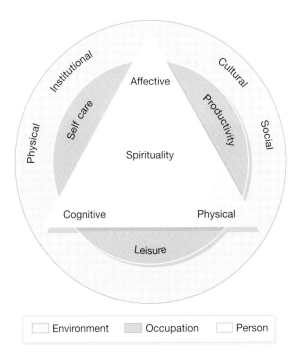

Environment ▢   Occupation ▨   Person ▢

Fig. 18.1 The Canadian Occupational Performance Model (COPM) (Reproduced by kind permission of Canadian Association of Occupational Therapists.)

Collins (1998) outlined the significant contribution that occupational therapy has to make to the enhancement of spiritual wellbeing through therapeutic interventions.

LOSS AND GRIEF

A diagnosis of HIV may result in many losses and fears for the future. There may be fears of deterioration in health and physical ability resulting in reduced independence and privacy. Relationships may end because of the death of friends or partners or because non-infected individual are concerned about routes of infection. Partners and carers also need to come to terms with changes in the relationship and their concerns for the future. Patterns of illness and limitations may result in changes in lifestyle and the end of previously enjoyed activities, leading to increased isolation. Plans, goals and intentions for the future may have to be abandoned or adjusted. It may no longer be possible to follow a planned career. Hopelessness and loss of choice,

feelings of uselessness and loss of options may all be evident. There may be expressions of anger, despair, guilt and unresolved issues around death.

PREJUDICE AND DISCRIMINATION

Many individuals continue to face discrimination associated with being HIV positive. They may be frightened by harassment and anxious over threats to their safety.

SERVICE PROVISION

ACUTE CENTRES

The hospital is the acute centre where a person receives their acute inpatient care, attends outpatient clinics, has regular reviews of their physical and psychological health and wellbeing and obtains their medication. The inpatient service will include the individuals outlined in Figure 18.2. The multidisciplinary team will adopt a collaborative approach to address the individual needs of the person.

HOSPICES

Many hospices in the UK are now designating a certain number of their beds for individuals with a positive HIV or AIDS diagnosis.

Hospices provide input related to symptom relief and pain control, respite for the individual and their carers, physical and psychological care, and support in the terminal stages of the illness. They can provide regular respite or rehabilitation admissions, inpatient or daycare input only or, in some instances, long-term care. Daycare services are frequently attached to hospices.

SOCIAL SERVICES

For people with a positive HIV or AIDS diagnosis, the main role of the local authority Social Services department is to provide assessment, information and advice and to provide or facilitate the provision of services that enable a

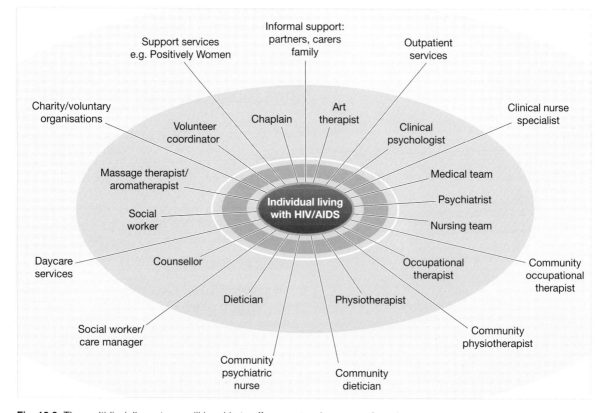

Fig. 18.2 The multidisciplinary team will be able to offer an extensive range of services.

person to live as safely and independently as possible in their own environment. The wider family or household, as well as the carer's needs, should also be evaluated.

An occupational therapist employed by a Social Services department will give practical assistance by assessing for and providing equipment and adaptations; giving energy conservation advice; and assessing rehousing needs as well as addressing occupational performance needs.

COMMUNITY HEALTH SERVICES

Members of primary care groups, including general practitioners, district nurses, health visitors, midwives and clinical nurse specialists in HIV and AIDS may be involved in caring for the individual and significant others, as may mental health teams and other specialists, for example, in wound care or tuberculosis. Individuals may

be reluctant to register with a general practitioner because they feel their acute centre is more familiar with their medication and has greater experience of their needs. Those individuals who wish to access community nursing services usually need to be registered with a general practitioner.

VOLUNTARY SERVICES AND SUPPORT SERVICES

These are based mainly in larger cities and contact details can be found by various routes, for example, the telephone directory, the National AIDS Manual Directory, Citizens' Advice Bureaux. Many organisations also have websites.

Particular benefit can be derived from such provision via individuals who share the experience of being positive or having an AIDS diagnosis. Such groups can also provide support for those affected by, as well as infected by, HIV or AIDS. Some services offer drop-in facilities, complementary therapies, counselling, advocacy and welfare and housing advice. They may also act as a focus for campaigning.

DAYCARE

Depending on the resources and setting, daycare may be available on a 5-day a week basis or at specific times only, which may include evening sessions. Professionals with a social work, nursing or occupational therapy background may be included within the team (Box 18.1).

Information sessions, activity-based groups and visits to places of interest may be organised with the aim of addressing psychosocial, psychological and social needs. Informal interaction with staff and others who attend provides an opportunity for support and may reduce stress and isolation. Daycare provision may be used by those with a positive HIV or AIDS diagnosis as a means of giving structure and purpose to their leisure time. Where leisure time becomes the main focus for an individual's daily routine they may seek a way of creating structure and meaning. This may be through voluntary work or taking up new or previous leisure interests,

---

Box 18.1 Services offered by a daycare facility

Daycare can:
- provide structure to the day and reduce feelings of isolation
- offer a safe environment where others are also HIV positive – their diagnosis being implicit not explicit
- provide access to a range of support networks – both peer and professional
- enable the individual to engage in previously enjoyed purposeful activities and skills, as well as introducing new ones, and so offer a sense of accomplishment
- stimulate interaction between daycare user and staff, with the benefit of continuity and consistency
- enable individuals to offer support and friendship to others and thus gain feelings of self-worth
- provide information and advice from a range of professionals
- allow the individual to engage in pleasurable activities and spend time with others in a social setting

---

although they may have to recognise that their capacity to engage in them could be affected by any changes in their health status.

THEORETICAL FOUNDATIONS FOR INTERVENTION

USING THE CANADIAN OCCUPATIONAL PERFORMANCE MODEL

The Canadian Occupational Performance Model (COPM; see Fig. 18.1) illustrates the relationship between persons, their environment and occupation.

Occupation is everything people do to occupy themselves, including looking after themselves, (self care), enjoying themselves (leisure) and contributing to the social and economic fabric of their communities (productivity) (Canadian Association of Occupational Therapists 1997) (see also Chapter 2). Occupational therapy based on this model involves the assessment of the abilities and disabilities – that is, the occupational performance – of the individual within his environment. It is an individualised measure and, within the three areas of self care, productivity and leisure, the person is encouraged to think about a normal day and identify activities that are difficult but that he would want to or need to continue. The person starts by identifying the importance of each activity using a scale of 1–10. He then rates what he considers to be his level of performance and satisfaction. This model recognises the person, not the therapist, as the one to identify needs and priorities. The individual rather than the therapist measures outcomes and satisfaction.

The occupational therapist's role is that of enabling, working in partnership to help people choose, organise and undertake occupations to an improved level of performance and satisfaction. Where the individual is unable to express his needs, such as when working with children and those with HIV-related brain impairment, then the primary caregiver or immediate friends/family will identify areas of need and goal setting (see also Chapter 2).

Evaluation of the COPM

The COPM encourages the individual to decide on difficulties experienced and prioritise areas of intervention. Being person centred, it encompasses the aims set out in the White Paper on Working for Patients (DOH 1989).

The person rather than the therapist will decide on how well they are achieving the task and how satisfied they are both before and after the occupational therapy programme. Being person centred and directed should lead to improved motivation and commitment to the programme. The overall aim is to maximise independence and maintain a person's self-worth through therapeutic and purposeful activities (Norris 1999).

For those who do not have English as a first language, the COPM can be difficult to explain and score. For those with a cognitive impairment who have limited comprehension and concentration, it may be necessary to seek assistance from the carer who has a greater knowledge and understanding of the person. For those at the late stages of the disease it may not be appropriate to consider performance and satisfaction, as there may be an ongoing deterioration in abilities that would only serve to highlight the difficulties being faced.

The use of the rating scale can help the individual recognise the changes in performance and lead to optimism about his ability to adapt to a changing situation. However, Norris (1999) has highlighted the fact that the outcome scores focus on what the person is unable to do, rather than the positive aspects of what he can do.

It is important to identify the appropriateness of the model with each person and be sensitive as to when and how it is used.

FRAMES OF REFERENCE

Primary frames of reference used in the field of HIV/AIDS address the physical and psychological needs of the individual. Given the wide range of issues present when working with people who have HIV/AIDS, it is not possible to identify all that may arise. However, given the nature of the issues most frequently encountered, experience shows that the occupational therapist is most likely to utilise the principles of the following frames of reference (see also Chapter 3):

- Biomechanical: to facilitate and encourage the remaining physical abilities. Neurological changes may be due to conditions such as progressive multifocal leucoencephalopathy or toxoplasmosis.
- Learning: an educational approach may be used to give information, skills and knowledge in order to assist informed decision making and problem solving.
- Cognitive behavioural: for those experiencing anxiety and depression.
- Compensatory: used to help the person adapt his existing skills to overcome a problem; for example, the use of equipment to help with visual loss as a result of an opportunistic infection such as cytomegalovirus affecting sight.

OUTCOME MEASURES

An outcome measure is the documentation of the person's progress following care intervention (Norris 1999). Hagedorn (1997) suggests that there is a need to measure outcomes so as to judge the efficacy of therapy. COPM is designed to allow outcome measures to be obtained. It does not replace the process of occupational therapy but helps to structure the assessment and intervention. There are five steps to the process which involve the use of a semi-structured interview. Based on the person-centred approach, the individual's perceived five most important problems are recorded in the areas of self care, productivity and leisure. The person then rates each problem on performance and satisfaction and the total scores are calculated by adding together the performance or satisfaction scores for all problems and dividing by the number of problems. Following intervention, reassessment can be carried out with the individual (or caregiver) again scoring each problem against performance and satisfaction. Subtracting the old score from the new score gives the changes (see the case studies in Boxes 18.2, 18.3 and 18.4).

Box 18.2 Case study: Sarah – based around the Canadian Occupational Performance Model

Social situation

Sarah is a 25-year-old woman with one child, aged 7, who is living with Sarah's family in Africa. Sarah is divorced and lives in shared accommodation (with one room of her own), attached to her job. She works in healthcare and is hoping to train as a nurse.

Health situation

Sarah was diagnosed HIV positive in 1998. She had TB and PCP, resulting in severe lung damage, and she is now unable to breathe independently without the use of additional oxygen, approximately 3 litres per minute.

Physical

Sarah has severe shortness of breath and depends on an additional oxygen supply. She experiences low mood, anxiety and fears for the future. She has been discharged from the acute hospital for a 4-week period of assessment and rehabilitation to identify her needs and the possibility of her returning to the community.

Psychological

Anxious, low mood.

Spiritual

Strong faith.

Canadian Occupational Performance Model

Self care: problems identified   *Importance*

1. Unable to carry out personal activities of daily living due to the need for
   continual additional oxygen, severe shortness of breath and extreme fatigue   10
2. No accommodation to return to – previous home provided with the job   10

Productivity: problems identified   *Importance*

1. Unable to return to study or previous work   5
2. Unable to manage any domestic activities of daily living   7

Leisure: problems identified   *Importance*

1. Unable to continue with any leisure activities that require movement away from the
   oxygen supply   6
2. Unable to continue with any sports, travel or outings   4

Occupational therapy intervention

Self care:

● Introducing a graded programme of self-care activities:
  – getting out of bed and sitting in chair
  – walking from chair to toilet in room
  – walking from bed to wash-hand basin to wash and clean teeth
  – dressing and undressing independently.
● Improving mood and feelings of self-worth:
  – having small achievable goals to boost confidence and self-esteem
  – obtaining charitable funds to purchase toiletries and new items of clothing
  – hairdresser visiting to restyle hair.
● Introducing a graded programme of self-care activities (without additional oxygen – following approval from medical team):
  – sitting in the kitchen preparing a drink and snack
  – using the bath with shower board and shower over the bath
  – sitting with others to watch television
  – using relaxation techniques to reduce the anxiety associated with reducing oxygen provision from cylinders
  – using a portable oxygen cylinder to increase independence
  – organising items/belongings in her room
  – liaising with the housing department and community occupational therapist regarding housing needs
  – liaising with the community care team and planning meetings with the interdisciplinary team around care
    in the community.

continued

Box 18.2 *continued*

Productivity:

- Organising belongings and clothing in her room
- Planning her programme for each day
- Having photographs taken and writing letters to send home to her family
- Making lists of items she would need in a bedsitting room.

Leisure:

- Reading magazines
- Undertaking art sessions and investigating community-based art courses to join
- Investigating support groups and local services
- Energy conservation: prioritising tasks, pacing self and spending time on enjoyable activities and those valued most.

Occupational performance problems (in order of importance as identified by Sarah)

	Initial assessment		Reassessment	
	Performance	Satisfaction	Performance	Satisfaction
1. Personal activities of daily living	1	1	7	9
2. Rehousing to property/return to the community	1	1	10	10
3. Ability to do some domestic ADL	1	2	3	6
4. Opportunity for some leisure activities	1	2	6	6
5. Unable to return to employment or study	1	2	5	6
Total	5	8	31	37
Number of problems	5	5	5	5
Score	1	1.6	6.2	7.4

Change in performance: $6.2 - 1 = 5.2$
Change in satisfaction: $7.4 - 1.6 = 5.8$

Summary

Sarah returned to the community to a property designed to wheelchair standards. She continued to increase in independence, gradually reducing the amount of additional requirements and increasing in energy and confidence. Cylinders of oxygen were delivered daily, including portable cylinders. A comprehensive care package was provided to help with domestic tasks and support her in her chosen activities. She was able to prioritise her needs and achieve goals, increasing both satisfaction and performance.

Box 18.3   Case study: Nikki – based around the Canadian Occupational Performance Model

---

Social situation

Nikki is 29 years old, married, and has two children, aged 8 and 6 years. She and her family live in a three-bedroomed local authority property. Nikki takes the primary childcare role and, as the children's school is some distance from their home, spends a lot of time walking the children to and from school. She is an asylum seeker and is planning to do a part-time degree in Business Studies.

Nikki is currently considering living apart from her husband because of his physical and verbal aggression towards her. Her husband is also HIV positive but is unwilling to acknowledge this and to address the issues this presents. It is unclear what physical, psychological and cognitive effects he experiences. He has input from Social Services regarding domestic activities of daily living of approximately 2 hours per week.

Health situation

Nikki was diagnosed HIV positive in March 1991 when she was being investigated for swollen glands and fevers. In 1990, TB of the lymph nodes and oral candida were diagnosed and Nikki was admitted to the Family Care Centre for 1 week.

continued

Box 18.3 *continued*

Physical

Nikki is well and self caring, independently mobile and performing all self-care and domestic care activities independently.

Psychological

Nikki is a strong believer in complementary therapies and has used massage, aromatherapy and reflexology in the past.

Canadian Occupational Performance Model

Self care: problems identified   *Importance*

1. Physical and emotional stress and fatigue related to primary childcare and domestic roles   9
2. Not currently on combination therapy regimen, in dialogue with medical team regarding this   6

Productivity: problems identified   *Importance*

1. Intends to start part-time Business Studies degree. Unsure whether or not she will be able to manage all areas of her life/activities from both a physical endurance and psychological stress aspect   9
2. Although she receives assistance from Social Services with domestic tasks, the primary responsibility remains hers   6

Leisure: problems identified   *Importance*

1. Has few opportunities for quiet or active recreation due to the various responsibilities that place demands on her personal time and energy   5

Occupational therapy intervention

- Offer space and time for discussion to enable her to explore priorities and possible options for the future.
- Provide support with the school run and domestic tasks. Validate her choices.
- Face-to-face sessions of training in relaxation techniques, using imagery and passive neuromuscular techniques.
- Prepared cassette of these techniques to enable her to practice them independently at evenings and weekends during her admission, and in the community on discharge.
- Offer the opportunity for personal time for relaxation and the learning of new skills which are within her control.

Occupational performance problems (in order of importance as identified by Nikki)

	Initial assessment		Reassessment	
	Performance	Satisfaction	Performance	Satisfaction
1. Physical/psychological stress and fatigue	7	6	8	8
2. Managing competing demands from physical and psychological aspects	7	7	8	9
3. Primary responsibility for domestic ADLs	6	7	8	9
4. Decisions re: combination therapy regimen	8	8	8	9
5. Few opportunities for quiet or active recreation or relaxation due to responsibilities and demands on self	6	5	9	9
Total	34	33	41	43
Number of problems	5	5	5	5
Score	6.8	6.6	8.2	8.6

Change in performance: 8.2 – 6.8 = 1.4

Change in satisfaction: 8.6 – 6.6 = 2.0

Summary

COPM enabled Nikki to identify and prioritise those aspects of her life that she realistically felt she could attain some mastery over and enhance, through utilising information, advice, energy conservation techniques and coping strategies. She also benefited from improved self-esteem through having honest and open discussion, recognising and reflecting the beneficial changes she had made in her life. It was also a realistic tool as numerous problems she identified were either longstanding in nature or not within her power to control or influence.

Box 18.4 Case study: Martin – Canadian Occupational Performance Model

Social situation

Martin, a 46-year-old man, is single and, until he was evicted, lived in a one-bedroomed council flat. He used to work in the field of press and publicity but is currently attending college to study Information Technology. Martin has been admitted to a specialist hospital for long-term rehabilitation or long-term residential care.

Health situation

Martin was diagnosed HIV positive in 1997. A brain scan showed cerebral atrophy and Martin suffered PCP pneumonia in 1997.

Physical

Martin has ataxia and shows signs of fatigue. He has sensory disturbance in his feet from peripheral neuropathy and is incontinent of urine and occasionally faeces.

Psychological

Martin is angry, agitated and shows signs of confusion and wandering.

Cognitive

Problems with orientation as Martin's short-term memory is affected. He displays irrational behaviour (hoarding food and other items found in the room), refuses to wash or change his clothing and refuses to take his medication. He is unable to concentrate for longer than 10 minutes and is very distractible.

Spiritual

The team is not able to discuss this with Martin at his present level of function.

Canadian Occupational Performance Model

Self care: problems identified by staff   *Importance*
1. Neglect of personal hygiene   10
2. Difficulty finding his way to the toilet; incontinence   10
3. Distractible, unable to dress without prompting   10

Productivity: problems identified by staff   *Importance*
1. Unable to return to the community; no property to return to   7
2. Unable to manage any domestic activities   6

Leisure: problems identified by staff   *Importance*
1. Concentration and attention deficits preventing ability to read
   books and journals on chosen subjects   7
2. Unable to use bike due to problems with balance and unsafe
   on main roads   3

Occupational therapy intervention

Self care:

- Time spent in talking to Martin and building rapport
- Walking round the ward identifying toilet, bath, kitchen, sitting room. Using memory strategies to help orientation. Point out objects, using senses (colour, smells, appearance), labelling to locate rooms
- Negotiating with Martin the timing and frequency of bathing
- Checking with Martin his preferred clothing. Encouraging organising of clothing on the bed. Clothes laid out to increase recognition of items and completion of the dressing sequence
- Having clothing that is quick and easy to put on within concentration levels
- Encouraging interaction with others on the unit and time spent one-to-one with named members of staff
- Setting boundaries around behaviour and language. Martin would be asked to stay in his room if these were not adhered to
- Setting small, achievable goals and acknowledging improvements and progress made.

continued

Box 18.4   *continued*

Productivity:
- Working within Martin's understanding to look at plans for the future
- Links with the community services. Regular reviews of progress being made and possibilities for return to the community.

Leisure:
- Spending time looking at journals, talking about areas of interest, using long-term memory
- Introducing Martin to daycare and encouraging him to make choices around activities in the programme
- Spending time out of the hospital. Martin was particularly interested in local architecture. Maintaining links with the community.

Occupational performance problems (in order of importance as identified by staff)

	Initial assessment		Reassessment	
	Performance	Satisfaction	Performance	Satisfaction
1. Personal hygiene	2	2	6	6
2. Orientation around ward/hospital	2	2	5	6
3. Ability to dress	3	3	6	6
4. No housing to return to	2	2	3	3
5. Concentration and attention	3	3	5	6
Total	12	12	25	27
Number of problems	5	5	5	5
Score	2.4	2.4	5.0	5.4

Change in performance: $5.0 - 2.4 = 2.6$

Change in satisfaction: $5.4 - 2.4 = 3.0$

Summary

This was the beginning of a rehabilitation process that lasted for a period of 9 months. Martin continued to make progress in areas of self care, productivity and leisure. New objectives were set at each review meeting and strategies to meet those were agreed with him. A property was identified and Martin was able to return to the community with support services. A year later he is still at home.

As Martin improved, he was able to take the lead in identifying difficulties and what was important to him (see chapter 2). He was often frustrated by his limitations and at times lacked insight into health and safety issues. His satisfaction levels increased as his long-term goal of returning to the community became a reality.

ASSESSMENT

Assessment needs to reflect the range of needs that the individual may experience, including physical changes, mental health needs or cognitive impairment.

Using clinical reasoning skills, the therapist will endeavour to get as full a picture of the person's level of occupational performance as possible. This can be achieved from specific questions to him but also by close working with family, friends and partners. It is essential to spend time listening to the individual before narrowing down the areas of difficulties and priorities for intervention.

PHYSICAL FUNCTION

Assessment may take place in a hospital, the home environment or the community. A comprehensive medical picture will help the therapist gain a clearer picture of the signs and symptoms and the potential for improvement. It is important to remember that housing and other physical environments can directly affect levels of independence. The type of housing will create very different needs. Use of the kitchen and bathroom may be limited by others in the property and affect the possibility of equipment or adaptations. The design and layout of the rooms will directly affect independence.

Access both to and within the property can enhance and inhibit performance. Fatigue is an issue for many individuals with HIV and coping with flights of stairs will reduce the available energy to carry out other tasks. Where shortness of breath is an issue, the distance between rooms may prove problematic.

The location of the residence will also affect level of independence. Distance to public transport, shopping areas, Post Office and pharmacy is all-important when an individual is returning to the community.

Occupational therapists assess the scope for adaptations to increase independence or the need for rehousing. Being able to identify suitable properties to meet individual need and advising on mobility and wheelchair standards will help increase independence. The occupational therapist may also feel it appropriate to undertake assessment of other frequently visited environments, such as work or leisure facilities and to consider private transport. Assessment related to frequently used equipment and furniture should also be included.

PSYCHOLOGICAL FUNCTION

Assessments may be standardised, such as rating scales used for those with depression, or non-standardised. Individuals may be asked to complete questionnaires, such as quality of life questionnaires, to give greater insight into psychological needs that will help guide the most appropriate forms of intervention. Non-standardised assessments may include stress and anxiety management questionnaires to identify the stresses, the impact on physical and mental wellbeing and the coping strategies used by the individual.

Verbal and non-verbal communication by the individual can all help in assessing their psychological situation. Contact with friends and family can help in identifying changes in the person's mood and behaviour.

PSYCHOSOCIAL FUNCTION
Risk assessment

This may relate to physical, psychological or cognitive areas of difficulty. For those with physical disabilities, there may be the risk of falling and reduced safety in carrying out daily living skills. For those with psychological problems, depression may lead to neglect, suicidal ideation and concerns around self-harm. Coping strategies may include alcohol and drug use, which increase the risk to personal safety. Cognitive impairment may result in forgetfulness, affecting safety in the kitchen and bathroom. Changes in personality may result in relationship difficulties and inappropriate behaviours create risks to both the individual and others. It is essential that the occupational therapist works with the interdisciplinary team to assess the level and areas of risk and agrees with the individual on action to be carried out for returning to, or remaining safely within, the community

Social skills

Social skills assessment includes elements of social behaviour such as verbal, non-verbal and assertion skills (Finlay 1997). For those with HIV-related brain impairment, there may be changes in personality and challenging behaviours while for those with specific neurological involvement, speech and language may be affected, requiring the need for non-verbal communication to make wishes known and alleviate frustration. Depression, anxiety and changes in appearance may all lead to lack of assertiveness and affect the ability to be independent in the community.

Life skills

This may encompass areas such as using public transport, budgeting, health and hygiene and time management. Assessment in this area will identify whether individual or group programmes may be helpful to increase independence or whether there is a need for support networks in the community.

COGNITIVE FUNCTION
Standardised assessments

Standardised assessments can be used to give a baseline and identify specific areas of impairment; retesting will indicate improvement or deterioration.

Assessment may start with the use of a screening tool to identify any deterioration in performance (Folstein et al 1975). This can be followed with more detailed assessment of any areas of difficulty encountered. Many of the tests have been standardised for the elderly with dementia or Alzheimer's disease, although not specifically for those with HIV/AIDS.

The tests may include the shorter of those used for severe impairment, which cover basic areas of function, such as the Middlesex Elderly Assessment of Mental State (Golding 1989). These cover areas such as orientation for time and place, remembering names, naming objects, comprehension, motor performance and spatial ability. The more advanced tests of cognitive function address the dysexecutive skills required for independent living (e.g. Behavioural Assessment of Dysexecutive Syndrome; Wilson et al 1996). These include problem solving, speed of thought and ability to cope with changing rules and competing demands. They require greater levels of attention and concentration and give an indication of the ability to undertake independent living.

It is important to consider a number of factors prior to conducting any cognitive assessment. Visual impairment can prevent certain assessments from being carried out. Language difficulties, due to dysphasia or when English is not a first language, will also affect the results. Some tests are not sensitive to cultural differences, using pictures of objects that may not be familiar in different cultures. Levels of attention and concentration need to be considered prior to starting a task, so that it is not too challenging. Fatigue affects most people with HIV and it is important to consider the timing and be sensitive to needs. Stress, depression, lack of sleep, alcohol use and drugs all affect performance and distort results (Jamieson 1999).

Well- and illbeing profile

Cognitive impairment may range from mild or moderate to severe impairment with varying levels of insight (Kitwood & Benson 1997). It is essential to recognise the effects of the impairment on the individual. Signs of illbeing may include despair, anger, grief, bodily tension, agitation and withdrawal. When working as part of a multidisciplinary team, it is important to recognise these signs and how they can be addressed. Observing individuals in different settings and social situations will help identify areas of difficulty and possible stressors.

INTERVENTION

Intervention needs to start with good communication and liaison with the individual, his family and the team of professionals in both health and social services in order to identify goals, draw up a plan of action and identify agreed outcomes.

Whilst it is clearly impossible to give an exhaustive outline of the areas of occupational performance with which the therapist can become involved, the following section documents some of those most frequently encountered and suggests ways in which occupational performance may be facilitated.

PHYSICAL FUNCTION

Agreeing priorities, achievable goals and strategies to help overcome difficulties in occupational performance can lead to improved motivation. The programme may include graded activity, starting with the personal activities of daily living (self care) and progressing to domestic (productivity) and social activities (leisure). Other areas such as employment, voluntary work or study may be included as appropriate. The intervention may start within a hospital, with retraining for improved performance, independence and confidence within the personal domestic environment and this should progress to observing function in both the home and local environments. The individual may be physically able to carry out personal and domestic activities but restricted due to fatigue. The use of energy conservation techniques and help with prioritising tasks, planning the day to build in time to rest, and identification of energy-saving devices and approaches will help towards the restoration of desired occupational performance.

Symptoms such as night sweats, diarrhoea and dermatological conditions can result in the need to wash regularly and the provision of equipment to maintain personal hygiene and reduce exhaustion. Decisions will need to be made in relation to the impact on other family members, for example, with the use of bathing equipment.

Sensory disturbance from peripheral neuropathy affecting the feet can create problems with mobility. Suitable shoes will be required and consideration will need to be given to the home environment, particularly will regard to stairs and floor coverings. Sensory disturbance affecting the hands can create problems with grip and awareness of temperatures (Fig. 18.3). Alternative methods which promote safety and the supply of equipment may need to be considered.

For a person with visual impairment, strategies for the identification of items and organisation in the home can assist with recognition and increased independence. Retraining in managing both personal and domestic activities may include the use of specific equipment for daily living, strategies such as colour contrasting and methods of labelling (Fig. 18.4).

Nausea, vomiting and disturbances with balance may be evident and require a carefully graded programme around times of symptom control.

Children and families

Parents with HIV/AIDS may face varying degrees of difficulty. Physical impairment, fatigue and generalised problems such as nausea, diarrhoea and night sweats all create additional demands in coping with self care and caring for

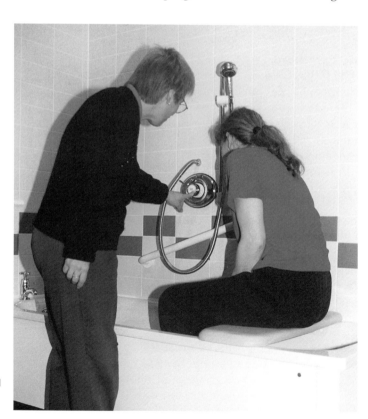

Fig. 18.3 The promotion of safety, the supply of equipment and adaptation to the environment will facilitate occupational performance for those who experience mobility and/or sensory disturbance.

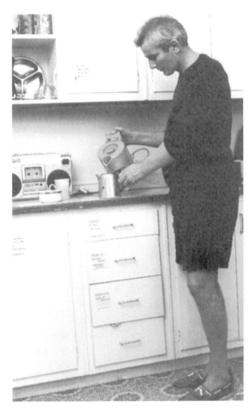

Fig. 18.4 Use of visual cues and colour contrasting can aid memory and can assist with object identification in a rehabilitation centre and later at home.

children and the home. There may be few opportunities to rest and families may feel unable to manage. Getting children up and ready for school or nursery may leave the individual with little energy to manage the rest of the day. The occupational therapist needs to work with the whole family to consider the options available to promote independence.

For many, their accommodation may present additional difficulties. Having flights of stairs to negotiate to reach the property while coping with carrying shopping, buggies and children can lead to exhaustion. Families may live in over-crowded situations, have inadequate heating, damp environments or have to share facilities with other families. Other family members may be unaware of the diagnosis, creating additional stresses and increased need for confidentiality at all times. Children who are not infected can be severely affected by HIV.

Children who are HIV positive also face varying levels of impairment. Difficulties may be mild to moderate and include neurological changes, developmental delay or failure to thrive. Fatigue and the effects of opportunistic infections may all increase the level of care and intervention required by families. Illness may lead to absence from school and the need for additional educational support.

Having access to services such as Family Care Centres where families can come for rehabilitation or respite together can help in supporting the family. The development of community-based family HIV services, community care and nursery provision for those with HIV/AIDS all help to support affected families.

A new generation of children born HIV positive is now reaching the teenage years. It is a time of life when there is great change physically and emotionally and a time when they will want to make individual choices and decisions on their health and future. For children born HIV positive, there may be a sign of developmental delay or opportunistic infections affecting function. A neurodevelopment frame of reference may be applied in the assessment of children with HIV.

PSYCHOLOGICAL FUNCTION

Low mood, lack of confidence and anxiety may lead to reluctance to engage in activities and of feelings of failure. It is important that activities are broken down to achievable and manageable components to boost morale and give a sense of achievement. Supervised practice in daily living and life skills after a period of hospitalisation can increase confidence in preparation for returning to the community.

Concerns around changes in health and the ability to care for families may be present. Thoughts of children going into care, fostering, adoption and the negative effects of HIV on the whole family are frequently present. One or more children may be HIV positive, having an impact on levels of care they require and the psychological effects on the other children. Relatives may be too far away to help or there may be fears around asking for help and the responses from relatives learning of the diagnosis. Guilt, blame and relationship difficulties with partners can all increase levels of psychological distress. Coping with secrecy, what to tell the children about the disease and how to tell them may all increase difficulties faced.

Stress management

It is suggested that everyone requires a certain degree of stress in their life to motivate and spur them into action. However, stress from both external or internal pressures can rise to levels that result in negative physical and psychological effects. The occupational therapist may be involved in helping an individual manage their stress (Box 18.5). This may be done through relaxation, which has three main aims (Payne 1995):

1. as a preventive measure: to protect the body from unnecessary wear, particularly the organs involved in stress-related disease
2. as a treatment: to help relieve stress, in conditions such as tension headache, insomnia and many others
3. as a coping skill: to calm the mind and allow thinking to become clearer and more effective.

The occupational therapist may be involved in teaching formal relaxation techniques in addition to guiding and advising the individual on managing identified stressors and encouraging beneficial lifestyle changes. Intervention may be on a one-to-one basis or delivered in group sessions. Techniques taught are then linked to daily occupations so that the individual learns how to use them as a tool during stress-provoking activities and/or to promote periods of calm during the planned daily routine.

HIV disease and its process may result in increased stress levels. Additionally, it can have an effect on any or all other areas of someone's life. These primary and secondary effects may fluctuate over time, with changes in health and personal circumstances, with age and in response to internal and external influences.

The level of stress that a person experiences does not necessarily correlate to the state of their physical, psychological or cognitive abilities. It is inevitably influenced by their individual and personal circumstances, personality type, responses, support networks and coping strategies. Stress, and the way in which the person deals with it, plays a significant part in their well-being and consequently it is an area that should be explored as fully as possible.

COGNITIVE FUNCTION

Problems with short-term memory, concentration and attention can all have an impact on the

---

Box 18.5 Stress management: aims, benefits and techniques as utilised with people who have HIV/AIDS

Aims

- Recognise levels of stress
- Identify what may trigger tension and anxiety
- Understand coping strategies
- Experience relaxation techniques
- Appreciate the importance of relaxation as part of daily life
- Channel and control anxiety during occupational performance

Benefits

- Reduced pain
- Focusing attention and strategies for managing stress
- Increased self-esteem and confidence
- Reduction in fatigue
- Improved sleep pattern
- Taking control of occupational performance

Formal relaxation techniques

- Breathing
- Imagery
- Tense release
- Passive neuromuscular
- Alexander technique
- Yoga
- Non-guided visualisation

Informal techniques

- Walking/exercise
- Listening to music
- Socialising
- Reading
- Sleeping
- Alcohol, drugs

ability to initiate and complete a task. Those with a cognitive impairment may forget whether they have eaten, forget medication and show signs of neglecting self care. Food may be left to burn and taps may be left running when attention to a task is lost. Going out shopping or to unfamiliar places may be impossible when there are orientation difficulties.

The intervention programme needs to use familiar tasks and methods graded to maintain interest and concentration. The use of memory strategies such as diaries and lists can help with remembering.

Some may not be able to express their wishes verbally but through observation and short direct questions requiring a yes or no answer, many individuals can make their wishes known. Those with severe impairment may be unable to cope with a large number of choices but giving the choice of two activities will give a sense of control within a person-centred, person-directed approach.

The use of worksheets, activities and games covering different areas of cognitive ability can help maintain interest. Prompts may be used to assist, ranging from demonstration of a task, such as picking up the jug of milk and pouring it into the cup, through to a question or gesture, such as pointing to the milk, to promote independence. Activity analysis can be helpful; breaking down tasks into small, achievable parts to maintain and gradually develop levels of concentration. Repetition and using the same sequence and cues can aid remembering. Sequencing and memory difficulties may result in problems with both personal and domestic daily living skills, such as dressing or meal preparation. Helping the individual keep things in the same order and using the same technique can all lead to increased independence.

There may be orientation problems resulting in difficulty finding rooms and routes around the home, outside the home or within a residential care setting. Using signs, colours and landmarks can help orientate the person. Encouraging people to make use of long-term memory, familiar tasks and routines will help build confidence. Individuals with a cognitive impairment may

have problems with sleep pattern and confusion around time. Having some regular routines and patterns can help reinforce whether it is the beginning or end of the day. The use of equipment should be kept to a minimum. Those with cognitive impairment may be unable to remember how to use the equipment safely, which may reduce its effectiveness unless supervised by a carer.

Such intervention, coupled with improvements in medication, have allowed many people with high levels of cognitive impairment to show significant improvements over a period of months. They can then return to the community and consider expanding their occupations into areas of productivity and leisure.

Previous predictions of life expectancy are changing. There will be large variations in abilities and community care needs to address the varying needs and changing patterns over time. The diagnosis of HIV brain impairment at present prevents people from returning to driving. Many are unhappy with this and doctors and therapists may be called upon to assess the person's ability to drive, especially when there have been significant improvements following combination therapy.

Daycare facilities can play a significant contribution in the continuing rehabilitation and support for those with HIV-related brain impairment and can support carers in maintaining the person in the community.

PRODUCTIVITY

The effects of the disease, the demands of employment and needing time off for hospital appointments may mean loss of employment for one or both partners and severely reduced levels of income. Coping with issues of confidentiality around medication and illness may lead to discrimination and problems in employment.

Some may consider starting back to previous employment; others may decide to start short educational or skill courses. These can help in developing new skills and friendships and can help improve quality of life and the possibility of employment. Some people may lack insight into the demands of employment and both occupational therapy programmes and Back to Work schemes can help in preparation for this.

CONCLUSION

There have been many advances since the first cases of HIV/AIDS were identified. Understanding of the disease process, ability to assess the effects on the individual and the effectiveness of medication have all increased knowledge and improved treatment. Advances in medication have led to vastly improved life expectancy and hopes for the future.

However, some aspects of HIV have not changed. The incidence of people infected by the disease continues to increase and to have an impact on all aspects of daily life. At present, the long-term effects of combination therapies are unknown and HIV/AIDS remains a disease without a cure.

Occupational therapy continues to have a valuable role to play at each stage of disease progression. Therapists can help people set priorities and use skills to improve both occupational performance and satisfaction in the areas of self care, productivity and leisure. Life expectancy for those with HIV is improving but many are facing increasing levels of impairment. Occupational therapists need to be continually developing their skills to meet the changing needs. They will meet individuals who have been recently diagnosed and also people who have been HIV positive for over 12 years – all will have differing needs. Occupational therapists need to use their range of assessment and problem-solving skills to promote independence and quality of life for a group with very complex and far ranging needs.

By enabling some of those needs to be met, the aim is to give improved quality of life even where quantity of life is reduced.

REFERENCES

All Party Parliamentary Group on AIDS 1998 Parliamentary Hearings for National HIV/AIDS Strategies. Summary and Recommendations. APPGA, London

AVERT 1998 AIDS dementia and HIV brain impairment. AIDS Education and Research Trust, Dr A Kocsis. AVERT, West Sussex

British Brain and Spine Foundation 1998 AIDS and the brain. BBSF, London

Catalan J 1999 Psychological problems for people with HIV infection. In: Catalan J (ed) Mental health and HIV infection. Psychological and Psychiatric Aspects.

Communicable Disease Report 28 January 2000 AIDS and HIV infection in the United Kingdom, monthly report. 10(4)

Collins M 1998 Occupational therapy and spirituality: reflecting on quality of experience in therapeutic intervention. British Journal of Occupational Therapy 61(6):280–284

Department of Health 2000 Developing an HIV/AIDS strategy for England. Progress Report. Department of Health and the HIV/AIDS Strategy Steering Group, April 2000. HMSO, London

Department of Health 2000/0306 HIV/AIDS and sexual health strategies merge.

Department of Health 1992 The health of the nation. HMSO, London

Department of Health 1989 Working for patients, Cm555. HMSO, London

Dew A, Ragni M, Nimorwicz P 1990 Infection with HIV and vulnerability to psychiatric distress: a study of men with haemophilia. Archives of General Psychiatry 47:737–744

Egan M, Delaat M 1997 The implicit spirituality of occupational therapy practice. Canadian Journal of Occupational Therapy 61(1):115–121

Entwistle V, Watt IS, Herring JE 1996 Information about healthcare effectiveness: an introduction for consumer health information providers. Kings Fund, London

Fee E, Krieger N 1993 Thinking and rethinking AIDS: implications for health policy. International Journal of Health Services 23(2):323–346

Finlay L 1997 The practice of psychosocial occupational therapy, 2nd edn. Stanley Thornes Publishers, Cheltenham

Folstein MF, Folstein S, McHugh PR 1975 Mini mental state: a practical method for grading the cognitive state of patients for the clinician. Journal of Psychosomatic Research 12:189–198

Golding E 1989 Middlesex elderly assessment of mental state. Thames Valley Test Company, Bury St Edmunds, Suffolk

Hagedorn R 1997 Occupational therapy perspectives and processes. Churchill Livingstone, Edinburgh

Jamieson S 1999 HIV related brain impairment. In: Cox S, Keady J (eds) Younger people with dementia. Jessica Kingsley, London

Kitwood T, Benson S 1997 The new culture of dementia care. Hawker Publications Limited, London

Law M et al 1997 Canadian Occupational Performance Model, 2nd edn. Canadian Association of Occupational Therapists, Toronto

Lloyd-Smith W 1998 The third way. Labour's white paper on the NHS. British Journal of Therapy and Rehabilitation 5(5):238–240

National AIDS Manual, May 2000 AIDS treatment update. HIV Treatment Publications, London

Norris A 1999 A pilot study of an outcome measure in palliative care. International Journal of Palliative Nursing, 5(1):40–45

Payne R 1995 Relaxation techniques. A practical handbook for the healthcare professional. Churchill Livingstone, Edinburgh

Refugee Council, December 1999. Information Service, London

Wilson BA 1996 Behavioural Assessment of Dysexecutive Syndrome. Thames Valley Test Company, Bury St Edmunds, Suffolk

World Health Organization 2000 Global World Statistics. WHO, Geneva

USEFUL CONTACTS

AIDS Treatment Project
020 7407 0777
Treatments helpline 0845 9470 047
Mon and Wed 3–9 pm, Tue 3–6 pm.
St Stephen's House,
115–129 Southwark Bridge Road,
London, SE1 0AX
Email: admin@atp.org.uk

DHIVA (Dietitians in HIV/AIDS Group)
Contact: Candice Philipps
01223 216655
Addenbrooke's NHS Trust Hospital,
Hills Road,
Cambridge
CB2 2QQ.
DHIVA can provide information on HIV specialist dieticians throughout the UK. The group has also developed an African diet sheet for HIV-positive people.

NAM Publications
020 7627 3200
NAM/BHIVA website:
Email: info@nam.org.uk
http://www.aidsmap.com
NAM Publications produces the *HIV and AIDS Treatments Directory*, the monthly newsletter *AIDS Treatment Update*, monthly factsheets, and information booklets about HIV/AIDS and treatments. NAM also runs monthly Information Forums and produces directories of HIV/AIDS services and community organisations throughout the UK, Europe and worldwide.

Positively Women
020 7713 0444
Helpline 020 7713 0222
Mon – Fri 10 am – 5 pm,
347–349 City Road,
London EC1V 1LR.
Email: poswomen@dircon.co.uk

Terrence Higgins Trust
020 7831 0330
Helpline 020 7242 1010
Daily 12 noon – 10 pm,
52–54 Grays Inn Road,
London WC1X 8JU.
Email: info@tht.org.uk

Vanguard AIDS Information Service
For African refugee communities
020 7627 5170
2b Thames House,
South Bank Commercial Centre,
140 Battersea Park Road,
London SW11 4NB.
Email:vanguard@dircon.co.uk

www.4aids.com This is a guide to HIV/AIDS from 4anything.com. The most interesting aspect of this Web site is the link to inspiring stories, with detailed and well-written accounts in plain English. Otherwise, it's a good-looking Web site. Packed with info and links to helpful sites.

www.aegis.com Aegis updates its Web site hourly, keeping you in the loop at any hour of the day. The site includes a daily briefing, which discusses topics ranging from scientific progress to exposure issues to nutrition and supplements that can help.

www.cdcnpin.com The Web site of the Centers for Disease Control (CDC) National Prevention Information Network, which is a national referral service on issues ranging from AIDS to STDs to TB. Stories are crisp and to the point, and the language is easy to read. Probably the best site to pick up the basics.

www.hivatis.com ATIS is a department of health and human services co-sponsored by big-time institutes such as the National Institute of Health and the National Library of Medicine. This Web site differs from the others by containing an updated list of all public service agencies, from the Food and Drug Administration to the Substance Abuse Administration. Also contains detailed articles on new developments.

www.yogagroup.org A helpful site for people with HIV/AIDS and healthcare providers interested in yoga. The Yoga Group is a non-profit organization based in Colorado, and provides free info and yoga classes to people with HIV.

19

Cerebrovascular accident

Linda Morgans   Stephanie Gething

INTRODUCTION

Cerebrovascular accident (CVA) or 'stroke' is the third leading cause of death and the major cause of adult disability in industrialised populations (Bonita 1992). A stroke is often a sudden and devastating event, causing major lifestyle changes to the individual and exerting major psychosocial and economic stress on the person and family members (Drummond 1998).

For example, the:

- businessman who is forced to retire 5 years earlier than he had planned
- young mother who can no longer bathe her baby safely
- grandmother who can no longer babysit for her grandchildren after school.

The person now not only has to cope with the physical, perceptual and emotional effects of the CVA but has to adapt to a different way of life and plan a new future.

IMPAIRMENTS CAUSED BY A CVA AND THEIR EFFECT ON OCCUPATION

The impairments associated with CVA can be motor, perceptual, sensory, cognitive and psychological and can have an impact on the individual's daily occupations (Fig. 19.1).

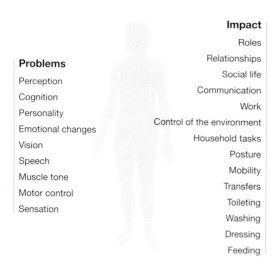

Impact

Roles

Problems

Relationships

Perception

Social life

Cognition

Communication

Personality

Work

Emotional changes

Control of the environment

Vision

Household tasks

Speech

Posture

Muscle tone

Mobility

Motor control

Transfers

Sensation

Toileting

Washing

Dressing

Feeding

Fig. 19.1 Examples of how impairments impact on daily occupations.

MOTOR

Muscle tone

Muscle tone can present as hypotonus (reduced tone) or hypertonus (increased tone) (Fig. 19.2).

Abnormal tone will affect performance in activities of daily living as the person no longer has a normal concept of midline. This results in uneven weight distribution in sitting or standing and impaired ability to transfer weight from left to right, forwards and back, e.g. whilst moving in bed, getting out of a chair or dressing. Impairment in reciprocal innervation results in the inability to stabilise one joint to enable movement at another, e.g. stabilise the shoulder to allow movement at the elbow to reach and retrieve a garment when dressing.

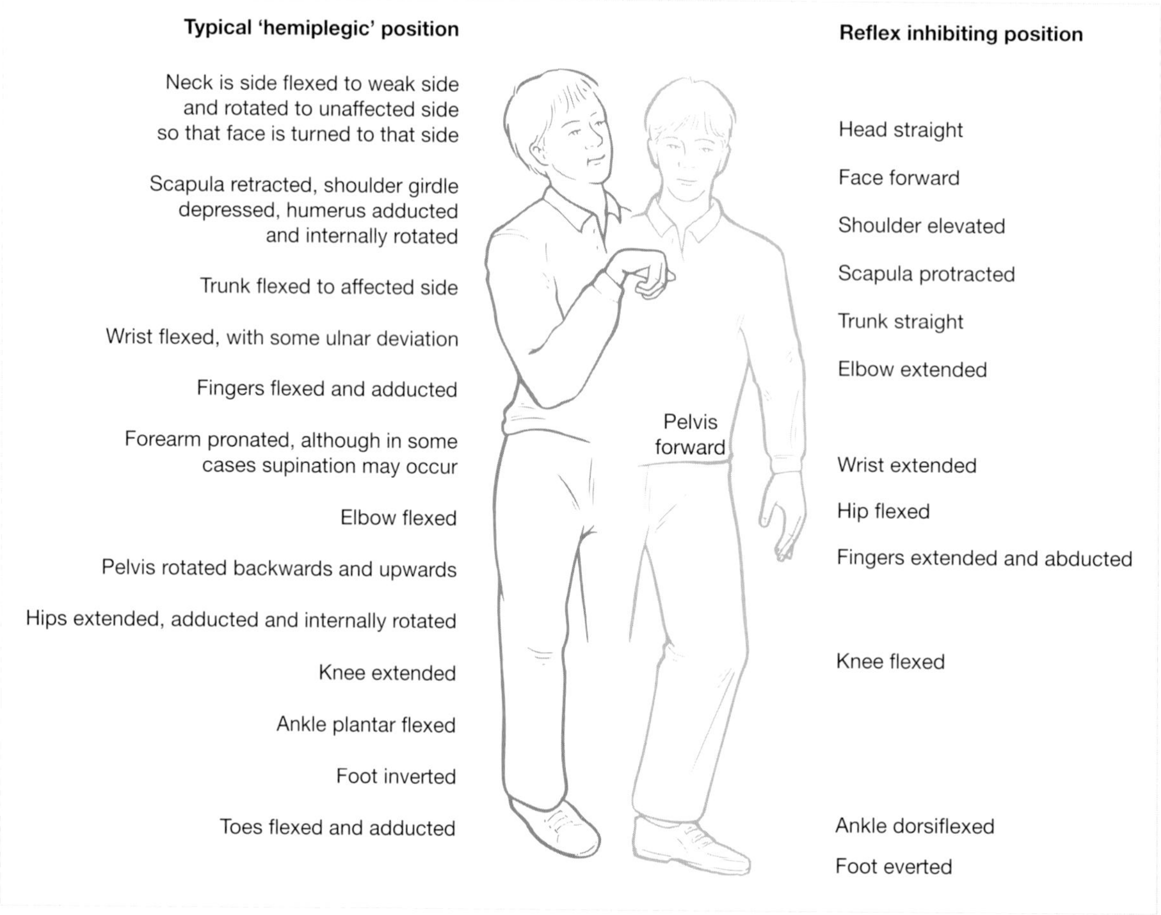

Typical 'hemiplegic' position

Neck is side flexed to weak side and rotated to unaffected side so that face is turned to that side

Scapula retracted, shoulder girdle depressed, humerus adducted and internally rotated

Trunk flexed to affected side

Wrist flexed, with some ulnar deviation

Fingers flexed and adducted

Forearm pronated, although in some cases supination may occur

Elbow flexed

Pelvis rotated backwards and upwards

Hips extended, adducted and internally rotated

Knee extended

Ankle plantar flexed

Foot inverted

Toes flexed and adducted

Pelvis forward

Reflex inhibiting position

Head straight

Face forward

Shoulder elevated

Scapula protracted

Trunk straight

Elbow extended

Wrist extended

Hip flexed

Fingers extended and abducted

Knee flexed

Ankle dorsiflexed

Foot everted

Fig. 19.2 Typical hemiplegic posture and its inhibiting position.

Muscle power

If a muscle is inactive because of hypotonicity, it will be weakened and deficient in power and movement even if muscle tone is restored. This will result in functional difficulties such as maintaining sitting or standing balance when dressing or preparing a meal.

PERCEPTUAL

Perceptual deficits can include:

- **Apraxia:** the inability to perform certain skilled, purposeful movements despite normal motor power, sensation and coordination. The person may know what a toothbrush is but does not perceive that it is used to brush his teeth.
- **Body scheme disorder:** a decreased awareness of the relationship of the body and its parts, often leading to neglect of the affected side. The person may sit on his affected hand or be unable to put his affected arm through a sleeve, unless shown how.
- **Spatial relations disorder:** the inability to recognise form, depth, and position of objects and to understand their relationship to oneself and the environment. The person may not be able to find a brush in a cluttered drawer, or pick certain items of clothing from a pile.
- **Agnosia:** the inability to recognise familiar objects using a given sense, although the corresponding sensory organ is undamaged. The person may be unable to recognise his own clothing or members of his own family. (Zoltan 1996)

SENSORY

Poor input from the proprioceptors on the affected side will result in an impaired motor response causing problems with balance, positioning and movement of the head, trunk and limbs. Loss of sensation such as light or deep touch, pain and temperature can be partial or complete. Visual disturbances can occur, the most common being homonymous hemianopia.

The person is unable to see half of their visual field on the affected side. Vision may be peripheral, sparing central sight, or lost in only one quadrant (quadrantanopia).

If a perceptual deficit is present in conjunction with a sensory impairment, the risk of injury to the individual will be greater. For example, if a left inattention exists with a total sensory loss, the person will be at greater risk from burns or scalds when cooking and at danger when negotiating stairs or when crossing a road.

DEFICITS IN COGNITION AND COMMUNICATION

Deficits in concentration, memory, decision making and sequencing, for example, will have a direct bearing on the individual's ability to respond to treatment and retain new information. Difficulty with speech or comprehension can cause the person to feel isolated and lacking in self-worth and to appear uncooperative to treatment. It is therefore important to identify cognitive deficits in order to discriminate them from perceptual or speech impairments, as the occupational therapy approach used may be different.

PSYCHOLOGICAL CHANGES

Disturbance in and difficulties with control of mood are common following a CVA. Many people become emotionally labile and exhibit uncharacteristic emotions, such as crying or laughing at inappropriate times (emotionalism). Mood changes may occur as a result of the person's realisation of his changed situation. Frustration and aggression can be present, particularly if the individual has communication difficulties. Anxiety is often provoked by situations such as fear of falling, e.g. when transferring to the toilet. Symptoms suggestive of depression are common and often highlighted by reduced appetite, social withdrawal and lack of motivation (Wade 1999). These changes can be distressing for the individual and the family, who may not understand that they are a result of the CVA itself.

THE ROLE OF THE MULTIDISCIPLINARY TEAM IN RECOVERY AND REHABILITATION

The majority of recovery after a stroke is believed to occur within the first 3–6 months (Chang & Hasselkus 1997). However, it is impossible to predict outcome, even with the presence of good prognostic signs, because there are those who improve unexpectedly and those who do poorly despite a good predicted prognosis (Carr & Shepherd 1998). In the acute phase, neurological deficits are assessed by the specialist neurorehabilitation team and treatment is provided to stabilise the individual's condition (Wade 1999). The use of a care pathway will ensure that the person receives care appropriate to his needs following the CVA.

Research-based evidence reinforces the importance of the multidisciplinary team approach in that rehabilitation and remedial therapy services should be provided at all stages in whatever environment (Health Evidence Bulletin Wales 1998).

Rehabilitation should commence as soon as the person is medically stable in order to avoid learning abnormal patterns of movement (Lettinga et al 1997), which may set in within 48 hours. Therapy at this acute stage involves promoting correct positioning in bed, or whilst sitting out of it, and assessment of the need to support the affected limb. As rehabilitation progresses, specific interventions will be dependent on the person's identified needs, stage of recovery reached and long-term goals (Fig. 19.3). At all stages of the individual's rehabilitation programme, the multidisciplinary team must maintain effective lines of communication and work together with the individual and family so that any transition is successful and seen as a positive step.

THEORETICAL FOUNDATIONS FOR OCCUPATIONAL THERAPY INTERVENTION

The therapist can refer to a number of approaches based on various frames of reference

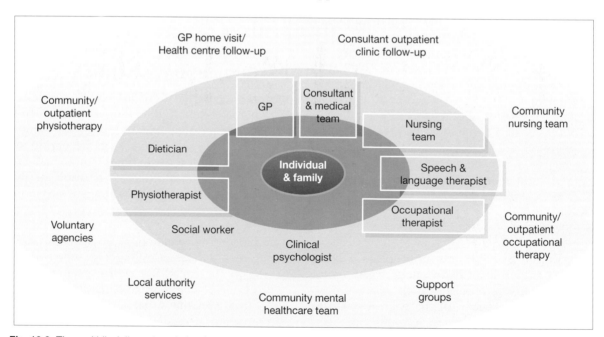

Fig. 19.3 The multidisciplinary team's involvement at acute (inner circle), short-term (middle circle) and longer-term (outer circle) stages of recovery.

Box 19.1 An example of the various approaches that may be adopted

Frame of reference

Humanistic frame of reference	**Physiological frame of reference**	**Cognitive frame of reference**	**Adaptive/compensatory frame of reference**
Client-centred approach: • client directs rehabilitation process • client selects and prioritises goals • works in partnership with the therapist	*Neurodevelopmental approach:* Techniques include: • Bobath • Ayres • Rood • PNF They all aim to prevent abnormal patterns of movement and facilitate normal movement	*Cognitive approach:* Assessment and training in: • perception • cognition	*Functional/adaptive approach:* Adaptation of: • the environment • roles • occupations • activities • the individual and other people relating to that person

---

to guide intervention with a person following a CVA (Box 19.1). The approaches chosen will depend on the problems identified during the assessment process and how they impact on the individual. For example, a problem due to an impairment in the central nervous system can be addressed using a neurodevelopmental approach and a problem due to a perceptual or cognitive impairment by using a cognitive approach (Hagedorn 1997). There is no evidence to support the use of one approach over another, although all members of the team should adopt the same approach (Wade 1999). The humanistic frame of reference underlies the rehabilitation process because it promotes a **client-centred approach**, which enables the individual to regain a sense of control over his situation and to work in partnership with the therapist.

A **neurodevelopmental approach** is based on principles of neuromuscular facilitation and sensory integration and is sequential in nature. Techniques include:

- *Bobath*: encourages normal movement patterns so as to inhibit the development of abnormal patterns of movement. This is achieved through correct positioning, equal weight bearing and movement across and around the midline of the body.
- *Proprioceptive neuromuscular facilitation:* utilises mass movement patterns that are spiral and diagonal and uses sensory, visual and verbal input to facilitate maximum output.

- *Rood*: emphasises the use of tactile stimulation (brushing, icing, tapping) to facilitate motor activity.
- *Ayres:* emphasises the importance of sensory input (touch, sound, smell, colour) to promote normal posture and reflexes.

Although these techniques are not directly related to occupational therapy, they can be adapted for use in functional activity where the task is secondary to the desired neurological outcome.

A cognitive approach is based on the individual's ability to benefit from education and experience using assessment and training in perception and cognitive skills, such as memory training and coping strategies so the individual can transfer these skills into activities of daily living.

A functional approach (Carr & Shepherd 1998) uses activity rather than abstract exercise with clear explanation to the person, accurate feedback, evaluation throughout each treatment and provision of an enriched environment to assist motivation and recovery of both mental and physical abilities.

A compensatory adaptive approach focuses on assessment and retraining of activities of daily living as part of a normal daily routine, with the aim of returning the person to a maximum level of independence as quickly as possible.

By using the appropriate approaches within the context of the occupational therapy philosophy and the occupational therapy models derived from it, such as the Model of Adaptation through

Occupation (Reed & Sanderson 1992), or the Canadian Model of Occupational Performance (Canadian Association of Occupational Therapists 1997), the therapist ensures that all areas of the person's life are considered, so that meaningful goals can be achieved.

ASSESSMENT

The therapist should have information about the individual before assessment can take place. This data collection can include details of:

- the CVA, for example, results of the computerised tomography (CT) scan to identify the area of brain affected, information about whether the person's medical status is stable
- secondary factors, that is, previous medical history
- the person's social background, for example, family, job, hobbies
- the person's previous level of function (premorbid status).

A baseline assessment of impairments caused by the stroke is carried out, ideally using a standardised tool such as AMPS (Assessment of Motor and Process Skills), Rivermead Perceptual Battery, COTNAB (for perception and cognition), FIM and Barthel ADL Index (function). Reference to an occupational therapy model will provide a checklist of occupations that are important to the individual so that the therapist can prioritise what needs to be done and select which approaches to use with the individual. This can be difficult because 'tension may exist between the idealism of the (therapist's) expectations and the realities of the stroke recovery as it is experienced within the context of the person's ongoing lifestyle' (Chang & Hasselkus 1997). The use of the Canadian Occupational Performance Measure, for example, will help the individual to set realistic, meaningful goals with the therapist. Goals may include:

- minimising the effects of CVA, for example altered muscle tone

- maximising the function of affected limbs
- maximising the level of independence in activities of daily living
- resettlement to/management of a suitable environment
- return to meaningful quality of life, that is, work, leisure, relationships.

EARLY INTERVENTION ACTIVITIES

Depending on the approach being adopted and the resources available, the therapist can use different types of activity within the treatment programme to enable achievement of agreed goals (Wade 1999). Activities of daily living and therapeutic activities such as games, craftwork and horticulture can be used throughout the rehabilitation process, as the therapist uses her skills in activity analysis to grade the activity according to the person's level of functioning and potential for improvement following the stroke.

Ideally, the therapist should not work single handed as this limits the scope for optimum intervention. Support staff should be experienced and skilled in the treatment of individuals following a CVA to assist the therapist in her work. Family can also be involved if the therapist takes care to explain what she is doing and their supporting role within the process. Joint treatment sessions with other members of the neuro-rehabilitation team make good use of often limited resources (Fig. 19.4).

The therapist can use her knowledge of the person's background to use an activity that is meaningful. However, use of a particular activity is not as important as the explanation given to the person by the therapist as to *why* the activity is being used and *what* is going to be achieved.

During early recovery, the individual is encouraged to move on the bed, to alter position for pressure relief and reach bedside objects, so regaining some control over his environment. Correct patterns of movement to promote proprioceptive awareness and discourage abnormal

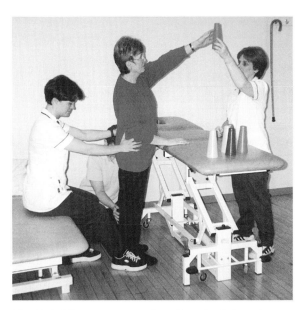

Fig. 19.4 Joint treatment session with a physiotherapist.

patterns of movement are facilitated using a neurodevelopmental approach (such as Bobath).

Dressing whilst sitting on the edge of the bed promotes sitting balance and trunk control. These help to maintain a functional position and are a prerequisite for standing up, for example, to pull up lower garments (Fig. 19.5).

Functional mobility can be addressed within the compensatory approach in the early stages of recovery by the provision of a wheelchair to enable the individual to regain further control of his environment, for example, accessing toilet facilities or day room whilst acquiring the skills and movements necessary for mobility.

If a self-propelling wheelchair is being used, the possibility of associated reactions must be considered and appropriate cushion support will facilitate stability and positioning of the pelvis and trunk. If the person has a flaccid arm or sensory impairment, provision of an armrest or perspex tray should be considered, but this should be withdrawn as soon as possible to encourage the person to sit freely and take responsibility for his own arm by placing it on a support (Fig. 19.6) (Adams Training & Advisory 1997).

Use of a therapeutic activity, such as playing a remedial game placed on a high–low table

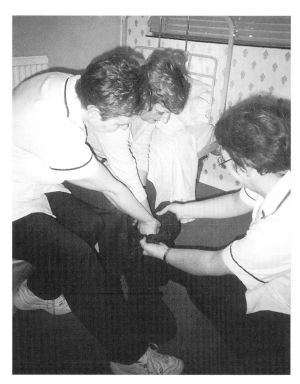

Fig. 19.5 Dressing on the edge of the bed.

(Fig. 19.7), allows the therapist to facilitate independent standing and weight transference, so encouraging normal body alignment. This activity will help further motivate the individual in the progression to walking, often a priority in his goals for recovery (Wade 1999).

Domestic activities, such as making a hot drink, can be used to promote movement beyond the midline of the body when reaching up to a cupboard, turning to move objects from one surface to another or bending, thus enabling the individual to exercise more refined control over his environment (Fig. 19.8).

Deficits in cognition and perception can have an effect on the rehabilitation process and a cognitive approach can be used to address the resulting problems with activities of daily living. Tasks requiring use of cognitive skills must be practised frequently with the individual to enable him to regain these skills or learn new methods of carrying out a desired activity. For example, the use of computer tasks to encourage scanning

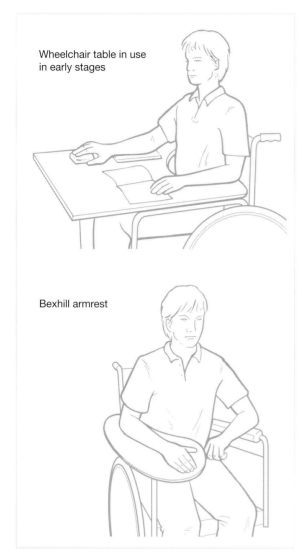

Wheelchair table in use in early stages

Bexhill armrest

Fig. 19.6 Wheelchair adaptations to support the affected upper limb.

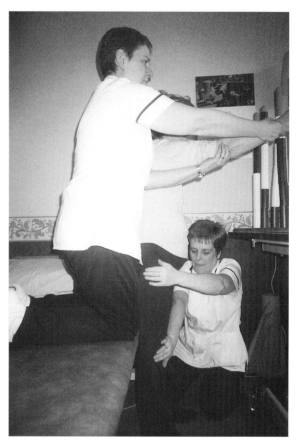

Fig. 19.7 Use of remedial game on a high–low table.

to overcome hemianopia (Fig. 19.9), meal preparation to encourage planning, sequencing and task completion. Visual cues such as signposting, setting out clothes in the correct sequence for dressing can be helpful.

At each stage of the rehabilitation process the therapist must evaluate what she is doing with the person to ensure that intervention is appropriate to his progress. This can be done by referring back to the baseline assessment to iden-

tify progress made and which areas are still impaired. If the necessary recovery to carry out an activity is not achieved, a compensatory approach can be introduced, such as use of a raised toilet seat, using adapted cutlery in the unaffected hand, use of a wheelchair and, if there is little or no return of function, considering the use of a hoist.

The individual's preferred environment, usually home, may need to be assessed and adapted to suit his needs following a CVA. This will ensure that he is able to carry out his desired occupations in his chosen environment, despite any limitations in function as a result of the CVA. Carers should receive the necessary equipment and training in moving and handling in order to position and transfer the individual safely (Wade 1999).

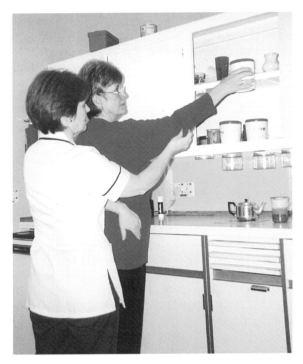

Fig. 19.8 Occupational therapist facilitating the upper limb and trunk.

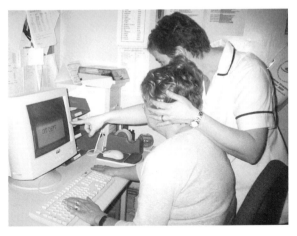

Fig. 19.9 Use of a computer activity.

LONGER-TERM INTERVENTION

There is strong evidence to support continued occupational therapy for longer than 3–6 months after CVA (National Clinical Guidelines for Stroke 2000 10.1d(iv) and 11.2c,d) and this has been found to result in a significant reduction in the number of individuals requiring readmission to hospital during the year post-CVA (Corr & Bayer 1995). The aims of intervention can include:

- to continue treatment to maximise function and independence
- to re-establish the person's role in the family/community as far as possible
- to highlight and address persisting problems and help maintain the person at home
- to help the individual to regain maximum quality of life, for example, to introduce new hobbies, retrain for return to work

Duration of treatment depends on the person's progress and the goals to be achieved, as well as on the resources available.

Regular review of the individual's progress is necessary to ensure intervention is still meeting the agreed goals. A close working relationship is forged between the therapist, the individual and his family, which they might be reluctant to forego at the end of intervention. In many areas, there is a network of social groups for people who have had a stroke and their families, with some input from professional or voluntary staff, which can provide continued support.

FAMILY AND RELATIONSHIPS

After the initial crisis of stroke, when family members may fear the death of the individual, they are often left with feelings of anxiety and a sense of powerlessness. They feel the need for factual information but also want to talk about what stroke means to them now and in the future (Thomas & Parry 1996). The Stroke Association provides multilingual booklets containing appropriate and accurate information. Carers must be allowed time with the multidisciplinary team to air their concerns and feel confident that these will be addressed; for example, provision of a sitter so that the carer can go out shopping or have time to herself.

The person's changed role within his environment, as perceived by himself or his family, can cause problems with relationships. The therapist is often dealing with personal, intimate aspects of daily living and may be the one the person or carer confides in. Her skills in interpersonal communication and knowledge of dynamics will help to address their concerns or, with agreement, she may refer them to the appropriate team member for counselling, education and support after a CVA (Blais 1994).

It is unlikely that the CVA will affect sexual function. Anxiety can cause problems, either for the person or partner, which can be addressed through counselling. Medication, such as drugs to lower blood pressure, can cause difficulties that can be resolved with a change of prescription. The couple may need to change their usual positions so that less physical effort is required of the person who has had the stroke. It may be important to advise them that intercourse is just part of a loving relationship, not something to feel pressured about. The 'Sex after Stroke Illness' pamphlet published by the Stroke Association answers many questions people may be too embarrassed to ask, and so should be readily available.

WORK

The therapist can help prepare the individual for return to work by simulating the work environment and expectations as far as possible. Her skills in activity analysis and grading can help the person progress to the level required to carry out his work. The use of remedial games, printing, woodwork, computer tasks and other activities are useful in this process. The therapist may visit the workplace to advise on positioning of furniture, equipment, wheelchair access or lighting to help the person be as effective as possible on his return to work. Specialist support is available for job seekers with a disability or for disabled people already in work.

DRIVING

The individual must be given accurate information on his responsibilities and advised to contact his insurance company and the Drivers' Medical Group at the DVLA. If he wishes to return to

driving, the therapist can assess his cognitive and motor abilities using the Stroke Drivers Screening Assessment (Nouri & Lincoln 1993) to rule out absolute contraindications and refer him to the nearest mobility/driving assessment facility.

LEISURE

Not everyone who has a CVA is in employment or wishes to work, such as those who have retired, been made redundant, or do not work because of other illness, disability or family commitments. The person is often unable to return to any form of employment because of residual effects of the CVA. Many studies have shown that involvement in leisure pursuits decreases after stroke as little help or advice is given about how to participate in leisure interests, although this could appreciably improve the individual's quality of life (Drummond & Walker 1995). The therapist can assist the person to adapt to his new situation positively by providing information and advice and encouraging him and his carer to try something new. Non-competitive sports and activities are beneficial in encouraging exercise without the corresponding rise in blood pressure; for example, walking, swimming, yoga and gentle keep fit.

Hobbies can be made easier by adapting the activity, for example, long handled tools, raised flower beds. The Hamilton Index (Disabled Living Foundation 2000) is a useful resource for information on equipment to facilitate all activities of daily living. Provision of a wheelchair for outdoor use can enable the person and his family to go out together and information regarding specialist holiday accommodation is also helpful. Research suggests that providing a leisure rehabilitation programme does increase involvement in leisure activities (Drummond & Walker 1995). Local stroke support groups provide a social and information network for the person and his family and help them to feel less isolated in the community.

LIFESTYLE

Although not specialised in areas such as dietetics or hypertension management, the therapist still has a wealth of knowledge she can pass on to the person who has had a stroke regarding his future lifestyle and prevention of further illness (Wade 1999). Risk factors such as hypertension, diet, obesity, smoking and excess alcohol can generally be addressed during treatment. For example, during a kitchen practice, the individual's daily eating habits can be discussed and advice given about using less salt or less sugar, and using low fat foods. The person may feel easily stressed, which can contribute to high blood pressure or the need for a cigarette or a drink. Relaxation techniques can be taught and a tape provided if helpful.

The benefits of time management, assertiveness and energy conservation can all be explained to help the person regain and maintain his stamina and wellbeing when he becomes more active. A balance of occupations can be encouraged so that the person finds time for leisure and exercise within his routine of work, eating and sleeping.

CONCLUSION

Initially, the person may just be concerned with getting well and able to return to a more normal

---

Box 19.2 Case study

Mrs D. was referred for occupational therapy at a multidisciplinary team meeting following admission with right hemiplegia, dysphasia and dysphagia. The cause was confirmed by CT scan as being a left temporal parietal infarct.

Past medical history

Mrs D. suffered from hypertension and insulin-dependent diabetes mellitus.

Social background

Mrs D. lives alone in a ground-floor flat. Her family are very supportive and two daughters who live nearby visit daily. She was previously independent and self caring. Her hobbies include swimming and watching television.

Current medical condition

A baseline assessment was carried out.
Mrs D.'s deficits were identified as:
• Communication: dysphasia
• Motor: poor sitting balance; unawareness of midline; low tone in right upper limb, trunk, right lower limb; dysphagia.

Problems affecting occupational performance (*using the Reed & Sanderson Model of Occupational Therapy*)

• *Self-maintenance*: requires the help of two people to carry out transfers, mobility and personal care
• *Productivity*: unable to prepare a meal, carry out desired domestic tasks
• *Leisure*: unable to enjoy previous hobby of swimming
• *Environment*: unable to manage ADL unaided in home environment. This upset Mrs D. because she enjoys her independence and does not wish to be a burden on her family.

Action taken

Using neurodevelopmental and functional approaches to regain maximum functional skills for safe discharge:
1. Mrs D. was referred to a speech and language therapist and to a dietician to address her dysphasia and dysphagia. The occupational therapist discussed Mrs D.'s previous functional levels with her family and explained to them the rehabilitation process.
2. The occupational therapist and physiotherapist worked together on anterior and posterior pelvic tilts to improve stability at Mrs D.'s hips and trunk and to encourage sitting balance. The occupational therapist provided a wheelchair and Bexhill board for correct postural sitting and identification of midline.

Activities used included dressing, Connect 4 at high–low table to encourage sitting balance and sit to stand. Also transfer practice on/off bed, chair and toilet. Kitchen activities were used to improve independence in domestic activities of daily living, as these were important to Mrs D. Mrs D. received daily 5/7 intervention for 5 weeks. An occupational therapy home visit was carried out with Mrs D., her family and her social worker, when problems in the home were addressed and a suitable care package was identified and discussed with Mrs D. and her family.

Following a multidisciplinary team meeting, Mrs D. returned home with twice-daily care for assistance with dressing and bathing and domestic help. She was able to make a hot drink and light snack safely and her family made her main meals.

Mrs D. was to continue with outpatient treatment to further improve her functional levels and independence in activities of daily living. She attended outpatient treatment sessions twice a week for 3 months and at the end of treatment was able to dress and strip-wash independently, cook main meals daily and resumed her swimming at the local Stroke Group sessions held at the leisure centre. Mrs D.'s care package was reduced and she feels positive about the future.

routine. Once this is established, his priorities may change as he looks to the future. The therapist uses specialist knowledge in neurodisability, in addition to her occupational therapy skills, to guide her intervention with the individual, to enable him to adjust to the consequences of the stroke and 'achieve a personally acceptable lifestyle with the goal of maximising health and function' (College of Occupational Therapists 1994). This is illustrated in the case study in Box 19.2.

REFERENCES

Adams Training & Advisory 1997 Course notes: O.T. for the physical rehabilitation of neurological disorders.

Blais MJ 1994 Using the evidence – stroke literature review. Northampton Health Authority, Northampton, ch8, pp 40–44

Bonita R 1992 Epidemiology of stroke. Lancet 339:342–347

Canadian Association of Occupational Therapists 1997 Canadian Model of Occupational Performance. CAOT ACE, Toronto

Carr J, Shepherd S 1998 Neurological rehabilitation: optimising motor performance. Butterworth-Heinmann, Oxford

Chang L, Hasselkus B 1997 O.T.'s expectations in rehabilitation following stroke. American Journal of Occupational Therapy 52(8):629–637

College of Occupational Therapists 1994 Conceptual foundation for practice care skill and a position statement. College of Occupational Therapists, London

Corr S, Bayer A 1995 O.T. for stroke patients after hospital discharge. Clinical Rehabilitation 9:291–296

Disabled Living Foundation 2000 Hamilton Index. Leisure activities. Remploy Print, Manchester

Drummond A 1998 Stroke – the impact on the family. British Journal of Occupational Therapy 51:193–194

Drummond A, Walker M 1995 A randomised controlled trial of leisure rehabilitation after stroke. Clinical Rehabilitation 9:283–290

Hagedorn R 1997 Foundations for practice in occupational therapy, 2nd edn. Churchill Livingstone, New York

Health Evidence Bulletin Wales 1998 Cardiovascular diseases. Welsh Office. SCG Printing, Merthyr Tydfil

Lettinga A, Mol T, Helders T, Rispens P 1997 Differentiation as a qualitative research strategy. A comparative analysis of Bobath and Brunnstrom approaches to treatment of stroke patients. Physiotherapy 83(10):536–546

Nouri F, Lincoln N 1993 Stroke drivers screening assessment

Reed K, Sanderson S 1992 Concepts of OT, 3rd edn. Williams & Williams, Baltimore

Thomas C, Parry A 1996 Research on users' views about stroke services: towards an empowerment paradigm or more of the same? Physiotherapy 82(1):6–12

Wade D 1999 National Clinical Guidelines for Stroke 2000. The Intercollegiate Working Party for Stroke. Publications Unit, Royal College of Physicians, London

Zoltan B 1996 Perceptual and cognitive dysfunction in the adult stroke patient. CV Mosby, St Louis, MO

FURTHER READING

Hagedorn R 1997 Foundations for practice in occupational therapy, 2nd edn. Churchill Livingstone, Edinburgh

Pedretti W 1990 O.T. practice skills for physical dysfunction, 3rd edn. CV Mosby, St Louis, MO, ch 34, pp 603–619

Shah S 1998 Current concepts and controversies in stroke recovery; rehabilitation implications. British Journal of Occupational Therapy 61(2):83–88

Stroke Unit Triallists' Collaboration 1997 Collaborative systematic review of the randomised trials of organised inpatient (stroke unit) care after stroke' British Medical Journal 314:1151–1159

USEFUL CONTACTS

Disabled Living Foundation, 380–384 Harrow Road, London W9 2HU

The Stroke Association, Whitecross Street, London EC17 8JJ

20

Motor neurone disease

Cath Doman

INTRODUCTION

Motor neurone disease (MND) is perhaps one of the most challenging conditions an occupational therapist will work with. Its relentless and rapid progress leaves little time for the person faced with it to deal with its implications. Diagnosis often takes many months, during which time the condition moves on and deterioration continues. In the meantime, the individual can only guess and worry at the cause of his problems and the professionals often have to respond to the person's fears about his deteriorating function.

This chapter will consider the occupational therapist's role in the treatment of MND and how this needs to adapt in a flexible manner to predict and respond to the person's changing needs. It will also illustrate that rigid adherence to particular treatment approaches, models or frameworks may inhibit an appropriate response to the problems at hand. Needs that can be dealt with from a rehabilitative or biomechanical approach in the early days after diagnosis would be inappropriate for later stages where palliative care is needed.

WHAT IS MOTOR NEURONE DISEASE?

Motor neurone disease is a fatal, progressive, neurodegenerative disorder. It is a collective name for four forms of the disease: amyotrophic lateral sclerosis (ALS), progressive bulbar palsy

(PBP), progressive muscular atrophy (PMA) and primary lateral sclerosis (PLS). The generic term used in the United States is amyotrophic lateral sclerosis (ALS) or Lou Gehrig's disease, after the famous American 'Yankees' baseball player who died from the disease in 1941. It was first described in 1869 by the French neurologist Jean-Marie Charcot and, as a result, is also sometimes known as Maladie de Charcot or Charcot's disease.

MND affects only the motor nerves. Sensory nerves and the autonomic nervous system remain unaffected, as are bladder, sexual functioning and sight. It does not cause pain directly, although pain is often experienced as a result of secondary symptoms such as immobility leading to joint stiffness and pressure problems

It is also often assumed that cognitive function remains unimpaired, unlike the other neurodegenerative conditions such as Alzheimer's disease, stroke and Parkinson's disease (Moore et al 1998). Recent studies now indicate that this is not the case and MND has been found to have an effect on executive functioning and memory (Newsom-Davis et al 1999). Emotional lability (pathological laughing and crying – PLC) is also a common symptom, particularly in the amyotrophic lateral sclerosis and progressive bulbar palsy forms of the disease.

EPIDEMIOLOGY

The incidence of MND in the United Kingdom is around 2:100 000 per annum. The prevalence of MND is about 7:100 000. World-wide, the incidence is about 1–1.5 per 100 000 of the population; the prevalence is 4–6 per 100 000. Figures on the incidence and prevalence vary according to their source. More men are affected than women, to a ratio of 3:2. In the United Kingdom about 1200 people are newly diagnosed each year Motor Neurone Disease Association (MNDA 2000). Although not proven, it is thought that the majority of people with MND have been very fit, have pushed themselves physically and have remained slim throughout their lives (for example, as competitive athletes) (Schiffman & Schiffman 1996, cited in Rowland 1998).

The average age of onset is in the mid-to-late 50s, with the incidence increasing with age (Jenkinson et al 1998). Only about 5% of cases are seen before the age of 30 (Rowland 1998). On average, the life expectancy is between 3 and 5 years.

AETIOLOGY

The cause of MND is as yet unknown. Around 5% of cases are familial. The current hypotheses being researched include the following:

- genetic: attempts to identify a gene for MND
- excitotoxicity: abnormalities of calcium and amino acids, which are vital for neurotransmission, causing damage to cell metabolism
- neurotoxic effects of heavy metals and trace elements
- deficiency of neurotrophic agents
- autoimmune dysfunction
- viral infection: little evidence yet of a potentially causative virus. (MNDA 1998)

PATHOLOGY

Progressive neurodegeneration occurs in three areas of the central nervous system. The resulting clinical features are dependent on the site of the lesion:

- The anterior horn cells of the spinal cord, causing degeneration of lower motor neurons. Degeneration here will cause flaccid weakness, muscle wasting and muscle fasciculation.
- Cells of the corticospinal tract (pyramidal tract), resulting in upper motor neuron degeneration. As 90% of the corticospinal tract decussates in the medulla, a lesion within the cerebral cortex will result in contralateral signs. Degeneration in the corticospinal tract will result in spastic weakness, stiffness, increased reflexes and extensor plantar responses.
- The motor nuclei in the brain stem (medulla) resulting in both upper and lower motor neuron lesions:
  - upper motor neurone degeneration: hypertonic tongue, explosive speech,

dysarthria, increased reflexes, emotional lability, wasting of tongue muscles
- lower motor neurone degeneration: fasciculation and wasting of the tongue, paralysis of the diaphragm, dysphagia, and slurred speech (MNDA 1998).

CLINICAL FEATURES

The onset of MND is insidious. It is thought that between 30 and 50% of the motor neurons have already been destroyed before any clinical signs become apparent (Phul et al 1998 pS87). Early signs and symptoms that may lead the person to seek advice from their general practitioner include unexplained falls, an altered gait pattern, stumbling, foot-drop, weakened grip, tiredness, slurred speech, asymmetrical muscle weakness and muscular atrophy, fasciculation, and abnormal reflexes and cramps (Swash 1998 pS35, MNDA 1998).

DIAGNOSIS

Motor neuron disease is notoriously difficult to diagnose. The wide variety of early clinical signs and symptoms and the lack of any diagnostic test make the process of diagnosis one of inclusion of clinical signs and exclusion of diseases that mimic MND. The 1994 El Escorial diagnostic criteria were developed principally for diagnosing the most common form: amyotrophic lateral sclerosis (Swash 1998). Diagnosis requires the presence of upper and lower motor neuron signs and progression of the condition. Diagnosis is categorised into suspected, possible, probable and definite ALS (Graham 1997). Diagnosis of primary lateral sclerosis, however, can generally only be made post mortem (Swartz & Swash 1991).

The impact of the diagnosis

The experience of diagnosis can have a major impact on how the person deals with living with MND. Borasio et al (1998) cite research that indicates that a poorly delivered diagnosis may result in psychiatric illness. It follows that profes-sionals involved in the person's postdiagnosis care may have more than a physical illness to deal with and a holistic approach is therefore vital. The research also identified that individuals may express relief at an end to uncertainty or resentment at the length of time taken over their diagnosis.

TREATMENT

There is no curative treatment for MND. Medical and therapeutic treatments are aimed at maintaining function, adapting to insidious disability and palliative care. Riluzole is the only pharmacological treatment that has a modest impact on the progression of the disease and was licensed for use in 1996. It has been shown to have some life-prolonging effects although these are minimal and the side-effects can outweigh the benefits. Side-effects include nausea, asthenia and dizziness, and these will affect carrying out activities of daily living.

Other medication is effective for relieving secondary symptoms like muscle cramps and spasticity and analgesia can be given for immobility-induced pain. The distress caused by dyspnoea when the respiratory muscles become weak can be relieved by morphine. Diamorphine, hyoscine and chlorpromazine are given by injection in acute respiratory distress or choking and in the terminal stages of the disease (MNDA 1998).

THE IMPACT OF MND ON OCCUPATIONAL PERFORMANCE

The combination and presentation of signs and symptoms vary according to the form of MND. The three most common forms of MND – amyotrophic lateral sclerosis, progressive bulbar palsy and progressive muscular atrophy – all present with distinct patterns and combinations of signs and symptoms. However, there is blurring and overlap of signs and symptoms, particularly as the disease progresses.

AMYOTROPHIC LATERAL SCLEROSIS

This is the most common variant of MND (around 66% of cases) involving upper and lower motor neurons.

Impact on function

A general progressive weakness and wasting of the upper and lower limbs and trunk is experienced, initially often asymmetrically. Dysarthria and dysphagia can also be present and about 15% of individuals develop dementia (Swartz & Swash 1991). This results in a negative impact on the ability to carry out the following activities:

- **Upper limb:** feeding and drinking, self care, grooming, dressing and undressing, pursuing hobbies, domestic activities, stroking pets, cuddling children, maintaining an active role in sexual relationships and work tasks.
- **Lower limb:** impairment of mobility, transfers difficult or impossible, decreased or no ability to weight-bear, falls, access indoors around the home and outdoors, driving, incontinence caused by inability to access toilet in time, taking part in physical leisure activities.
- **Trunk and antigravity muscles:** maintaining an upright posture, head/neck control, sitting balance, standing balance, maintaining posture for all of the above and many more activities of daily living. A neck collar (Fig. 20.1) may be needed to support the weight of the head, particularly when the person is being transported in a wheelchair or car. The design needs to ensure that the front of the throat is not compressed, causing further difficulties with breathing or swallowing.
- **Bulbar muscles:** communication, chewing and swallowing.

PROGRESSIVE BULBAR PALSY

This variant of MND accounts for around 25% of cases. Upper and lower motor neurons may be involved, particularly those that innervate the larynx, pharynx, lips, tongue and facial muscles. Weakness, fasciculation and atrophy of the

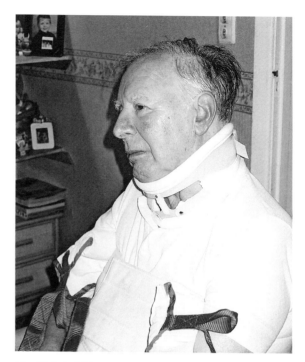

Fig. 20.1 A rigid neck collar with adjustable height chin support and open front.

tongue are evident. Progressive dysarthria occurs, sometimes leading to anarthria.

Impact on function

Speech becomes progressively impaired, with slurring and difficulty articulating words and producing adequate speech volume. This has a serious impact on communication, leading to frustration at not being understood and hindering the person playing an active role in their own treatment. Discussing their fears and emotions, attracting help or attention and communicating with family and friends become extremely difficult, leading to increased anxiety and isolation.

Difficulties swallowing food, liquid and oral medication, combined with excessive salivation and drooling due to poor lip-seal, a dry mouth and slow eating because of poor upper limb control and dysphagia can all result in malnutrition and reduced hydration and nutrition. This is often resolved by a percutaneous endoscopic gastrostomy (PEG), which provides an alternative route for nutrition and hydration without the risk of aspiration of food, drink or saliva. Respiratory and nutritional complications will determine the rate of progression of the disease (Swartz & Swash 1991).

PROGRESSIVE MUSCULAR ATROPHY

Accounting for around 7.5% of cases, progressive muscular atrophy causes mainly lower motor neuron degeneration, resulting in progressive muscle weakness.

Impact on function

The impact of PMA is similar to that of ALS. However, the younger onset of this form will include people with younger families. It is also more likely that the person will be employed and therefore contributing to a greater or lesser degree to the household budget. The impact of lost roles may therefore be felt more strongly than the older person who has perhaps already experienced and relinquished certain roles.

PRIMARY LATERAL SCLEROSIS

This is a rare form of the disease (around 1.5% of cases) and affects only the upper motor neurons, therefore producing symptoms such as high muscle tone in all the limbs and spastic dysarthria (MNDA 2000). It is also unusual in that the survival rate is around 20 years.

THE GENERAL IMPACT OF ALTERED MUSCLE TONE ON FUNCTION IN ALL FORMS OF MND

Limb and joint stiffness and oedema occur secondary to the symptoms listed above. For instance, the impact of spending long periods of time in a sitting position will result in a fairly typical pattern of flexor tendon shortening. If someone is unable to move out of a sitting position, his knees and hips will remain flexed at 90°. The tendons are not stretched through the natural extension caused by standing and therefore shorten to the length required for a sitting position.

Elbows and wrist flexors also shorten to the natural, relaxed, slightly flexed, position. Hypertonic upper limbs caused by upper motor neuron lesions will result in a spastic pattern of shoulder elevation and protraction, and elbow, wrist and finger flexion. Passive movement and careful positioning need to be employed to inhibit this position, preventing flexor tendon shortening. For this reason, a supportive sling should not be used as it will encourage a flexor pattern.

Conversely, hypotonic limbs, particularly the arms, do not have the requisite muscle tone to retain the head of humerus in the glenohumeral joint. An unsupported arm can cause painful subluxation at this joint with the resultant implications for decreased function, moving and handling and oedema. Careful supported positioning using cushions or bean-bag supports and simple support devices, such as a collar and cuff sling, can be employed to support the weight of the arm. A neoprene shoulder brace keeps the shoulders in a supported, retracted position.

Mobile arm supports

A mobile arm support can take the weight of the arm allowing movement to be achieved with minimal muscle strength. Figure 20.2 shows an elevating mobile arm support being used to enable an individual with ALS to feed himself. (Without it, he is unable to elevate his hand to his face.) He is also able to shave using an electric razor. Mobile arm supports require careful assessment and setting up, and also persistence from the individual, but they can enable him to retain independence in certain activities of daily living, such as feeding himself, writing, typing or turning pages of a newspaper, for longer than he would without one.

Sensation

Although MND does not affect the body's sensory systems, pain and discomfort are common as a result of immobility, constipation, muscle spasms and the weight of unsupported limbs overstretching atrophied joints.

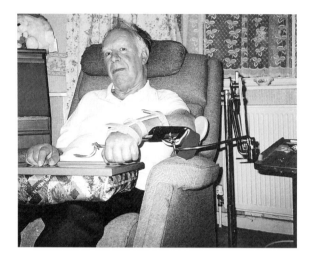

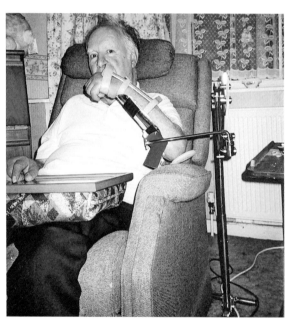

Fig. 20.2 An elevating mobile arm support to enable independent feeding and other activities of daily living.

THE MULTIDISCIPLINARY TEAM AND WORKING TOGETHER

The multiprofessional involvement in a condition like MND can be overwhelming for the individual and their immediate family. Skilled case-management from an appropriate team member is therefore the key to coordinated care and support because of the numerous professionals involved (Table 20.1). The point at which a particular professional gets involved, and their intervention, will vary according to the type of MND, the individual and local services. The case manager (or key worker) is likely to be someone with a major input to the case already, for example, the occupational therapist or district nurse. When the individual is at home, the social services care manager may be best placed to be the key worker, maintaining an overview, coordinating all the agencies and being a single point of contact for the individual.

The individual with MND and his carer/family need to have an assurance and tacit understanding that all the agencies and professionals involved are a source of coordinated expertise, which can respond as required. An uncoordinated and piecemeal service will only add to stress levels, leaving the individual and family feeling isolated and unsupported (Young 1998).

Professional roles blur. The occupational therapist and the physiotherapist may be equally adept at providing advice on mobility, transfers, positioning, orthotics, moving and handling and so on, but it is a professional necessity and responsibility that close liaison occurs to ensure that the person gets the services they need from the professional best able to provide them. Assumptions that other professionals involved in the care package will deal with a particular issue must be avoided to prevent omission or duplication of a service. The professionals involved have a responsibility to ensure that they are explicit about what they are able to offer to the person with MND and what lies within the remit of others. In the latter instance, it is their duty to refer the individual to other appropriate professionals.

LIAISON

Whilst an independent professional assessment is key to planning effective intervention, close team working can limit multiple and repetitive assessments, many of which seek at least some of the same information. This is particularly the case with social information, medication, symptoms and welfare benefits.

Regular liaison and planning is required so that intervention can be provided in a coordinated and timely manner. This fosters understanding of the variety of professional roles involved and ensures that the most appropriate professional(s) deals with a particular issue(s). It is a tool to prevent overlap, duplication or omission of services. Liaison meetings also serve an educational function for professionals with little or no experience of treating MND.

CASE MANAGEMENT

The responsibility for case management, particularly when providing services at the individual's home, may shift in response to the dominant service provider. Initially, homecare services are likely to be assessed for and arranged via the local Social Services department. At the point on the care continuum where the individual's care needs develop from those manageable by a care assistant to those requiring expert nursing care, the lead coordinating role will be better placed with the district nurse or general practitioner (Box 20.1).

OCCUPATIONAL THERAPY INTERVENTION

A diagnosis of MND has wide-ranging physical and psychological consequences for the person diagnosed and for his carer and family. It has no cure and it is fatal. Every person's experience of the disease is unique to them and this is the occupational therapist's prime concern.

Although the symptoms and course of the disease may be similar from person to person, the life that the disease enters is not like anyone else's. This section considers occupational therapy intervention from two approaches: firstly through the Model of Human Occupation, which facilitates ongoing assessment of the impact of the disease throughout the human system and the impact it has on occupational performance, patterns and order of behaviour and choices and motivation. Secondly, by considering occupational therapy assessment and intervention designed to enhance or compensate for deteriorating function.

THE MODEL OF HUMAN OCCUPATION

The Model of Human Occupation (MOHO) provides a good position from which to assess the individual's social, physical and temporal context, emphasising the experience of the individual and the uniqueness of their life. The occupational therapist's role is to work within the context of that unique life, defining the deficits within the human system caused by the disease.

MOHO is a comprehensive approach to analysing the effects and impact of MND on occupational performance because it considers how the human system, the environment and the task interact in a fluid and dynamic way to produce occupational behaviour. The human system is a continuously evolving and adapting one and is shaped by its occupational behaviour. It not only produces occupational behaviour but also is shaped and organised by it. For example, someone with an active and physical lifestyle will have good muscle strength, a healthy cardiovascular system and high levels of stamina. Those physical abilities enable the person to produce active and physically demanding occupational behaviour. In other words: we are what we do.

MOHO describes three subsystems that contribute to our innate drive to act on the environment:

- **volition**: the motivations, values, interests and choices that drive our will to act on and engage with the environment
- **habituation**: the automatic patterns, habits and roles that shape our occupational behaviour
- **Mind–brain–body performance**: the musculoskeletal, neurological, perceptual and cognitive structures and systems required to produce the behavioural output (Kielhofner & Forsyth 1997).

Table 20.1 Multidisciplinary team intervention throughout the course of MND

	Medical personnel				Rehabilitation	
	GP	**Consultant neurologist**	**District nurse**	**Palliative care team**	**Occupational therapist (Health and Social Services)**	**Physiotherapis**
Prediagnosis/ diagnosis stage	Referral for investigations /diagnosis Medication prescription 'Special rules' Attendance Allowance	Diagnostic process Medication			Initial functional assessment Emotional and psychological support Establish relationship	Assessment of mobility Advice on breathing/cou Advice on exerc to maintain ra of movement
Independent function, early stages	Symptom control Referral to specialist services	Outpatient review		Emotional and psychological support for whole family ongoing throughout care	Energy conservation techniques Environmental needs Maintenance of ADL skills Transfer techniques Orthotics (collars and splints)	Orthotics: collar ankle–foot orthoses Active/passive range of mov to maintain independent movement
Increasing dependence and loss of function	Access to hospital-based respite Breathing space programme implementation	Symptom control via medication Facilitates access to other specialist services	Pressure care assessment Bowel and bladder management Gastrostomy nursing care	Symptom control	Assisted transfer techniques Wheelchair assessment Access issues Mobile arm supports Environmental control systems Positioning and posture	Passive movem to prevent contractures Advice on techniques to maximise respiratory function and to assist coughing
Total dependence/ end stage	End-of-life decisions		Increasing nursing care May act as case coordinator	Ventilation decisions Palliation Gastrostomy management End-of-life decisions	Moving and handling advice Ongoing emotional support	Passive range o movement exercises Chest physiotherapy
After death				Bereavement care for the family	Sensitive removal of equipment Emotional support for the family	

health professionals		Social services personnel		Voluntary sector	
ch and language ist	Dietician	Social worker/care manager	Domiciliary care staff	MNDA Regional Care Advisor	Voluntary sector
ng/swallowing essment sment of munication els entative ices if essary	Initial feeding assessment with speech and language therapist Advice on modification of food consistency when necessary	Counselling/support at diagnosis Benefits advice		Support at diagnosis Information resource Ensures access to services	MNDA volunteer visitors
ng monitoring assessment cation of munication ices		Initial assessment of care needs and introduction of care package when appropriate May act as a case coordinator	Minimal assistance to assist with personal care Possible domestic assistance	Organises volunteer visitors Loan of special equipment/access to charitable funding	
ng assessment e on techniques educe excessive vation problems e to family on munication/ ding issues	Advises on strategies to ensure adequate hydration/nutrition Trains carers in the use of gastrostomy system	Increase of care package Respite care Sitting service Ongoing support and counselling for whole family	Increasing assistance, washing and dressing, handling, feeding, emotional support and daily contact	Advice to professionals involved May act as a case coordinator on occasions	Living wills and advanced directives Voluntary Euthanasia Society Carers National Association
es when oral ding is no longer e	Monitors nutrition	Counselling in end-of-life decisions			
		Postbereavement care		Postbereavement support	CRUSE: bereavement counselling

Box 20.1 Case study: the shift from social care needs to healthcare needs

Mrs J. was diagnosed with the progressive bulbar palsy form of motor neuron disease after presenting with increasing difficulties with her speech and swallowing. She was also finding it increasingly difficult to walk, and managing the stairs was becoming particularly hard. Her upper limbs were also becoming weak, although she was able to hold a pen to write as her communication levels deteriorated.

Her husband made a referral to social services when Mrs J. was unable to access her shower unit. Up until this point, there had been no occupational therapy intervention. Mrs J. was already in touch with a speech and language therapist who provided support as required.

Problems identified on assessment

- Mrs J. was finding it increasingly difficult to access the shower unit adjacent to her bedroom.
- Mr J. was having to assist his wife to the toilet during the night.
- Mr J. was becoming exhausted due to restless nights and the increasing amount of care he provided for his wife. He felt unable to leave her alone and therefore never had the opportunity to take a break or go shopping. He was no longer able to pursue his golfing hobby.
- Mrs J. was experiencing difficulty getting in and out of her deep armchair, which had been raised with cushions.
- Mrs J. was a very keen jazz pianist and was now unable to pursue this activity.

Predicted problems

- Access to the first floor facilities including the bathroom and bedroom.
- Access in and out of the property.
- Mr J. was becoming exhausted providing increasing amounts of care for his wife.
- Communication was becoming increasingly poor.
- Mrs J. was having more and more difficulty chewing and swallowing food and drink.
- She was beginning to have problems using the 'Lightwriter' communication aid as it was too heavy for her to hold and operate.

Mr J. was extremely keen to have a stairlift installed as soon as possible.

Occupational therapy intervention

- Establish rapport and the level of understanding Mrs J. and her husband had about her condition. From their description of the course of events leading up to the recent diagnosis, it was apparent that the condition was progressing very rapidly.
- Liaison with other relevant professionals:
  - an immediate referral was made to the care manager to investigate opportunities for practical help and respite for Mr J.
  - contact was made with the speech and language therapist to advise of the increasing difficulties

with swallowing, aspiration and using the Lightwriter
  - contact was established with the district nurse
  - a referral was made to the Motor Neurone Disease Association Regional Care Advisor.
- A functional assessment was carried out and the following intervention was arranged:
  - Transfers in and out of the armchair were resolved by the installation of an electric riser–recliner chair. Although Mrs J would be able to manage to transfer successfully from a chair raised to the optimal height, the occupational therapist predicted that this would not solve long-term transfer problems. The riser–recliner chair enabled Mrs J to adjust her position independently, transfer independently, ease assisted transfers, as they became necessary, recline to support her head as her neck muscles became weaker.
  - Advice was given to avoid the installation of a stairlift as Mrs J's transfers were already becoming difficult and it would be dangerous to assist her on and off a stairlift seat. Alternative options were discussed, including living on one level of the property (ground or first floor) to avoid using the stairs. There was adequate room to turn the rarely used dining room into a ground-floor bedroom. Mrs J decided that she would go ahead with the installation of a stairlift and was able to use it for a few weeks. When she became unable to use it she preferred to remain upstairs.
  - Options around managing personal care were discussed. The ground-floor toilet was adapted using a combined raised seat and frame. This enabled independent use in the short term. The occupational therapist also identified that the ground-floor cloakroom was large enough to wheel a commode into and over the toilet if necessary at a later date.
  - The installation of a shower facility was discussed and decided against as Mrs J.'s condition was progressing so rapidly. She was also experiencing extreme fatigue and decided that an assisted wash would be a less exhausting option.

Care needs

The social services care manager arranged a package of care to provide personal care assistance to Mrs J. A sitting service was also arranged once a week to enable Mr J. to play golf. The care was continuously reviewed and adjusted to meet Mrs J.'s changing needs. Regular liaison meetings between the district nurse, occupational therapist and care manager were arranged to ensure close working.

As Mrs J.'s condition progressed, it became more appropriate for the district nurse to take a lead in the care management process as Mrs J.'s needs became more health-orientated. Mrs J. began to have breathing difficulties and needed very careful handling. She was also unable to speak or eat and had a PEG feed tube inserted.

continued

Box 20.1 *continued*

Her positioning had to be adjusted frequently through the night, resulting in sleepless nights for Mr J. A night sitting service was arranged through the Marie Curie nursing service, arranged and funded by the GP. Mrs J. was also admitted to the local Macmillan ward for symptom control. The hospital-based occupational therapist assessed for a collar to support Mrs J.'s head,

although Mrs J. was not willing to wear one as she found it too uncomfortable around her neck. She preferred to recline in bed or in her chair to keep her head upright.

At the end stage, Mrs J. was admitted to the Macmillan unit where she was treated palliatively. With her palliative care consultant, she decided against ventilation.

All three subsystems work in a coordinated and complementary manner, resulting in the behavioural output or action of the person. The task in hand will determine the subsystem that dominates: a fight or flight response to danger, for instance, will result in the dominance of the mind–brain–body performance subsystem. A typical activity of daily living such as brushing the hair or teeth is so automatic that it is a habitual process that does not require thought or choice in particular and therefore the habituation subsystem leads. The volition subsystem will take the lead when choice, motivation and decision making are required, such as choosing which car to buy or conducting an orchestra.

The rapid clinical development of MND and the emerging signs and symptoms can encourage a medically orientated approach from the professionals involved in the case. The instinct is to alleviate the problem and the resultant suffering it causes. This is rightly the priority for medical intervention, for example, administering opiates to relieve an acute respiratory attack. However, this approach concentrates on the treatment of pathology and symptoms to preserve life and not on the unique illness experience of the individual. The occupational therapist's approach is different, focusing on enabling continued interaction and mastery of the individual's environment in the face of deteriorating function.

MOHO provides a reasoned approach to framing the presenting problems in the context of the individual's unique experience of them. It is therefore a starting point to fully understand the impact and experience of MND for the individual. Intervention techniques can then be chosen from a wide variety of other models of practice and theoretical frameworks, depending on the

problem to be tackled. For instance, a problem-solving approach may be most appropriate for designing wheelchair-accessible bathroom facilities, whereas reduction of spasticity to enable easier dressing may require a neurodevelopmental approach.

Resonance

The three subsystems in the model of human occupation 'resonate' throughout each other. An interruption in the mind–brain–body performance subsystem, such as that caused by muscle wastage in the quadriceps resulting in the inability to weight-bear and therefore to stand to transfer, will resonate through the other subsystems. Occupational behaviour led by the habituation subsystem, such as getting out of a chair and going to the toilet, is interrupted. The effect further resonates to the volitional subsystem, impacting on the individual's ability to choose to walk out of a room or to perform tasks involving his lower limbs to exert choice and control over his environment. His inability to partake in his own occupational choice is curtailed, leading to frustration, anger and even depression at his inability to be master of his body and his environment.

Awareness and understanding of the process of resonance is key to skilled, reflective and holistic occupational therapy practice. When planning intervention, the occupational therapist must fully consider its resonance throughout the three subsystems. Without due regard to the potential resonating effects, unforeseen outcomes may arise. For example, the need for a wheelchair in the near future may be predicted. Considering this at the mind–brain–body performance subsystem level, a wheelchair would restore mobility and enable the carer to move the individual around indoors and out: problem solved. What may not have been considered, however, is the impact the arrival of a wheelchair will have on the individual's volition. It may be against his will, it is symbolic of disability and it reminds him of his deteriorating condition. It could reinforce his inability to kick a ball around the garden with his children or to continue to work, mow the lawn or drive a car.

ASSESSMENT

Assessment flows through the entire episode of input. It is a reasoning process that guides intervention appropriate to the individual's unique circumstances, ensuring that it remains appropriate and focused on the individual's changing needs.

The first assessment takes a 'snapshot' of the current extent and impact of the disease. It is not simply an identification of occupational performance deficits with a view to introducing a piece of equipment or an adaptation to resolve them, it is an evaluation of the resonance of the disease throughout the human dynamic system.

The initial assessment may take place over several days or weeks at a pace led by the individual and his presenting problems. Time needs to be given to establish rapport and trust between those involved. This is crucial so that the therapist can respond quickly if necessary. If emergency intervention is needed at a later date, a therapist who knows the situation, person and family well should not add to the distress.

The individual must have an active role in the assessment process. Although this sounds obvious, it can be very easy to be so focused on solving the latest problem quickly that the individual's volitional needs are ignored. The intervention is much more likely to be received in a positive and constructive way if the person's opinions and preferences are considered. A thorough initial assessment should include the following:

- Identifying problems that require immediate resolution, which are a priority for the individual and his family. A lengthy assessment, perhaps taking a number of visits to the home or ward, is inappropriate if the individual cannot get to the toilet. This needs to be resolved first. The solution of an emergent problem will also help to establish trust in the professional's abilities.
- Establishing what the individual and his carer/family know about the condition. Some people are referred before they are aware of their diagnosis and this needs sensitive, tactful handling as it is not within the remit of the occupational therapist to divulge a diagnosis.
- Providing a clear explanation of the reason you are involved and your role as an occupational therapist.
- Assessing the physical and psychological impact MND has had on the individual and his carer/family.
- Assessing the individual's functional abilities and activities of daily living, taking the form of activity analysis wherever possible. The occupational therapist must be able to observe the activity and analyse its components, so that the performance problem can be identified and modified. She should programme her observations so that unnecessary repetitions are avoided. It is important to remember that demonstration of activities is tiring and may leave the individual with no energy left to tackle other crucial activities of daily living.
- Assessing the home environment needs, or the current environment needs if in hospital or respite care, to identify obstacles to performing activities of daily living, for example, getting in and out of the house, accessing the toilet and bathroom, accessing a room for sleeping in. This assessment must also consider future, predictable needs, for example, whether the bedroom has adequate space for a hoist to be used or whether there is adequate circulation space for walking aids or a wheelchair.
- Establishing details of occupation, past and present roles, leisure interests, ambitions and motivating forces for the individual and the carer.

- Establishing the needs of the carer and/or family.

The occupational therapist must be able to negotiate with the individual to agree a plan of action based on the identified assessed needs. Where alternative, equally appropriate solutions are possible, the individual's preference should be respected. However, this may not always be possible if the costs of the solutions vary widely or if the preference is likely to put carers at risk. For example, a person may be having great difficulty transferring. He is not able to stand without significant support and finds it very difficult to step to turn. The occupational therapist identifies that the safest option to carry out this manoeuvre is to hoist the individual. If carers continued to assist the individual to stand and turn, they would put themselves and the person at significant risk of injury. The occupational therapist must be able to explain the rationale behind the decision very clearly to assist the individual to understand the potential risks to all concerned.

The environment

This can refer to any setting in which occupational behaviour takes place and may therefore include the home, workplace and other places with which the individual interacts, for example, a hospital ward, church or supermarket.

Occupational therapists recognise the impact the environment has on the individual's ability to interact with it. A detailed environmental analysis, particularly of the home setting, will identify environmental press, that is, which features facilitate and enhance occupational performance and which limit or prevent it (Hagedorn 1992).

The environmental analysis of a building will include a wide range of aspects, including the physical and spatial properties of the building, such as the size and number of rooms, access into and out of the property, general state of repair, heating and lighting. It also identifies what the rooms are used for and their meaning for the individual concerned, including social, cultural or emotional significance (Hagedorn 1992).

For example, a ground floor spare room could be changed into an easily accessible bedroom but it may not be spacious enough to accommodate a double bed or twin beds to allow lifelong partners to remain sleeping together. Although this would be a safe and functionally ideal solution allowing easy wheelchair access, it may be entirely unacceptable to the individual with MND and his partner to contemplate sleeping apart at such a highly emotional and fearful time. Goldstein et al (1998) found that the level of strain experienced by the partners of people with MND correlated with the loss of intimacy they felt.

Occupational therapists analyse the environment to identify which elements of it contribute to the individual's dysfunction. In the absence of illness or disability, the person has an understanding of his own efficacy in relation to the world around him. The introduction of illness or acquired disability will challenge that perception, as it will affect the manner and degree to which he can act on his surroundings.

The occupational therapist's role, in this respect, is to consider ways of changing the person's method of interaction with his surroundings, changing the surroundings themselves, adding to the surroundings, or a combination of all three. In other words: teaching a new technique, adapting the physical elements of the property or changing their original use, or introducing a piece of equipment. Examples of these might include: teaching a new way to transfer in and out of bed, relocating the bedroom to the ground-floor dining room to prevent having to use the stairs, or installing a hoist to lift the person in and out of bed.

Environmental adaptations

Environmental adaptations range from the very simple, for example, a grab rail fixed adjacent to a toilet to enable a safe and controlled transfer on and off the toilet, to extensive reorganisations of the home environment, which may include extending the property.

Predicting the need for adaptations is fraught with difficulty. By its very nature, an adaptation of any size can take a great deal of time to come to fruition. Aside from securing funding for an adaptation, building work may take several weeks, particularly if the works are outdoors and the weather conditions are poor.

Funding systems such as the United Kingdom's Disabled Facilities Grant can be unresponsive to the needs associated with rapidly progressing conditions like MND. The application procedure can be lengthy, funding is currently limited to £20 000 and strict guidelines define what can and cannot be provided. Funding for the installation of a stairlift, for instance, may not be forthcoming if a ground-floor room is usable for sleeping in. The guidelines for the grant do not take into consideration social, cultural or emotional factors.

However, good practice exists in various local authorities to allow fast-track grant applications for rapidly progressing conditions such as MND. Occupational therapy managers need to work closely with local Environmental Health departments to ensure that good working practices are fostered.

Although time is of the essence, time spent on careful assessment and planning of an adaptation will result in a usable facility. Any adaptation for someone with MND needs to be appropriate for changing and deteriorating needs. It must be suitable for the person as they are now and for any eventuality and combination of needs the condition may bring. A stairlift, for example, may provide access to first-floor facilities whilst the person can transfer safely on and off it at both the top and the bottom. However, once the person is unable to weight-bear and needs assistance to get on and off the stairlift seat, it will be extremely dangerous for the carer to attempt to transfer the individual from the seat to a wheelchair, in a restricted space at the top of a flight of stairs. Alternative solutions are a through-floor lift that can take a wheelchair, moving the bedroom to the ground floor or deciding to live on only one level (upstairs or downstairs).

Moving and handling

The key principles of moving and handling individuals are contained in Chapter 7. However, there are some issues specific to handling an individual with MND.

The progressive nature of the condition means that the individual is likely to progress from totally independent mobility and transfers through to complete dependence, possibly in a very short space of time. As discussed earlier, the occupational therapist must predict the manual handling needs of an individual so that advice can be given on techniques or equipment can be made available immediately it is required. This should avoid any serious risk of the individual injuring himself by falling, of carers being injured by attempting to help by using dangerous techniques.

Once a care package is in place, the occupational therapist must ensure that all of the carers have received adequate training to enable them to perform the manual handling task with the individual. This may be without equipment initially, relying on special techniques only and the residual ability of the individual. As his function deteriorates, small handling devices such as a handling belt or transfer board may be introduced, followed by turning devices and finally a hoist when the person is no longer able to weight-bear.

Moving and handling techniques must consider the needs of the person carrying out the task as well as the individual being moved. For example, a ceiling track hoist (Fig. 20.3) may be a necessity if the main carer is unable to manoeuvre a mobile hoist.

The occupational therapist must review and document the manual handling techniques very regularly to ensure that no-one is placed at risk as techniques become redundant.

The psychological implications of equipment and adaptations

Equipment or adaptations typically arranged by occupational therapists can be associated with illness or disability. A wheelchair symbol, for instance, designates parking bays for disabled people. A ramp outside a public building is instantly recognised as the entrance for disabled people. When such adaptations begin to enter the home they provide a very strong reinforcement of illness and disability. With a condition like

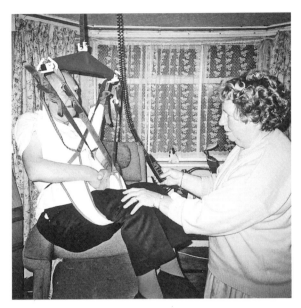

Fig. 20.3 A ceiling track hoist and toileting sling being used to transfer the person between a riser–recliner armchair and a commode. This type of sling is unlikely to remain suitable as the individual deteriorates.

MND, each new piece of equipment or adaptation symbolises further deterioration and further loss of function and control over one's environment. Goldstein et al (1998) found that this was associated with anxiety, depression and loss of self-esteem.

The onus is therefore on the occupational therapist to introduce any new resource with care and tact. Where possible, equipment and particularly adaptations should be provided to meet a wide range of dysfunction that will suit the changing needs over a period of time, rather than having to replace it when it no longer meets the need. A ceiling track hoist, for example, could potentially be used independently by the person initially when they are unable to weight-bear. This could allow them to access the toilet in privacy, or get in and out of a wheelchair. At the other end of the functional continuum, it can still be used (with a change of sling) when the person is totally dependent for all care.

An electric riser–recliner chair will meet a wide range of the person's needs, from providing head support (Fig. 20.4), to assisting him to rise safely to a standing position, to enabling him to adjust his position independently (Fig. 20.5). It will also allow him to elevate his legs to reduce ankle oedema. This approach, of course, is not always feasible and the occupational therapist has a duty to guide the individual and his family through the options and their associated pros and cons so

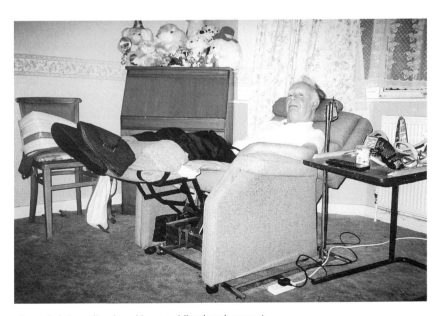

Fig. 20.4 Riser–recliner chair in reclined position providing head support.

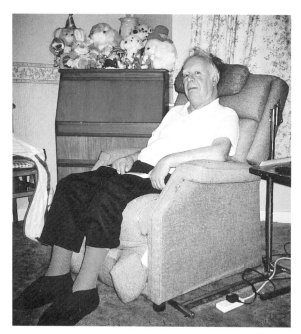

Fig. 20.5 Riser–recliner chair in a slightly elevated position, giving an upright posture.

that an informed choice can be made. This is particularly the case when people wish to fund adaptations or equipment privately.

Predicting need

Motor neuron disease can progress very swiftly. Symptoms may appear and then pass before the occupational therapist has been able to assess, advise on alternative techniques, order and deliver the requisite piece of equipment or arrange even a minor adaptation to the property.

When to introduce the likely need for future change, including adaptations or special equipment, presents a dilemma. The therapist needs to work in partnership with the person, firstly in raising the issue of the need for change, such as an adaptation or piece of equipment, and, secondly, in explaining why it will be needed. This needs to be handled very sensitively and the therapist must be fully conversant with the degree of knowledge the person has about his condition. This will necessitate discussion about the likely course of the condition.

Research has shown that people with MND appreciate a direct and empathetic style when being given the diagnosis and that they are also able to see positive aspects of such a diagnosis (Borasio 1998). A similar approach is therefore appropriate when presenting options for meeting predictable future needs. The individual's level of understanding about the reasoning behind the proposals will have an impact on their acceptance of them.

The occupational therapist must be clear in her reasoning behind the decision to provide a piece of equipment, an adaptation or any other part of her intervention:

- What will it achieve?
- What is its purpose?
- What are its drawbacks?
- What are its benefits?
- How long will it remain appropriate?
- Under which circumstances will it become inappropriate?
- What will the impact be on the carer/family?
- What will the impact be on the home?
- What will it cost?
- How will it be funded?
- How long will it take to put in place?
- What are the alternatives, if any?

The rate of progression and pattern of loss of function is variable according to the individual, his unique experience of living with MND and the type of MND that he has. This only serves to emphasise the need for individual assessment, intervention and prediction whenever possible.

CONCLUSION

The occupational therapist has a key role in the assessment, treatment and efficient management of people with MND (Corr et al 1998). The dual hospital and community role offered by the health and social services can fully consider the physical, social and emotional impact of the disease on activities of daily living. It is able to offer solutions to these in the form of rehabilitative or compensatory techniques, adaptations or equipment that will adapt to meet the shifting demands of the condition. A timely, direct and empathetic manner is fundamental to the occupational therapist's approach.

ACKNOWLEDGEMENT

I would like to thank Mr Nigel Lester and Mrs Joan Lester for allowing me to use the photographs in Figures 20.1–20.5.

REFERENCES

Borasio GD, Sloan R, Pongratz DE 1998 Breaking the news in amyotrophic lateral sclerosis. Journal of the Neurological Sciences 160 (Suppl. 1):S127–S133

Corr B, Frost E, Traynor BJ et al 1998 Service provision for patients with ALS/MND: A cost-effective multidisciplinary approach. Journal of the Neurological Sciences 160 (Suppl. 1):S141–S145

Graham DI 1997 Greenfield's Neuropathology, 6th edn. Arnold, New York, vol 2

Goldstein LH, Adamson M, Jeffrey L et al 1998 The psychological impact of MND on patients and carers. Journal of the Neurological Sciences 160 (Suppl. 1):S114–S121

Hagedorn R 1992 Occupational therapy: foundations for practice. Churchill Livingstone, Edinburgh

Jenkinson C, Swash M, Fitzpatrick R 1998 The European amyotrophic lateral sclerosis health profile study. Journal of the Neurological Sciences 160 (Suppl. 1):S122–S126

Kielhofner G, Forsyth K 1997 The model of human occupation: an overview of current concepts. British Journal of Occupational Therapy 60(3):103–110

Moore MJ, Moore PB, Shaw PJ 1998 Mood disturbances in motor neurone disease. Journal of the Neurological Sciences 160 (Suppl. 1):S53–S56

Motor Neurone Disease Association (MNDA) 1998 Motor neurone disease. A problem solving approach for general practitioners and the primary healthcare team. MND Association, Northampton

Motor Neurone Disease Association (MNDA) 2000 MND resource file. Motor Neurone Disease Association, Northampton

Newsom-Davis I, Abrahams S, Goldstein LH et al 1999 The emotional lability questionnaire: a new measure of emotional lability in amyotrophic lateral sclerosis. Journal of the Neurological Sciences 169(1,2):22–25

Phul RK, Smith ME, Shaw PJ 1998 Expression of nitric oxide synthase in the spinal cord in amyotrophic lateral sclerosis. Journal of the Neurological Sciences 160 (Suppl. 1):S87–S91

Rowland LP 1998 Diagnosis of amyotrophic lateral sclerosis. Journal of the Neurological Sciences 160 (Suppl. 1):S6–S24

Schwartz M, Swash M 1991 Motor neurone disease. In: Swash M, Oxbury J (eds) Clinical neurology. Churchill Livingstone, Edinburgh, vol 2, p 1356

Swash M 1998 Early diagnosis of ALS/MND. Journal of the Neurological Sciences 160 (Suppl. 1):S33–S36

Young C 1998 Building a care and research team. Journal of the Neurological Sciences 160 (Suppl. 1):S137–S140

21

Multiple sclerosis

Liz Tipping

INTRODUCTION

Multiple sclerosis (MS) is the most common cause of neurological disability in young adults. Onset usually occurs between the ages of 20 and 40 years and affects women more than men, in a ratio of 3:2. Life expectancy is not significantly reduced and, due to its progressive nature, it has a great impact on individuals throughout their lifespan – affecting their physical, mental and social health and that of their family and carers.

The disease is characterised by the demyelination of the central nervous system. The sites of the demyelination can occur in patches in the brain and spinal cord but there is no pattern to the location of these sites. The resulting weakness and disability will therefore vary greatly between individuals.

The course of the disease can also vary depending on the type of MS diagnosed. It has been classified into four main types:

- Relapsing/remitting. This is the most common form, affecting about two-thirds of people. Relapses are interspersed with periods of remission where temporary or prolonged improvement may take place. There is no set pattern between one remission and another but following a relapse there is usually some residual damage leading to an increase in disability.
- Primary progressive. This affects about 10% of people. The symptoms gradually increase over the years with no form of remission.

Onset tends to be later and there is a poorer prognosis.

- Secondary progressive. Of the people experiencing a relapsing/remitting course, 75% go on to develop this chronic progressive form of the disease.
- Benign. The individual has little or no disability after 15 years, although some cases may develop the progressive form later in life.

Multiple sclerosis is therefore unpredictable and no two people ever present in the same way. The degree and type of disability is variable, although the pattern of the first 5 years can give an indication of the eventual prognosis. Some factors are thought to precipitate a relapse, such as increases in emotional and psychological stress. Recent studies have also identified clinical viral infections as triggers of new attacks. Further factors include trauma and surgery, although the evidence is not conclusive (Thompson et al 1997). Pregnancy, too, was thought to precipitate a relapse; however, research indicates that it does not affect the final outcome of the disease (MS Research Charitable Trust 1998).

The range of signs and symptoms, and when they occur, will be specific to the individual and consequently there is no prescriptive intervention. As the causes of multiple sclerosis are still being explored, treatment is focused on symptom alleviation and management of the condition.

IMPACT OF MULTIPLE SCLEROSIS

The initial episode may last for only a short period of time, with the individual experiencing isolated symptoms or several in combination, which may then be followed by a remission. However, as the condition progresses the subsequent disturbances will become apparent, depending on the areas of the brain and central nervous system affected. The range of symptoms is extensive but it is important to note that severe disability is not the norm, with most people experiencing only a few of these symptoms (MS Society 1990).

PHYSICAL IMPACT
Visual

Lesions in the optic nerve may give rise to visual disturbances. These are the most commonly experienced initial symptoms and therefore tend to occur at a time when there is uncertainty and anxiety about the possible diagnosis. Optic neuritis, which leads to loss of vision and eye pain, blurred vision, nystagmus (abnormal eye movements) and diplopia (double vision) may be present. These impairments can be very distressing and disabling and are very difficult to treat.

Motor and sensory

- General weakness, stiffness and clumsiness in one or both lower limbs in the early stages is common, frequently leading to tripping and falls. This may also be associated with a feeling of heaviness. Walking becomes difficult due to ataxia (lack of coordination) and hypotonus (reduced muscle tone). People with MS have reported that the ensuing unsteady gait can be misinterpreted by observers who do not understand the person's condition.
- Spasticity is also a common problem and can be very disabling. It can affect the ability to walk and balance, thus increasing the amount of effort needed. It can lead to contractures causing pain, deformity and reduced function, and to exaggerated reflexes. It may be brought on by tiredness, or placing the limbs in certain positions. Clonus, regular sustained shaking, particularly of the lower limbs, can also occur.
- Paraesthesia gives rise to numbness and tingling in the extremities, causing pain.
- Tremor is common and affects tasks that demand accuracy, such as eating, drinking and writing. It can occur in the head (titubation), neck and trunk but is more common in the limbs especially on movement (intention tremor).
- Pain. Until recently pain was considered an unusual symptom of MS (Gilmore & Strong 1998). However, approximately 50% of people experience some form of pain during the course of their disease. This can be acute, for

example, due to trigeminal neuralgia or Lhermitte's sign; subacute, due to pressure sores or urinary tract infections; or chronic, due to the demyelinating process or musculoskeletal abnormalities. Chronic pain affects the person both physically and psychologically – the mental health of people experiencing pain was found to be significantly poorer than those who were pain free (MS Research Charitable Trust 1998).

Bladder and bowel

Urinary symptoms such as frequency, urgency and incontinence are very common in people with MS and are often described as being the most distressing part of their condition. They are due to the pathology of the disease but poor mobility will also contribute to the problem due to the inability to hurry to the toilet. Bowel problems such as constipation and faecal incontinence also have a high prevalence. These symptoms can have a significant impact on the individual and the family and result in social isolation.

Speech and swallowing difficulties

Dysarthria leading to slurred, slow deliberate speech is not uncommon. Dysphasia is less common but can be recognised by difficulties such as word finding. Chewing and swallowing may become a problem and the person may experience episodes of coughing and choking when eating or drinking.

Sexual problems

Partial or complete impotence may be experienced. Lack of sensation and vaginal lubrication, spasticity and fear of incontinence can result in reduced libido, further increasing the pressures and stresses on the relationship between the individual and his partner.

Fatigue

Fatigue is the most common symptom of MS. It has been shown that over 85% of people with MS suffer from fatigue on a daily basis to such an extent that it becomes the main disabling

symptom of their condition (MS Research Charitable Trust 1998). It has been described as an overwhelming sense of tiredness, lack of energy and feelings of exhaustion and can therefore be distinguished from the normal fatigue experienced by adults. People become exhausted more quickly and take longer to recover, and this can affect their concentration and memory. They may feel that these symptoms are the start of another relapse and so increase their anxiety levels. It is very much a 'hidden' symptom and is difficult to explain to others. Family and employers may misunderstand the signs and brand the person as lazy or work-shy.

Other features

- Prior to a definite diagnosis, there is often a long period of uncertainty when the presenting problems appear to be inexplicable. At this time, the person can be labelled as anxious or neurotic and may have feelings of 'I must be going mad' and frustration at not being taken seriously. This can lead to distress and depression.
- Once the diagnosis has been made it is often greeted with relief, although the experience of the whole diagnostic process can affect the way the person copes with the ensuing course of the disease for many years to come. Feelings of anger – 'Why me?', denial, sorrow and grief may all be experienced as part of the process of coming to terms with MS. The prospect of a very uncertain future with fears of increasing disability, possible dependency and loss of control can bring on feelings of isolation and rejection by family and friends.
- Depression is a common symptom and may be part of the reaction to the disease process. It may also be associated with loss of roles within the family, community and work or as a secondary symptom to pain.
- About 50% of people with MS develop cognitive symptoms, which can vary from mild to severe (MS Research Charitable Trust 1998). However, these do not appear to be associated with the degree of disability. In severe cases these problems can affect the person's ability to work and, if they are not

acknowledged or identified, the resulting behaviour can easily be misunderstood by employers, family and carers. Signs include memory loss, reduced concentration and reasoning skills and difficulties with decision making and problem solving.

- Irritability and insensitivity may be evident. These behaviours can be hurtful and upsetting for the family and have a significant impact on their ability and tolerance to maintain support and care.

IMPACT ON THE INDIVIDUAL

Multiple sclerosis has an impact on the person throughout its course. At the onset, the individual will probably be in the prime of health and functioning at an optimum level. Psychosocial development theories also highlight this time as being one of making choices and relationships and being productive, usually through work or parenthood.

The course of the disease will therefore affect the person's physical health and psychological wellbeing, which, in turn, will affect his choices, relationships and decisions about the future. It will affect his roles within the family, such as being a parent, breadwinner or homemaker. Social and leisure activities and the ability to work may be affected due to reduced function, poor mental state and body image.

Although middle adulthood is often seen as a time of personal crisis, it should not bring about great changes in the health status of the individual. It could be seen as a time for the changing of roles, such as becoming an in-law or grandparent, and a time for rewarding relationships with family and friends. As one reaches late adulthood, remaining in contact with others is considered important and can contribute to greater satisfaction and quality of life (Berger 1998). The ageing process brings with it issues around self-image for many adults; for the person with MS, poor self-image is further exacerbated by the disease process, and opportunities for role change and rewarding relationships may be reduced. Social activities may be severely restricted and this, as surveys suggest, can lead to poor quality of life (Aronson 1997).

IMPACT ON OTHERS

The impact of MS on the immediate family can be devastating and the condition seriously affects the lives of all concerned. In the initial stages, the individual may be denying that there are problems and refusing to accept any help. He may be trying to 'normalise' the situation by, for example, not accepting the use of a walking aid, and consequently falling; then, when offered help by the family, reacting angrily towards them.

The disease may affect decisions such as whether to start a family – not just due to fear of a relapse but because of doubts about the ability to look after a child. It can have an impact on the family's social and leisure activities and any change in financial status could place further restrictions on them. Ultimately, it can be responsible for the break-up of the family – divorce and separation rates in families where one member has MS are high (MS Society 1990). Where this is not the case, it has been shown that poorer quality of life is associated with being the spouse of someone with this condition and with being in the caregiving role over a long period of time (Aronson 1997).

THE INTERVENTION TEAM

People with MS, their families and carers, need access to regular support, information and specialist knowledge throughout the stages of the disease. It is therefore of paramount importance that a team approach is adopted. Coordinated services will ensure that there is no overlap, which can lead to confusion and frustration for all concerned, and that the individual is not overwhelmed by the number of professionals involved. Effective communication between organisations and health and social care professionals is vital to ensure that services are appropriate and acceptable to individuals and their families. High quality services for people with MS can only be assured if all members of the team work in an integrated way using interventions based on sound evidence. Figure 21.1 shows some of the resources that are available –

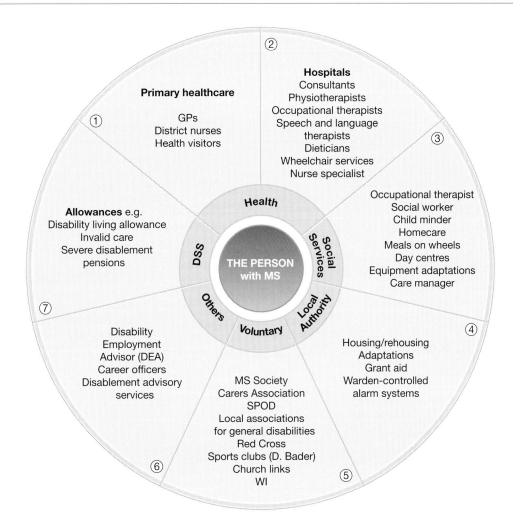

Fig. 21.1 Likely resource needs for people with multiple sclerosis.

but it is important that the individual and his family are seen as central and that a client-centred approach is adopted.

The team consists of a wide range of people from the statutory, voluntary and private sectors. It should aim to provide:

- ongoing support of the individual, family and/or carers throughout the course of the disease
- ongoing continuous education and information about the disease
- access to and advice about appropriate treatment and self-management options

- improvement and/or maintenance of the person's physical, mental and social capacity and quality of life
- advice on adapting the environment to suit the individual needs of the person and carers.

The roles and responsibilities of some of the members of the intervention team are as follows:

- Consultant neurologist and general practitioner. The consultant neurologist is responsible for confirming the diagnosis and, together with the general practitioner, will prescribe the appropriate drug therapies to alleviate symptoms and monitor the person's health throughout the course of the disease. They can prescribe steroids, which may reduce the severity and length of a relapse, drugs such as baclofen and dantrolene, which can reduce the effects of spasticity, and amantadine to help the symptoms of fatigue. Ongoing research continues to improve drug management regimens.

- Nurses. The specialist MS nurses have a role in coordinating the overall care and providing ongoing support, both in hospital and in the community. They are often designated as the key worker, and are involved increasingly with drug therapy and its administration. They are able to provide education about the condition not only to the individual and family but also as a specialist resource to other professionals on the team. Nurses monitor the general health of the person to reduce the risk of complications such as pressure sores and urinary tract infections. They also have a role, alongside other members of the team, in providing long-term emotional support.

- Continence adviser. Expert advice is needed to manage distressing bladder and bowel problems. The continence adviser can ascertain the reason for the particular symptoms and recommend the most appropriate interventions. This may be in the form of alternative continence management techniques.

- Physiotherapist. Physiotherapy is essential in helping the individual to maintain balance, normal patterns of movement and mobility skills. Physiotherapists provide advice and education on positioning to help control muscle tone and deformity, and appropriate exercise, so allowing the person some influence over their condition.

- Speech and language therapist. Speech and language therapy may be ongoing throughout the course of the disease if there are any speech or swallowing problems. Therapists will offer advice, specific techniques and equipment to help overcome the difficulties.

- Dietician. The dietician is another member of the team who can help the person take some control over his condition. Many individuals have very specific ideas about which foods or supplements make a difference to them. Dieticians,

however, generally advise the person to follow a 'healthy' regimen of a low intake of saturated fats, plenty of fish and lean meats, vegetables and fresh fruit.

- Care manager. Legislation within the United Kingdom requires that community services should be flexible and tailored to the individual, and requires close working partnerships between health and social care services. A care manager, who could be one of any of the professionals within the care team, is required to offer a needs-led assessment and to arrange and coordinate a comprehensive 'package' of care. This will be designed to support the individual and his family within the community, and will also represent 'best value' for the commissioning authority.

- Social worker. The social worker can offer advice, support and assistance with a wide range of issues, including finance and employment, but particularly where there may be personal and/or family relationship problems to address. They can offer counselling skills for ongoing psychological and emotional support to help the person and family come to terms with his condition. Where the situation is very complex, family therapy may be offered by social workers, some of whom are trained family therapists.

- Clinical psychologist. Clinical psychologists can help the individual with the management of any cognitive, behavioural or emotional problems he may be experiencing. They are able to assess and advise the family and other professionals on a wide variety of coping strategies.

These professionals form part of the statutory health and social care services for people with MS but the individual may choose to seek-out alternative therapies and ways of coping such as homeopathy, herbal remedies, hyperbaric oxygen treatment and massage. There are several voluntary agencies that can offer welfare, support and practical help, such as provision of specialist equipment, for example, Action for Research into Multiple Sclerosis (ARMS) and the Multiple Sclerosis Society, which has a strong advocacy role through its welfare officers, and works closely with both carers and professionals.

OCCUPATIONAL THERAPY – THEORETICAL FOUNDATIONS FOR INTERVENTION

Multiple sclerosis affects an individual's physical, mental and social health and wellbeing. The potential complexity and diversity of each person's needs requires the therapist to draw on a wide range of theoretical knowledge in order to choose and use the most relevant approaches and techniques.

To make sense of the problems with which she is presented, the occupational therapist must have knowledge and understanding of the condition. The fact that it is progressive means that the individual's needs and priorities can change and different approaches will need to be taken throughout the stages of the disease. Continuous problem solving and clinical reasoning are therefore essential in helping the person to improve or maintain their quality of life.

A study has shown that whereas therapists predominantly address self-care problems, people with MS see productivity and leisure as being very important in their lives (Bodium 1999). This needs to be addressed by the therapist, who must use a strong client-centred approach if intervention is to reflect the individual's values, beliefs, needs and priorities. Participation in the intervention process can also help to increase motivation, which may be reduced due to fatigue or cognitive dysfunction.

A number of models are currently used to underpin practice with people who have progressive disorders. Using a model can help guide the therapist in her thinking, particularly in complex situations. However, it is important that her thinking is not restricted by following a 'recipe' for assessment and intervention. Problem solving and clinical reasoning should be incorporated into the process so that the broader contextual issues are addressed. Mattingly and Fleming (1994) state that when therapists treat people as whole beings, they use several different types of reasoning:

- procedural reasoning is used to identify and solve problems and difficulties and is closely linked to the occupational therapy process
- conditional reasoning is used when therapists try to understand the individual in the broader context of their own world
- interactive reasoning actively engages the individual in the problem-solving and reasoning process and the therapist is able to pick up and interpret cues in order to understand his views and wishes.

Whichever model of practice is adopted, the range of approaches must allow for all the individual's needs to be addressed. The ability to identify and clarify their problems and to agree clear goals will lead towards successful outcomes.

The Canadian Model of Occupational Performance (CMOP; Fig. 21.2) allows client-centred intervention to be implemented. It places the individual in a social–environment context and recognises, clearly, the dynamic relationship between persons, environment and occupation (Sumsion 1999). The individual is placed at the

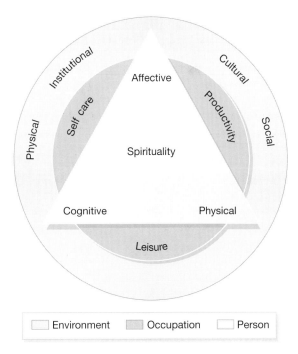

Fig. 21.2 The Canadian Model of Occupational Performance.

centre, together with the performance components that he uses to perform activities within the occupational performance areas of self care, productivity and leisure. All these activities take place in the context of the social, physical, cultural and institutional environments.

Within this framework, several frames of reference (see p53) may be used throughout the intervention; for example, a learning frame of reference may well be utilised, with a cognitive behavioural approach, to provide education about the disease itself. This is important as it has been shown that, despite being diagnosed for several years, many people do not consider themselves to be well informed about their diagnosis (Campion 1996). New behaviours may need to be learned to conserve energy and simplify tasks, and it may be appropriate to introduce preventive techniques such as back care and ways of reducing risk for the family and carers.

A biomechanical frame of reference may be used to maintain range of movement, strength and endurance using graded activities and exercise. There is evidence to suggest that controlled aerobic exercise can lead to improved mobility and general health, although this requires careful prescription in order not to exacerbate fatigue.

The other key frame of reference would be compensatory, with its rehabilitative and adaptive approaches, and the sequence in which these two approaches are used will vary according to the individual. In the initial stages, functional techniques may need modifying but, as the condition progresses, alternative support will be needed, for example, daily living equipment and changes to the personal, family and physical environments – perhaps role modification or adaptations to the work or home environment.

Woven through these approaches is problem solving, adopted to identify strengths and needs, and to select, modify and teach differing ways of management and living. These guide the occupational therapist's intervention and interaction throughout her contact with the individual and will ensure a flexible individual approach with them and their family.

INTERVENTION

The overall aim of intervention is to enable optimum function, self-satisfaction, quality of life and accomplishment within a person's usual living environment. Incorporating a model, frames of reference and a wide range of approaches into mutually agreed goals and the subsequent programme will enable the therapist and the individual to understand the impact of MS on himself, his family and carers, his home and other relevant environments.

ASSESSMENT

The assessment process will be ongoing and will take place in environments of relevance to the individual, for example, his home, workplace, local clinic. A range of assessment tools may be used depending on the stage of the disease and where the assessments take place.

The initial assessment may take the form of an informal interview. It is very important that the occupational therapist plans the interview and allows sufficient time to discuss problems, fears and anxieties. From the outset, it is paramount that a good working relationship is formed as this relationship may continue over many years. The therapist must use her observational and listening skills to gain a clear picture of the immediate family set-up, social networks, interests and, if appropriate, work circumstances. It is vital that the person's abilities and difficulties within their own environment are established.

Using the elements of the Canadian Model of Occupational Performance (Table 21.1), the therapist will gather information to form the baseline for the subsequent intervention. This information will highlight not only the physical performance of tasks but also the person's motivation to participate in these tasks. The performance components – affective, physical, cognitive and spiritual – are interdependent, although spirituality is seen as the core of the person. The concept of spirituality is defined in its broadest sense and refers to the 'innate essence of self; the expression of will,

Table 21.1 Components of the Canadian Model of Occupational Performance

Performance components	Occupation components	Environment
• **Spiritual** – innate essence of self, core of the model • **Physical (doing)** – sensory, motor, sensorimotor • **Affective (feeling)** – social and emotional functions, inter- and intrapersonal factors • **Cognitive (thinking)** – perception, concentration, memory, judgement, reasoning	• **Self care** – occupations involved in looking after the self, e.g. grooming, functional mobility, organising space and time • **Productivity** – occupations that make social and economic contributions: play, work, parenting, homemaking **Leisure** – occupations for enjoyment: socialising, sports, games, creative activities	• **Social** – social groups, roles • **Physical** – natural and built surroundings • **Cultural** – values and beliefs shared by groups of people • **Institutional** – economic, legal and political practices

drive and motivation' (Canadian Association of Occupational Therapists 1997 p43). Sumsion (1999) refers to this as the 'inner strength of individuals to cope with adversity', and the occupational therapist needs to acknowledge this unique aspect of the individual and to respect their beliefs and goals. Ideally, the therapist should attempt to address the person's most pressing problem and consider completing her full assessment in stages. This will not only assist the therapeutic relationship but will ensure that the therapist works at the individual's own pace. It is important, however, that the occupational therapist not only helps him and his family towards adopting a realistic attitude to the future, but also conveys hope and acceptance (Sumsion 1999).

As the therapist gains insight into the impact of the condition, she may want to use more structured methods to guide the intervention process. The Canadian Occupational Performance Measure (COPM; Law et al 1998) reflects the concepts of the model. This measure can be used as an initial or an ongoing assessment of changes in occupational performance over time. It is client centred, that is, it is based on self-evaluation, and addresses the areas of self care, productivity and leisure. It takes into account the person's perspective in identifying and prioritising the problems and concerns he has with performing everyday tasks. Initially, it can help formulate these problem areas and, following a period of intensive rehabilitation, can then be used to measure the effectiveness of the intervention, that is, it provides an outcome measure. As the COPM allows the person to score his performance and his level of satisfaction with the performance areas, the results can assist the

individual in making decisions about which activities give satisfaction and which cause distress and excessive frustration. This may help him to decide how he wishes to reorganise the balance of his work, leisure and social interests.

Many other assessment tools are available to the therapist, such as ADL and specific functional assessments, and she needs to ensure that all areas are considered, as the COPM is not designed to be used exclusively throughout the occupational therapy process (Sumsion 1999).

The initial assessments should highlight the most urgent problem or priority and, once this has been addressed, the individual may decide that ongoing intervention from the occupational therapist is not required for the present. It is important that lines of communication remain open and that the individual and his family are aware of potential sources of advice, services and support.

However, it is likely that contact will be maintained on a regular basis and the occupational therapist's overall aims should now be to:

- offer education, advice and support to the individual, family and carers
- assess and maintain the individual's level of personal independence in accordance with his own priorities
- enable the individual to maintain his dignity despite increasing disability
- advise and assist the individual regarding employment or alternative productive use of time
- maintain, and restore where possible, the individual's optimal physical, mental and social wellbeing and quality of life.

EDUCATION

The occupational therapist needs to establish early on how much the person and his family understand about the disease and be prepared to answer questions. Availability of written information should be considered as it has been shown that this can be a major resource and a source of empowerment for the individual. Appropriate and adequate information at this stage can assist the person to cope with their uncertain future (Campion 1996).

Advice about general health, diet and exercise and information about the consequences of overexertion and raised body temperature will enable the person to take control over their symptoms. Group therapy involving the multidisciplinary team is widely used in this education process.

ENERGY CONSERVATION/WORK SIMPLIFICATION

The individual will need to use his problem-solving skills to find ways of conserving energy and simplifying tasks. Fatigue is experienced by the majority of people with MS and therefore, given the effect it has on day-to-day activities, must be an area of concern. There is evidence that energy conservation is the most common intervention used by occupational therapists (Welham 1995) and its aims are to conserve physical resources and to improve functional endurance. The principles of energy conservation can be found in Box 21.1.

Box 21.1   Principles of energy conservation

- Avoid rushing
- Plan and organise tasks effectively
- Prioritise tasks
- Keep a diary to identify levels of fatigue following exertion
- Eliminate unnecessary tasks
- Maintain good posture
- Use correct body mechanics
- Avoid unnecessary energy expenditure
- Use assistive devices
- Take frequent breaks – balance activity and rest

SPECIFIC ACTIVITY PROGRAMMES

Specific activity programmes may be appropriate for some people and occupational therapy should include graded activities to increase range of movement, strength, coordination and balance and to improve mobility and endurance.

Some people may benefit from learning stress management or relaxation techniques to enable them to adjust their lifestyle. These techniques must be carefully selected, as methods appropriate for musculoskeletal problems may be contraindicated for those experiencing neurological pain. Pacing activities and relaxation may also be useful strategies when coping with pain (Gilmore & Strong 1998) and, given its effect on the health and wellbeing of individuals, pain management techniques may be of benefit. This may be particularly relevant to people experiencing chronic pain that affects their ability to carry out everyday activities.

Periods of intensive rehabilitation and subsequent improvements in function not only have a positive effect on the quality of life of the person, they can also reduce the amount of help required within the home. Changes in techniques, routines and habits take time to occur (Kielhofner 1992) and therefore a coordinated team approach is needed to assist the individual in transferring these skills into their relevant environment.

SELF CARE

It is likely that personal independence will begin to be affected from the onset due to lack of coordination, loss of sensation and general weakness. Early advice and assistance will enable the person to tackle difficulties, not only as they arise but also in preparation for future problem solving. Problems can often be solved by learning new methods and/or using labour-saving techniques, and these should be tried in the first instance. However, as a last resort, a compensatory approach may be needed and equipment or adaptations prescribed to assist independent living. The timing of the introduction of these will vary depending on each individual but the philosophy of this stepped approach will allow the person to adjust to each stage without being overwhelmed with an array of equipment. In some cases, however, it may be necessary to use a combination of all the above solutions at the same time.

Dressing

Light-weight, loose-fitting clothes that have 'give' and are strong enough to withstand pulling and stretching are advisable. Sports clothing such as track suits are particularly suitable, as long as the individual finds them acceptable. Choice of clothing will also play a part in the person maintaining continence and appropriate equipment, for example, a dressing stick, may encourage independence.

Eating and drinking

Lack of coordination, intention tremor and loss of sensation can affect the person's ability to cope with eating and drinking and this can lead to embarrassment and an unwillingness to participate in family meals or social occasions. Good posture and support whilst eating are essential in helping to reduce the risk of spasms and assist with control of upper limbs. Weighted bracelets may help the person overcome the difficulties of tremor and adapted utensils may be useful.

Personal hygiene

To overcome problems of general weakness and fatigue, the individual should be encouraged to carry out activities such as washing and cleaning his teeth whilst seated, using the basin for support. A range of adaptive equipment is available for tasks such as shaving and hair care and advice about alternative techniques for applying make-up is available in many high street stores.

The therapist may also advise on suitable protection and ways of coping with hygiene during menstruation. The use of self-adhesive pads and a portable bidet may allow continuing independence and dignity.

Use of the toilet

Initially, the person may only experience difficulty when rising from the seat. If a change of technique cannot be achieved, the correct toilet height and possible installation of grab rails may be sufficient to help the person overcome any difficulties. As the condition progresses, the use of a commode on wheels, which can be pushed over the toilet, may help to eliminate the need for some transfers.

When the condition reaches a stage where transfers are becoming a more obvious problem, the therapist and the person may need to consider changing the layout of the toilet and bathroom to ensure that there is sufficient space for wheelchair use and for assisted transfers. Installation of a ceiling track hoist or use of a mobile hoist may need to be discussed.

Bathing/showering

General weakness, lack of coordination and fatigue will make it increasingly difficult for the individual to get in and out of the bath. The temperature of the water will also affect the person's ability to transfer in and out safely. Use of a bath board and seat and well-positioned grab rails may be sufficient initially but, if this is too tiring, strip washing while sitting may be preferable. More complex equipment may be needed as the person's condition deteriorates and he may wish to choose an in-bath lift, static bath hoist or ceiling track hoist.

Showering is the recommended option from the occupational therapist's perspective, as the person is likely to experience difficulties with transferring on and off a bath lift in the longer term. It is therefore important that the therapist provides sufficient information to help the person make a realistic decision. The advantages of installing a level-access shower or 'dished' floor finished with a slip-resistant surface, used in conjunction with a wheeled shower chair, would need to be stressed. A thermostatically controlled shower unit, rather than one that works directly from the domestic hot water system, will be imperative, as loss of sensation could lead to scalding.

Mobility

Initially, the use of simple walking aids may be required. While the person is still ambulant, the normal heel–toe gait and good posture should be maintained. Walking should be encouraged for as long as possible but, whereas it may still be safe to walk within the home, the use of a wheelchair outdoors may be appropriate to avoid fatigue and the risk of falling. The timing of the introduction of a wheelchair is crucial, not only in terms of safety but also from the psychological point of view. Very often, people with MS see the introduction of a wheelchair as unacceptable and depressing. However, if the approach is both tactful and well timed, with the benefits of using a wheelchair stressed, it may be easier for the person to accept. Careful wheelchair and seating assessments must be viewed as a priority, and carried out through all the stages of the disease. Supportive seating and good posture, which enhance cardiac and respiratory functions, discourage potential deformity and offer pressure relief and effective skin care, are vital.

Other areas of general mobility will need to be assessed, such as the heights and accessibility of the bed, chair and toilet. A change of technique and/or the provision of adaptive equipment will enable continued independence and safe transfers. Instructions for safe assisted transfers while the person is still weight bearing will need to be given to all his carers. Regular review of risk assessments may have to be completed to ensure everyone's safety and to ensure compliance with health and safety legislation. The occupational therapist should adopt a hierarchical approach to teaching moving and handling techniques and the prescription of handling aids, as described in Chapter 7.

PRODUCTIVITY

Home management

All aspects of general home management will need discussion, including household cleaning, food preparation, cooking and shopping. The general problems of fatigue will be in evidence with all daily routines so it is important that the therapist advises and encourages the person to use energy conservation and work simplification principles. However, any alterations to the home must take into account the needs of all family members.

As far as possible all food preparation should be undertaken sitting down. Provision of a few well-chosen labour-saving items, many of which do not have the 'disability' label attached to them and are commonly available, may be all that is needed. Safety in the kitchen is paramount and cooker guards and slip-resistant flooring may be necessary. Convenience foods used in conjunction with a microwave may be a very acceptable alternative and enable the person to maintain independence for a longer period of time.

Planning is vital if fatigue is to be avoided. Heavy tasks, such as shopping and cleaning, need to be balanced with lighter ones, and other family members may have to be involved. Supermarkets and other retail outlets are increasingly aware of the needs of wheelchair users and these resources need to be investigated. Internet and home delivery services may appeal to many who regard shopping activities a chore.

Transport will become more difficult as the condition progresses and location will dictate how the problems may be solved. There are many national schemes to facilitate easy transport and access to toilet facilities for people with disabilities and the therapist needs to advise accordingly (see Chapter 7). The person will also require guidance on financial benefits and information about the availability of all appropriate services and facilities.

Work

The ability to continue to work will allow the person to maintain one of his normal roles. It is increasingly being recognised that enabling people to remain in the workplace is beneficial and there are many national and European schemes to enable this, such as partnership schemes between employers and disability organisations.

The employer may be able to transfer the person internally to an alternative job and an ergonomic workplace assessment will need to be completed to ensure that the person is able to carry out the job safely and efficiently. The Disability Employment Advisor, based within a job centre, will be able to advise about finance for adaptations to the workplace and the availability of retraining schemes. However, the employer may have legal responsibilities to ensure that the employee is treated fairly and that reasonable adjustments are made to the premises.

Some people may decide to find alternatives to paid employment so that they can learn new skills and meet new people.

LEISURE

Special interests and leisure activities will become increasingly important as the condition progresses. If the individual is unable to continue to work, he will have more time to fill. Activities that involve the whole family will prevent him from feeling isolated and being a burden, and encourage interaction within the family unit. Pursuing new interests will not only depend on the person's physical and cognitive abilities and interests but also on local amenities and financial resources.

ENVIRONMENT
Physical environment

Throughout her intervention, the occupational therapist must be aware of the problems that may arise from the layout of the home and its locality. The physical environment can hinder or facilitate the individual's ability to perform everyday activities. Minor or major adaptations may be needed to maximise the person's abilities and minimise the barriers to occupational performance.

Planning adaptations can only occur when the therapist has established, very clearly, what the person and his family want to achieve. There will often be a range of solutions but the rationale for the final decision must be thought through carefully. For example, provision of a level-access shower facility may enable the individual to be independent in his personal care. However, this may not be appropriate if this task takes him so long to complete that it leaves him feeling exhausted, and he may wish to choose alternative means.

In the short term, solutions may include safe access to and within the property, use of rails in hallways, extra banister rails on the stairs and careful positioning of furniture. If the person lives in a house, the day's routine will need to be planned so that he does not have to climb the stairs more than once a day in order to avoid fatigue. It may be necessary to consider a ground-floor toilet, if one is not available.

Long-term planning for eventual wheelchair use will need to be broached at a time when the individual and family are psychologically attuned to accepting that he will need a wheelchair. It is imperative that the physical needs of the individual are taken into account, but not in isolation from the whole family. When considering major adaptations, the therapist will need to discuss what is the usual practice and routine of the household in order to maintain normality as far as possible. If the major problem is one of gaining access to a first-floor bedroom, a single bedroom on the ground floor would immediately split partners, which would not only be detrimental to their relationship but enforce feelings of isolation on them both. If they have young children, it would also lead to the person's exclusion from normal bed-time reading and seeing the children 'tucked up'. Installation of a through-floor lift would allow access to all parts of the house and cut down on the numbers of transfers that are needed.

General access to the home and garden, as well as changes to internal fixtures such as the electric sockets, light switches, window openers and appropriate door handles will all need to be addressed.

Social environment

Relationships with family, friends, neighbours and volunteers who form part of the person's social environment may be affected by his reduced abilities and it is essential that the person's normal roles are maintained as far as possible.

However, as social contacts become more difficult, the person may be more dependent on other means of contact to keep him in touch. The occupational therapist can advise on a range of alternative communication aids or, if the individual has a specific impairment, speech and language therapy may be indicated. Word processors or personal computers enable written communication and may also facilitate work and leisure interests too. Resources may be available for loans of computers and word processors and access to the Internet can open up a whole range of opportunities.

Telephones and alarm systems designed with people with disabilities in mind to ensure their personal security are widely available. As the condition progresses and the individual is unable to manage tasks such as using the phone, the prescription of an environmental control system may enable him to retain his independence. It is important to ensure that, if the person lives alone, his security and independence do not exclude social contact.

Where couples are experiencing problems with interpersonal relationships, it may be appropriate for the therapist to offer counselling to allow feelings, thoughts and issues to be explored. This may need to be undertaken with, alongside or by referral to, other organisations such as the Association to Aid Sexual and Personal Relationships of People with Disability (SPOD).

Cultural environment

The cultural environment can influence the way the individual deals with the challenges of increasing disability and the therapist may encounter a range of coping strategies, such as denying the need for assistance or refusal to undergo some treatment procedures. Changes in the person's 'cultural norms', such as inability to remain 'head' of the family, will have an impact on how he will cope with the disease. The therapist must be aware of these issues, which she may find challenging, particularly if they conflict with her own cultural background.

Institutional environment

Economic

The family will need advice on all possible financial help to assist with adaptations, whether it be a disabled facilities grant from the local authority and/or local social services schemes, or other national and local sources of assistance. The occupational therapist must be aware of all local arrangements, policies and priorities if she is to be an effective advocate for the family, as difficulties may arise where these arrangements conflict with the priorities of the individual and his family.

Legal

Whilst it must be remembered that many people with MS experience only minimal disability, it is most likely that the occupational therapist will be involved with people in the advanced stages of the disease. The impact of severe disability and cognitive dysfunction can affect the person's judgement and this may bring about legal and professional dilemmas for the occupational therapist. In the later stages, for example, it is likely that major pieces of equipment (such as a ceiling track hoist) or adaptations will need to be introduced to facilitate safe transfers. The therapist has a clear duty to ensure the health and safety of all those involved with assisting the person and, although the installation of a hoist may be contrary to the person's, and family's, wishes, she may feel that health and safety issues demand it. She must listen to their concerns and take time to explore all the issues in order to relieve their anxieties. It must be acknowledged that the person and his family are the experts on how the disease affects them and they need to feel that they have some control of the situation. It is vital that the occupational therapist works in partnership with the individual and his family if acceptance is to be achieved.

CONCLUSION

The course of MS continues over very many years and each individual needs to learn to cope with, and accept, his levels of function at each stage of the illness. It is important that he is empowered to make decisions and decide priorities based on his own values and beliefs and not those of the team involved with his care. The occupational therapist will play a key role in the management of the person with MS. She must give clear information and reasons for her advice – but it is the person's choice as to when, and if, he accepts it (Campion 1996).

A model of practice has been suggested that allows the therapist to work in partnership with the individual and his family. It provides a tool to help clarify the ongoing assessment and evaluation necessary to cope with the changing needs experienced over a long period of time. The importance of a client-centred approach has been emphasised, although the therapist also needs to take into account the requirements of the family in all aspects of daily living (Box 21.2).

Box 21.2 Case study

Mr A. is 49 years old and was diagnosed with MS 18 years ago. At the time he lived with his wife and two sons in a three-bedroom Housing Association property. He was very angry about the way he was diagnosed and remains very bitter about the way he was treated. Initially, his GP thought his symptoms were related to anxiety and referred him to a clinical psychologist. It took 18 months for the diagnosis to be confirmed and the result was that Mr A. refused any involvement with the statutory services.

Mr A.'s mobility deteriorated over time and he eventually referred himself to the social services occupational therapist. All he wanted was an extra banister rail for the stairs. On the initial home visit, the therapist identified other problems – Mr A. admitted he was falling regularly, which was clearly distressing his wife and family but he was not prepared to accept any of the options proposed to him.

Over a period of time, the occupational therapist built up a relationship with Mr A. and his family and was able to start addressing some of his difficulties. However, the family dynamics were so fraught that the occupational therapist referred Mrs A. to the social worker, as she felt she was unable to be advocate for both Mr A. and his wife.

Mr A. finally agreed to major adaptations to his property. Several options were discussed but Mr A. was very clear that his priority was to have access to all parts of his home and to maintain their normal sleeping arrangements. He felt that a stairlift would solve his difficulties. Following extensive discussions, Mr A. agreed that a through-floor lift would ensure his independence, even when transfers became difficult.

A Disabled Facilities Grant (DFG) application was made for ramped access to the house, a through-floor lift, removal of the bath and the installation of a level-access shower tray and thermostatically controlled shower unit and appropriate grab rails. Social services would provide a mobile shower chair and a ceiling track hoist in the bedroom and bathroom.

The adaptations met Mr A.'s needs, although the timescale for their completion has not helped the relationship with his wife. Mr A. is coping well at the moment and, following attendance at a rehabilitation unit, is taking on desk-top publishing work. He attends the local ARMS (Action for Research into Multiple Sclerosis) centre for hyperbaric oxygen treatment, which he says helps to reduce his feelings of fatigue. Currently he feels well, although he now spends most of his time in his wheelchair, but he is fearful about his future.

REFERENCES

Aronson KJ 1997 Quality of life among persons with multiple sclerosis and their caregivers. Neurology 48(1):74–80

Berger KS 1998 The developing person through the lifespan, 4th edn. Worth, New York

Bodium C 1999 The use of the Canadian Occupational Performance Measure for the assessment of outcome on a neurorehabilitation unit. British Journal of Occupational Therapy 62(3):123–126

Campion K 1996 Meeting multiple needs. Nursing Times 92(24):28–30

Canadian Association of Occupational Therapists (CAOT) 1997 Enabling occupation: an occupational therapy perspective. CAOT Publications ACE, Toronto, Ottawa

Gilmore R, Strong J 1998 Pain and multiple sclerosis. British Journal of Occupational Therapy 61(4):169–172

Kielhofner G 1992 Conceptual foundations of occupational therapy. FA Davis, Philadelphia, PA

Law M, Baptiste S, Carswell A, McColl MA, Polatajko H, Pollock N 1998 Canadian Occupational Performance Measure, 3rd edn. Canadian Association of Occupational Therapists Publications ACE, Toronto, Ottawa

Mattingly C, Fleming MH 1994 Clinical reasoning: forms of inquiry in a therapeutic practice. FA Davis, Philadelphia, PA

MS Research Charitable Trust 1998 Multiple sclerosis information for nurses and health professionals. MS Research Trust, Letchworth

Multiple Sclerosis (MS) Society of Great Britain and Northern Ireland 1990 An information pack for professional carers. MS Society, London

Sumsion T 1999 Client-centred practice in occupational therapy. Churchill Livingstone, Edinburgh

Thompson AJ, Polman L, Hohlfeld R (eds) 1997 Multiple sclerosis: clinical challenges and controversies. Martin Dunitz Ltd, London

Welham L 1995 Occupational therapy for fatigue in patients with multiple sclerosis. British Journal of Occupational Therapy 58(12):507–509

FURTHER READING

Bowcher H, May M 1998 Occupational therapy for the management of fatigue in multiple sclerosis. British Journal of Occupational Therapy 61(11):488–492

Cohen H (ed) 1999 Neuroscience for rehabilitation. Lippincott Williams and Wilkins, Baltimore, MD

Disability Discrimination Act (1995). Her Majesty's Stationery Office, London

Fearing VG, Las M, Clark J 1999 An occupational performance process model: fostering client care and therapist alliances. Canadian Journal of Occupational Therapy 64(1):7–15

Grant D, Lundon K 1999 The Canadian Model of Occupational Performance applied to females with osteoporosis. Canadian Journal of Occupational Therapy 66(1):3–13

Hagedorn R 1997 Foundations for practice in occupational therapy, 2nd edn. Churchill Livingstone, Edinburgh

Hansen RA, Atchison B 2000 Conditions in occupational therapy: effect on occupational performance, 2nd edn. Lippincott Williams and Wilkins, Baltimore, MD

Jones M et al 1996 The effectiveness of occupational therapy and physiotherapy in multiple sclerosis patients with ataxia of the upper limb and trunk. Clinical Rehabilitation 10:277–282

Pedretti LW 1999 Occupational therapy: practice skills for physical dysfunction, 4th edn. Mosby, St Louis, MO

Weiner WJ, Goetz CG 1994 Neurology for the non-neurologist, 3rd edn. JB Lippincott, Philadelphia, PA

22

Spinal disorder (back pain)

Sarah Jane Kelly

INTRODUCTION

Back pain generally refers to any pain occurring in the thoracic, lumbar, sacral and coccygeal regions of the spine. This chapter will focus on low back or lumbar pain, as it is most frequently referred to in occupational therapy literature and has been the focus of most research. The treatment of low back pain is considered a good model for the treatment of any such pain and, for the purposes of this chapter, pain is defined as acute if it is present for up to 3 months and chronic if it continues after 3 months (Merskey & Bogduk 1994).

EPIDEMIOLOGY AND RISK FACTORS

Over 60% of the population will report back pain at some time in their life, although back pain is no more common now than it was in the 1960s. However, reduced function as a result of back pain has increased substantially and is now one of the most common causes of disability in adults. In any month approximately 10% of adults report some restriction of activities due to back pain. The increasing number of people who go on to develop chronic disability is of particular concern. The reasons for this appear to include 'changed attitudes and expectations, changed medical ideas and management, and changed social provisions in the second half of the twentieth century' (Clinical Standards

Advisory Group (CSAG) 1994). Lifestyle factors associated with increased risk of low back pain include heavy manual work, sedentary work, driving, smoking and pregnancy.

While back pain may occur from childhood to old age, the proportion of people reporting back pain increases from the late teens to early 50s and then remains constant until the mid-60s. The vast majority of back pain is simple mechanical backache, pain that is 'musculoskeletal in origin and in which symptoms vary with different physical activities' (Waddell 1998). A very small proportion of back pain is due to other conditions. For example, less than 1% is the result of serious pathology such as tumour, less than 1% as a result of inflammatory or systemic disorder and less than 5% is sciatica with nerve root entrapment. Of these, only a small proportion requires surgery. However, a diagnosis of simple mechanical backache does not mean that the pain is necessarily mild. Someone with a prolapsed disc may not experience any pain while an individual with simple mechanical backache may find himself with extreme pain and unable to move. It is important to be clear that pain does not always mean an injury has occurred. In the case of chronic pain, faulty pain mechanisms are more likely to give rise to pain than a tissue injury. It is important to communicate this to individuals with back pain as early as possible, because many people believe that more intense pain reflects more serious injury or disease. This is not the case and an individual who continues to believe this is less likely to make a good functional recovery than one who understands that the pain they are experiencing does not mean damage is occurring in their back.

PROGRESS OF THE CONDITION

Some people experiencing an acute episode of back pain will rest. Rest is no longer considered a treatment but it is a potential response to extreme discomfort on movement. Though the individual may be restricted in activities of daily living during this period, most people recover and resume normal activities. Back pain becomes disruptive to function if the individual fails to resume normal activity. The reasons why people fail to regain normal function are multifactorial and a clear understanding of this is critical for the therapist assessing and planning intervention.

As already mentioned, back pain often resolves spontaneously, while physical therapies, surgery and drug therapy may resolve or control symptoms for others. However, many individuals with chronic, unresolving back pain are assessed and treated by a bewildering succession of medical professionals and complementary therapists. Seeking a cure is an obvious course of action for many people but the longer the pain is sustained, the less likely it is to resolve with or without treatment. Some individuals, realising their pain is unlikely to respond to treatment, look for advice on managing it in a way that maximises their quality of life. Others may continue to seek a cure and become increasingly frustrated with healthcare services that continue to provide unsuccessful treatments.

IMPACT ON FUNCTION

The majority of functional limitation in back pain conditions is a result of avoiding specific positions and activities because of pain, fear of pain and/or fear of reinjury, rather than mechanical restriction due to structural changes in the spine.

This avoidance of certain activities (Box 22.1) has a marked impact on the physical confidence and fitness of the individual (Harding et al 1998). As a person with chronic pain becomes less active, he tires more easily and, even on a 'good day', manages less than he used to. Moreover, many people report that their pain increases with activity. They commonly carry on until they can tolerate movement no longer and finally rest to allow the pain to subside. When up and about once more, the individual often resumes activities, again up to their maximum pain tolerance.

This swing between overactivity and rest is called 'activity cycling' (Fig. 22.1). As time goes on, the level of activity the individual can manage before aggravating his pain gradually decreases and he finds himself increasingly

Box 22.1 Activity avoidance: as physical condition and confidence decline, the individual may become increasingly limited in the activities they feel confident and able to carry out

Restricted activities include:
Lifting and carrying heavy objects
Jumping
Running
Walking outdoors
Bending, reaching and stretching
Tasks in standing
Tasks in sitting
Lifting and carrying light objects
Walking without aids
Walking indoors
Self care
Transferring

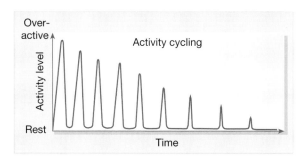

Fig. 22.1 Activity cycling: the swinging between overactivity and rest; a maladaptive behaviour frequently observed in people disabled by back pain. The individual strives to reach a peak of activity until pain drives him to rest. Over time, the maximum peak of activity declines steadily as physical fitness and confidence are eroded. Many people become increasingly fearful of the pain as they notice their physical deterioration. This is often accompanied by increasing episodes of low mood or anxiety.

restricted in functional activities. Work, domestic tasks, leisure and sexual activity may all be affected. The individual's tolerance to walking, sitting or standing and other sustained postures is reduced. He may report difficulties with personal care activities, requiring help or equipment to carry out these tasks.

Activity cycling makes planning future events difficult. Many people find their flare-ups of pain are unpredictable. This may cause difficulties at work but also adversely affects the individual's confidence in committing to social events and other activities such as holidays. As a result, many

people with chronic pain report they have lost touch with friends and feel socially isolated. Sexual difficulties, increased irritability and withdrawal can result in relationship problems with partners and family.

Individuals who are activity cycling and avoiding activity find their life spinning out of control. In a multidimensional context, this is sometimes described as the downward spiral of pain (Fig. 22.2). Individuals may find their normal occupational roles eroded, so the 'income earner', 'parent', 'partner' and 'friend' that they viewed themselves as change as they become increasingly dependent financially, physically and emotionally on others. Many people report decreased self-confidence and a sense of increasing disability but also feel frustrated by others implying that they are malingering. This may come from friends, family and the public, but equally from healthcare professionals. Implied blame or psychogenic causes of disability are particularly destructive and give rise to a sense of personal hopelessness and distrust of healthcare professionals. This can adversely affect rehabilitation and therapists should be sensitive to concerns individuals may have about this.

Ultimately, disability as the result of back pain can have a devastating affect on the individual's quality of life. Sleep disturbance, low mood and anxiety are frequently associated with ongoing pain. As well as affecting physical and psychological wellbeing, the individual's earning capacity may be restricted, with all the associated social ill-effects for them and their family. For society, lost time at work has a practical and financial impact for employers and the wider economy. The cost of providing medical services and social support to people disabled by back pain is also rising.

THE TEAM

When an individual with back pain approaches a healthcare professional for the first time they should receive diagnostic triage. This distinguishes between simple backache, nerve root

How does pain affect you?

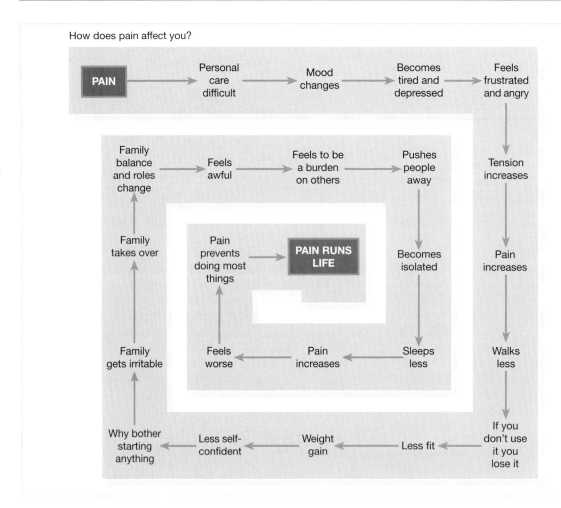

Fig. 22.2 The downward spiral of pain as described by participants of the November 1998 and January 1999 Pain Management Programmes at the King's Mill Centre for Healthcare Services National Health Service Trust.

problems and more serious spinal pathology or cauda equina syndrome (Box 22.2). Signs and symptoms of serious spinal pathology, known as red flags, are rare. However, if red flags or cauda equina symptoms are present they require urgent medical investigation.

Whatever the results of the assessment, the most effective intervention at this point is good communication. The message should be optimistic but realistic. Most back pain will resolve over a few weeks; back pain with nerve root entrapment may take a few months and recovery will be aided by returning to normal activity and work. If red flags are present, they only indicate further tests. Often these tests are negative. If back pain continues beyond 3–4 weeks, health professionals must be alert to potential long-term disability. Risk factors for long-term disability are called yellow flags and are covered in more detail on page 529.

Back pain is increasingly treated in the context of pain management programmes, usually run within a group setting. The Pain Society (1997) recommends that a pain management team include a 'medically qualified specialist in pain; clinical psychologist; physiotherapist; occupational therapist and nurse'. Table 22.1 gives an overview of these professionals and their roles in pain management teams. The composition of the team will be influenced by the client group for whom the programme is designed, such as prevention or early intervention for back pain,

---

Box 22.2 Diagnostic triage of low back pain (with permission from The Royal College of General Practitioners 1997)

Diagnostic triage is the differential diagnosis between:
- simple backache (non-specific low back pain)
- nerve root pain
- possible serious spinal pathology

Simple backache

Specialist referral not required:
- Presentation 20–55 years old
- Lumbosacral, buttocks and thighs
- 'Mechanical' pain
- Patient well

Nerve root pain

Specialist referral not generally required within first 4 weeks, provided resolving:
- unilateral leg pain worse than low back pain
- radiates to foot or toes
- numbness and paraesthesia in same direction
- straight leg raise reproduces leg pain
- localised neurological signs

Red flags for possible serious spinal pathology

Prompt referral (less than 4 weeks):
- presentation under age 20 or onset over 55
- non-mechanical pain
- thoracic pain
- past history – carcinoma, steroids, HIV
- unwell, weight loss
- widespread neurology
- structural deformity

Cauda equina syndrome

Immediate referral:
- sphincter disturbance
- gait disturbance
- saddle anaesthesia

Table 22.1 The core and extended team members in pain management programmes and their roles

Team member	Core skills	Shared skills
Doctor	Medical screening and provision of appropriate treatment under the medical model	Doctors are rarely directly involved in pain management programmes, although they sometimes attend as 'invited speakers' on topics such as medication
Psychologist	Facilitating identifying and addressing dysfunctional thought processes such as catastrophising, overgeneralisation, low frustration tolerance, external locus of control, mislabelling somatic sensations and irrational beliefs about pain Facilitating identifying and addressing cognitions, affect behaviour associated with low mood and anxiety	Education on physiological and psychological aspects of pain Relaxation techniques Goal setting Sleep strategies Facilitating identifying and addressing incorrect and unhelpful beliefs about pain Facilitating and supporting helpful adaptive behaviours to manage pain
Physiotherapist	Graded exercise programme Education on exercise, anatomy, posture and conservative pain relief modalities	
Occupational therapist	Pacing in ADLs Education on ergonomic techniques and ergonomic adaptation of the environment Functional goal setting Facilitating return to work	
Specialist nurse	Education and information on TENS, nerve blocks and epidurals Support with appropriate medication use and reduction	

Other team members and invited speakers may include:

- pharmacist
- dietician
- Disability Employment Advisors
- past programme members and self-help group members
- complementary practitioners such as T'ai chi and yoga instructors

management of chronic pain or special focus on people with profound physical disability, affective changes or limited social support.

Individually and collectively, team members bring unique professional skills to the treatment of both acute and chronic back pain. They enable the individual to develop skills in the management of his pain. Team members' roles frequently overlap, as described in Table 22.1, and this can be used to ensure consistent messages are given to group participants.

Depending on the clinical setting and resources available in the area, one-to-one interventions may be offered, usually as part of a wider team, such as a surgical, rheumatological or community team.

FOUNDATIONS FOR PRACTICE

From the beginning of the 20th century, therapeutic intervention for spinal disorder and back pain has focused on resolution of the spinal disorder and relief of pain. Since the mid-1970s, there has been a growing awareness that the simple presence of a spinal disorder does not account for back pain and that a biomedical approach cannot always provide adequate relief from pain. Instead, research has focused on why back pain is increasingly associated with disability and what interventions may be offered to prevent disability or help people regain functional activity.

The following section provides an overview of current theories on pain, disability as the result of pain and treatment approaches. A list of books providing a more in-depth understanding of these theories is found in the Further reading section (see p538).

GATE CONTROL THEORY OF PAIN

This theory, put forward by Melzack and Wall in 1965, describes a mechanism by which pain impulses could be modulated. Previous to this, impulses from a painful stimulus, such as stubbing a toe, were described as following a pain

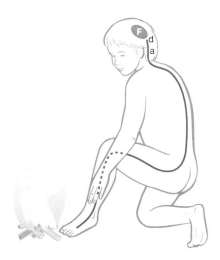

Fig. 22.3 The traditional Cartesian model of specific pain pathways.

If for example fire comes near the foot, the minute particles of this fire, which as you know have a great velocity, have the power to set in motion the spot of the skin of the foot which they touch, and by this means pulling upon the delicate thread which is attached to the spot of the skin, they open up at the same instant the pore against which the delicate thread ends, just as by pulling at one end of a rope one makes to strike at the same instant a bell which hangs at the other end. (Foster 1901, as translated from Descartes 1664)

pathway from the nociceptors directly to the brain, where the stimulus would be perceived as pain (Fig. 22.3). Melzack and Wall (1965) described a conceptual gate, lying in the dorsal horn of the spinal cord and receiving impulses from the nociceptors. This pain gate regulates the transmission of impulses to the brain. The intensity of impulses transmitted on up to the brain depends on the activity of other afferent nerve fibres entering the gate and also on descending fibres from the brain (Fig. 22.4). The more 'open' the gate, the more intensely pain is perceived by the individual. If the gate is closed, no pain will be perceived. Different physical and psychological conditions that open and close the pain gate are described in Box 22.3. An understanding of gate control theory can help individuals take greater control of their pain through the conscious use of cognitive and behavioural techniques to close the pain gate.

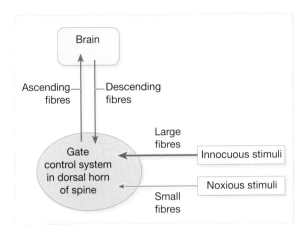

Fig. 22.4 Gate control theory of pain.

Box 22.3   Cognitive, affective and physical factors thought to open and close the pain gate

Factors thought to close the pain gate:

- emergency/life-threatening situation
- distraction
- exercise
- relaxation
- massage
- transcutaneous electrical nerve stimulation (TENS)
- acupuncture.

Factors thought to open the pain gate:

- thinking about/concentrating on pain
- lack of exercise and immobility
- stress and tension
- fear of pain
- fatigue.

PAIN MECHANISMS

Pain is multidimensional in nature, a fact that becomes obvious when it is seen that the initial experience of pain triggers a response at several levels (Fig. 22.5). When tissue damage occurs, the inflammation process is activated. This inflammation sensitises nerve endings in the tissues so that they fire spontaneously, producing ongoing discomfort, such as a throbbing pain. The nerves fire more easily to mechanical stimulation, making the tissues markedly more sensitive to pain. Pain helps to induce behavioural change, such as resting and guarding the injured area, thus providing the best possible conditions for healing. If this were the only active pain mechanism, it would follow that pain would cease once healing was complete. However, other mechanisms are also triggered, which, in the acute stages of injury, promote recovery. If these mechanisms continue beyond healing they may maintain behavioural changes such as resting and interfere with functional recovery. In brief, these mechanisms are (Gifford 1998):

- nociceptive mechanisms – pain derived from the tissue response as described above
- peripheral neurogenic mechanisms – pain arising from abnormal impulses generated by peripheral nerves
- central mechanisms – neuroplastic changes in the brain resulting in alterations in the processing of afferent information, perceived as pain
- sympathetic motor mechanisms – sympathetic and motor responses capable of enhancing pain
- affective mechanisms – negative and emotional responses reinforce pain and affect capacity to cope with pain.

Figure 22.5 demonstrates the interactive nature of the pain mechanisms. Pain mechanism theories suggest that the individual may more effectively manage his ongoing pain by maintaining or regaining functional activity, pacing those activities and exercising. Reducing emotional distress and addressing other factors that increase sympathetic nervous activity may also be helpful.

PAIN BELIEFS

There is considerable evidence (Waddell 1998) that an individual's understanding and beliefs about the pain he is experiencing strongly influence his risk of becoming chronically disabled. Reduced physical function in people with ongoing back pain is highly correlated to beliefs that pain is evidence of spinal damage and that spinal damage inevitably leads to disability. These beliefs can be reinforced by healthcare professionals through the language they use and advice they give. For

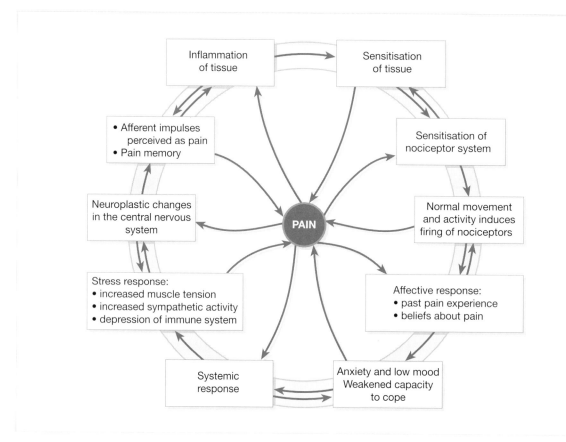

Fig. 22.5 Pain mechanisms triggered by pain and their interaction (inspired by Gifford 1998 description of pain mechanisms).

example, expressions such as 'crumbling spine' and 'slipped disc' can cause alarm in individuals who envisage catastrophic damage to the spine. This impression can be reinforced with advice to 'be careful' and 'rest', which is still sometimes advised (although it is not recommended practice). Addressing the individual's beliefs about back pain is pivotal in rehabilitation. An individual who still holds a belief that his pain is the result of catastrophic spinal damage exacerbated by movement will have little confidence in a therapist who appears to be 'ignoring the severity of his disorder'. This will give him little motivation to comply with advice to become more active.

FEAR AVOIDANCE THEORIES

Fear avoidance means that an individual tends to avoid activities because he fears increased pain

or reinjury. There may be many factors reinforcing this fear. Clearly, pain beliefs as described above are significant. For example, someone with back pain who believes it to be benign and unthreatening is more likely to confront his pain and engage in activity. However, if he believes that his pain, and any activity that aggravates it, indicates further spinal damage, he is more likely to avoid activity. Vlaeyen et al (1995) described a cognitive–behavioural model of fear of movement/(re)injury that shows how the individual's cognitive response to the pain experience was found to affect functional recovery (Fig. 22.6). A 'catastrophising response', that is, reading the pain as catastrophic, resulted in poor functional recovery. A non-catastrophic response resulted in confrontation of the pain and recovery.

The individual's ability to set realistic goals is also influential. If advised to exercise by his

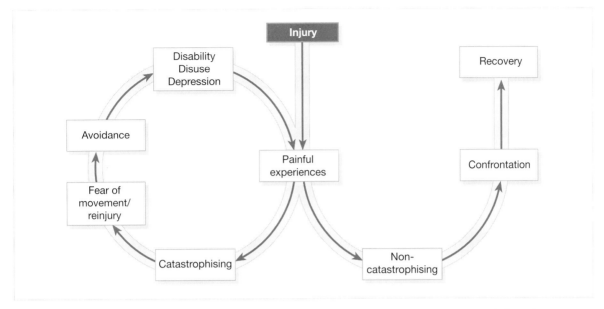

Fig. 22.6 Cognitive–behavioural model of fear of movement/(re)injury (reprinted from Vlaeyen et al (1995) Fear of movement/(re)injury in chronic low back pain and its relation to behavioural performance, Copyright 1995, pp363–372, with permission from Elsevier Science).

therapist, the individual who immediately begins to swim several lengths and then has a flare-up is less likely to attempt the exercise again. The individual who gradually builds up their swimming stamina will experience less pain and is more likely to maintain the activity. These responses are operantly maintained behaviours and are discussed in more detail below. As well as addressing pain beliefs, fear avoidance may be reduced by graded exposure to the feared activity as will appropriate goal setting and pacing.

PAIN BEHAVIOUR

Pain behaviours are the verbal and non-verbal ways that an individual uses to communicate his pain. This includes resting, guarding, use of sticks and aids, sighing and grimacing. These behaviours may have the effect of eliciting help from other people. This is a very useful response with an acute injury, providing optimal conditions for recovery. If pain continues beyond healing, these behaviours become unhelpful and self-reinforcing. The caring response of other people discourages the individual from carrying out activities independently, resulting in a loss of physical confidence. The individual may also become increasingly perceived as 'disabled', reinforcing his fears of the inevitability of disability. The concern and caring of others may be reassuring and rewarding for an individual. Unconsciously, this shapes the individual's behaviour through operant learning.

COGNITIVE–BEHAVIOURAL APPROACH

Many pain management programmes use a cognitive–behavioural approach. Avoidance of activities and pain behaviours can be reinforced by operant learning. Operant learning refers to the process by which the frequency of a given behaviour is modified by the consequences of that behaviour. An individual who feels rewarded – intrinsically or extrinsically – following an activity is more likely to engage in that activity again. Strategies such as pacing, goal setting and ergonomic assessment may all help to achieve a rewarding experience, rather than a punishing flare-up of pain.

Pain behaviour, meanwhile, may be extinguished by ignoring the pain behaviour and reinforcing 'well behaviour'. Individuals who feel disempowered by an overcaring family might not be aware of how their behaviour is eliciting this response. The individual could ask his family and friends to avoid offering help unless it is explicitly asked for.

Thoughts (cognitions), including beliefs, attitudes and expectations also shape behaviour. A cognitive approach explores the individual's fear of pain and expectations of disability. Individuals with ongoing pain have a higher risk of depression and anxiety and this may also increase pain perception, resulting in a vicious circle of increased pain, reduced activity and increased anxiety and depression. Identifying and addressing dysfunctional thought processes, such as catastrophising, can boost psychological coping skills.

STAGES OF CHANGE MODEL AND MOTIVATIONAL ENHANCEMENT THERAPY (MET)

Back pain management necessitates the individual actively changing maladaptive behaviour, such as activity cycling, to adaptive behaviours such as pacing. While these behaviours are rela-tively straightforward to learn, often the greatest challenge for the individual is recognising the need for, and following through, the process of change. Prochaska et al (1992) identified specific stages of change as people move from maladaptive behaviour to adaptive behaviours (Fig. 22.7). In brief, these are:

- precontemplation – the individual does not see a need for change and is not considering any change in his behaviour
- contemplation – the individual recognises the need to change, is thinking about carrying out that change in the near future but is still weighing up the pros and cons
- preparation – the individual has decided to make the change and begins to make some preparations to take action
- action – the individual adopts the new behaviour
- maintenance – the individual endeavours to sustain the new behaviour
- relapse – an individual who is unable to sustain the new behaviour enters the relapse stage from where he may continue the cycle of change again at the contemplation stage.

Relapse in this model is seen as part of the process of change. An individual may relapse several times before this behaviour is incorpo-

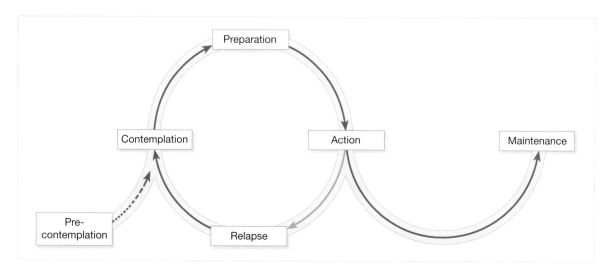

Fig. 22.7 A representation of a cycle of change (inspired by Prochaska et al's (1992) description of specific stages of change).

rated into his lifestyle and requires little effort to sustain.

Motivational enhancement therapy (MET) works on the premise that the therapist's interaction with the individual can enhance or hamper his motivation to change maladaptive behaviour (Jenson 1996). If the individual is strongly motivated to change, he alone will take responsibility for initiating and implementing that change. MET sets out five principles of therapist–client interaction that augment the individual's motivation to change:

- expressing empathy – reflective listening
- developing discrepancy – reflecting back to the individual the discrepancy between his behaviour and his goals in an empathic and supportive manner
- avoiding argumentation – the therapist should avoid argument for a behavioural change at all costs. This will only compel the individual to defend his current behaviour and inhibit motivation to change
- rolling with resistance – if the individual makes resistive statements, the therapist should not argue the point. Other strategies are recommended, including reflective listening.
- supporting self-efficacy – making statements and asking questions that promote the individual's hope and belief that they can change.

The therapist's task is to identify the individual's current stage and facilitate their advancement through the stages towards maintenance. Further information about MET and specific motivational strategies is listed in the Further reading section (see p542).

DEVELOPMENT OF DISABILITY AND YELLOW FLAGS

Most of the research (Waddell 1998) into the progression of disability with back pain has focused on loss of work time. The overwhelming consensus of these studies is that the longer an individual is off work, the less likely he is to return. This has important implications for intervention. If an individual is already off work when he consults a doctor for the first time he has a 10% chance of still being off sick 1 year later. This rises to 20% if still off sick at 1 month and to 50% at 6 months. Time off sick is therefore an important predictor of long-term disability and intervention at an early stage can be important in the prevention of chronic back pain and disability.

Waddell (1998) has shown that psychosocial factors are much better predictors of future disability than physical factors. For example, the nature and severity of the original injury seems to have little influence on whether that person becomes disabled by back pain. The same applies to the intensity of pain a person reports on first consultation. However, once an individual has lost 3 or 4 weeks at work due to back pain, whatever the cause, psychological and social factors become important in predicting his risk of becoming chronically disabled. These psychosocial risks are referred to as yellow flags. Some are described in Box 22.4. They are similar to the red flags described earlier in that they signal the need for appropriate intervention. In the case of yellow flags, this would be cognitive–behavioural management. The presence of yellow flags does not mean that the individual's

---

Box 22.4 Psychosocial yellow flags

- Unhelpful attitudes and beliefs about back pain, such as pain indicates tissue damage and back pain inevitably results in disability.
- Disproportionate illness or pain behaviour.
- Compensation or medicolegal proceedings.
- Diagnostic and treatment issues, such as poor understanding of diagnosis and its implications and an expectation that a cure lies in receiving treatment rather than self-management.
- Psychogenic distress and depressive symptoms, both as a result of major life events and anxiety in response to back pain.
- Personal problems, including alcoholism, marital and financial problems.
- Low job satisfaction.
- Total work loss (due to back pain) in past 12 months.
- Family beliefs and attitudes about the problem, such as 'pain should be ignored' or encouraging the individual to be 'careful and rest', and family taking on caring roles.
- Family's reinforcement of pain behaviour.

pain is any less real, only that the individual is at higher risk of developing chronic disability. An awareness of yellow flags and their implications is important when assessing and planning intervention.

ASSESSMENT AND INTERVENTION

A BIOPSYCHOSOCIAL MODEL FOR ASSESSMENT

Figure 22.8 illustrates a biopsychosocial model of the clinical presentation and assessment of people with low back pain and disability. The model combines the elements that contribute to the state of disability an individual is experiencing at any one time. All these elements, described above, should be included when assessing and planning intervention.

ASSESSMENT MEDIA

The precise focus of the occupational therapy assessment will depend on context of the referral, such as work-related or ADL functional difficulties, or following surgery. All assessment, however, should reflect the elements of the biopsychosocial model illustrated in Figure 22.8. There

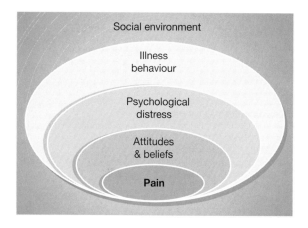

Fig. 22.8 A biopsychosocial model of the clinical presentation and assessment of low back pain and disability at one point in time (after Waddell et al 1984, with permission from BMJ Publishing Group).

are many standardised assessments and approaches covering these elements and the reader is advised to refer to Chapter 5 and the Further reading section (see p542). Occupational therapy assessments frequently occur in tandem with other members of the team, providing a complete picture of the individual's pain and disability.

Standardised functional assessments include the Canadian Occupational Performance Measure (Law et al 1994), which can be used clinically to aid goal setting and also as an audit tool. The Assessment of Motor and Process Skills (AMPS) measures the quality of a person's overall ability to perform domestic and personal activities. The 5-minute walk test and sit-to-stand test (Harding et al 1994) are physical function measures that can also provide feedback to an individual on their progress. Standardised self-report questionnaires are frequently used outcome measures and include the Oswestry (Fairbank et al 1980) and the Roland and Morris (1983) versions. Specific non-standardised assessments include ergonomic assessment of the home or work environment and ADL function.

INTERVENTION FOLLOWING SPINAL SURGERY

A small proportion of people with back pain are offered spinal surgery. In these cases, clinical signs and symptoms usually relate to investigation results and often involve neurological disturbance. The most common surgical interventions include spinal discectomy and decompression for disc prolapse and spinal fusion.

Following a discectomy, most people are able to return to activities of daily living without restriction. A soft corset may be issued by the occupational therapist to provide increased comfort postoperatively. Individuals should gradually reduce wearing time and cease using the corset by 6 weeks. Individuals awaiting spinal fusion or decompression may be assessed by an occupational therapist preoperatively. The assessment includes an initial interview followed by explanation of the postsurgery rehabilitation process. A 'spinal information booklet' not only provides a reference but might also include a height measurement sheet for home furniture, so potential transfer difficulties may be identified and dealt with quickly after surgery.

Following surgery, the general assessment covers cognitive function, mobility, transfers, personal and domestic ADL. Adaptive equipment may be issued for between 1 and 3 months to help the individual maintain a good posture and increase functional independence. He is encouraged to return to normal activities as soon as possible and a goal-setting approach may be used to aid this.

BACK SENSE AND ERGONOMICS

Ergonomics is the study of human characteristics and limitations that affect the design of equipment, environments, products, systems and jobs (Wilson 1995). Back care techniques are ergonomic approaches that help people understand 'how to perform safely, effectively, and comfortably within the environment' (Khalil et al 1993). These techniques are not primarily aimed at avoiding injury/re-injury, and this should be emphasised to people. Back care may then be better referred to in a more positive context, which does not imply that the back is fragile in any way. The authors prefer the use of 'back sense' to convey a sensible approach to carrying out activities that will reduce additional pain or discomfort brought on by poor or sustained postures and repetitive movements. This approach emphasises enabling the individual to engage in activities more confidently, over longer periods and of a wider range, rather than avoiding activities as a result of fear that the 'wrong' movement may cause an injury.

An understanding of ergonomics can help occupational therapists to support individuals in employment or in preparation for their return to work, and to liaise effectively with employers. Figure 22.9 shows the main risk factors associated with back pain at work. These are influenced by the organisation and design of people's work, as well as factors such as seating, work heights and the work environment.

Posture

A good posture is one that can be sustained with a minimum of static effort (Pheasant 1996). Static

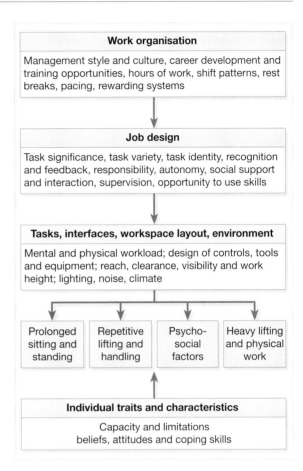

Fig. 22.9 An ergonomic model of back pain.

effort is characterised by prolonged muscular contraction. It requires higher energy consumption and heart rate, and longer rest periods. Activities should provide adequate rest breaks to allow tissue recovery and changes of posture so that different muscle groups are used.

Most people either stand or sit at work. Standing is more common where workers need to move around frequently, such as in the service industries and in handling heavy or large objects when the strong muscles of the lower body are needed to exert force. The upright standing position is more efficient, because little spinal muscular energy is required. However, standing for long periods can lead to aching legs and feet caused by venous congestion and oedema in the lower limbs, and to immobility of the joints of the feet, knees and hips (Kroemer & Grandjean

1997). A seated workplace is therefore usually preferred, although prolonged sitting can increase the risk of back pain. Sit–stand workplaces are sometimes a good compromise and dual-purpose seating is being developed for this purpose.

The height at which we carry out activities affects our posture. The most suitable height for a work surface will depend on the particular task and on the height of the worker. For example, heavy manipulative tasks such as sawing involve downwards pressure and a working height of 100–250 mm below elbow height is recommended (Pheasant 1996). However, for lighter tasks this would be too low. The trunk, neck and head would be flexed forwards, which would result in fatigue of the muscles if the position were held for long. Stooped postures can also result from inadequate reach and clearance, for example, lack of toe recesses, having to reach over obstacles or not being able to see clearly.

Sitting provides stability for carrying out fine manipulative tasks, uses less energy than standing and is less fatiguing for the lower limbs. However, in relaxed unsupported sitting, the pelvis rotates backwards. To allow the trunk to remain vertical, the lumbar spine compensates by flexing forwards, which 'flattens out' the lumbar lordosis or curve. Initially, this position is more comfortable because the back muscles are relaxed. Over long periods, however, this posture can lead to stretching of the posterior ligaments of the spine and can raise intradiscal pressure (Oliver & Middleditch 1991). This effect can be decreased by slightly inclining the backrest and increasing the lumbar support. Forward-tilting seats can also encourage good spinal posture by reducing the angle of flexion.

Seating should be matched to the demands of the activity and the dimensions of the individual user, for example, hip width, popliteal height, and thigh length. Prolonged sitting prevents variation in movement, reducing the flow of nutrients to the discs. So the design of seated work and activity should encourage frequent changes in posture, whether this is driving, video display unit (VDU) work, operating an industrial sewing machine or simply watching television.

European Community legislation has imposed strict guidelines on seating and work surface heights (Directive 89/654/EEC). In the United Kingdom this is implemented through the Workplace (Health Safety and Welfare) Regulations (1992), which require all employers to arrange workstations and provide seating that is suitable for the work being carried out. Guidance is available through the Health & Safety Commission Approved Code of Practice L24 (1992). Students and therapists practising in regions other than the EU are advised to consult their own national requirements for seating and workstations, as their implications are important for assessing and planning intervention.

Workstations where VDUs, process control screens and the like are used are also subject to the Health and Safety (Display Screen Equipment) Regulations (1992), again in response to EC legislation (Directive 90/270/EEC). Guidance is available through the Health & Safety Executive document L26 (1992).

Manual handling, lifting and heavy physical work

The European Community Directive guiding the reduction of manual handling risks (90/269/EEC) is implemented in the United Kingdom through the Manual Handling Operations Regulations (1992). These regulations are made under the Health & Safety at Work Act (1974). Guidance is available through the Health & Safety Executive document L23 (1992). No specific weight limits are set because, in reality, there is no such thing as a 'safe' lift. Safe manual handling entails consideration of several characteristics – those of the individual worker, the working environment, the load itself and the particular task. Basic guideline figures for lifting and lowering are given but need to be adjusted according to the interaction of these characteristics.

Manual handling risk factors include pushing, pulling, sudden exertion of force, bending and twisting, and lifting. Poor posture and excessive repetition are influencing factors. Holding a load closer to the body requires less effort by the back muscles than holding it away from the body. The load can be more easily counterbalanced by the weight of the body and is less likely to get out of control. Symmetrical lifting avoids torsional or twisting loads on the spine.

Psychosocial factors

Despite greater understanding of biomechanical influences on the spine, and the introduction of extensive legislation to minimise manual handling risks, reports of work-related back pain continue to rise. Failure to explain the reasons for this rise simply through physical factors has led to a change in focus, looking at the influences of psychological, organisational and sociological factors. A number of studies have shown that individual, subjective perceptions of the organisation of work are also thought to be closely associated with reports of back pain. Factors thought to be most influential include: the amount of social support available, the amount of control, the mental demands of the job, responsibilities, the variety of the work, recognition for work done and supervisor support. Individuals need to feel that their work has some significance or value and, if possible, to complete whole jobs rather than small parts of them. Job satisfaction very much depends on whether individual needs are being met and individual values fulfilled. A job that is seen as boring, unfulfilling and unrewarding may strongly affect a worker's readiness to report a back problem.

Although the ergonomic model outlined above is linked to the workplace, the same principles can be applied to any purposeful activity. For example, gardening can be a heavy activity and can provoke back pain but if we can exercise choice and control over when and how we do it, pace ourselves, and vary the different parts of the activity then we can minimise the risk of pain. Using well-designed and maintained tools and equipment will also help. Admiration from friends and family and a personal sense of pleasure and achievement may affect our response to discomfort.

PAIN MANAGEMENT PROGRAMMES

Pain management programmes are usually implemented by a multidisciplinary team. There is often a blurring of roles between team members and some of the more generic interventions are described below. Those more specific, though not exclusive, to occupational therapists are described in more detail, including goal setting, pacing, ergonomics, workshop and return to work.

Education

Providing information on pain and the development of disability is key in addressing people's misperceptions about pain and tissue damage, often referred to as 'hurt versus harm'. Topics include basic back anatomy, diagnosis, pain gates and mechanisms of pain. The overall message should reinforce the fact that the spine is a strong structure and that back pain does not mean catastrophic spinal damage has occurred, or is occurring.

Stress and depression management

Ongoing pain and disability often contribute to heightened anxiety and vulnerability to depression. In turn, stress and depression tend to open pain gates, increasing pain perception. The importance of tackling negative thoughts, especially catastrophising, is often emphasised during the management of stress and depression. Such maladaptive cognitions increase not only the individual's risk of stress and depression but also the risk of becoming and remaining disabled by pain.

Relaxation

Relaxation is often used as an aid to stress management but, in the case of pain management, it also helps to teach conscious reduction of muscle tone, which is frequently increased as an automatic response to pain. Some individuals are able to use self-suggestion techniques to 'close' their pain gate, providing partial or complete pain relief for a while.

Sleep management

Sleep management includes standard strategies for tackling insomnia but may also embrace pacing for intolerance to specific lying positions, advice on supportive beds, mattresses and pillows, and positioning. A pain nurse or pharmacist may provide advice on appropriate medication use.

Goal setting

Goal setting is a useful technique in both prevention of disability and rehabilitation from chronic disability. It allows the individual to set a realistic timetable to return to normal activity and provides milestones by which the individual can monitor his progress.

Those experiencing an acute or subacute episode of back pain are encouraged to return to previous levels of activity, ideally including exercise in their lifestyle if this has been missing. To prevent activity cycling as described earlier, activity levels should be built up gradually and goals set accordingly. If activity cycling is already established, goal setting should include pacing. When setting a goal, the individual should ask if the goal is:

- Relevant – to increase motivation, the goal set must be important to him
- Realistic – if he believes the goal to be beyond his ability, he will be disinclined to attempt it. Long-term goals can be broken down into short-term goals, turning a mountain into a series of molehills
- Time-limited – just as a short-term goal increases motivation, an achievable time limit motivates action rather than just contemplation
- Measurable – what exactly does he intend to achieve within the time limit? How would others be able to observe that he had achieved it?

The individual also needs to consider how he will reward his achievements. An extrinsic reward may help to reinforce intrinsic satisfaction when a goal is achieved. This may be especially relevant for people with chronic disability, as motivation and self-efficacy are often low.

Pacing

Pacing activities is a behavioural adaptation to overcome activity cycling (as described in Fig. 22.1) and disuse syndrome. Pacing aims to flatten-out fluctuations in rest and overactivity, gradually increasing the level of activity the individual can tolerate without causing flare-ups. Pacing is implemented in two stages. First the individual learns to pace his activity in two ways:

1. to limit the time spent in one posture such as standing, sitting and walking
2. to limit the total time spent on any one functional activity such as shopping, playing golf or vacuuming.

Setting-up a pacing schedule

The individual should be clear what he is trying to achieve by discussing activity cycling and pacing. The difference between increased pain and aching as a result of activity or exercise and flare-ups of pain needs to be explored with the individual. The aim of pacing is to reduce prolonged periods of inactivity as a result of flare-ups of pain. Both the therapist and individual setting up the pacing schedule should keep this in mind.

A baseline pacing time then needs to be set for individual postures. This usually includes sitting, standing and walking, but may be expanded to include postures required for specific activities important to the individual. Some examples include:

- kneeling to play with grandchildren
- stretching with arms above head to clean the windows
- lying in a certain position in bed that is normally painful and wakes the individual.

Finding the baseline

Once the individual has decided which postures and activities he wants to start pacing (using the goal-setting process), he must set a baseline for each one. Initially, he should keep a diary (Fig. 22.10) of how long he can tolerate the activity or posture for. For example, he could time for how long he can 'comfortably' walk. He may need advice or a definition of 'comfortable', as many people report immediate pain on walking.

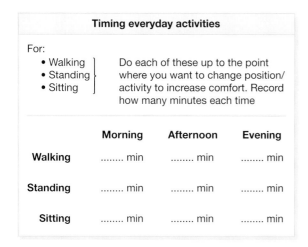

Timing everyday activities			
For: • Walking • Standing • Sitting	Do each of these up to the point where you want to change position/activity to increase comfort. Record how many minutes each time		

	Morning	Afternoon	Evening
Walking	.... min	.... min	.... min
Standing	.... min	.... min	.... min
Sitting	.... min	.... min	.... min

Fig. 22.10 Diary to record time able to tolerate a sustained activity or posture.

Most people recognise there is a point at which they would rather 'sit down' or 'stand for a moment', even if they could push on for a bit longer. This inclination to change posture should be taken as the end of the 'comfortable' time.

This measurement should be taken at least three times, preferably on 'bad pain' and 'better' days. Find the average of the times measured and subtract between 20% and 50%. The percentage subtracted depends to some extent on the clinical setting. If the individual has a physiotherapist, liaise with them to agree a percentage. This will make it easier for the individual to use in both settings.

The baseline represents a level of activity that can be maintained, even on bad pain days. A lower baseline that the individual can easily achieve on a bad pain day will boost his self-confidence and sense of achievement.

Pacing by time

Once the baselines have been set, the individual can begin to use pacing. Goal setting allows the individual to focus on and pace one or two functional activities. Once the basic skill and discipline of pacing has been practised, many people find it easy to generalise to other activities of daily living.

The individual should consider what postures their selected activity involves and how they might break the activity up to ensure they do not maintain any one posture for longer than their baseline time. The total length of time carrying out the activity should also be considered and included in the pacing schedule.

For example, pricking out seedlings might involve standing at a worktop for about half an hour. The pacing plan might be:

- stand and work: 2 minutes
- sit on stool and work: 5 minutes
- stand and work: 2 minutes
- go for a drink: 10 minutes
- stand and work: 2 minutes
- sit on a stool and work: 5 minutes
- stand and work: 2 minutes
- finish for today and repeat routine over next 2 days.

Once the individual has tried out and successfully used the pacing baselines, they can gradually increase their pacing time. Gradual increase is the key and, as a rule of thumb, the time should not be increased by more that 20% a week; less than this is acceptable. The individual must have time to both build his confidence and adapt physically to the new level of activity. A large increase that results in a flare-up of pain is counterproductive and feeds into the overactivity/rest cycle. The individual must take active responsibility for preventing this.

To aid pacing by time, countdown timers and alarm clocks are often helpful. Some models have a vibrating alarm, which may be used more discreetly in social situations.

Other methods of pacing

Pacing is often a difficult behaviour to adopt, especially if the individual is accustomed to pushing themselves to their pain limit. Most people find 'pacing by time' a clear and unambiguous method to learn this new behaviour but it does not suit everyone. In this situation, it is preferable to ask the individual, armed with an understanding of activity cycling and pacing, to decide how they might use pacing in a way that suits their temperament. For example, other pacing methods include quantity, for example, ironing only two shirts, washing up four cups, digging a square foot of garden, washing the wheels, bonnet and doors of a car at separate times. Alternatively, time could be used in a more general way. For example, take a break every 10 minutes, don't hold a posture for more than 20 minutes.

Successful pacing and increased activity tolerance will build the individual's confidence when carrying out activities of daily living. This increases the likelihood that he will go on to broaden the activities he is prepared to attempt, including his eventual return to work.

Workshop activity

Workshops are used in the context of pain management and as a media for work hardening. The workshop provides a supportive environment for individuals to engage in and increase their confidence in heavy work activity. It also provides a setting to practise pacing and back sense (Fig. 22.11), initially under the guidance of the therapist. Ultimately, the individual should aim to develop the adaptive techniques as habitual behaviours. Distraction is also a powerful cognitive technique for closing the pain gates. Individuals should be encouraged to consider how they may expand activities they enjoy to capitalise on this benefit.

RETURN TO WORK

The occupational therapist's role in facilitating return to work is becoming ever more important. Many people with chronic back pain will be being paid by their employer, in receipt of benefits or unemployed. To many the possibility of return to work seems like a distant dream. With increasing time spent away from work there is a loss of self-confidence, self-esteem and self-worth. Thoughts of being 'no use to anyone' are common. The individual becomes isolated, lacks motivation, and is also physically less active.

It is generally accepted that work is an essential part of life (MacDonald 1976). It provides people with economic, psychological, physical

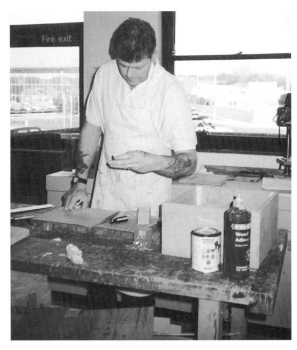

Fig. 22.11 A participant of a back pain programme uses a timer to pace his activity in the workshop. He alternates between sitting and standing to work, and may include timed rest breaks or walks in his pacing schedule.

and social benefits (Anthony & Blanch 1987). There has been a trend towards the therapist intervening in the workplace (Hook 1985–1986). The therapist is able to view the exact role of the individual, their tasks, their ability to complete those tasks and look at the other pressures that might have an effect on their general wellbeing. Job analysis of this sort is termed an ergonomic assessment.

The occupational therapist can identify potential problem areas that can be resolved easily. If time can be spent observing the individual in their work role, additional aspects can be observed, such as attitudes of other colleagues towards the individual with back pain, and treatment approaches such as pacing can be encouraged. Communication with the individual's manager, occupational health or human resources department can also help to integrate the individual into work. Planning a graduated return and providing support will all help. Back pain is little understood by the general population and information about it should be provided to those working with the individual. An ergonomic report or job analysis report can be forwarded to the employer who can then action the recommendations. Alternatively, funding for equipment may be available from government or voluntary sources.

Work tolerance screening (Hook 1985, 1986) is another approach to help with the return to work. This has been used within reports of therapists for compensation claims. This screening may involve the therapist spending some time observing the individual carrying out several tasks in order to reflect the demands of a job. To

a degree, it is often difficult to make an accurate assessment as this is in a simulated environment and people with back pain may be able to carry out a task in this situation but experience pain several hours after the activity without the therapist's knowledge.

If an individual is currently unemployed due to their back pain, they may need to look at retraining options, job search skills, work placements and other supported employment options. It is important to motivate the individual to search out these options so that he is empowered to make his own choices.

ACKNOWLEDGEMENTS

I would like to thank my colleagues who have contributed to the writing of this chapter, including Carol Coole (Ergonomics), Alison Biggs (Return to work), Susan Brennan and Jessica Harrison (Surgery), and Amanda Farr (AMPS). Many colleagues have read the draft and offered much-appreciated comments, suggestions, amendments and material including Pat O'Hara, Louis Gifford, Jenny Radcliffe, Dr David Walsh, Deirdre Madeley, Meg Birch, Margaret Wheeler, Jackie Adams and Louise Aylwin. Many thanks to the members of the East Midlands Special Interest Group in Pain for their contributions and to the members of King's Mill Centre NHS Trust Back Pain Team for their full support and encouragement. Finally, thank you to my husband, Dermot, who encouraged me throughout and my daughter, Brigid, who was born during the writing of this chapter.

REFERENCES

Adams N 1997 The psychophysiology of low back pain. Churchill Livingstone, New York

Anthony WA, Blanch A 1987 Supported employment for persons who are psychiatrically disabled: a historical and conceptual perspective. Psychosocial Rehabilitation Journal 11:5–23

Callaghan DK 1993 Work hardening for a client with low back pain. American Journal of Occupational Therapy 47:645–649

Clinical Standards Advisory Group (CSAG) 1994 Back pain. HMSO, London

Directive 89/654/EEC. Commission of European Communities (CEC) 1989 Council Directive concerning the minimum safety and health requirements for the workplace. Official Journal of the European Communities, No. L 393 1–12, Brussels

Directive 90/270/EEC. Commission of European Communities (CEC) 1990 Council Directive on the minimum safety and health requirements for work with display screen equipment. Official Journal of the European Communities, No. L 156 14–18, Brussels

Directive 90/269/EEC. Commission of European Communities (CEC) 1990 Council Directive on the minimum health and safety requirements for the manual handling of loads where there is a risk particularly of back injury to workers. Official Journal of the European Communities 33 No. L 156 9–13, Brussels

Fairbank J, Couper J, Davies J, O'Brian J 1980 The Oswestry Low Back Pain Disability Questionnaire. Physiotherapy 66:271–273

Foster M 1901 Lectures on the history of physiology during the sixteenth, seventeenth and eighteenth centuries. Cambridge University Press, Cambridge (translated from Descartes R 1664 L' homme)

Gifford L (ed) 1998 Topical issues in pain: whiplash: science and management. Fear-avoidance behaviour. NOI Press, Falmouth

Harding V, Simmonds M, Watson P 1998 Physical therapy for chronic pain. Pain VI (3):1–4

Harding V, C de C Williams A, Richardson P, Nicholas M, Jackson J, Richardson I, Pither C 1994 The development of a battery of measures for assessing physical functioning of chronic pain patients. Pain 58:367–375

Health & Safety Commission 1992 Workplace health, safety and welfare. Approved code of practice L24. HSE Books, Sudbury, Suffolk

Health & Safety Executive 1992 Display screen equipment work. Guidance on the health and safety (display screen equipment) regulations. L26. HSE Books, Sudbury, Suffolk

Health & Safety Executive 1992 Guidance on manual handling operations regulations L23. HSE Books, Sudbury, Suffolk

Health and safety (display screen equipment) regulations 1992 UK Government statutory instrument no. 2792. HMSO, Norwich

Hook TW 1985–1986 A private practice work evaluation unit. Occupational Therapy in Health Care 2(4):59–65

Jenson M 1996 Enhancing motivation to change in pain treatment. In: Gatchel R, Turk D (eds) Psychological approaches to pain: a practitioner's handbook. The Guilford Press, New York, ch 4, p 78

Khalil TM, Abdel-Moty EM, Rosomoff RS, Rosomoff HL 1993 Ergonomics in back pain: a guide to prevention and rehabilitation. Van Nostrand Reinhold, New York

Kroemer KHE, Grandjean E 1997 Fitting the task to the human, 5th edn. Taylor & Francis, London

Law M, Baptiste S, Carswell A, McColl M, Polatajko H, Pollock N 1994 Canadian Occupational Performance Measure, 2nd edn. CAOT Publications Ace, Toronto, Ottawa

MacDonald EM (ed) 1976 Occupational therapy in rehabilitation, 4th edn. Baillière Tindall, London

Manual handling operations regulations 1992 UK Government statutory instrument no. 2793. HMSO, Norwich

Melzack R, Wall PD 1965 Pain mechanisms: a new theory. Science 150:971–979

Merskey H, Bogduk N 1994 Classification of chronic pain, 2nd edn. IASP Press, Seattle, WA

O'Hara P 1996 Pain management for health professionals. Chapman & Hall, London

Oliver J, Middleditch A 1991 Functional anatomy of the spine. Butterworth-Heinemann, Oxford

Pheasant S 1996 Bodyspace: anthropometry, ergonomics and the design of work, 2nd edn. Taylor & Francis, London

Prochaska JO, DiClemente CC, Norcross JC 1992 In search of how people change: applications to addictive behaviours. American Psychologist 47(9):1102–1114

Roland M, Morris R 1983 Roland and Morris Disability Questionnaire. Harper & Row, New York

Royal College of General Practitioners (RCGP) 1997 National low back pain clinical guidelines. RCGP, London

Strong J 1996 Chronic pain: the occupational therapist's perspective. Churchill Livingstone, New York

The Pain Society 1997 Desirable criteria for pain management programmes. Report of a Working Party of The Pain Society of Great Britain and Ireland

Turk D, Melzack R 1992 Handbook of pain assessment. The Guilford Press, New York

UK Government 1974 Health and Safety at Work Act. HMSO, Norwich

Vlaeyen JWS, Kole-Snijders AMJ, Boeren RGB, Eek HV 1995 Fear of movement/(re)injury in chronic low back pain and its relation to behavioural performance. Pain 62:363–372

Waddell G, Bircher M, Finlayson D, Main CJ 1984 Symptoms and signs: physical illness or illness behaviour? British Medical Journal 289:739–741

Waddell G 1998 The back pain revolution. Churchill Livingstone, Edinburgh

Wilson JR 1995 A framework and a context for ergonomics methodology. In: Wilson JR, Corlett EN (eds) Evaluation of human work, 2nd edn. Taylor & Francis, London, pp 1–39

Workplace (Health, Safety and Welfare Regulations) 1992. UK Statutory Instrument No. 3004. HMSO, Norwich

FURTHER READING

Pain mechanisms, psychosocial aspects of pain and pain management

Gifford L (ed) 2000 Topical issues in pain 2: biopsychosocial assessment and management. Relationships and pain. CNS Press (formerly NOI Press) Falmouth

HMSO The Back Pain Book. The Stationery Office, London

Occupational therapy assessment and intervention

Turk D, Melzack R 1992 Handbook of pain assessment. The Guilford Press, New York

Motivational enhancement therapy

Jenson M 1996 Enhancing motivation to change in pain treatment. In: Gatchel R, Turk D (eds) Psychological approaches to pain: a practitioner's handbook. The Guilford Press, New York, ch 4, p 78

USEFUL CONTACTS

achesandpainsonline:
http://www.achesandpainsonline.com/
The International Association for the Study of Pain:
http://www.halcyon.com/iasp/index.html

Fighting Back: http://www.fightingback.co.uk/
The Royal College of General Practitioners:
http://www.rcgp.org.uk/

23

Rheumatoid arthritis

Alison Hammond   Paula Jeffreson

INTRODUCTION

The major concerns of people with rheumatoid arthritis (RA) are frustration in performing everyday activities, fears about disability and dependency on others, pain and loss of self-esteem. RA is a chronic, progressive inflammatory disease primarily affecting joints, characterised by pain and fatigue. People can experience multiple joint and other systemic effects for decades. The disease course is extremely variable between individuals and psychological status and social support affect its progress.

RA develops from early adulthood onwards, affecting three times as many women as men. It usually starts between 25 and 55 years and may cause difficulties with: establishing or consolidating long-term relationships, childcare and family obligations, running the home, developing a career, maintaining a job and wider social roles. Fatigue and pain can mean there is little energy left for leisure after day-to-day commitments. The disease and its effects can increase life stress, further worsening disease symptoms. There is an established link between stress and RA outcomes.

ONSET, PATHOLOGY AND PROGRESS

RA often starts intermittently with flitting hand and foot pain, general fatigue, diffuse aching and morning stiffness. Over time, disease activity becomes sustained, spreading to other joints. Some have an acute, severe onset. There are periodic exacerbations or 'flares', that is, periods of multiple, severe joint swelling and pain. Between these, the disease is varyingly active and it can go into remission.

Inflammation of the synovial lining of joints, tendon sheaths and bursae leads to thickened synovium and excess synovial fluid, increasing pressure on nerve endings and causing pain. Swelling stretches and weakens joint capsules and ligaments. Inflammation directly infiltrates and erodes joint capsules, ligaments, cartilage and subchondral bone. Joint erosion and deformity occur progressively. About 15% of people have mild, self-limiting disease, which can be reversible; 25% have persistent disease with mild to moderate joint damage; 50% have progressive deformity and disability; and 10% become severely disabled (Pincus 1996). Advances in drug therapy mean outcomes are improving but many people are reticent to take disease-modifying drugs long term because of concerns about side-effects.

IMPACT OF RA

The largely 'hidden' nature of pain and fatigue mean problems may be poorly appreciated by family, friends or work colleagues at first (Box 23.1).

Box 23.1 Possible reactions when coming to terms with living with RA (adapted from le Gallez 1993, Ryan 1996, Williams & Wood 1988)

- Frustration and anger at increasing difficulties with ordinary activities.
- The need for more information about the disease, drug and self-management strategies and open communication with health professionals.
- A fear of 'appearing different' and losing one's standards.
- Lowered self-esteem and self-efficacy.
- Feelings of loss of control and helplessness as greater functional problems develop.
- Living with uncertainties: about disease progression, fear of disability, losing meaningful roles.
- Fear of burdening others and distressing loved ones.

PHYSICAL EFFECTS

These include painful and swollen joints. Muscle wasting develops as the disease affects muscle fibres and pain reduces activity levels, causing deconditioning. There is a reduction in range of movement and structural joint changes, combined with mechanical stress during daily activities, produce deformity over time. In the hand, metacarpophalangeal (MCP) and proximal interphalangeal (PIP) swelling, wasting of the interossei and dorsal swelling (tenosynovitis of the common extensor tendon sheath) are early features, causing difficulty with pinch and dexterity. Later, wrist dorsal subluxation and radial deviation develop, reducing grip strength, which is on average only 20% of normal. Ulnar deviation and dorsal subluxation develop at the MCPs, and swan-neck and boutonnière deformities are seen in the fingers. Over one-third of people with RA have hand deformities with impaired hand function within 4 years of onset. Almost half develop MCP ulnar deviation in 5 years (Bishop et al 1991).

The feet are affected early. Common deformities are: metatarsal head subluxation, in which the fibrofatty pad protecting the ball of the foot displaces – reported as 'walking on marbles'; hallux valgus (bunions); and toe clawing. Deformities, along with foot pain and weakened longitudinal arches, cause difficulty walking and in prolonged standing. As the disease progresses, range of movement in the hip, knee, neck, shoulder and elbow becomes limited, causing more problems with outdoor mobility, driving and using transport, reaching and carrying and with household and self-care tasks.

Systemic features include vague ill-health, undue fatigue and decreased stamina, poor appetite and weight loss. Fatigue is reported by 90% of patients (Belza 1996) and its effect is often underestimated and not perceived as being due to RA (Box 23.2).

RA can also affect the heart, liver, blood vessels and lungs.

FUNCTIONAL AND SOCIAL EFFECTS

RA is generally worse in women and can have a major impact on a sufferer's life (Box 23.3).

Box 23.2   Factors contributing to fatigue

- Higher disease activity.
- Sleep patterns disturbed by pain.
- Pain and stiffness causing psychological distress.
- Deconditioning – cardiorespiratory and muscular systems are less efficient at producing and using energy because of inactivity.
- Anaemia, either due to RA or as a side-effect of medication.
- Depression and stress.
- Poor nutrition.

Box 23.3   Percentage of women with RA experiencing role/functional difficulties

RA for less than 2 years (Eberhardt et al 1990)

- 50–60% housework, shopping, leisure, social activities
- 35% family and parent roles; early retirement due to ill health.

RA for 10 years or more (Reisine et al 1987)

- 89% leisure
- 88% housework
- 66% shopping
- 53% work (giving up, reduced hours or increased sick leave)
- 42% cooking
- 42% family and social roles.

Disruption of homemaking, nurturing and work roles affects an individual's sense of identity and reduces satisfaction, self-esteem and the work–social support network. Declining financial status can cause difficulties and limits social and leisure opportunities. On average, income is reduced by 50% and money worries can contribute to stress. Three-quarters of people with RA are forced to alter leisure activities because of this disease and half are dissatisfied as a result (Fex et al 1998). Loss of valued activities, particularly leisure, is significantly associated with depression and poorer quality of life.

Sexual difficulties can result from joint pain and reduced mobility affecting positioning. Fatigue, systemic symptoms causing vaginal dryness and drug side-effects also affect sexual performance. Hand and upper limb pain can limit touching and caressing. Depression can reduce sexual drive and people may have feel-ings of unattractiveness; partners may feel less physically and emotionally wanted.

Family roles can change. A partner may become the sole breadwinner or have to seek work. Partners may need to do more childcare and housework than they have done previously. The family's social activities may become limited and friends and relatives visit less often. Families with well-developed structures adjust but people with RA have a higher rate of divorce and separation. Positive social support is significantly associated with better outcome in RA.

PSYCHOLOGICAL EFFECTS

Many experience psychological distress at some point. Depression is estimated at 20%, three times higher than in the general population, and can have a significant effect on pain and disability. Higher levels of social support (e.g. providing needed assistance and information, listening to concerns, care and affection) are associated with better psychological, social, home and family functioning (Blalock & de Vellis 1992).

Psychological status directly effects the health of people with RA. Those with greater perceived control of their disease symptoms have a more positive mood, greater satisfaction with physical and functional abilities, better dexterity, a better sense of psychological wellbeing, greater belief in their ability to control pain and perform everyday activities, less functional impairment and less pain. Those with more flexible cognitive and behavioural coping responses, for example, information seeking, problem solving and self-management, have greater psychological adjustment (Blalock et al 1993). Psychological status can be improved through structured therapy. The interrelationship between problems and symptoms is illustrated in Figure 23.1.

ADJUSTING TO LIVING WITH RA

Shaul (1995) summarised three stages in the process of learning to live with RA:

- **'Becoming aware'**: symptoms are ignored until persistent and causing difficulties with

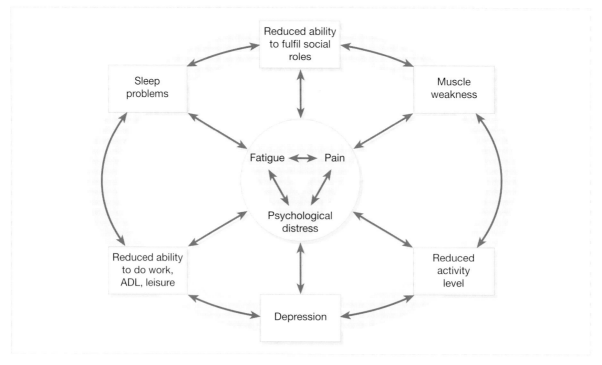

Fig. 23.1 The relationship between problems and symptoms.

work (paid or at home). The first few years are often the worst, grappling to live with symptoms and their effects on daily life.

- **'Learning to live with it'**: the first few severe flares lead to frustration, despair and feelings of being overwhelmed. Gradually people learn what strategies work best for which problems and incorporate the illness into their self-image.
- **'Mastery'**: people gain a different perspective on their health, illness, family relationships, work, leisure and everyday abilities and gain a satisfying quality of life. They are able to manage symptoms more, recognise cues signalling symptom worsening or flares and able to change activities and routines to manage this.

Adjusting to living with RA can take many years and is influenced by many factors, including personality, psychological status, emotional and social support and disease severity. Eberhardt et al (1993) identified that, at 2 years post-onset, two-thirds of sufferers still did not appreciate

that they had a chronic disease and had difficulty accepting being unable to do many of their leisure activities and that one-third felt guilty for varying reasons (e.g. inability to keep the house tidy, not being a good sexual partner, not being able to fulfil their family and parental roles). Le Gallez (1993) suggests that it takes at least 5 years for most people to come to terms with the physical and emotional effects of the disease. The varying progression of the disease also means that people may move between different stages of adjustment if their disease worsens.

AIMS OF MANAGEMENT

The main aims of occupational therapy and team care are to assist people in:

- learning to manage to live with RA
- improving and maintaining their psychological status
- maintaining valued life activities and roles.

Multidisciplinary team management is essential and includes:

- education in the disease, its treatment and in self-management
- sustained long-term psychosocial support
- relief of symptoms (pain, stiffness and fatigue) and prevention or slowing of disease progression
- maintaining optimal joint function
- modifying the environment and activities to suit the individual's needs.

THE TREATMENT TEAM

The core team includes the person with RA and their family, the rheumatologist, nurse practitioner, physiotherapist and occupational therapist. The wider team is shown in Figure 23.2. Specialist rheumatology care increased during the 1990s and early treatment is crucial to limit functional loss; most damage occurs within the first 2 years. The longer RA goes untreated, the worse the disease outcome and GPs should refer rapidly if RA is suspected. Rheumatologists prescribe slow-acting antirheumatic drugs (SAARDs), such as methotrexate and sulfasalazine, to try to control joint erosions. However, difficulties in diagnosis, drug side-effects, concerns about long-term drug effects and complicated dose regimens can affect maintaining intensive drug treatment.

Treatment is usually provided in a hospital outpatient department, with regular review by consultants, rheumatology nurse practitioners or clinical assistants, and referral to other team members. There is a steady growth in community-based services, with outreach clinics in local community hospitals, greater liaison with primary care nurses to provide local disease monitoring and greater provision of home-based therapy services. The emphasis is on shared team care and teaching people early to self-manage their disease more effectively. Patient education is a key activity.

The person with RA and their family are central in the team. Better outcomes result from effective self-management combined with effective team interventions. Self-management is the process of gaining better control of disease symptoms through recognising disease fluctuations,

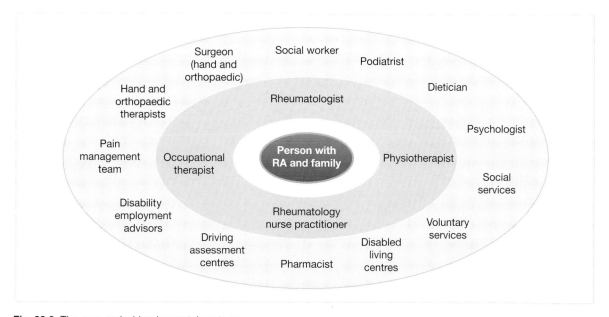

Fig. 23.2 The core and wider rheumatology team.

altering activities accordingly and maintaining as healthy a lifestyle as possible. It includes using a wide range of positive behavioural and cognitive coping methods:

- information seeking
- appropriate use of health behaviours, for example, rest, relaxation, exercise, joint protection, energy conservation, pain relief methods, orthoses, medication, good diet
- communicating effectively with others and health professionals
- problem solving
- positive self-thoughts
- keeping socially active.

Kate Lorig is a major proponent of self-management and has done much to promote this through the development of the Arthritis Self-management Program (called 'Challenging Arthritis' in the United Kingdom).

The consultant is responsible for diagnosis, identifying and managing appropriate drug therapy and surgery needs, referral to other team members and overall coordination of disease management. Hospital admissions are infrequent unless the person is in severe flare or requires intensive rehabilitation or monitoring of less common drug therapy procedures.

Rheumatology nurse practitioners and clinical assistants (who are physiotherapists and occupational therapists working in an extended capacity) play a pivotal role. Increasingly, following diagnosis and initiation of medical management, ongoing drug monitoring and care is provided in clinics run by these specially trained staff. Hill et al (1994) have demonstrated that such clinics lead to better patient satisfaction with care, understanding of the disease and its management, less pain and depression and better referral to and use of team care than medically run clinics. Rheumatology nurses and clinical assistants have more time to spend with patients, freeing up consultant time to focus on diagnosis and complex cases. Following training, nurses and clinical assistants can initiate and interpret clinical and laboratory investigations, referring back to consultants when problems arise. They can also give intra-articular steroid injections,

alter existing drug prescriptions within strictly agreed protocols and in future may have limited prescribing abilities to further increase their role in pain management. They can:

- identify psychological, social, functional, physical and educational needs
- provide ongoing education about the disease, drug therapy, side-effects and self-management strategies
- provide ongoing psychosocial support to the person and their family
- refer on to physiotherapy, occupational therapy and other team members
- coordinate shared care
- work closely with therapists in developing and delivering patient education programmes.

They may also run telephone helplines to provide ready access for support and advice to clinic attendees (Hill 1998).

Physiotherapists reduce inflammation, pain and maximise function by using a range of modalities. Superficial heat and cold therapy, electrotherapy (ultrasound, short wave diathermy, laser and interferential therapy and transcutaneous electrical nerve stimulation) are used to reduce pain and swelling. Mobility and function are improved through home exercise programmes; range of movement, strength, aerobic and hydrotherapy exercises; help in taking up recreational exercise; and assessment and provision of walking aids with gait and postural training. Static and serial splinting (particularly for the lower limb), traction and mobilisation techniques are used to reduce contractures (Lloyd 1999).

The wider team increasingly becomes involved if the disease has a greater impact and if surgery becomes necessary.

The team may be involved with people from disease diagnosis, with relatively few physical and functional needs but many educational, psychosocial and preventive care needs, through to people with severe disability. It is also involved pre- and postsurgically following joint replacements and tendon repairs that need specialised rehabilitation and social services.

THEORETICAL FOUNDATIONS FOR INTERVENTION

Team management aims to empower people with RA to understand, adjust to and self-manage their disease and its effects in order to maximise quality of life. Mutual goal setting based on the person's priorities is essential and this also enhances adherence with treatment and self-management advice. Within an occupational performance framework, self-management education and treatment focuses on enhancing feelings of control, self-efficacy, improving use of health behaviours and maximising self-care, productivity and leisure activities (Fig. 23.3).

FRAMES OF REFERENCE

A person-centred approach is vital, exploring the person's and the family's difficulties and psychosocial concerns. In the early stages, a learning frame of reference is adopted, including educational and cognitive–behavioural approaches, to teach self-management strategies such as joint

protection and energy conservation. The compensatory approach is applied progressively as the person is trained in alternative ADL methods, in the use of assistive devices, and in task and environment modification. The biomechanical approach is used through selected activity and home exercise programmes and provision of orthoses to maintain joint function and muscle strength and provide pain relief.

PATIENT EDUCATION AND SELF-EFFICACY

Patient education and enhancing self-efficacy are essential. Self-efficacy is the person's belief in their ability to achieve a specific goal. This is influenced by their degree of certainty in their physical and functional abilities and their ability to control thoughts, feelings and their environment. People with high self-efficacy are more likely to start and continue with self-management methods than those with low self-efficacy. People who give up on self-management behaviours often do so because they lack confidence in doing them.

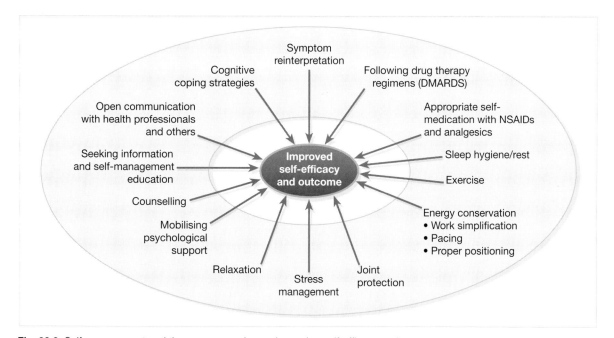

Fig. 23.3 Self-management and therapy approaches to improving self-efficacy and outcome.

Self-efficacy varies for different behaviours and can be improved. Approaches include (Boutagh & Brady 1998, Lorig 1996, Taal et al 1996):

- *Skills mastery* – breaking activities or behaviours into small, manageable actions or goals so each step is achieved successfully before progressing. For example, in joint protection a person is taught ways of opening a jar, then lifting a kettle. They practise these separately first, then progress to integrate multiple techniques into making a cup of tea. Contracting and feedback is used to encourage people to practise at home between therapy sessions.
- *Modelling* – teaching methods to groups of people with similar difficulties so they can solve problems and practise together. Seeing others achieve, and learning from each other, reinforces people's confidence in their own skills and enhances perceptions of 'I can do that'. Leaflets with pictures of 'real people with RA' should be used.
- *Reinterpreting symptoms* – exploring people's beliefs about what makes them worse and why they react as they do. People may believe the best response to fatigue is rest. If fatigue results from disease activity, resting and activity pacing are most appropriate. However, fatigue can also occur because of depression or deconditioning, when exercise and involvement in leisure and social activities would help; poor nutrition, when a balanced diet would help; work and family stress, when relaxation, cognitive coping methods and communicating effectively would help. Helping people see that problems have multiple causes encourages use of a wider range of self-management methods. Educating about the benefits of these is essential as people will not use techniques they do not perceive as beneficial.
- *Persuasion* – encouraging people to do just a little more than they can now and not setting unrealistic goals. Being a better persuader is helped by showing respect for the person and their beliefs and abilities, giving correct information about treatment and its efficacy and being flexible in negotiating therapy goals.

Facilitating improved self-management is best done by using educational, cognitive and behavioural approaches. These include teaching and learning principles to aid recall, motor learning strategies to train motor skills (e.g. joint protection and exercise) and self-efficacy enhancing techniques. Small group programmes of 2 hours per week over a 4–6-week period, with four to eight people attending, are a good way to apply approaches because they enable time to be used more efficiently, than in one-to-one sessions, allow people to gain additional support from meeting others with RA and encourage adherence to self-management methods at home by enabling people to learn through modelling and with peer support. Educational methods that facilitate behavioural change in group and individual therapy include:

- regular repetition of information (verbal and written)
- teaching the main points only
- repeat demonstration of behaviours in as near realistic a setting as possible (or in the home)
- repeat practice of techniques (for longer and in more complex sequences as the programme progresses) with feedback on performance
- providing written information
- weekly goal setting and contracting to practice strategies
- weekly review of goals with repeat demonstrations by the person and feedback on ability.

Inviting a relative or friend to attend may also help increase practice and support at home. Arthritis education programmes teaching multiple self-management strategies but not using these approaches have been shown to be ineffective in changing behaviour (Hammond & Lincoln 1999a). It may also be better to encourage people to attend separate, short education programmes targeting one or two self-management strategies at a time (e.g. joint protection, energy conservation, exercise, relaxation or pain management). This enables the person to build-up a repertoire of habitually adopted skills.

Verbal information should always be supported with written information. The Arthritis Research Campaign and Arthritis Care provide a wide range of high quality patient education materials either free of charge or at low cost. Arthritis Care runs an excellent community-based programme called Challenging Arthritis, which has proved highly effective at enhancing self-efficacy and use of exercise, relaxation, cognitive coping strategies and assertive communication with health professionals.

Understanding patient education theory and methods is important to help maximise adherence with therapy and self-management; a good introductory text is Lorig (1996).

PROBLEMS WITH ADHERENCE

People are encouraged to use many self-management methods and treatments which require time to perform and changes to normal routine. At least 50% of people with RA are non-adherent, irrespective of the intervention. Adherence is less when too many behaviours are targeted for change at the same time. People may feel overwhelmed by the changes demanded of them, that the disease has come to rule their life and react by avoiding using these. Coordinated team care and effective education should help people make changes gradually and use methods proven to enhance adherence.

THERAPY PROVISION

As RA is a chronic disease, occupational therapists may be involved in treating a person intermittently over many years. Ideally, people should be referred early. Taking time to establish a good rapport is vital if individuals are to self-refer back as and when necessary. A comprehensive therapy programme identifying the individual's needs and concerns, providing self-management education, psychosocial support

and therapy over four or five sessions is more likely to be effective in helping people change than short, one-off appointments. Review appointments (every 6 or 12 months as necessary) may help people continue to develop self-management skills, discuss psychosocial issues and solutions to new difficulties and identify if splints need replacing. Such regular assessment identifies if further ADL training, more intensive rehabilitation or surgery is needed.

Little research exists as yet to support the preventive benefits (both physical and psychological) of early stage therapy. However, when RA has become moderate to severe, occupational therapy has been proven effective. Helewa et al (1991) evaluated a comprehensive occupational therapy programme provided over a 6-week period, including assessment and appropriate provision of ADL training, assistive devices, joint protection and energy conservation, home adaptation, rest and work orthoses, advice on footwear and care, advice on foot orthoses and supports, psychosocial counselling, vocational and leisure counselling and support, stress management and use of community resources. Significant functional improvement and quality of life was identified in those receiving this programme in comparison to those who did not.

OCCUPATIONAL THERAPY INTERVENTION

ASSESSMENT

This should focus on what is problematic from the person's perspective. The assessments selected will depend on the time and resources available and the person's priorities. There are many arthritis-specific outcome measures for use in audit and research covering functional, physical, educational, psychosocial and quality of life aspects (Bowling 1997, Lorig et al 1996).

Person-centred assessments

- The Canadian Occupational Performance Assessment (see Chapter 5) is an interview of performance in self care, productivity and leisure in which the person rates their most important problems.

- The Disease Repercussion Profile (Carr 1996) is a self-report questionnaire of daily activities, social activities, financial/work status, relationships, psychological state and appearance.

Self-administered outcome measures

- The AIMS2 (Arthritis Impact Measurement Scale 2; Meenan et al 1992) includes 12 subscales: mobility, self-care, household tasks, upper limb function, social support, work, social activities, pain, psychological status, health perceptions and arthritis impact, along with satisfaction with abilities. It takes 20 minutes.
- The HAQ (Health Assessment Questionnaire; Kirwan & Reeback 1986) includes 24 functional activities and takes 5 minutes.

Functional assessments

- The Evaluation of Daily Activities Questionnaire (EDAQ; Nordenskiold et al 1998) includes 102 items divided into 11 areas of personal and instrumental daily activities. It is completed at home over a 1–2 week period.
- The Functional Status Index (Jette 1987) measures dependence, pain and difficulty in 45 functional and role activities.
- A detailed, non-standardised checklist is described by Backman (1998). It lacks reliability and validity, but is helpful in treatment planning.
- Home assessments evaluate ADL ability in the home, help from others, home and local circumstances.
- Driving assessments: people with RA rely heavily on their cars. Simple problems can be assessed by the therapist, otherwise referral to a specialist mobility/driving assessment centre is needed.

Work assessment

- Work Assessment Questions (Melvin 1998) includes items on preparing to get to work,

transport, work setting, breaks, work activities and work relationships.

Leisure

- Interest checklists may be used to identify past and current patterns of leisure and to explore areas that might offer new leisure opportunities.

Upper limb assessment

How detailed this is depends on its purpose and may include:

- grip and pinch strength (using the Grippit measure (Nordenskiold 1993) or Jamar dynamometer)
- joint range of movement, hand span and deformities, for example, using the method described by Treuhaft et al (1971)
- pain, for example, using visual analogue scales
- joint indices (e.g. EULAR articular index)
- hand and grip function during simulated ADL, for example, using the Sollerman Hand Function Test, Grip Ability Test, Sequential Occupational Dexterity Assessment or Arthritis Hand Function Test.

Foot assessment

Feet and walking should be observed to provide simple footcare advice and insoles and identify the need for referral to podiatry.

Joint protection and energy conservation in daily activities

- Joint Protection Behaviour Assessment (Hammond & Lincoln 1999b) helps identify which movement patterns people need to change to reduce joint stress and evaluates outcomes of education.
- NIH Activity Record (ACTRE; Gerber & Furst 1992) is a daily log recording daily activities in half-hour blocks over 2 days. Each is rated for pain, fatigue, difficulty and rest breaks. The record helps identify problem activities and evaluates daily life patterns.

Psychological assessment

This is usually done through informal means, although if there is concern in this respect it may be useful to select a comprehensive measure such as AIMS2, which includes this aspect.

INTERVENTIONS

Improving functional ability in home, work and leisure activities

Initially, problems relate to dexterity and activities requiring power and pinch grips, such as meal preparation, fastenings, using tools and computers, writing, active sport and leisure. Foot problems cause difficulty walking. Operating hand and foot controls when driving becomes difficult. As upper and lower limb joints are increasingly affected then self-care, household and mobility problems develop.

Therapy should focus on the person's priorities and the amount of therapy should increase as the disease progresses. Some may consider focusing on kitchen and household activities is important; others will be happy to buy readymade meals and to hire domestic help and will want to focus on leisure and work. Function can be improved through observation of the problem and activity analysis to identify the cause and to select and implement relevant solutions:

- Teaching alternative techniques and giving advice on modifying routines, joint protection and energy conservation.
- Providing/recommending assistive devices. The most common required are:
  - kitchen aids (electric can opener, easy vegetable peeler, ergonomic knife, tap turner, jar opener are most useful)
  - for transfers: bathboards, raised toilet seats, chair raises
  - to reduce standing: perch stools
  - for dressing: long shoe horns, sock/tight aids, easy fastenings, dressing stick
  - enlarged and/or longer handles: for cutlery, comb, razor
  - lightweight power tools
  - helping hands and universal turning aids

  - driving adaptations: key adaptations, additional mirrors, power steering, automatic gear box.
- Use of orthoses and exercise to maximise ability to perform activities.
- Teaching principles of selecting ergonomically well-designed household, work and leisure equipment and furniture. This enables people to make long-term decisions about what is best to purchase for easier use in the future when items need replacing and if function deteriorates. This needs handling sensitively.
- Environmental modifications: people may progress to need adapted bathrooms (e.g. level-access shower), ramps, additional stair rails, toilet rails, stairlifts and rearranging furniture to allow wider access for mobility aids. Kitchens may need to be redesigned to reduce the working triangle, lower wall cupboards, ensure storage is easy to access and enable tasks to be performed whilst seated. It may be necessary to consider discussing moving to adapted, one-level housing with ergonomically designed fixtures.

The section on ADL for people with osteoarthritis in Chapter 27 is also applicable for people with more established RA.

At work, work heights need adjusting and supportive seating provided. Those using computers may experience hand and upper limb pain, and wrist splints help. Health and safety recommendations should be applied and appropriate equipment provided; for example, wrist support pads and ergonomic keyboards and the workstation should be ergonomically assessed and altered to reduce neck and upper limb strain if necessary. For those in manual jobs, work task analysis helps identify how to apply joint protection principles and correct lifting techniques. The person may need to change to lighter work in the long term. Liaison with Disability Employment Advisors can help in obtaining grants for work adaptations, equipment and negotiating reducing work hours or changing tasks with employers. Arthritis Care manages a scheme to help people gain confidence in applying for jobs and getting back into work. A social worker can assist in identifying the financial implications of changing jobs and can advise whether additional benefits can be claimed. Home-based employment may be another realistic possibility.

Leisure activities should be discussed, especially if people have had to give up work. Active leisure (sports such as football, golf, racket games) are lost early. Encouraging people to take up swimming, gentle exercise classes and maintain walking are important for general health, joint mobility and to prevent deconditioning. Regular exercise also promotes better psychological status. Interests in more sedentary and passive leisure need exploring, such as Internet use, crafts, painting, puzzles, board and card games, social visits (cultural events, cinema, museums, visiting friends, going to the pub), joining social clubs and other interest groups to develop or resurrect past interests. A good knowledge of a range of leisure activities and local community facilities is needed to help people (and their family/friends) make goals to try new activities and appreciate the importance of pursuing a meaningful leisure life to reduce psychological effects of the disease and increase family enjoyment.

Joint protection

The aims of joint protection are to reduce pain, inflammation and internal (i.e. muscular compressive forces) and external (e.g. pressure from lifting heavy weights) joint stresses in order to preserve the integrity of joint structures and reduce the risk of deformities (Cordery & Rocchi 1998).

Ignoring pain may lead to further joint damage and pain. Being too sensitive to pain may lead to reduced activity, muscle wasting and further promote joint instability. Individuals should therefore be aware of pain levels and moderate their activity accordingly. If pain continues for more than 1 hour after ceasing the activity, that activity should be moderated in future. To help identify what activities may need to be altered, it is useful to ask individuals to self-monitor them:

● informally, taking the time to be aware of pain on selected days and during selected activities (e.g. housework, work, cooking)

● formally, by keeping a record of activities and pain/fatigue levels over one weekday and one weekend day (the ACTRE).

Joint protection can be brought about by altering movement patterns and by the use of assistive devices (Fig. 23.4). The principles of joint protection include:

● Distributing load over several joints. As much surface area of the hands and/or both hands should be used when lifting. Examples include:
− using the palms of both hands to carry plates, mugs, trays and so on with fingers in extension (not deviated)
− using two hands to lift objects with handles, for example, pans, kettles and jugs. The wrist holding the handle should be maintained in extension (if achievable), or neutral, and the other wrist should take the weight on the flat of the hand.

● Using stronger, larger joints. The stronger the joint, the more able it is to tolerate a given amount of load. Examples of this are to:
− use the hip to close drawers or doors
− use the palm of the hand or side of the fist to push in a plug, rather than holding it with the fingertips
− lift bags and other large items with the forearms and trunk, holding the weight close to the chest
− carry a bag over the shoulder or forearm.

● Using joints in their most stable and functional positions. Most joints are more stable in straight alignment, enabling greater efficiency of muscles and leverage to be applied during action. Flexed or deviated positions, and applying rotational force during activity, increases stress on ligaments. For example:
− to stand, feet should be flat and facing forwards, the person should stand up straight, avoiding twisting the knees
− the wrist should be maintained in extension when lifting and gripping to maximise grip strength
− correct lifting techniques should be taught.

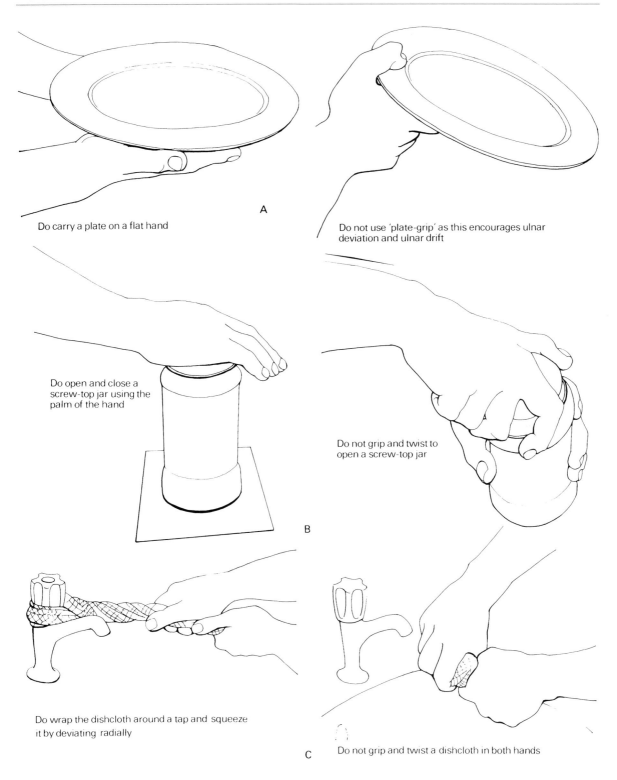

Do carry a plate on a flat hand

Do not use 'plate-grip' as this encourages ulnar deviation and ulnar drift

A

Do open and close a screw-top jar using the palm of the hand

Do not grip and twist to open a screw-top jar

B

Do wrap the dishcloth around a tap and squeeze it by deviating radially

Do not grip and twist a dishcloth in both hands

C

Fig. 23.4 Hand joint protection techniques in rheumatoid arthritis. (A) Carrying a plate, (B) opening a jar, (C) squeezing a dishcloth.

- Reducing effort. Using less muscular effort to perform daily tasks reduces internal joint stress. Examples include:
  - using assistive devices
  - labour-saving gadgets, for example, food processors, dishwasher machines, tumble driers or combined washer/driers, lightweight power tools
  - employing leverage, for example, by extending handles, using a knife to flip off ring-pulls
  - avoiding lifting and carrying by using wheels (a small hostess trolley to move items round the house, mounting a laundry basket on castors, using a shopping trolley, using 'cabin baggage' to transport briefcases and laptops), sliding objects along work surfaces or the floor or tipping (for instance, raising a jug kettle on a block of wood and tipping to pour or using a kettle tipper).

Using assistive devices reduces pain during activity (Nordenskiold 1994). However, a substantial proportion are not used (between 18% and 59%). Attitudes to and appearance of devices should be carefully considered when prescribing. People with RA have a greater need for assistive devices (particularly kitchen gadgets) than other groups. Care should be taken to prescribe these appropriately and over a period of time to enable the person to adjust to them gradually. Preferably, gadgets that are available from high street stores and which are used by people without arthritis (e.g. electric can openers, Good Grip peelers), should be recommended. Many prefer to do an activity in a modified way rather than use an aid as this can reinforce perceptions of being disabled and different to others. The opportunity to 'try before you buy' should be given.

- Avoiding positions of deformity. Stresses contributing to common patterns of deformity should be avoided. These may be external pressures, for example, pushing joints sideways or downwards when lifting objects, or internal stresses from muscular compressive forces. For example:
  - strong power, pinch and tripod grips promote anterior subluxation at the MCP

joints and strong pinch promotes IP joint deformities. Handles, pens, and so on can be enlarged and padded
  - finger-twisting actions promote ulnar deviation. The palm should be used to turn taps and open jars, with the fingers held straight
  - lifting heavy items with a flexed wrist promotes wrist anterior subluxation. The wrist should be extended or neutral.

Adherence

Adherence with joint protection is problematic. Joint protection is usually taught over one or two sessions for at most 2 hours, focusing on principles and discussing alternative methods, with limited time for demonstrations and supervised practice. This approach has been proved ineffective in changing behaviour and outcomes (Hammond & Lincoln 1999a). Barriers to behaviour change include difficulty recalling methods and making changes habitual. Group education using a four-session, educational–behavioural programme including self-monitoring, modelling, supervised practice, feedback, problem solving, goal setting and home practice has been found to improve adherence and to reduce pain, swelling, numbers of flares and duration of early morning stiffness (Hammond et al 1999c; Hammond & Freeman 2001). Group education also provides peer social support, which is extremely important. Using effective teaching techniques is essential if people are to gain the benefits of joint protection.

Rest

Acutely inflamed and painful joints should be rested. However, prolonged rest can have deleterious effects, with 3% of muscle strength lost daily. Remaining in bed should not be encouraged unless prescribed but people should rest for 10 hours in 24, if possible (unless in remission), including an hour during the day, to assist natural recovery processes, improve overall endurance for activity and enhance muscle function. This should be accompanied by a regular exercise programme. People may perceive resting as 'giving in' and education on the benefits of rest and its contribution as part of a package of lifestyle changes is necessary.

Correct positioning

Advice should be given on correct resting positions. Joints should be well supported when sitting and lying. Chairs should have an adequate seat depth to support the upper legs and to allow the hips, knees and ankles to be positioned at 90 degrees. Chairs should have a supportive back, which may include a lumbar back support, and should also support the head. They should have firm arms to assist with rising. Beds should be flat and firm, providing even support. This can be assisted by providing bed boards. Positioning should support and preserve the anatomical curves of the spine. A neck pillow (or soft towel) is more supportive than a regular pillow, which causes neck flexion and tension. People should spend part of the night on their back, maintaining the hips and knees in extension. A pillow should not be used to support the knees as this can encourage flexion contractures in more severely affected joints. If there are nodules and skin involvement, sheepskin pads and foam protectors help reduce pressure.

Sleep management

Sleep problems can be common, see Box 23.4.

Duvets are easier to pull up during the night than sheets and blankets. For those wearing night resting orthoses, a shorter design extending just beyond the finger and thumb PIP joints may be an option. These leave the finger-tips free to pull up bedclothes, switch on/off the bedside light and radio and turn pages of bedtime reading. Orthoses that limit these activities and cause sleep disturbance and annoyance are unlikely to be worn as recommended.

For those with early morning stiffness, setting the alarm early, taking medication and rising when it starts to take effect can help. This should be discussed with the doctor because certain drugs must be taken with food.

Box 23.4 Sleep management

- Ensure the bedroom is comfortable (firm bed, dark, quiet, comfortable environment and temperature).
- Avoid drinks containing caffeine, alcohol, large meals and smoking several hours before bedtime.
- Relax using relaxation methods or a hot bath; an electric underblanket (on a low setting) can assist with pain relief.
- Regular daily exercise. A few gentle range of movement exercises in bed before sleeping can also help reduce pain and discomfort.
- A regular sleep schedule of going to bed and rising. As people get older, they require less sleep. Rest need not be equated with sleep. A regular bedtime ritual helps.
- Medication should be taken as prescribed before bedtime. The doctor or pharmacist can advise on the best time to take these to minimise nocturnal pain if this is the cause of sleep problems.

Energy conservation

This helps reduce fatigue and enables the person to save energy during daily tasks, giving greater control in distributing energy to more meaningful activities. The main principles are to:

- Balance rest and work with regular short 'microbreaks' for a few minutes every 20–30 minutes. This may be difficult for some, particularly if they consider rest is 'giving in'. It may be helpful to get people to compare energy levels (using the ACTRE) during their normal activity patterns versus using regular rest periods.
- Use correct body positions. Good posture balances the weight of the head and limbs on the bony framework so that the force of gravity helps keep a correct joint position. More energy is used to maintain poor postures as muscles have to work against the effect of gravity to maintain position. Hunched shoulders, a craned neck and bent back cause muscle tension, pain and tiredness. Standing requires approximately 25% more energy than sitting, so tasks should be performed seated if possible.
- Avoid staying in one position for long periods, which can lead to stiffness. It is recommended to change position every 20–30

minutes, for example, taking a short walk round the house, rather than remaining seated for the whole evening; stretching the hands regularly rather than writing continuously.

- A correct work height allows the head and neck to be held as straight as possible whilst sitting or standing. Work surfaces should be approximately 2 inches below the elbow when the shoulders are relaxed. Work surfaces can be altered (by reducing height or raising with blocks) or a high stool with a back support may be used (ensuring the feet are supported).
- Avoid activities that cannot be stopped if they become too stressful, that is, cause sudden or severe pain. Some tasks, for example, carrying a heavy package along a corridor, cannot be stopped readily and could therefore strain weakened ligaments.

It is helpful to teach people work simplification analysis so they can apply these principles themselves to functional problems at home. Wilden (cited in Melvin 1989) suggested questions that can be used to help make changes (Box 23.5). Not all activities can be changed to reduce energy consumption but altering some reduces fatigue. Furst et al (1987) demonstrated that using regular rest periods sustains daily activity for longer.

Box 23.5 Work simplification: task analysis

- How many trips were made between two points?
- Could the number of trips be reduced?
- Could the order of performing different parts of the job be reduced?
- Are the materials and needed equipment within easy reach? Can storage areas be reorganised?
- Do storage areas contain only the required equipment or are they cluttered with seldom-used things?
- Can any part of the task be omitted or changed and still produce the desired results?
- Are good body mechanics used in posture, sitting, standing and lifting?
- Are two hands used to the best advantage?
- Would the use of wheels be helpful?
- Are sitting facilities comfortable? Are these and work surfaces of the proper height?
- Are the materials pre-positioned and ready for use?
- Is the rate of work too fast?
- Should someone else do part of the task?

However, no differences in self-reported pain, functional disability or fatigue were shown but this was likely to be because the study was too small with too short a follow-up to demonstrate effectiveness.

Exercise and activity

Muscle strength and joint range of movement should be maintained through exercise, full ranging of joints during daily activities and therapeutic activity programmes. Exercise programmes are prescribed by physiotherapists and aerobic exercise should be incorporated two to three times per week to improve stamina, such as cycling, swimming and walking. The occupational therapist may be concerned with reinforcing information as to how and when to exercise and in providing hand exercises. Combinations of range of movement and resistive hand exercises are most effective (Brighton et al 1993). Lorig and Fries (1992) describe exercise programmes and principles for their use. The activities selected should be done at a slow, steady rhythm, with rests to allow muscles time to recover and prevent fatigue. Therapeutic home activity programmes can also be recommended by incorporating leisure activities as hand exercises, for example, baking, light gardening and art.

Increased physical activity promotes bone and muscle strength, aids in weight reduction (thus reducing stress on lower limb joints) and increases endorphin levels in the cerebrospinal fluid, leading to an increased sense of wellbeing and reduction in pain perception. Exercise activity that fits in with an individual's lifestyle and provides social interaction is more likely to be sustained. It is best to exercise when medication is at its most effective and at periods in the day when the person experiences least pain, stiffness and fatigue. Warm-up activities should always be incorporated to avoid straining soft tissues.

Orthoses

These support the joint, reduce stress to the joint capsule, reduce pain during motion and help decrease inflammation. There is no objective evidence as yet that any splint designs prevent or limit progress of deformities. It is essential any orthosis is well-fitting, well-made and that clear instructions on wear and care are given (see Chapters 7 and 17). Adherence with splint wearing varies at between 25 and 65%. Careful attention should be paid to assessing attitudes to splint wearing, education on splint function and wear regimens, and quality and comfort of the splint provided in order to maximise adherence.

The most commonly provided orthoses are:

- hand resting orthoses (Fig. 23.5). These are worn continually in acute flares and have been found to reduce inflammation in the short term. For chronic synovitis, they are worn regularly at night or for a few hours during the day. Most people gain pain relief from these orthoses but there is conflicting evidence as to whether they help with stiffness, range of movement or swelling. They must be easy to put on and off and comfortable (for the user and their bed partners). Lined, softer splints are worn more often.

- Wrist working orthoses (Fig. 23.6). These immobilise or partly immobilise the wrist (depending on the design). Pain is reduced during activity and grip strength improved (Kjeken et al 1995) but these orthoses do restrict dexterity, palmar grip or slow hand function. A period of adjustment of 1 to 2 weeks is needed to notice benefits. Elastic wrist splints are preferable in many cases.

- MCP orthoses. A variety of designs is available to provide pain relief and improve function in those who already have ulnar deviation, improving correct alignment of the fingers for grip (Rennie 1996).

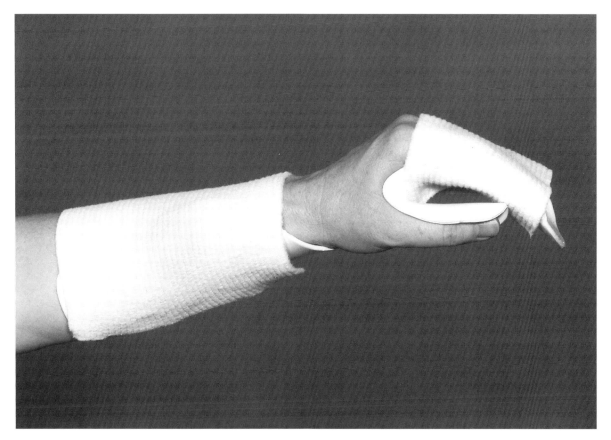

Fig. 23.5 Hand resting splint.

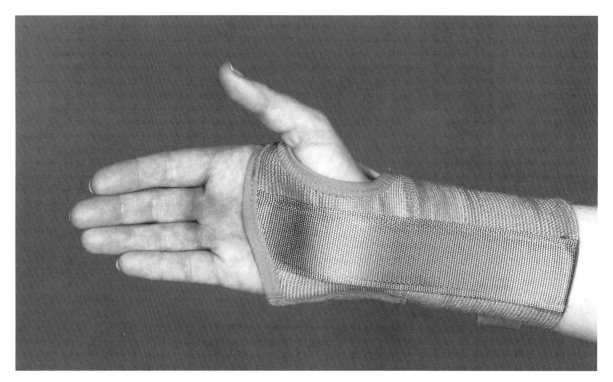

Fig. 23.6 Working wrist splint.

- Thumb orthoses may be required to stabilise the carpometacarpal (CMC) or MCP joints of the thumb during function. The thumb is held in palmar abduction in a position enabling finger opposition. In cases of CMC involvement, a wrist–thumb orthosis will be necessary.
- Finger orthoses. Small figure-of-eight orthoses can be fitted to hold non-fixed boutonnière or swan-neck deformities in correct alignment. Worn continually over a 6-week period there is some evidence these reduce deformity, although it can recur when use discontinues.
- Dynamic orthoses are used post-MCP replacement to retain correction of ulnar deviation. These may also be used following extensor tendon repair to overcome MCP extension lag.
- Foot orthoses. Provision of insoles (with metatarsal pads, bars or domes), can reduce foot pain and increase mobility.

Commercially manufactured shock-absorbing insoles (as used for sports shoes) can also reduce foot joint stress. Advice on footwear should include the wearing of flat, well cushioned shoes that support the fore- and mid-foot and around the ankle. If insoles are fitted, shoes need greater depth to accommodate the foot adequately without excess joint pressure developing.
- Other orthoses may include: cervical collars; knee supports; and long leg resting orthoses.

Particular attention should be paid to the straps and fastenings on an orthosis because people with poor reach or manual dexterity may not wear them if they are difficult to put on and take off. Regular review is essential, especially in the first 2 weeks, to ensure correct fit, application and improvement in function. If hand deformities progress, the orthoses may no longer fit adequately and further review is needed.

Relaxation, pain and stress management

Pain is a major concern of people with RA. It is a primary determinant of physical dysfunction and is associated with psychological symptoms such as helplessness and depression. Pain can be partly modified in its perception and affective and behavioural responses. Various cognitive–behavioural approaches have been proven effective:

- Relaxation training. Common methods used are guided imagery and progressive relaxation methods.
- Teaching cognitive coping strategies, for example, attention refocusing (thinking about some other activity), vivid imagery (thinking about a pleasant scene or event), dissociation (mentally separating from the painful body part) and relabelling (thinking of the pain as a nuisance). These should be applied with care and within the context of the person receiving education on joint protection. It is important that individuals do not learn to ignore pain that is indicative of joint stress.
- Cognitive restructuring: identifying, challenging and modifying automatic negative thoughts.
- Behavioural coping strategies: exercise, joint protection, energy conservation, activity pacing.
- Problem solving. Identifying activities that cause pain or events that increase stress, and identifying methods of resolving these.

Most cognitive–behavioural pain management programmes typically include an education phase, a skills teaching and acquisition phase, and a skills maintenance phase. The person will be taught how psychological factors influence pain. Specific skills are taught and methods of enabling the individual to maintain these at home are built into the programme. This is not an alternative to medication, as these methods only reduce perceptions of pain, not the underlying disease processes.

Management of severe RA

With improved understanding of RA and its management, there should be fewer people with severe forms of the disease in the future. However, 10% of people now affected have severe symptoms and represent a relatively large proportion of those seen by occupational therapists because they require more regular extensive intervention.

It is also still possible to see people with multiple problems who have never seen an occupational therapist. These people have multiple joint involvement and deformities, often with systemic involvement such as heart, respiratory, kidney and liver problems, poor skin prone to ulceration, osteoporotic bones and widespread muscle weakness.

Intervention in severe RA uses the same strategies described earlier, but focuses more on ADL training, assistive devices, environmental modification, splinting and possibly wheelchair provision than preventive strategies such as joint protection. Many cope well despite severe deformity and have developed compensatory actions. Others may be severely disabled, with limited leisure and social activities.

Surgery, particularly joint replacements, is an important part of the management of severe RA. People may have hip, knee, shoulder, elbow and MCP replacements, as well as ankle, toes and wrist arthrodeses, neck and spine surgery, tendon repairs and correction of hand deformities. With advancing techniques and improved prostheses, joint replacements are lasting longer and are easier to revise when these eventually fail. However, surgical rehabilitation is often challenging because therapy must be provided within the context of multiple joint pathology. For example, following a total hip replacement, a person may have difficulty managing crutches or a walking frame because of painful or deformed shoulder, elbow, wrist or finger joints. Rollators with forearm gutter supports take the strain off the hands and wrists but direct it towards the shoulders and neck, so careful planning is essential to identify which mobility aids and assistive devices are of most benefit.

Surgery options are usually discussed in joint clinics run with rheumatologists, orthopaedic and hand surgeons, with the close involvement of physiotherapists and occupational therapists. Preoperative assessments by occupational therapists are often required and are essential if multiple joint surgery is planned to help determine the appropriate order for surgery to maintain and maximise functional ability and facilitate rehabilitation. Depending on individual circumstances, it may be better to replace the elbow before the hip, to enable a person to mobilise with walking aids more successfully after a hip replacement (see also Chapter 27 on surgical rehabilitation following hip and knee surgery).

The functional success of most surgery, particularly for the upper limb, depends as much on the motivation and hard work of the person as the quality of postoperative rehabilitation. Preoperative assessments must consider not only physical ability and function but psychological and social circumstances. If the person is insufficiently motivated to pursue their rehabilitation, the outcome is unlikely to be successful.

Surgical rehabilitation is a specialised area; an information discussion appears in Melvin and Jensen (1998 volumes 4 and 5).

CONCLUSION

Rheumatoid arthritis cannot be cured but people can be helped to adopt self-management techniques that reduce disease symptoms to some extent, allow them to adjust psychologically to the changes the disease can impose and enable them to maintain roles and activities, thus maximising quality of life (Boxes 23.6 and 23.7). Education is an important component of therapy to enable people to make informed decisions on how to manage their disease most effectively.

Box 23.6   Case study: early RA

Rajiv Singh is 34, married and has 3 sons under 10 years of age. He works in the family business fitting kitchens. Ten months ago he had acute onset RA affecting his wrists, MCPs, knees and toes. Pain and fatigue were worsened by his job, which requires him to lift heavy loads, bend to work in awkward positions and grip tools tightly. He was moody and short-tempered and unable to play football with his sons. His wife was having to help him undress and he was worried about supporting his family if he had to give up work. He was continually frustrated with difficulties doing small jobs like opening jars and fastening buttons.

Occupational therapy was provided over 4 weeks. To

reduce pain and joint swelling, information was given about RA, along with education and training using rest, pacing and joint protection. Mr Singh attended a joint protection programme. To improve hand function he was fitted with working wrist splints (see Fig. 23.6) and taught hand exercises. Assistive devices to help grip were recommended. Exacerbating factors for pain and fatigue were identified and activities were discussed to modify and eliminate tasks and to pace and plan the working day to save energy for family activities. A work assessment was conducted to explore work adaptations. Mr Singh felt he was unable to adapt his work and is now planning to change to business administration.

Box 23.7   Case study: severe RA

Maggie Alders has longstanding, severe RA. During the early stages her husband cared for her. When he died, she was unable to manage alone and was admitted for rehabilitation and surgical assessment. Her problems included reduced mobility, difficulties with transfers and environmental controls, poor upper limb function, pain, sleep disturbance, social isolation, low mood and psychological dependency.

ADL assessment, training and assistive devices were provided to help her practice self-care and meal preparation. Joint protection advice was given to help reduce pain. An upper limb assessment was conducted, wrist splints provided to reduce pain and improve function and a programme of upper limb activities initiated to help improve range of movement.   Time was spent exploring Maggie's goals and interests to help plan future therapy. A home visit was conducted to modify the environment to

facilitate safe mobility and independence. The Home Care Organiser attended to arrange help for personal care and meal preparation.

Over the next few years, Maggie was admitted for a series of operations to upper and lower limb joints. Therapy included reassessment, education about surgery and precautions to reduce anxiety, postoperative rehabilitation and home visits. She was referred for a driving needs assessment and encouraged to become involved in social activities.

Now Maggie is independently mobile, can manage self-care and meal preparation, operate environmental controls and drive her car. She has developed social interests, has learnt computing and uses the Internet to communicate with others. She has less pain, better function and feels happier and more fulfilled.

Many people develop their own methods of coping with the disease, which should be respected. Comprehensive occupational therapy rehabilitation can make a significant difference in maintaining a person's functional status, particularly as the disease progresses, and is vital before and after surgery.

Multidisciplinary teams providing comprehensive care, planning education and treatment to dovetail, with regular monitoring, review and re-referral to therapy, result in better long-term outcomes than ad hoc referral systems with irregular review. All team members should aim to provide shared care.

REFERENCES

Backman C 1998 Functional assessment. In: Melvin J, Jensen G (eds) Rheumatologic rehabilitation series. American Occupational Therapy Association: Bethesda, MD, vol 1: assessment and management, ch 8, pp 157–194

Belza BL 1996 Fatigue. In: Wegener ST, Belza BL Gall EP (eds) Clinical care in the rheumatic diseases. American College of Rheumatology, Atlanta, GA, ch 20, p 117

Bishop AT, Hench PK, La Croix E, Millender LH, Opitz JL 1991 Keeping the rheumatoid hand working. Patient Care 25:74–111

Blalock SJ, DeVellis RF 1992 Rheumatoid arthritis and depression: an overview. Bulletin on the Rheumatic Diseases 41:6–8

Blalock SJ, DeVellis MB, Holt K, Hahn P 1993 Coping with arthritis: is one problem the same as another? Health Education Quarterly 20:119–132

Boutagh ML, Brady TJ 1998 Patient education for self management. In: Melvin J, Jensen G (eds) 1998 Rheumatologic rehabilitation series. American Occupational Therapy Association: Bethesda, MD, vol 1: assessment and management, ch 10, p 219

Bowling A 1997 Measuring disease. Open University, Buckingham, UK

Brighton SW, Lubbe JE, van der Merwe CA 1993 The effect of a long-term exercise programme on the rheumatoid hand. British Journal of Rheumatology 32:392–395

Carr A 1996 A patient-centred approach to evaluation and treatment in rheumatoid arthritis: the development of a clinical tool to measure patient perceived handicap. British Journal of Rheumatology 35:921–932

Cordery J, Rocchi M 1998 Joint protection and fatigue management In: Melvin J, Jensen G (eds) Rheumatologic rehabilitation series. American Occupational Therapy Association: Bethesda, MD, vol 1: assessment and management, ch 12, p 279

Eberhardt KB, Rydgren LC, Pettersson H, Wollheim FA 1990 Early rheumatoid arthritis – onset, course and outcome over 2 years. Rheumatology International 10:135–142

Eberhardt K, Larsson B-M, Nived K 1993 Psychological reactions in patients with early rheumatoid arthritis. Patient Education and Counselling 20:93–100

Fex E, Larsson B, Nived K, Eberhardt K 1998 Effect of rheumatoid arthritis on work status and social and leisure time activities in patients followed eight years from onset. Journal of Rheumatology 25:44–50

Furst GP, Gerber LH, Smith C, Fisher S, Shulman B 1987 A program for improving energy conservation behaviors in adults with rheumatoid arthritis. American Journal of Occupational Therapy 41:102–111

Gerber LH, Furst GP 1992 Validation of the NIH activity record: a quantitative measure of life activities. Arthritis Care and Research 5:81–86

Hammond A, Lincoln N 1999a The effect of a joint protection programme for people with rheumatoid arthritis. Clinical Rehabilitation 13:392–400

Hammond A, Lincoln N 1999b Development of the joint protection behaviour. Assessment. Arthritis Care and Research 12:200–207

Hammond A, Lincoln N, Sutcliffe L 1999c A crossover trial evaluating an educational-behavioural programme for people with rheumatoid arthritis. Patient Education and Counselling 37:19–32

Hammond A, Freeman KE 2001 One year outcomes of a randomized controlled trial of an educational–behavioural joint protection programme for people with rheumatoid arthritis. Rheumatology (in press)

Helewa A, Goldsmith C, Lee P, Bombardier C, Hanes B, Smythe HA, Tugwell P 1991 Effects of occupational therapy home service on patients with rheumatoid arthritis. The Lancet 337:1453–1456

Hill J, Bird H, Lawton C, Harmer R, Wright V 1994 An evaluation of the effectiveness, safety and acceptability of a nurse practitioner in a rheumatology out-patient clinic. British Journal of Rheumatology 33:283–288

Hill J 1998 Rheumatology nursing: a creative approach. Churchill Livingstone, Edinburgh

Jette AM 1987 The Functional Status Index: reliability and validity of a self-report functional disability measure. Journal of Rheumatology 14 (Suppl. 15):15–19

Kirwan JR, Reeback JS 1986 Stanford Health Assessment Questionnaire modified to assess disability in British patients with rheumatoid arthritis. British Journal of Rheumatology 25:206–209

Kjeken I, Moller G, Kvien TK 1995 The use of commercially produced elastic wrist orthoses in chronic arthritis: a controlled study. Arthritis Care and Research 8:108–113

le Gallez P 1993 Rheumatoid arthritis: effects on the family. Nursing Standard 7:30–34

Lloyd J 1999 Rheumatoid arthritis. In: David C, Lloyd J (eds) Rheumatology physiotherapy. Churchill Livingstone, Edinburgh, ch 8

Lorig K (undated) arthritis self-management program: program leader's manual. Arthritis Foundation, Atlanta, GA

Lorig K 1996 Patient education: a practical approach, 2nd edn. Mosby, St Louis, MO

Lorig K, Fries J 1992 The arthritis helpbook: a tested self-management program for coping with arthritis, 3rd edn. Addison-Wesley: MA

Lorig K, Stewart A, Ritter P, Gonzalez V, Laurent D, Lynch J 1996 Outcome measures for health education and other healthcare interventions. Sage: Thousand Oaks, CA

Meenan RF, Mason JH, Anderson JJ, Guccione AA, Kazis LE 1992 AIMS2: the content and properties of a revised and expanded Arthritis Impact Measurement Scales Health Status Questionnaire. Arthritis and Rheumatism 35:1–10

Melvin J 1998 Work assessment questions. In: Melvin J, Jensen G (eds) Rheumatologic rehabilitation series. American Occupational Therapy Association: Bethesda, MD, vol 1: assessment and management, ch 8, pp 192–194

Melvin J, Jensen G (eds) 1998 Rheumatologic rehabilitation series. American Occupational Therapy Association Bethesda, MD, vol 4: the hand: evaluation, therapy and surgery; vol 5: surgical rehabilitation

Nordenskiold U, Grimby G 1993 Grip force in patients with rheumatoid arthritis and fibromyalgia and in healthy subjects. A study with the Grippit instrument. Scandinavian Journal of Rheumatology 22:14–19

Nordenskiold U 1994 Evaluation of assistive devices after a course in joint protection. International Journal of Technology Assessment in Health Care 10:294–305

Nordenskiold U, Grimby G, Dahlin-Ivanoff S 1998 Questionnaire to evaluate the effects of assistive devices and altered working methods in women with rheumatoid arthritis. Clinical Rheumatology 17:6–16

Pincus T 1996 Rheumatoid arthritis. In: Wegener ST, Belza BL, Gall EP (eds) Clinical care in the rheumatic diseases. American College of Rheumatology, Atlanta, GA, ch 26, p 147

Reisine ST, Goodenow C, Grady KE 1987 The impact of rheumatoid arthritis on the homemaker. Social Sciences and Medicine 25:89–95

Rennie HJ 1996 Evaluation of the effectiveness of a metacarpophalangeal ulnar deviation orthosis. Journal of Hand Therapy 9:371–377

Ryan S 1996 Living with rheumatoid arthritis: a phenomenological exploration. Nursing Standard 10:41, 45–48

Shaul MP 1995 From early twinges to mastery: the process of adjustment in living with rheumatoid arthritis. Arthritis Care and Research 8:290–297

Taal E, Rasker JJ, Wiegman O 1996 Patient education and self-management in the rheumatic diseases: a self-efficacy approach. Arthritis Care and Research 9:229–238

Treuhaft PS, Lewis MR, McCarty DJ 1971 A rapid method for evaluating the structure and function of the rheumatoid hand. Arthritis and Rheumatism 14:75–87

Williams GH, Wood PHN 1988 Coming to terms with chronic illness: the negotiation of autonomy in rheumatoid arthritis. International Disability Studies 10:128–133

FURTHER READING

Brattstrom M 1987 Joint protection – rehabilitation in chronic rheumatic disorders. Wolfe Medical, London

Disability Information Trust 1997 Arthritis: an equipment guide. Disability Information Trust, Mary Marlborough Lodge, Oxford

Holroyd J 1990 Arthritis at your age? Grindle Press, Scottsdale, AZ

Klippel JH, Dieppe PA 1994 Rheumatology. Mosby, St Louis, MO

le Gallez P (ed) 1998 Rheumatology for nurses: patient care. Whurr: London

Melvin J, Jensen G (eds) 1998 Rheumatologic rehabilitation series. American Occupational Therapy Association: Bethesda, MD, vol 1: assessment and management; vol 2: adult rheumatic diseases; vol 3: paediatric rheumatic diseases; vol 4: the hand: evaluation, therapy and surgery; vol 5: surgical rehabilitation

Newman S, Fitzpatrick R, Revenson TA, Skevington S, Williams G 1996 Understanding rheumatoid arthritis. Routledge, London

Nordenskiold U 1996 Daily activities in women with rheumatoid arthritis: aspects of patient education, assistive devices and methods for disability and impairment assessment. PhD thesis. Department of Rehabilitation Medicine, Goteborg University, Goteborg, Sweden

Palmer P, Simons J 1991 Joint protection – a critical review. British Journal of Occupational Therapy 54:453–458

Schwartz SP 1997 250 Tips for making life with arthritis easier. Arthritis Foundation, Atlanta, GA

Unsworth H 1992 Coping with rheumatoid arthritis. Nottingham Rehab: Nottingham

Wegener ST, Belza BL, Gall EP 1996 Clinical care in the rheumatic diseases. American College of Rheumatology, Atlanta, GA

USEFUL CONTACTS

Patient education resource material

Arthritis Research Campaign
St Marys Court, St Marys Gate, Chesterfield, Derbyshire S41 7TD

Arthritis Care
18 Stephenson Way, London NW1 2HD

Arthritis Foundation
PO Box 1616, Alpharetta GA 30009–1616, USA

Useful websites for information on rheumatic diseases

Arthritis Research Campaign, UK: www.arc.org.uk

The Arthritis Society of Canada: www.arthritis.ca

Arthritis Foundation, USA: www.arthritis.org

American College of Rheumatology: www.rheumatology.org

24

Oncology

Jill Cooper

INTRODUCTION

WHAT IS ONCOLOGY?

Oncology is the study and practice of treating benign and malignant tumours, that is, cancer. It is important to appreciate that 'cancer' is a disease process and is a general term relating to tumours and growths. Cancer can be unpredictable and many questions are as yet unanswered. There is uncertainty about the disease, its causes, treatments, symptoms and future. However, a clear understanding of what is happening helps all concerned to cope with decisions and choices. No generalisation can be made with regard to prognosis or timescales. Each person has to be assessed and monitored individually and many people live free of the disease, without any problems, following successful treatment.

Prognosis is determined by the stage at which the disease is discovered. The more advanced the cancer is when it is diagnosed, the poorer the prognosis.

There are over 200 types of cancer and all start in the same way – when the normal, continuous, process of body cell regeneration and death becomes abnormal, resulting in an uncontrolled increase in the growth rate of the cells. This results in a mass, tumour or growth; this tumour may be benign or malignant. Benign tumours grow slowly, are usually curable if treated early and do not recur after excision. They may be life threatening if they affect vital organs. Malignant tumours can infiltrate and destroy the normal tissues surrounding them and spread to other sites. Malignant cancers can be cured but they might recur. The primary site, or tumour, is where the cancer begins.

Metastases or metastatic spread occurs when the primary malignant tumour spreads by invading surrounding cells via the bloodstream or lymphatic system. These tumours are also known as secondaries, and are composed of the same tissue as the primary. For example, if the primary cancer is breast and it spreads to the liver, the tumour(s) in the liver are secondary cancers of the breast.

'Cure' means that all evidence of cancer has been eliminated and there is no chance of it returning. Recurrence occurs when some primary tumour cells remain undetected and grow again later, which may be in a few months or several years. Quite often a secondary cancer may appear in the lymph nodes, or be seen on an X-ray, with no sign of a primary site. The primary source must be detected by specific investigations, such as surgery. When treated, it may be cured or enter remission. If the primary is not identifiable, it is unlikely to be cured and treatment is aimed at controlling or preventing symptoms.

It is important to remember that there is always a future after a diagnosis of cancer, though timescales may vary.

CAUSES OF CANCER

More is not known than is known about the causes of cancer. Possible causes include a tendency for cells to grow abnormally, which may be congenital, and triggers, such as exposure to radiation, asbestos, smoking and other inhaled or ingested carcinogens. Cancer is a disease of older age and as increasing numbers of people live longer, the incidence of cancers rises (Fig. 24.1).

Initial signs of cancer may include:

- a lump
- a sore that does not heal
- a mole that changes in shape, size, colour or bleeds abnormally
- persistent problems, such as cough, change in bowel movements, menstruation, urinary habits or weight loss.

There is no finite line between the acute, palliative and terminal stages. The focus may change from one to another as the disease progresses or goes into remission. Symptoms are approached in a problem-solving manner. Treatment depends on the individual's functional status and holistic view of the circumstances.

'Palliation' refers to alleviating symptoms rather than aiming to cure disease and is associated with the advanced stages of all diseases. The World Health Organization (1990) defines palliative care as 'the active total care of patients and their families by a multiprofessional team when the patient's disease is no longer responsive to curative treatment'.

'Terminal care' refers to an important part of palliative care and usually to the management of the person during their last few days, weeks or even months of life, from a point at which it becomes clear that he is in a progressive state of decline (National Council for Hospice and Specialist Palliative Care Services 1995).

THE FOCUS OF OCCUPATIONAL THERAPY

The functional difficulties with which the occupational therapist helps the individual might be the result of the disease process itself and/or the treatment. As it is a constantly evolving and changing field of medicine, the occupational therapist needs to investigate the specific disease, treatment process and prognosis with which the individual presents. It is impossible to generalise on all cancers so specialist advice should be sought as situations arise.

The effects of the disease and the side-effects of treatments can be acute in physical, psychological, emotional and social terms and, if there is recurrence, these may be longer term, which can influence the individual in their functional roles in the family and can affect their educational and/or career opportunities. There are often financial implications. The home environment might need to be altered and there can be an effect on relationships, cultural influences and spirituality.

Effective communication between the members of the multiprofessional team as well as the family and the individual is a key factor, as none of the

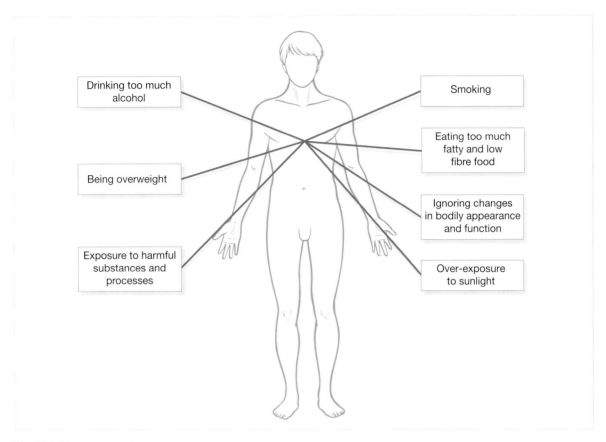

Fig. 24.1 Major causes of cancer.

above problems is seen in isolation. Robinson (1992) describes how it is the family rather than the isolated person who experiences the illness and family members should not be treated as bystanders but as an influencing, organising and creative agent.

TREATMENT SETTINGS AND THE TREATMENT TEAM

Early detection of cancer is vital for optimum success in treatment. National screening programmes are in place, for example, cervical smear tests and mammograms. Treatments offered to persons with cancer include radiotherapy, surgery, chemotherapy and specific treatments such as biological therapies or bone marrow transplantation. The person will be treated by a team of multidisciplinary professionals, including:

- healthcare professionals, such as occupational therapists, physiotherapists, dieticians, speech and language therapists, social workers, art therapists, lymphoedema therapists
- doctors, for example, GPs, surgeons, oncologists, radiologists
- nurses, for example, district nurses, clinical nurse specialists, Macmillan and other palliative care specialist nurses.

THEORETICAL FOUNDATIONS FOR INTERVENTION

Due to the complex nature of the disease process, it is vital to establish a supportive team. It is also essential for the occupational therapist to be skilled in the occupational therapy process and be able to access and use a wide range of assessment and intervention approaches to address the person's physical, psychological, emotional and social needs. These will not be unique to the cancer setting, as many will apply to other clinical areas, but they are influenced by the unique disease process of the cancer. Calman-Hine (1995) recommends the need for 'specialist cancer centres with multiprofessional teams to meet the patients' needs'. These needs are varied and demand immediate attention for intervention to be effective.

The goal of occupational therapy is to enable the individual to be autonomous, authentic and self-actualising. A humanistic, person-centred approach allows the individual to function as a free, self-directing, honest person whose life brings self-satisfaction and contains personal meaning. It is a dynamic, holistic, flexible approach that can deal with psychological, developmental and physical dysfunctions and with deteriorating and terminal conditions.

MODELS OF PRACTICE

Models of practice serve to provide a theory to underpin practice and reinforce the benefits of occupational therapy input. Hagedorn (1993) describes the rehabilitation model of occupational therapy as maximising existing functions and compensating for deficits. It promotes personal independence and restores normal or near normal function. The problem-solving model (Hagedorn 1993) complements the rehabilitation model, stating that interventions should be directed towards specific goals and be flexible. The problem-solving model works on the assumption that any problems should have several applicable solutions, be tackled in an order of priority decided by the person with cancer and the occupational therapist, and that progress should be monitored and evaluated.

Bray (1997) and Bayliss (1998) discuss using the Reed and Sanderson's Personal Adaptation through Occupation Model particularly in the assessment, preparation, planning, coordination and follow-up of people with cancer who wish to

return home. It focuses on wellness and takes into account the motor, sensory, cognitive, intra- and interpersonal skills, self-maintenance, productivity and leisure activities of the person with cancer, and enables the occupational therapist to define her role with each individual. It focuses on the analysis of activities and the individual's 'wellness' so that the occupational therapist can address capabilities and disabilities.

FRAMES OF REFERENCE AND APPROACHES

Cooper (1997) believes a biomechanical frame of reference is needed to address many of the physical limitations caused by the disease process. This frame of reference works on the assumption that the application of a graded programme of activities, linked to the individual's identified occupational needs, will work towards restoration or maintenance of normal or near normal function.

Use of a compensatory frame of reference serves to overcome any residual disability. This is the theoretical basis that underpins the provision of mobility or adaptive equipment and orthoses.

Within the learning frame of reference, both educational and cognitive approaches can be used to help the individual and his family make informed decisions regarding the issues in hand and to address their changing roles, functions and aspirations.

For the occupational therapist to reflect on how her input helps the person with functional difficulties, a combination of principles from a variety of frames of reference and approaches is taken, as the difficulties are multidimensional and complex.

OUTCOME MEASURES

Outcome measures are still being assessed in oncology. Norris (1999) studied the use of the Canadian Occupational Performance Measure in palliative care and found that the results focused on the individual's role in the intervention, thereby ensuring that issues important to him are emphasised. However, it was noted that the concept of self-rating proved difficult to use in practice – the final scores were subjective and interpretation using the score system alone proved difficult. An all-encompassing outcome measure that suits all requirements has yet to be established. Before choosing an outcome measure, the goals need to be established.

All these aspects in turn affect the occupational therapist's performance and coping abilities, so it is essential to ensure one's own needs are addressed in support, supervision, caseload and time management and prioritisation (see Chapter 8).

Soderback and Hammersley Paulsson (1997) state that quality of life may be negatively affected by cancer because of irreversible functional and occupational impairments. It is of great importance that occupational therapy is begun as early as possible.

INTERVENTION

Short and brief episodes of assessment and treatment are required due to the overwhelming fatigue that is nearly always present, with continuing reassessment and evaluation as conditions may change rapidly. Consequently, the person with cancer is unlikely to be able to tolerate a long session of assessment because the treatment causes such extreme fatigue. Once the individual becomes fatigued, it worsens other symptoms, for example, pain.

ASSESSMENT

By using the Human Occupations Model, the person can be assessed under the headings of self care, productivity and leisure. This encompasses functional and social aspects of personal and domestic activities of daily living, the home situation, transfers and mobility. This model reflects the belief that areas identified as important to the individual will provide the motivation that drives occupational performance. Emphasis is placed on the concept of person-centred treatment and joint goal setting so that the goals are meaningful to the individual.

TREATMENT

Following assessment, experience shows that the occupational therapist is likely to be involved in the following areas of intervention:

- assisting individuals fulfil prioritised occupational performance needs that have been interrupted by physical dysfunction
- facilitating individuals to perform personal and domestic activities that fall within their roles
- assessing seating needs and the prescription of wheelchairs
- retraining individuals with cognitive and perceptual dysfunctions arising from brain dysfunction
- using splinting in the prevention of joint deformities from immobility and decreased use of limbs
- assessing and providing equipment in the person's home
- assisting with psychological adjustment and goal setting related to loss of roles and functions
- supporting and educating carers
- lifestyle management based around stress and anxiety management and energy conservation
- breathing exercises and anxiety management for shortness of breath as well as anxiety (Cooper 1997).

PRINCIPLES UNDERPINNING THE INTERVENTION PROCESS

Occupational therapy enables individuals to set goals and priorities and to achieve those that are important to them. In retraining areas of functional independence, arranging homecare support or in symptom control, the occupational therapist works as part of the multiprofessional team to facilitate and not take over or interfere.

In all aspects of intervention, the carers and family are integral to the assessments and treatments and should not be treated as a separate entity. However, if the individual with cancer does not wish them to be included, that should be respected and addressed as appropriate.

Issues such as coping with role change, body image and loss are broad concepts that become part of the intervention process and the individual's cancer journey. Depending on the person's situation and problems that arise, it may be the occupational therapist who becomes a key worker, or other members of the multiprofessional team may be more involved. Loss, grief and bereavement are likely to be addressed by all team members to some extent, not as a separate issue but as part of their intervention. Some oncology services may have a specific bereavement officer whose role is to help people with cancer and their carers. This does not prevent other team members contributing to the adjustment and adaptation to loss, or preparing for imminent loss. The team and the individual decide the areas in which help is needed, the approach to be taken and how best to use each team member's specialist skills. Support for individuals and their families may include emotional support through problem solving and active listening, self-help groups, carers' support groups and bereavement support.

The skills employed by the occupational therapist range from teaching breathing control and relaxation techniques to providing certain items of equipment in the home which facilitate independence. The psychological and physical approaches contribute towards helping persons with cancer reach their optimum functional independence. Other team members have their own areas of expertise to help the individual and support colleagues.

Areas of dysfunction are not always physical sequelae to treatment and the disease process. Problems are multifaceted and multidimensional. They overlap with each other and have profound effects on the individual, carers and the team caring for them.

SPECIFIC SYMPTOM CONTROL WITHIN INTERVENTION

Individuals with cancer experience a variety of symptoms depending on the origin of the cancer, so it is difficult to highlight the most common. Cancer is a continuous and ongoing situation;

symptoms are hastily replaced by others. The percentage of symptoms commonly seen in metastatic lung cancer differ from those experienced, for example, in brain tumours. Variants may include age, presence of other illness and premorbid status. The individual may have mental illness, cardiac or neurological disease, arthritis and psychosocial difficulties as well as the cancer. The case studies illustrated in Boxes 24.1 to 24.3 aim to show how the occupational therapy approaches to symptom management are rarely carried out in isolation and many aspects of occupational therapy skills are used to address dysfunctions.

As there are over 200 types of cancers, a list of cancer sites together with occupational therapy interventions would be endless. Table 24.1 shows examples of presenting problems and the cancer sites at which they might be seen and suggests possible solutions. A pattern of aims and interventions can be seen in the table but it is by no means definitive and serves purely as an indicator of those areas in which occupational therapy becomes involved and therapists will develop their own areas of expertise. It does illustrate that there are no set answers to functional difficulties as all individuals and their circumstances vary.

The following areas show in detail how the occupational therapist working in oncology uses her range of skills to assist in the following areas:

- spirituality
- culture
- management of pain
- management of fatigue
- sexuality
- anxiety and stress management
- management of breathlessness.

Spirituality

Spirituality can mean allowing people to express themselves and helping provide meaning, a sense of fulfilment and purpose to their lives. Stoter (1996) felt that although religion is a component of spirituality, there are many other aspects. Egan and Delaat (1994) discuss how illness creates a block to spiritual expression and

---

Box 24.1 Case study: Mr X.

Mr X. is a 59-year-old retired civil servant who has been diagnosed with myeloma. Mr X. invested his retirement money in a sports clothing business. He is a very keen football supporter and sportsman. Married, with two adult children and five grandchildren, his family is managing his business successfully for him.

Two years ago Mr X. was admitted to hospital with spinal cord compression presenting with bilateral leg weakness, altered sensation but no urinary or bowel problems. He had decompression laminectomy and was advised to commence walking and increase trunk strength gradually with carefully planned physiotherapy exercises. Physiotherapy referred him to occupational therapy for relaxation and breathing exercises as he was very anxious about his distressing symptoms. He attended occupational therapy for five sessions and coped well using structured relaxation and breathing exercises.

Six months ago, Mr X. was admitted with pathological fractures to the ribs. There was no further evidence of spinal cord compression. He underwent radiotherapy to ribs to relieve pain and aid healing.

Areas of occupational therapy assessment

- To assess personal and domestic activities of daily living.

- To assess home environment.
- To review breathing and relaxation exercises.

Occupational therapy intervention

No functional problems were identified other than in personal activities of daily living:

- a thorough assessment and discussion took place regarding coping at home
- showering equipment was identified as necessary to decrease the effort of movements involved. Mr X. discussed with his wife whether they would prefer a social services referral or proceed with private purchase of the equipment.
- breathing exercises were reviewed. The rapport that had been established previously enabled the occupational therapist to introduce relaxation again and Mr X. was keen to pursue this.

There then followed a pattern of ongoing and increasingly frequent admissions to hospital for management of pain and constipation by the medical and nursing team. Ongoing occupational therapy evaluation was required to ensure that functional problems were anticipated and planned for. Equipment was in place as soon as required without intruding on and taking away the control from Mr X. and his family.

Box 24.2 Case study: Mrs Z.

Mrs Z. is 40 years old and works as a Project Manager for a multinational company. She had no hobbies prior to taking 10 months off sick for treatment of colorectal cancer (she received a colostomy, which would be reversed in 8 months). Mrs Z. was married, with no children. She was referred by her consultant oncologist for relaxation because she was extremely restless and anxious. She underwent chemotherapy and 5 weeks of daily sessions of radiotherapy.

Aims of occupational therapy assessment

- To assess for relaxation and anxiety management.
- To establish a programme of relaxation sessions.

Occupational therapy intervention

The initial appointment was made with a view to seeing Mrs Z. five times. During the first session, no breathing or relaxation exercises were carried out because Mrs Z.

talked extensively about losing control of her life. A timetable was drawn up to look at the structure of her days. She had, in fact, taken up several hobbies – gardening, computer skills and painting – about which her husband was concerned because he felt his wife was not resting. The approach taken by the occupational therapist was to persuade Mrs Z. and her husband to view the activities as constructive and positive but to monitor them so that she did not exhaust herself, particularly as radiotherapy progressed and she became more tired.

Relaxation techniques were taught over the next four sessions and Mrs Z. was encouraged to put aside time to practise these as an active exercise rather than a passive relaxation. Mrs Z. felt able to follow the relaxation exercises and benefited both from these and from seeing her weekly timetable set out on paper. She began to accept the changes in her lifestyle and view them as purposeful by looking at the range of skills being developed.

---

how examining one's values and beliefs may cause a spiritual crisis. Illness causes a change in life roles and the occupational therapist can help the individual regain some control by optimising functional independence. Occupational therapy can allow expression and adaptation to dysfunction. Reminiscence work, in the form of diaries, letters or life stories, as well as the use of creative

---

Box 24.3   Case study: Mrs P.

Mrs P. is now aged 76. Breast cancer was originally diagnosed and treated 27 years ago. Upon admission she presented with lung, liver and bone metastases resulting in shortness of breath and pain on walking.

Mrs P. is now widowed and lives alone but she has a caring adult family, all living locally, who help with domestic chores. A package of carers is already in place to assist with self care. Her family leaves meals already prepared. Mrs P. was coping well until the bone metastases started to cause increased pain. She was admitted to hospital for a course of radiotherapy to alleviate bone pain.

Areas of occupational therapy assessment

- To liaise with the multiprofessional team as part of the overall assessment and review of input including dietetics, physiotherapy and occupational therapy.
- To assess Mrs P.'s safety and independence in activities that are important to her.
- To assess Mrs P.'s functional independence including transfers on/off furniture in hospital and at home.

Occupational therapy intervention

Occupational therapy assessment identified increased difficulties with mobility, especially all transfers on/off bed, armchair, toilet, and bathing as a priority. A home assessment was carried out prior to discharge from hospital with Mrs P., one member of her family and a key worker from the care team were also present. The main issues addressed were:

- Stairs: Mrs P. was no longer able to manage the stairs, even with additional rails, and did not want to have a

stairlift installed even if charitable monies could pay for it. She agreed to use one of the downstairs rooms as a bedroom; there was a downstairs toilet next to this room. The bed proved to be too low and nursing services preferred to have an adjustable-height bed with a pressure-relieving mattress overlay in place, which would help them in caring for her. A commode was installed by her bed.
- Bathroom: As Mrs P. could no longer manage the stairs, the bathroom was inaccessible. Care workers agreed to help her have a strip wash daily.
- Furniture heights: chair raisers were fitted to her armchair to enable safe and comfortable transfers. A pressure-relieving cushion was supplied and a Mowbray frame (toilet frame and raised toilet seat combined) was fitted round the toilet to facilitate safe transfers.

Although moving the bedroom downstairs proved to be a major change in Mrs P.'s living accommodation, the disruption and introduction of equipment to aid daily living was kept to a minimum. Further functional difficulties were addressed as they arose and the occupational therapist provided solutions as necessary, including a hoist to help the carers transfer Mrs P. with minimum effort.

A 6-week programme of daycare attendance once a week at the local hospice was also organised. This aimed to reduce Mrs P.'s social isolation, encourage decision making and active participation in creative activities, and gently increase exercise tolerance in attending the daycare. It also enabled the palliative care team to monitor Mrs P.'s progress and stabilise medication.

---

writing, may help the person reflect on the past and contribute a memento for the future. However, not everyone dies having come to terms with their mortality. Issues might not be addressed or resolved and it is the individual's right to cope in this way. Not everyone can die happy and at peace; anger at a life-threatening illness is understandable. The occupational therapist may be part of the close team who can help resolve some issues and is likely to become involved in practical issues such as those listed previously. Becoming involved in practical areas does create an intimacy, particularly relating to personal care, washing, dressing, toileting, bathing and showering. The professional rapport that develops allows the occupational therapist to help in more emotional matters. If the occupational therapist does not feel equipped to deal or help with these, there are professionals available

who can, so it is vital to recognise one's limitations and boundaries. No one single person or healthcare professional can deal with all the individual's problems. It is not a failing but a valuable professional strength to know when one can help and when to ask others for their professional expertise.

Culture

Major body image issues may be influenced by different cultures and religions. As the individual feels so tired and may suffer nausea and vomiting, the family roles are often changed and this can have a devastating effect on the family unit. In a society with either strongly male- or female-dominated boundaries it can be extremely difficult for the family to cope, particularly as healthcare professionals may have a poor understanding of the family's cultural expectations.

Table 24.1 Occupational therapy aims and interventions in presenting problems in people with cancer

Presenting problems	Disabilities result from	Occupational therapy aims	Occupational therapy interventions
Lymphoedema, accumulation of lymph in the interstitial space of subcutaneous tissue	Any areas in which lymph nodes become compromised and damaged resulting in reduced efficiency in lymphatic system, for example, upper limb in breast cancers, lower limb in pelvic, gynaecological and prostate cancers Radiation-induced brachial plexopathy (Cooper 1998)	To optimise functional independence within limits of affected limb(s) To work with lymphoedema therapist in reducing and maintaining limb volume To educate person regarding care of lymphoedematous limb Assess for independence in all areas important to the individual	Arrange for provision of adaptive equipment; teach alternative techniques as appropriate Splinting to avoid joint deformity and provide support and comfort Establish routine to help person manage compression hosiery or bandaging Reinforce educational elements of lymphoedema treatment programme such as advice on skin care
Cognition	Brain tumours Advanced stages of cancers with brain metastases Confusional states resulting from hypercalcaemia	To assess how cognitive dysfunction affects functional independence To assess person's abilities in problem solving, sequencing, memory, attention span, initiating activities, recognition and orientation. Standardised assessment such as Chessington Occupational Therapy Neurological Assessment Battery, Middlesex Elderly Assessment Mental Score, Rivermead, or using part of these as appropriate to the level of the individual's stamina and concentration	Working with individual and carers to support them and help them cope with the altered person Identify areas in which the person wishes to retain and/or regain optimum independence Facilitate compensation of dysfunctions by practising activities chosen by the individual Support integration of the relearned functions, skills and the compensation technique in the person's daily life in relation to activities of daily living, work, leisure and social life
Hemiplegia	Brain tumours Advanced stages of cancer with brain metastases	To assess functional independence To establish realistic treatment programme with physiotherapist and speech and language therapist within limitations of fatigue To provide appropriate equipment to compensate for dysfunction To facilitate individual and carer's acceptance of limitations and establish coping strategies	Establish routine of incorporating assessments and practice of identified areas of importance Evaluate these with other team members, the individual and carers to focus on abilities and strengths but avoid overtiring him Introduce equipment to aid functional independence, plan ahead and anticipate any likely needs if condition appears to be deteriorating Work with team, individual and carers to discuss their concerns, practical and emotional difficulties and how to address these

continued

Table 24.1 *continued*

Presenting problems	Disabilities result from	Occupational therapy aims	Occupational therapy interventions
Sensory impairment Neuropathies	Brain tumours Myeloma Sarcoma Temporary or permanent side-effects of chemotherapy (Cook & Burkhardt 1994) Breast cancer resulting in lymphoedema Radiation-induced brachial plexopathy (Cooper 1998)	Ongoing assessment of function To provide appropriate equipment to adapt and compensate for sensory loss To assess for treatment programme over a set period of time To help the individual cope with adaptation to loss of function	Arrange for provision of equipment to enable optimum functional independence Treatment programme to incorporate functional practice to retrain for sensory loss and impairment, including advice on coping with and adapting to functional loss
Spinal cord compression	Primary tumour of spine Advanced stage of any cancer, for example, lung or breast with spinal metastases Advanced stage of any cancer resulting in crush fracture due to weakened vertebrae	To assess functional independence To provide equipment to aid optimum independence in the short and long term To work with multiprofessional team, individual and carers to cope with physical and psychological trauma of disability	Establish routine of optimum independence in functional activities that are important to the individual Immediate provision of appropriate equipment to optimise independence and comfort. If wheelchair dependent, establish routine of safe transfers or hoisting. Ensure pressure care issues are addressed by all team Educate individual and carers about pressure care and importance of skin, bowel, urinary care Make plans with individual and carers regarding future requirements to return home with appropriate levels of care and equipment Anxiety management, breathing and relaxation exercises Liaison and advice regarding safe and appropriate return to work and driving

Communication is essential because the multi-professional team might have preconceived ideas regarding the extent of family and community support that is available and make incorrect assumptions about this. A background knowledge should be established, therefore, about how the disease is viewed within specific communities and how it affects status. The team needs to establish the individual's and carers' views on autonomy versus others caring for them. Furthermore, assumptions should not be made that the individual follows their religion or cultural norms devoutly – the person might not wish to have traditions followed. Occupational therapists should communicate with the family and carers to ensure

that appropriate assessment and treatment programmes are followed, just as any treatment plan is negotiated with the individual. Areas of particular concern are often focused around:

● hair loss, of particular importance to men and women in many cultures
● amputation of a body part, for example a breast or limb
● stoma care in colostomies, ileostomies and urostomies, which may create difficulties for people whose religion does not permit them to worship if the stoma is functioning or if the individual will need to leave to carry out ablutions.

Management of pain

Pain is a multidimensional symptom and varies between individuals. Pain associated with cancer can result from the tumour pressing on, or infiltrating, pain-sensitive structures. It can also be caused by injury to the nerves, bone and soft tissue as a result of chemotherapy, radiotherapy or surgery. There may also be tumour- or radiation-induced vascular occlusion. Acute pain may be associated with anxiety and fear, and chronic pain is not merely an extension of this but continues long term and may result in depression and fatigue. Pain control in palliative care does not have the same behavioural and cognitive elements as chronic pain control in other pain clinics. Medication needs to be established, using the basic principles of pain control as recommended by the World Health Organization analgesic ladder for cancer pain management (1986; Fig. 24.2).

The concept of 'total pain' is encompassed in the World Health Organization Cancer Pain Relief Programme, which states that pain cannot be considered in isolation and should be seen as a comprehensive programme that encompasses the physical, psychological, social and spiritual aspects of both pain and suffering. Individuals may experience more than one type of pain. If there are secondaries causing bone pain, for example, this will be quite different to constipa-tion pain or nerve pain. Thorough and precise assessment is needed, therefore, to assess the type of pain, the nature of the pain (niggling, aching, sharp, disabling), its duration, what exacerbates it and what relieves it. Various pain assessments exist to enable the occupational therapist to undertake a thorough assessment. Box 24.4 illustrates Foley's (1996) Components of Pain questionnaire.

Occupational therapy intervention can contribute in pain relief by:

- Using a problem-solving approach to look at the structure of the day. This is a foundation for planning and changing lifestyle

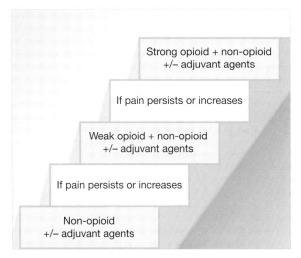

Fig. 24.2 World Health Organization (1996) analgesic ladder for cancer pain management.

Box 24.4 Components of pain questionnaire (Foley 1996 in The Oxford Textbook of Palliative Medicine (© Derek Doyle, Geoffrey WC Hanks and Neil MacDonald (1993) (eds) by kind permission of Oxford University Press)

Wisconsin Brief Pain Questionnaire

- Self-administered, easily understood, brief method to assess pain.
- Addresses history, intensity, location and quality of pain.
- A drawing of a human figure is provided for the person to shade the area corresponding to his pain. Pain is rated at its worst, usual pain, pain now and how it interferes with mood, relations with other people and functional ability. Pain scales consist of numbers 0–10, 0 being no pain, 10 being the worst pain imaginable.

The McGill Pain Questionnaire

- Categories divided into four dimensions: sensory, affective, evaluative and miscellaneous.
- Offers a methodological approach to assess these dimensions of pain but may be difficult and cumbersome for individuals to understand and complete and may be limited by its language constraints.

The Memorial Pain Assessment Card

- Comprises three visual analogue scales, which measure pain intensity, pain relief and mood, and a set of pain severity descriptors adapted from the Tursky Rating Scale.
- Provides valid, multidimensional information for the evaluation of pain and distress in cancer patients.
- Can distinguish pain intensity from pain relief and from global suffering and can be used to study the subtle interactions of these factors.

management so that adaptations can be made to levels of fatigue and coping with pain.

- Analysing activities that result in an increase in pain. The occupational therapist and the individual can aim to change components of the activity to avoid pain being exacerbated.
- Assessing for and arranging provision of items of equipment to improve the safety and comfort of transfers, for example, in and out of bed and bath or shower, on and off the toilet or armchair. Pressure relief and correct positioning in bed or chair will also alleviate pain and discomfort.
- Splinting to prevent painful joint deformities.
- Incorporating relaxation and stress management into the individual's programme to help him cope with or avoid anxiety attacks, which can affect pain levels. The relaxation programme includes recognising situations that evoke anxiety and learning how to prevent the situations escalating.
- Addressing emotional pain at the loss of function by exploring the individual's feelings and rationalising them, helping the person to adapt to and cope with the loss. Relaxation and breathing exercises can help the person take back some control over their life when it may appear that things are spiralling out of control.
- Supporting and educating the individual and his carers and enabling them to manage these aspects of pain control themselves.

Management of fatigue

The most common factor seen in both acute and advanced stages of cancer is fatigue. It may be related to weight loss, pain and decreased mood and affects the individual's wellbeing, daily living, valued relationships, roles and functions and compliance with treatment. People who have undergone radiotherapy report an increase in fatigue over a 5- or 6-week course and those undergoing chemotherapy report an increase for around 14 days after treatment. It is also natural for surgery to cause fatigue.

Fatigue can diminish, although it remains in a small number of people. Prolonged or chronic fatigue can be very distressing and the team needs to plan ongoing care and support. A structured plan of treatment may improve stamina but the approach needs to be flexible as there may not be significant improvement. A programme to increase exercise tolerance is not likely to be successful in cancer-related fatigue. A thorough assessment is required as tiredness may be linked to cachexia, anorexia, pain or breathlessness and should be treated appropriately. A treatment programme should be based around the individual and his therapist scheduling activities (Box 24.5) by:

- making priorities and choices
- deciding which activities to shed
- organising remaining tasks at manageable level
- looking at the structure of the day
- compiling a weekly diary or timetable.

Simply giving the individual a sheet of instructions on energy conservation is rarely effective as such major changes to lifestyle need close attention to detail. By using the above techniques, the occupational therapist can enable the individual to take control of his fatigue by working with him to establish exercise and activity tolerance levels. An overall balance of activities in the day needs to be considered and related directly to the person's identified occupational needs and priorities. The individual is helped to look at the amount of activity he can tolerate and his posture when exercising as well as when working and resting. This can also affect his pain levels so alternative seating in the workplace, home and car could be considered.

The individual will need to work through his daily timetable of activities to have an objective view of what he can and cannot manage and what can be omitted. It is very difficult to carry out this exercise subjectively. Encouraging frequent rests and doing tasks differently, delegating and eliminating non-essential activities can take a lot of persuasion. Planning ahead for tasks ranging from shopping, preparation of meals, arrangements for childcare and returning to work or studies are complex tasks that require a

---

Box 24.5 Scheduling activities

A weekly timetable in which a 42-year-old woman undergoing radiotherapy daily for 6 weeks has focused her energies on activities she wishes to continue. The woman works part-time, has a partner who works full-time and two sons at school. She has parents-in-law and parents who can help with some jobs, for example, childcare.

Monday

a.m. Attend hospital for radiotherapy
Relaxation session in occupational therapy
Lunch
p.m. Rest for 2 hours
Collect children from school
Tea and TV

Tuesday

a.m. Attend hospital for radiotherapy
Lunch
p.m. Attend massage therapy session
Grandparents to collect children and give them their tea
Practice relaxation at home
Rest before evening

Wednesday

a.m. Attend hospital for radiotherapy and clinic appointment
Lunch
p.m. Sleep for 2 hours
Practice relaxation at home
Grandparents to collect children and give them their tea
Light housework if able

Thursday

a.m. Go into work for 2 hours
Lunch
p.m. Attend hospital for radiotherapy
Grandparents to collect children and give them their tea
Rest before family at home for the evening, make shopping list

Friday

a.m. Go into work for 2–3 hours
Lunch
p.m. Attend hospital for radiotherapy
Grandparents to collect children, give tea and take to Scouts
Shopping with partner, regular rests

Weekend

Regular rests, no appointments, limit visits by friends to 20 minutes. Partner and parents to take telephone calls and ensure visits do not exceed this.
Timetable a session to practise relaxation at home.

---

programme of sessions in which the individual and occupational therapist work through issues using a flexible problem-solving approach. Individuals with fatigue also experience poor and disturbed sleep patterns, which can be affected by medication, so the medical team needs to be consulted about changing times and dosages of drugs. Anxiety affects sleep and a programme of sessions can be introduced to teach the individual how to incorporate relaxation techniques into his daily life to avoid stress.

Sexuality

Cooper (1997) reports that fatigue is a major factor in problems relating to sexuality, as are anxiety, pain, altered body image and depression. Whether the underlying problems relating to dysfunction are physical or psychological, the individual needs to be able to discuss these and the occupational therapist needs to be able to give appropriate advice or refer on to specialist help. Physical help for side-effects such as vaginal dryness, impotence or erectile dysfunction may be managed medically, but more emotional issues will require a structured and problem-solving approach. Communicating these fears and worries with a partner may avoid difficulties in relationships. The occupational therapist's role is to establish trust so that issues are discussed and recognised. Advice on sexual functioning could be facilitated by the clinical nurse specialist in gynaecology, for example, or referral to a counsellor. A relationship may require renegotiating if the sexual problems persist so that each partner understands the other's feelings and worries. A close and trusting rapport needs to be established so that the individual feels secure in addressing these issues. The occupational therapist might find limitations in her skills. This is dealt with by acknowledging this and seeking advice from more appropriately qualified colleagues.

Anxiety and stress management

Anxiety is a normal biological defence mechanism warning the body of potential danger and allowing it to react quickly in times of stress.

Individuals with cancer may feel out of control because they have the diagnosis imposed on them and have to comply with treatment that makes them feel very ill; this can spiral into episodes of anxiety. Prolonged stress over a period of time can result in decreased energy, initiative and motivation as well as the physical manifestations of tense muscles, excessive fatigue, tension headaches, palpitations, dizziness, blackouts, stomach churning, tightness in the throat and chest, restlessness, excessive sweating, shaking and stammering. Psychological symptoms may include apprehension, insomnia, loss of confidence, depression, short temper, irritability, self-consciousness, sexual difficulties, fears, phobias and difficulties in personal relationships and in formulating thoughts.

Significant areas of muscular tension, known as trigger points, may include the forehead and eyes, shoulders and neck, clenched hands and chest pains. If a person can recognise tension in these areas and implement relaxation techniques, accumulation of anxiety and tension may be avoided. Stress management programmes offer a practical way to change maladaptive responses, using cognitive and physiological components. The occupational therapist and the individual need to establish a set number of sessions during which they will explore issues and practise dealing with this. Identifying negative thoughts, understanding the meaning of them and changing and modifying thoughts can help stressful situations become manageable. By incorporating relaxation techniques and breathing control into daily living, individuals can counteract stressful responses and replace these with relaxed posture and controlled breathing. Techniques should be selected on an individual basis to suit specific needs. Progressive muscular relaxation may not be suitable for individuals with bone or muscle pain; people with limited concentration and extreme fatigue may need shorter techniques.

As with all intervention, thorough assessment and intervention must be planned. Relaxation and stress management can be in a group or individual setting but group members may have varied and diverse needs so the dynamics have to be carefully considered.

Box 24.6 Aims of relaxation (Cooper 1997)

- To understand and recognise your level of anxiety.
- To understand the need for relaxation and recognise certain situations that may trigger tension.
- To experience a variety of relaxation techniques thus enabling you to choose the most appropriate one.
- To appreciate the importance of planning time for relaxation as part of your daily activities and lifestyle.
- To improve quality of sleep.
- To lessen pain caused by inappropriate muscle tension.
- To encourage peace of mind.
- To improve performance of physical skills.
- To increase self-esteem and confidence.
- To ease relationships with others.
- To channel and control effects of anxiety.
- To avoid unnecessary fatigue.

As with all intervention, clear therapeutic aims and objectives are required and the occupational therapist must ensure that the person with cancer does not become dependent on her for relaxation. The aim of the sessions is to teach the individual coping techniques so that he can deal with anxiety-provoking situations in his daily life. The techniques may also be used to help him deal with episodes of nausea and vomiting, which, in turn, result in anxiety and distress.

Specific relaxation techniques do not help with specific symptoms. A relaxation programme teaching a range of exercises enables the individual to take a balanced approach to dealing with anxiety. He can practise and experience these and use them to facilitate his occupational performance (Box 24.6).

Management of breathlessness

Like pain, shortness of breath (dyspnoea) is a sensation that can be subjective as well as a physical medical symptom. It can be exacerbated by fatigue and anxiety, limit function and restrict normal activity. It can be described as ranging from tightness in the chest, needing to gasp or pant to extreme fear or 'suffocation' or 'drowning'. It occurs as an acute or chronic symptom. Primarily, it is essential that the individual is made comfortable and reassurance given by the medical and nursing team, possibly using oxygen and other medication as appropriate to reduce the distress.

Possible causes of breathlessness are primary or secondary lung cancer, pulmonary asthma, chronic obstructive airways disease, pleural effusion, pneumothorax, bronchial asthma, pulmonary embolism or chest infection. Cardiac disease such as heart failure can cause shortness of breath, as can hyperventilation. When considering the causes of breathlessness it is important to consider the chronic and other incidental diseases, which are perhaps unrelated to the main condition, whether this is malignancy or another terminal condition.

Once the acute symptoms are managed, the occupational therapist can begin to investigate coping mechanisms and lifestyle management. As well as considering the breathlessness, the occupational therapist can advise how to reduce unnecessary exertion that may exacerbate the symptom, for example, by placing a commode by the bed or moving the bed downstairs. Carers can assist with personal care so that basic activities do not become too difficult and can explore other ways of changing the daily routines to prevent breathless attacks. Relaxation and anxiety management techniques may assist the individual once a trusting rapport has been established. Focusing on breathing exercises when someone is having breathing problems may seem contradictory, but by slowing the breathing pattern and reducing the anxiety levels, the individual can feel in control of his breathing. Breathlessness is often associated with weight loss, so dietetic support is essential. It is often impossible to separate the physiological components from the frequently accompanying psychological, social and spiritual dimensions. The longer the episode of breathlessness, the increased likelihood of overriding fear and anxiety. Muscle fatigue related to breathlessness may be significant, particularly with pleural tumours such as mesothelioma. No gold-standard measurements exist for this symptom although the occupational therapist can help the individual identify his own exercise tolerance through functional assessment and practice. By establishing when the person becomes short of breath, he can prearrange activities to avoid episodes of distress.

CONCLUSION

The occupational therapist working in oncology will use all her core skills and will need to work in, or at least have access to, a supportive, established, multiprofessional team. There is no 'check-list' for intervention with individuals with a diagnosis of cancer because presenting symptoms are constantly changing and multifaceted. The diagnosis of cancer is not necessarily one of death in the immediate future. Timescales vary, depending on:

- the stage at which the disease is diagnosed and the course of the disease
- the person's response to treatment
- whether the cancer is cured, goes into remission or progresses.

The Personal Adaptation through Occupation Model helps the occupational therapist underpin her professional practice in oncology. Clear therapeutic aims and objectives need to be set with a flexible problem-solving and person-centred approach. The occupational therapist has a clear role in enabling the individual to achieve optimum functional independence and it is a challenging clinical area which demands the highest standards of care and expertise.

REFERENCES

Bayliss S 1998 Planning for home – the role of the occupational therapist. Palliative Care Today 3(1):8–9
Bray J 1997 Occupational therapy in hospices and daycare. In: Cooper J (ed) Occupational therapy in oncology and palliative care. Whurr, London, ch 10, p 174

Calman K, Hine D 1995 A policy framework for commissioning cancer services. Department of Health, London
Cooper J 1997 Occupational therapy in oncology and palliative care. Whurr, London

Cooper J 1998 Occupational therapy intervention with radiation-induced brachial plexopathy. European Journal of Cancer Care 7:88–92

Egan M, Delaat MD 1994 Considering spirituality in occupational therapy practice. Canadian Journal of Occupational Therapy 61(2):95–101

Foley KM 1996 Pain assessment and cancer pain syndromes. In: Doyle D, Hanks GWC, MacDonald N (eds) Oxford textbook of palliative medicine. Oxford University Press, Oxford, ch 4.2.2, pp 151–154

Hagedorn R 1993 Occupational therapy foundations for practice. Churchill Livingstone, Edinburgh

National Council for Hospice & Specialist Palliative Care Services (NCHSPCS) 1995 Specialist palliative care: a statement of definitions. NCHSPCS, London

Norris A 1999 A pilot study of an outcome measure in palliative care. International Journal of Palliative Nursing 5(1):40–45

Robinson SN 1992 The family with cancer. European Journal of Cancer Care 1(2):29–33

Soderback I, Hammersley Paulsson E 1997 A needs assessment for referral to occupational therapy. Cancer Nursing 20(4):267–273

Stoter D 1996 Spiritual care. In: Penson J, Fisher R (eds) Palliative care for people with cancer, 2nd edn. Edward Arnold, London, ch 11, p 158

World Health Organization (WHO) 1986 The analgesic ladder. WHO, Geneva

World Health Organization (WHO) 1990 Palliative care. WHO, Geneva

---

FURTHER READING

BBC/Macmillan Cancer Relief 1997 The cancer guide. BBC Learning Support, London

Buckman R 1995 What you really need to know about cancer. Macmillan, London

Cook A, Burkhardt A 1994 The effect of cancer diagnosis and treatment on hand function. American Journal of Occupational Therapy 48(9):836–839

Cooper J 1997 Occupational therapy in oncology and palliative care. Whurr, London

Fisher SN 1998 Multidisciplinary teamwork. In: Guerrero D (ed) Neuro-oncology for nurses. Whurr, London, ch 9, p 233

Doyle D, Hanks GWC, MacDonald N 1996 Oxford textbook of palliative medicine, 2nd edn. Oxford University Press, Oxford

Guerrero D 1998 Neuro-oncology for nurses. Whurr, London

Kaye P 1995 Breaking bad news. EPL Publications, Northampton

Penson J, Fisher R 1995 Palliative care for people with cancer, 2nd edn. Edward Arnold, London

Royal College of Radiologists (RCR) 1995 Management of adverse effects following breast radiotherapy. RCR: London

Salter M 1997 Altered body image, 2nd edn. Baillière Tindall, London

Souhami R, Tobias J 1995 Cancer and its management, 2nd edn. Blackwell, Oxford

Tobias J 1995 Cancers: what every patient needs to know. Bloomsbury, London

25

Cardiac and respiratory disease

Kim Oliver Louise Sewell

INTRODUCTION

Coronary heart disease has been called the plague of the 20th century (Kavanagh 1998) and the World Health Organization identified it as the number one cause of death worldwide. Coronary heart disease is the highest cause of death in the United Kingdom, where it accounts for 22% of all deaths (Murray et al 1993).

Coronary heart disease is a condition that impacts on every aspect of daily life and significantly affects quality of life, future employment and personal relationships, as well as increasing the risk of premature death (National Service Framework – Coronary Heart Disease). It is estimated that in England more than 1.4 million people have angina, 300 000 people have heart attacks every year and 110 000 people die from heart-related problems.

Chronic respiratory diseases are also increasingly being cited as major causes of disability. Respiratory diseases (not including respiratory malignancies) currently account for 17% of deaths in England and Wales and are the third main cause of death (Office for National Statistics 2000). Individually, asthma is the most prevalent respiratory disease and is thought to affect approximately 4% (approximately 2.5 million people); chronic obstructive pulmonary disease (COPD) affects 1% (600 000 people). However, COPD carries a higher mortality rate than asthma and it is thought to be the fifth most common cause of death in England and Wales (Calverley & Sondhi 1998).

THE EXTENT OF THE PROBLEM

Coronary heart disease can affect people of all ages, each gender and all social classes. However, its prevalence is unequal. The National Service Framework for coronary heart disease (DoH 2000) identified that:

- Rates of coronary heart disease vary according to social circumstances.
- Morbidity rates differ with angina.
- Myocardial infarction and cardiovascular accidents are most common amongst people in the manual social class.
- Differences in the social spectrum are increasing, including changes in ethnic variations.

Advances in the medical management of coronary heart disease, which have reduced the mortality rates, have led to greater numbers of people with chronic cardiovascular disease.

Subtle changes in the functioning of the heart occur naturally as part of the ageing process. These, combined with an increasing prevalence of chronic cardiovascular disease, have led to considerable impact on the demands of the health services (McMurray & Cleland 2000).

Recent studies (Katz 2000) have identified that one in 20 new hospital admissions are due to coronary heart disease. Individuals with coronary heart disease should be managed across the number of medical specialities in different areas of health and social care provision.

Respiratory diseases can also affect people of all ages and all social classes. Activities of daily living are typically limited by problems of dyspnoea and fatigue. Common problems for people with either chronic respiratory disease or coronary heart conditions include physical deconditioning, anxiety, depression and social isolation.

This chapter concentrates on chronic conditions associated with coronary heart disease and respiratory impairments and the impact of these with an ageing population. For specific guidance on the acute management of coronary heart disease, respiratory conditions and respiratory and cardiac rehabilitation, please refer to the references provided at the end of the chapter.

TYPES OF RESPIRATORY DISEASE

The main respiratory diseases fall into one of two categories: obstructive disease and restrictive disease. These descriptions reflect the pathological mechanisms that lead to respiratory insufficiency. Obstructive diseases are more prevalent than restrictive disorders because of the wider incidence of COPD and asthma. Secondary problems caused by these two major disorders are most commonly encountered by the occupational therapist working in the area of general physical medicine.

OBSTRUCTIVE RESPIRATORY DISEASE

Chronic obstructive pulmonary disease

COPD is the most common term used to describe two main conditions: chronic bronchitis and/or emphysema. COPD is a slow and progressive disease and is characterised by airflow obstruction that does not change over months. Cigarette smoking is regarded as the primary cause of COPD. Occasionally, COPD is found in non-smokers, but this rare.

Chronic bronchitis

This is characterised by excessive mucus production in the bronchial tree, which causes an excessive expectoration of sputum that is often accompanied by a productive smoker's cough. Individuals have usually had a productive cough on most days for at least 3 months a year for at least two successive years. Inflammation causes narrowing of the airways and eventually chronic inflammation leads to fibrotic changes in the airways, leaving scarring and permanent lung damage.

Emphysema

Primarily emphysema is a disease of the terminal air spaces (alveoli) in which the alveoli are actually destroyed, resulting in hyperinflated lungs, increased expansion of the rib cage and a barrel-shaped chest. Reduced oxygen diffusion across the damaged alveolar capillary membrane results in inefficient gas exchange. Emphysema is commonly caused by smoking but may occur at a much earlier age as the result of a congenital molecular defect.

Asthma

Asthma is a chronic inflammatory condition of the airways and is characterised by a heightened response to a trigger or stimulus. Common triggers include allergens such as pollen, mould, animal hair, dust mites, dairy foods, nuts, exercise, chest infections, stress, smoking and certain drugs. The overreaction to these stimuli or triggers, known as bronchial hyper-reactivity, causes the normally smooth muscles in the bronchial walls to constrict and may result in changes in the mucus glands. These changes cause obstruction of the airways and this can become chronic. Asthma is primarily treated by drugs that prevent and/or reverse bronchoconstriction.

Bronchiectasis

Bronchiectasis is a disease involving irreversible dilation of the bronchi, usually as a consequence of an earlier infection of the bronchus, often during childhood. The elastic composition of the walls of the airways is destroyed and the warm, moist environment within the lung encourages infection to develop, so excess mucus is produced. This results in persistent infection, inflammation and obstruction.

Cystic fibrosis

This inherited disease presents as a chronic obstructive disorder that significantly reduces life expectancy. It is caused by a faulty gene, which affects the epithelial surfaces and results in impairments in numerous body systems, including a malabsorption deficiency in the digestive system. In the lungs, mucus becomes thick and sticky, thus encouraging bacterial infection. There is often a chronic cough and dyspnoea and malnutrition can add to an already impaired respiratory disease system.

RESTRICTIVE DISEASES

Interstitial lung diseases

This umbrella term covers a number of diseases resulting in impaired gas transfer, reduced compliance of the lung (i.e. a stiff lung) and reduced lung volumes.

Fibrosing alveolitis is the most common interstitial lung disease and has a poor prognosis (50% of people with fibrosing alveolitis die within 5 years of diagnosis (Bois 1992)). It features widespread fibrosis with severe respiratory impairment. Other diseases in this category include sarcoidosis and asbestosis (Hough 1997).

Neuromuscular/skeletal disorders

Disorders that impair the movement and mechanics of the lungs will clearly impair lung function. This may be due to arthritic changes in the spine and ribs (as seen in ankylosing spondylitis) or from weakness or paralysis of the diaphragm and respiratory muscles. These disorders restrict the way in which the lung expands and so reduce lung capacity. They also affect the ability to cough and clear secretions effectively. This may result in an increased risk of contracting chest infections.

IMPACT OF CHRONIC RESPIRATORY DISEASE

The overall impact of any chronic respiratory condition is often far reaching. The disease will affect not only the individual diagnosed with the respiratory impairment, but will also impact on that person's family and friends, and on the community, for a significant length of time. The next section will outline the main clinical problems and consider how these impact upon the person, family, carers, friends and society.

MAIN CLINICAL PROBLEMS

Dyspnoea (breathlessness)

This is the most predominant clinical feature of chronic respiratory disease. A large natural reserve of lung function and modern sedentary lifestyles often mean that dyspnoea does not inhibit daily occupational performance until a substantial portion of lung function has been lost. Daily activity is commonly limited by increasing levels of breathlessness upon exertion. This sensation of breathlessness is uncomfortable and frightening, so the individual typically begins by reducing the overall level of activity.

Fatigue

The breathless individual often reports high levels of fatigue at different times during the day, which limits his ability to plan the day effectively. Lareau et al (1999) suggest that this problem may limit occupational performance as much as dyspnoea.

Recurrent exacerbations

Some individuals experience frequent chest infections, which may be accompanied by dyspnoea at rest and a cough with some difficulty in expectorating purulent sputum. Individuals with a chronic respiratory disease have an increased risk of contracting infections because of an inability to effectively clear the chest of secretions. These exacerbations are often managed medically by oral antibiotics and steroids.

Physical deconditioning

This may be a primary or secondary consequence of chronic respiratory disease. There is often noticeable atrophy of large muscle groups and individuals report decreased levels of exercise tolerance.

IMPACT UPON THE PERSON

The main clinical features of most chronic respiratory diseases, as discussed above, have a profound impact upon the person's daily life. Effects range from being unable to climb stairs to feeling unable to go out with friends. The impact of a chronic respiratory disease can be examined under the following four components: physical,

psychological, social and cognitive/intellectual. However, it should be noted that these components are clearly linked and cannot be viewed in isolation. Physical limitations will inevitably have psychological and social consequences for the person. This is evident in the disability spiral (Fig. 25.1).

Physical impact

Common physical, functional restrictions include decreased ability to walk outside, walk uphill, climb stairs, attend to personal care and complete domestic tasks. Many people find activities involving upper limb mobility and strength particularly difficult. This is because there is an increased metabolic demand to overcome gravity in tasks that involve elevation of the upper limbs. In addition, there may be some impairment in the respiratory muscles, which are involved in both respiration and upper limb activities.

Dyspnoea and fatigue are the major causes of physical limitation in individuals with chronic respiratory disease. Recognition that common physical tasks are becoming more difficult is a frequent reason for seeking medical help. This is common in COPD, where the progressive onset of the disease often results in a gradual decline in function. However, the impact may be less gradual for people with other respiratory diseases. Children with cystic fibrosis may have always been aware of limitations in competing in some energetic sports with their friends.

An important feature of chronic respiratory conditions is the variability of physical functioning and individuals will often state that they have 'good' days and 'bad' days. Recurrent chest infections also result in fluctuating levels of physical functioning. The impact of chronic respiratory diseases will change as the individual grows older because, for most people, a decrease in lung function is a natural part of the ageing process. Therefore, individuals who already have a substantial degree of lung impairment may notice physical limitations at an earlier age than their healthy peers. People with a respiratory insufficiency are often forced to make decisions such as taking early retirement or moving home

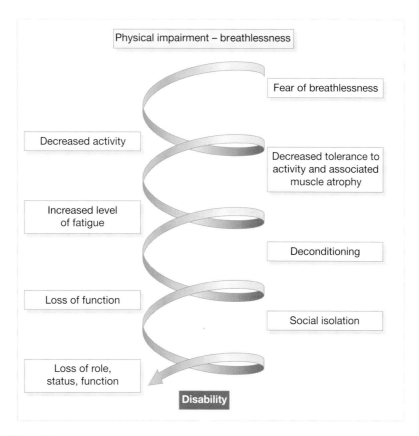

Fig. 25.1 The disability spiral.

to be closer to family or carers. A person with cystic fibrosis may be limited in the number of suitable career options on health grounds.

Psychological impact

Psychological adjustment to chronic respiratory disease will also vary from person to person. It is known that individuals with COPD are more likely to have a higher level of clinically significant depression than a healthy population (McSweeney et al 1982). Higher than average levels of anxiety have also been reported (Angle & Baum 1977). The cumulative effects of reduced daily activity will often result in a continuing spiral of disability (see Fig. 25.1). Breathlessness on exertion often causes anxiety and individuals are frequently convinced that further exertion

will result in an inability to recover control of their breathing. As they progress down the disability spiral it may simply be the thought of exertion, such as walking outside, that induces feelings of anxiety. This quickly becomes a self-fulfilling prophecy, with anxious thoughts causing the individual to become breathless. This process can also be true for depression. For example, the physical effects of a chest infection might initially curtail the individual's functional independence but it is a residual level of depression that will steal the motivation to regain this independence. This process can be compounded by low levels of self-efficacy and self-esteem.

Any chronic respiratory condition brings with it the fact that, by definition, the condition is unlikely to improve but very likely to deteriorate. This introduces important issues such as the fear of dying, which may need to be addressed. The person with cystic fibrosis may be aware that life expectancy is substantially reduced and might have had to adjust to this from an early age. Individuals with any chronic lung disease can enter a period of grieving at any time. Frequently, this occurs at the time of initial diagnosis or perhaps when a significant change in treatment is offered, for example, the introduction of long-term oxygen therapy.

Cognitive impact

Chronic respiratory diseases do not normally result in any loss of cognitive or intellectual function. However, there may be instances when chronic hypoxaemia (for people in respiratory failure) or sleep apnoea may lead to impaired cognition. The occupational therapist should be aware of this and tailor the assessment accordingly.

Social impact

Chronic respiratory diseases may affect the degree to which an individual can take up their normal social roles. The physical impact of respiratory insufficiency can mean changes to an individual's life stages. This will inevitably impact upon social roles, and vice versa. If someone is physically forced to retire early, this will impact upon their role as a breadwinner in the family. Increasing breathlessness may impact upon a partner's ability to maintain a sexual relationship.

The psychological component is also interrelated with social roles. The effects of anxiety, depression and loss of self-esteem following a prolonged exacerbation may restrict a person's motivation and ability to continue involvement in social clubs or visits to family or friends. Deterioration in the respiratory disease may add to physical and psychological problems and further restrict social roles. This gradual erosion of social roles may result in the individual perceiving that the only available primary role is that of client or patient – the sick role.

Impact upon family/carers/friends

The impact of respiratory insufficiency is clearly not confined to the person with the diagnosis. Psychological and social limitations are likely to have a profound effect upon members of the family, friends, colleagues, carers and peers. The degree to which other people are affected is related to the actual specific characteristics of the respiratory disease in question. For instance, the parents of a child with cystic fibrosis could have individual issues of grief, anxiety and perhaps guilt, which need to be recognised and addressed. Likewise, the wife of a man with asthma is likely to make lifestyle adaptations to minimise any possible triggers. This may mean such changes as entering a smoking cessation programme.

An important and common concern of the family and friends of a person with chronic respiratory disease is how to respond to episodes of severe breathlessness. Family members and friends often feel useless when watching someone trying to regain control of their breathing. A common response to this is to encourage the person with breathing problems to curtail all activities that are likely to induce dyspnoea. However, this well-meant approach tends to compound the problems caused by the disability spiral, as discussed earlier. Issues regarding the terminal stages of chronic lung diseases and dying are clearly important when considering the effect upon family, friends and carers. This may need to be considered at the time of diagnosis when some families need reassurance as to the exact prognosis of the disease, or may come to light when important decisions are taken by the medical team and the client regarding changes in management or treatment.

Impact upon society

Exact social and economic costs of all the chronic respiratory diseases have not been comprehensively calculated. It has been estimated that COPD alone accounts for over 200 000 hospital admissions each year in the United Kingdom, with a medical cost of treating COPD at around £154 per person per year and estimated figures of

$23.9 billion as the annual cost of treating COPD in the United States (Sullivan et al 2000). However, these figures do not reveal the whole story. Consideration should also be given to the impact in terms of lost working days, loss of potentially skilled personnel and demands upon hospital and social services resources. The impact upon other areas of society is, arguably, immeasurable. In particular, it is difficult to put a price on the loss of a volunteer worker to the community or the loss of a grandfather to a family.

TYPES OF CORONARY DISEASE

HEART FAILURE

An exact definition of heart failure is difficult to ascertain. In its broadest sense, heart failure, according to Timmis et al (1997), is 'a syndrome in which a cardiac disorder prevents the delivery of sufficient output to meet the perfusion requirements of metabolising tissues'. Contributing factors include coronary artery disease, cardiomyopathy, hypertension and irregular heart rhythm. In some instances, heart failure may be due to a congenital defect of the heart. The prevalence of heart failure increases with age, affecting 1–2% of the population at 50 years of age and rising to 10% of people at 80 years of age. The prognosis is poor, with a 30% mortality rate within 1 year, which rises to 60–70% at 5 years (McMurray & Cleland 2000). Diagnosis of heart failure can be difficult but the New York Heart Association classification (Zaret et al 1992) can be utilised to categorise the severity of the condition (Table 25.1).

Heart failure rarely occurs in isolation and comorbidities include peripheral vascular disease, diabetes, respiratory disease and renal insufficiency. There can also be evidence of depression and cognitive deficits (Rich 2000).

ANGINA

Angina is defined as a 'sense of suffocation' or as 'a suffocating pain'. Pain radiating to either arm,

Table 25.1 Classification of heart failure

Class	Description
Class I	No undue symptoms associated with ordinary activity and no limitation of physical activity
Class II	Slight limitation of physical activity, patient comfortable at rest
Class III	Marked limitation of physical activity, patient comfortable at rest
Class IV	Inability to carry on any physical activity without discomfort. Symptoms of cardiac insufficiency or chest pain possible even at rest

throat or jaw is the result of myocardial ischaemia and can be accompanied by shortness of breath. Angina is due to the imbalance between the myocardial oxygen supply and demand, and the oxygen restriction is often related to coronary artery disease. Angina can be stable, variant or unstable.

Stable angina occurs when a stimulus (effort) increases the myocardium oxygen demand. Such an increase is generally provoked by exertion and relieved by rest. The severity of the symptoms of angina is not directly related to the extent of the coronary artery disease but individuals with stable angina have similar risks of developing associated comorbidities as people with coronary artery disease.

Unlike stable angina, variant angina occurs in unprovoked situations. An exaggerated increase in coronary arterial tone has been evident and is thought to be a major factor leading to myocardial ischaemia. Individuals with variant angina are at a higher risk of developing irregular heart rhythms and prolonged spasms may result in myocardial infarction.

Unstable angina is primarily caused by the rupture of atheromatous plaques causing coronary thrombosis. It presents as recurrent and prolonged episodes of chest pain with minimal exertion or at rest. Myocardial infarction leading to death occurs in up to 30% of cases within 3 months of diagnosis and the management of unstable angina is considered to be a medical emergency.

IMPACT OF CORONARY DISEASE

MAIN CLINICAL PROBLEMS

Dyspnoea

As with chronic respiratory disease, dyspnoea is also a common feature of heart failure and angina, and is a distressing symptom for individuals and their carers. Dyspnoea in heart failure is due to a change in arterial pressure and occurs predominantly when supine. Unlike in chronic respiratory disease, the sensation can be alleviated through correct positioning and reduction in the pressure on the heart due to gravity. In advanced heart failure, dyspnoea is constantly present and daily activities are compromised by increasing levels of breathlessness.

Oedema

Fluids and salt are retained in the body as the result of the inefficiency of the heart. This results in an imbalance in tissue pressure with fluid building up in the interstitial spaces. Gravity adds to the problems, causing fluid to collect in particular areas of the body, especially the legs, feet and ankles, which further restricts mobility. Oedema can also affect the liver and abdominal cavity, causing discomfort and weight gain. The overall impact of oedema can be very limiting and perpetuates the spiral of disability.

Fatigue

Exertional fatigue is an important factor in the activity levels of people with heart failure. The body's capacity to exercise is limited because the heart is unable to supply sufficient oxygen to skeletal muscles. Recent research (Katz 2000) has identified that fatigue is due to structural and molecular changes in the muscles. The desire to perform daily activities can be heavily outweighed by the effort required.

Pain

Pain is totally subjective and is multidimensional. It is affected by mood, morale and the meaning attributed to the pain. It may be related to grief for lost activities or opportunities. Pain is not only problematic for the person with angina but also affects people in the later stages of heart failure (Gibbs et al 1998). Total pain and the threshold to which each individual is able to tolerate pain can be affected by many factors, including fatigue, mood, isolation or fear, and should be addressed in relation to physical, psychological, social and spiritual beliefs.

IMPACT OF CORONARY HEART DISEASE

Coronary heart disease has a profound impact on a person's life and on the lives of their family and friends. In many instances the impacts are similar to those of respiratory disease but the differences will be discussed in the next section.

Physical impact

Progression of coronary heart disease is not a consistent level of functional deterioration. Individuals have to cope with fluctuations in functional capacity. Medical advances have increased life expectancy, although longevity does not always guarantee quality of life. Common physical limitations result from reduced tolerance to activity, particularly activities that require exertion, such as dressing, bathing or walking uphill. Dyspnoea and pain are common factors in limiting functional levels and particularly affect the energy expended on such basic activities as toileting. In the management of oedema, diuretics increase the need to urinate, this results in regular energy expenditure on this basic activity, which cannot be reduced.

Psychological impact

Living with a condition that cannot be cured and will almost certainly deteriorate has a profound impact on some individuals. Depression and anxiety are common factors in people with coronary heart disease and the adjustments they are required to make to their lifestyle are a constant reminder of their clinical condition. The prognosis for individuals with coronary heart disease, and in particular heart failure, is difficult to define, and many medical interventions are aimed at 'therapeutic hopefulness'. This can result in a gulf between the individual's hopes and aspirations and the reality of living with heart disease. Psychological impacts include reduced motivation, anger, denial and grief processes for the losses the individual is experiencing.

Cognitive impact

There is little documented evidence of heart failure being linked to cognitive deficits. However, because it affects a predominantly elderly age group, heart failure is frequently associated with comorbidities such as dementia, and normal ageing processes are frequently evident. As with respiratory disease, where there is an inability for the body to provide sufficient oxygen to the cells, an individual's reaction times can be reduced.

Impact upon family/carers/friends

The effect of caring for an individual who has coronary heart disease is demanding and the lifestyle of everyone involved will be compromised. The medical treatment of heart failure can be particularly difficult to manage, with altered dietary habits, frequent micturition, fatigue and dyspnoea, which can all result in the individual becoming housebound. Family members can feel isolated as a result and the support networks for carers is limited in certain areas. As a result, grief processes similar to those experienced by the individual with the disease may be evident in family members, resulting from the loss or change of roles, loss of future aspirations, changes in status and limitation of choices.

Social impact

The impact that heart failure has upon society and the individual within society is similar to that of people with chronic respiratory disease. The overall management of people with heart failure consumes 1–2% of total healthcare expenditure in developed countries (Stewart & Blue 2001). In the United Kingdom this equates to £360 million, a figure that does not take into account lost earnings, social care costs or family contributions to care. The most significant impact for those with heart failure is the value of the life lost. As the incidence of heart failure is increasing, it is likely that everyone will have a relative or someone close with the condition and, as a result, all aspects of society will be affected.

THE INTERVENTION TEAM

Medical

Throughout the progression of cardiac and respiratory disease, management within primary and secondary care is dependent upon a close working relationship between general practitioners and physicians. Their roles are similar in as much as they aim to stabilise disease exacerbations and monitor the individual's physical condition. Medical practitioners also have a key role in coordinating a whole-team approach to an individual's care.

Pharmacist

An important factor in controlling the effects of cardiac and respiratory disease is correct use of medication. The pharmacist has an educational role, providing individuals with information and support to understand how each drug works and, more importantly, how to use the drugs effectively.

Physiotherapist

Physiotherapists are key members of the intervention team, giving education and practical guidance on how to breathe comfortably and effectively. They teach techniques on how to maximise and maintain breathing patterns, how to expectorate and how to maximise levels of cardiovascular and physical fitness.

Clinical nurse specialists

Specialist nurses have developed knowledge of the progression of the disease and the impact on individuals and their families. Clinical nurse specialists tend to be based in secondary care but provide an essential link with primary care settings and the community. A significant aspect of their role is to support and maintain individuals in their own home, educating them on how to recognise exacerbations and, where necessary, providing a rapid access service to specialist physicians.

Social worker

Social workers are well placed to follow the individual through the disease progression. They can assist with the provision of home care and support the individual when making the transition from hospital admission to discharge and community support.

Dietician

It is important for the individual with respiratory or coronary disease to maintain a good nutritional state – as poor nutrition is associated with morbidity. The dietician provides practical advice and treatment as to the most suitable ways for individuals to maintain a balanced diet. Where necessary, food supplements or food substitutes may be prescribed.

Voluntary organisations

Self-help groups and voluntary organisations have a valuable role to play. In many instances, group memberships include individuals who have some type of respiratory or cardiac disease, or have been involved in caring for others with these diseases. Voluntary organisations can provide practical advice and support to individuals and their families. In some situations they may be able to provide practical care, such as sitting services or help completing benefit claims. The availability of voluntary organisations or groups is dependent upon location, although the national groups, such as the British Lung Foundation and the British Heart Foundation, provide published literature.

OCCUPATIONAL THERAPY INTERVENTION

Interventions for individuals with chronic cardiac or respiratory disease have common themes and utilise similar strategies, so they will be addressed together in the following section.

ROLE OF THE OCCUPATIONAL THERAPIST

The contribution of occupational therapy is focused upon enabling adaptation and promoting the pursuit of purposeful, meaningful occupation in daily life. The therapist plays a pivotal role in encouraging individuals to take responsibility and ownership of their health. Through a combined approach of education, rehabilitation and compensation, the therapist aims to enable individuals to manage their condition with the least distress and disruption to daily life.

THEORETICAL APPLICATIONS

The possible impact of respiratory and cardiac insufficiency upon individuals, their families, friends and carers is diverse. Occupational therapists have a number of theoretical approaches at their disposal to address these wideranging problems and these will be discussed in the context of the three major aims of occupational therapy in the treatment of respiratory and cardiac insufficiency, which are:

- management of current, permanent functional limitations
- optimisation of physical functioning
- prevention of future functional problems and individuals' (and their family/carers) understanding of these problems.

Management of permanent functional limitations

Compensatory approach

Any current physical limitations may well be permanent. The compensatory approach is well placed to address these problems. Possible interventions signalled by this approach include:

- the provision of appropriate equipment to enable individuals to regain or maintain independence in activities of daily living
- liaison with social services regarding the provision of homecare services.

Educative approach

It is often appropriate to teach individuals and their families the principles of energy conservation and pacing activity. This will enable individuals to maintain independence in a selection of activities of daily living by spreading the energy cost across the day.

Optimisation of physical functioning

Biomechanical approach

Reduction in physical functioning in chronic cardiac and lung disease is complicated by possible systemic problems of poor exercise tolerance and reduced muscle bulk. This deficit can be approached by assessing a person's current level of functioning and then formulating a graded programme of activities, which will improve overall strength and stamina. This may be achieved as part of a formal cardiac or pulmonary rehabilitation programme or on an individual basis. Pulmonary rehabilitation programmes are normally completed on an outpatient basis, with individuals completing formal exercise training and also undergoing a comprehensive education programme. There is hard evidence to suggest that pulmonary rehabilitation is effective in improving exercise performance (Goldstein et al 1994, Griffiths et al 2000). There is less evidence and a paucity of research to support the theory that this will lead to improvements in levels of independence in activities of daily living. It is therefore crucial that occupational therapists explicitly address these issues of improving exercise tolerance, as a basis for optimising independence in activities of daily living, working in conjunction with any group rehabilitation interventions.

Prevention of future problems

Cognitive behavioural approach

The process of modifying people's behaviours by changing their perception of their illness has been pioneered in other areas of physical dysfunction, such as pain management programmes. However, the approach is applicable to addressing some negative consequences of cardiac or respiratory insufficiency. The management of breathlessness is one such area. Pulmonary or cardiac rehabilitation programmes that reinforce the message that being breathless is a normal consequence of exertion have found that people's negative perceptions of breathlessness can diminish (Griffiths et al 2000). It is thought that this fear is a common barrier to participation in physical functioning in chronic respiratory and cardiac disease. It therefore follows that a reduction in this negative perception may lead to an increase in physical functioning and may possibly prevent future problems caused by the spiral of disability.

This approach is important in addressing the common anxieties of both individuals and carers regarding future prognosis and possible functional difficulties.

Individual strategies will also be important in situations where a formal group-based approach (such as pulmonary rehabilitation) is not appropriate. Interventions completed on a one-to-one basis, such as energy conservation or anxiety management techniques, may be more suitably employed within this approach.

OCCUPATIONAL THERAPY INTERVENTIONS

In the early stages of respiratory or cardiac disease, individuals experience minimal impact on their everyday life. The occupational therapy intervention comprises education and adaptation to maximise functional capacity.

Whether in primary or secondary care, it is important for people with respiratory or cardiac disease to have access to a multidisciplinary educational programme, focused intervention for health promotion and teaching of self-management techniques. The aim of intervention is to maximise functional performance in an effort to minimise deconditioning. Hoffman et al (1989) concur with this rationale. By providing people with information on how to improve their functional ability and limit the impact of the disease, it is possible that they can learn to cope using positive strategies by:

- balancing work, rest and play activities
- using stress management techniques
- using energy conservation methods
- applying pulmonary/cardiac rehabilitation.

An important aspect of the occupational therapist's role is coordinating the level of rehabilitation against the support that individuals receive. It is essential for people to continue to participate in normal everyday activities to maintain physical health and wellbeing. Natural disease progression means that individuals are likely to have acute episodes where hospitalisation may be necessary. Functional capacity during these times may decrease significantly. It is therefore important for the occupational therapist to enable individuals and carers to recognise that the acute problems may be resolved and that with a period of rehabilitation, functional capacity may return to almost previous levels. Any compensatory intervention during an acute phase should therefore be considered initially as a short-term measure. For example, it may be necessary to provide homecare support upon discharge. However, within 3–4 weeks this should be reviewed to ensure that individuals do not become too dependent upon external assistance at the expense of continued functional improvement.

The chronic nature of cardiac and respiratory disease does, however, eventually lead to increasing levels of functional loss. The occupational therapist's skills in problem solving and rationalising are necessary to foreplan what will be needed to enable individuals to continue productive occupational performance. It may be necessary in the later stages to consider major adaptations to the home environment, or the use of adaptive equipment such as stairlifts, electric wheelchairs or level access showers with the aim of conserving energy.

Assessment

Upon initial contact with someone with respiratory or cardiac disease it is important to establish three areas of information:

1. How does the disease impact upon the individual's life? The extent to which daily life is affected depends upon the person's lifestyle and the progression of the disease. At all stages of the disease, information about how individuals are affected should include:

- what triggers exacerbations?
- how long does an exacerbation usually last?
- are there any residual problems?
- does the severity of symptoms vary throughout the day?
- which symptoms cause distress?

2. What coping strategies is the individual using? As most people have lived with their disease for a considerable length of time before being referred to occupational therapy, the individual will already have adapted some aspects of daily life to make them easier to manage. People employ positive and negative coping strategies and it is important to ascertain what techniques the individual is using.

3. Detailed assessment of occupational performance. The three components to be addressed are work, rest and play. During initial interview (Fig. 25.2) it is important to establish how disease affects these occupational performance areas:

- Work – what activities does the individual undertake, including self-care tasks, voluntary/paid employment, care of others?
- Rest – when does the individual rest, including sleeping patterns? How does the individual combine rest with work and play?
- Play – what does the individual do for enjoyment? How does the individual spend free time? Is the individual involved in any leisure pursuits?

Fig. 25.2 Initial interview – home situation and patient capabilites prior to admission.

Initial interview – home situation and patient capabilities prior to admission

Key:
1) Independent
2) Independent with equipment
3) Independent with difficulty
4) Supervision required
5) Prompts required
6) Physical assistance
7) Unable
8) Declined
9) Not assessed

Introduction of occupational therapist and role ☐   Patient consent: Yes ☐   No ☐   Heights form issued ☐

Information from: *Patient, carer, other*   **Accommodation**: *Type, situation, environment, ownership*

Social situation: *Who do they live with? Alone or others, any pets?*

Significant visitors: *Any contact with others, how frequent?*   Alarm/phone: *where is it situated?*

	Equipment in situ
Access: *Are there steps, driveway, slope? Is the property on or off the street? How long does it take to gain entrance to property?*	
Mobility: *Distance, length of time able to walk, any aids used, problems encountered indoor and outdoors, severity of breathlessness?*	*What type of equipment?*
Stairs: *Where and what are the stairs like, presence of handrails and situation, how frequently stairs are used, severity of breathlessness?*	*Who provided the equipment?*
Chair: *Any problems with transfer? What height is the chair/sofa? Assistance needed during the day to get in or out of chair?*	*When was the equipment provided?*
Bed: *Where do you sleep, up or downstairs? What type of bed? Any problem getting in or out? Height of the bed? How many pillows do you use?*	*Do they find the equipment useful?*
Toilet/commode: *Where is the toilet? How often do you need to use the toilet, including overnight? Any problem getting on or off?*	
Bath/shower: *Location, frequency of use, problems and effect of activity, including drying self? Need of assistance? Preference for bath/shower?*	
Washing: *When, where, how, frequency, effect and duration of washing. Any aspect more difficult? Need of assistance for aspects of task?*	
Dressing: *When, where, how? Effect of dressing or undressing? Any differences in time of day? Types of clothing preferred, e.g. loose fitting?*	
Feeding: *Level of appetite, frequency of eating/drinking? Ability to eat/drink when breathless/fatigued?*	
Meal preparation: *Who does the cooking, including drinks? Types and frequency of meals? Location of the kitchen? Access within the kitchen, e.g. height of work surfaces? Do they enjoy cooking? Can they eat after cooking? Where do they eat the meal? Do they need to transport items?*	
How long does it take to make the meal/drink? Gas ☐ Electric ☐ Microwave ☐ Fridge/freezer ☐	

Heating: *Type of heating, how is it controlled?*   Shopping/pension: *Who does the shopping, where and how often? Do they enjoy this?*

Domestic tasks (e.g. laundry/cleaning): *Who, how often and what domestic tasks are undertaken? Do they have any specific problems, e.g. pegging out laundry?*

Leisure/interests: *What do they enjoy doing? Have they been limited by their health? What would they like to be able to do with their leisure time?*

Transport/wheelchair: *Do they drive, use public transport or rely on friend/family? Do they possess a wheelchair? What type, how often do they use it and for what purpose?*

Social/day hospitals: *Do they or others attend organised groups? If so when, type and duration?*

Additional information: *What symptoms affect daily life, how do they cope with them? What makes the symptoms better or worse? What medication do they currently use, e.g. GTN spray or oxygen?*
What do they want to be able to do when they are at home?
Do they feel there has been a change in their level of ability?
Agreed plan of action with the person.

Therapist: Date: © GLENFIELD HOSPITAL, LEICESTER, 2001

Through structured observation a clear picture can be gained of how disease affects the individual during daily life. Aspects that need to be examined include intensity of dyspnoea, activity tolerance, fatigue, pain and recovery rates.

Intervention

Energy conservation

Many individuals with chronic cardiac or respiratory disease experience dyspnoea, fatigue and reduced physical tolerance to activity, which limits their occupational performance. Additionally, as many of these people are also elderly, they could have problems of ageing, with comorbidities and reduced range of movement. The disability spiral becomes evident as the effort to remain independent is outweighed by the physical cost.

A compensatory approach can enable people to perform activities in a more efficient way. Specific intervention at an early stage can enable people to manage priority activities using positive coping strategies. Functional activities of daily living can be adapted to minimise the impact of exacerbations through identification of trigger factors. Each aspect of daily life should be examined with regard to the three Ps – prioritisation, planning and pacing.

Prioritisation

A detailed list of occupational areas within work, rest and play should be made and rated in order of importance to the individual. The schedule in Table 25.2 can be used as a guide.

Table 25.2 Prioritising schedule

	Important	Unimportant
Self	1	3
What can I do?		
What do I want to do?		
Others	2	4
External assistance		
Paid/voluntary		

Planning

Once activities have been prioritised, each separate activity should be examined using a simplified form of activity analysis to determine the actions needed to perform the activity and the physical cost of undertaking it. When this has been established, consideration should be given to adaptive techniques or the use of adaptive equipment to enable the individual to perform the tasks in a less energy consuming but efficient way. Activity checklists (Fig. 25.3 and Box 25.1) can be helpful in assessing and planning activities, for example, using the kitchen trolley and collecting all the ingredients to prepare a meal.

Pacing

The key to maintaining functional abilities is to have a good balance between activity and rest. The aim of the three Ps is to enable individuals not only to cope with daily life but also to enjoy life. Pacing gives the body time to recover from physical and mental exertion. The inclusion of regular rest periods into the day can markedly increase the level of activity achieved by many people.

Dyspnoea significantly impacts upon the ability to perform activities, particularly functional activities of daily living. Hoffman et al

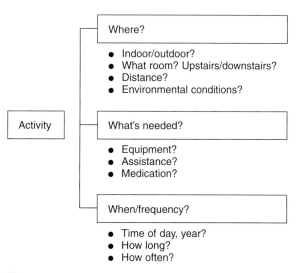

Fig. 25.3 Activity checklist.

Box 25.1   Case study: Mrs M.

Mrs M. is 62 years old and has been an outpatient at the local hospital for 3 years with a diagnosis of emphysema. She retired 2 years ago because of her respiratory problems but has since been able to help out on a voluntary basis at local luncheon club. Mrs M. was widowed 3 years ago and lives alone in her house. Mrs M. was recently admitted to hospital with a chest infection. She has since made excellent medical progress but, during a recent outpatient appointment, reported that she was finding it increasingly difficult to manage at home and was also feeling increasingly nervous when she left home alone. With Mrs M.'s permission, the respiratory physician referred her to the hospital's occupational therapy department.

The occupational therapist spent some time completing an activity checklist and undertaking a thorough assessment of Mrs M.'s recent difficulties with activities of daily living and was able to recommend some items of equipment, including a perching stool and shower seat, that Mrs M. felt would be of assistance to her. During the following session the occupational therapist discussed some other areas of daily life that Mrs M. may have also been finding difficult. Mrs M. reported that since her recent admission to hospital she had felt very anxious about being in social situations. Her main concern was not being able to cope if her breathlessness suddenly worsened. Mrs M. also stated that she now felt unable to carry on with her voluntary work and had not felt able to visit her son's family for some 6 months. The occupational therapist was able, over the following sessions, to discuss some anxiety management techniques with Mrs M. and also taught Mrs M. some relaxation skills. By the end of the course of intervention, Mrs M. had planned to return to her voluntary work, initially for 2 hours a week. She had also been able to visit her son and his family.

Mrs M. still reports feeling tired during the day and still occasionally feels anxious about managing her breathlessness. The occupational therapist has referred her to the local hospital's pulmonary rehabilitation programme with the aim of improving her exercise tolerance and confidence in managing her breathlessness. She will be reviewed following completion of the rehabilitation programme in 3 months' time.

Advice on washing

- Over-bath showers and bath boards reduce exertion when getting into the bath and shower.
- Increased room ventilation and avoidance of direct water onto the face reduce the risk of hyperventilation.
- Having all necessary washing items nearby, preferably on a shelf at shoulder height, reduces the need for bending and prevents overreaching.
- Using a warm towel robe to dry is easier than rubbing with a towel.
- Using a perching stool at the washhand basin reduces the need for standing.
- Long-handled equipment facilitates reaching to wash the feet and lower legs.

Advice on dressing

- Wear loose fitting clothes, especially at the waist and neck.
- Sit down to dress, put skirts on over the head to eliminate bending.
- Use dressing aids, such as a tights aid and long-handled shoe horn, to avoid bending to the feet.
- Be organised and collect all clothes together before starting to dress.

These same techniques can be applied to a range of activities. However, there are three important factors to consider at all times:

- maintenance of good posture whether sitting or standing
- maintenance of good breathing techniques
- allowing the body to recover from physical exertion before attempting further activity.

Coping with fear

Breathlessness is frightening. A fear of choking or suffocating has been expressed by many people with cardiac or respiratory disease. Fear can affect many individuals and exacerbate the sensation of breathlessness.

Fear can also inhibit the therapeutic process. Unnecessary avoidance of activity can prevent rehabilitation and contribute to further deconditioning. The spiral of disability is particularly

(1989) state that hyperinflation of the lungs particularly hampers activities that require bending or prolonged standing. Adaptation to the techniques for performance of occupational activity to reduce reach or standing time can enable individuals to cope more effectively. Examples for occupational therapy intervention in the performance of self-care tasks include:

evident in the later stages of the disease process. A multidisciplinary approach is important when combating the effects of fear and breathlessness. Pulmonary rehabilitation can be undertaken to address the symptoms of respiratory disease and to aim to increase physical conditioning and address the psychological aspects of coping with breathlessness and fatigue in daily life.

Individuals need to learn to recognise fear-driven aspects of breathlessness, and the cause and effect relationship that these have, in order to begin to break the cycle of fear. A combined approach of education, activity and rehabilitation can enable individuals to begin to cope and remove fear of breathlessness (Table 25.3).

Table 25.3 Occupational therapy intervention

Problem	Solution
Sensation of breathlessness	
Physical reaction to sensation	Education with aim of normalising sensation of breathlessness
Social isolation	In-depth examination of the individual's belief system
Reduced tolerance to activity	What is the individual's understanding of the mechanisms of breathing?
Anxiety/depression either individual or carers	What will the consequence of being breathless mean to the individual?
	Desensitisation programme increasing duration of activity balancing demand (physical and mental tolerance to activity) and effect (level of fatigue, breathlessness and anxiety)
Expectation of self realising the gulf between hopes, aspirations and reality of loss	
Reduced motivation	Graded therapeutic programme, e.g. leisure task to encourage motivation and enjoyment
Grief	
Reduction of self-efficacy	Adapting approach to daily life, balancing previous levels of independence with current levels. Focusing intervention on what can be achieved
Low self-esteem	Relaxation techniques to reduce tension and promote wellbeing
Expectation of others	
Guilt of not being able to have 'normal' relationship	Encourage communication of fears to normalise situation and neutralise stigma
Guilt/resentment of good health	Educate others about the mechanism of breathing and consequences of being breathless
Reduced understanding of disease	Support groups, voluntary organisations to facilitate support from people who are in similar circumstances
Conflict between individual and carers	Discuss relationships between individual and others. Do these interactions affect how the individual copes with breathlessness? Validation of possible conflict can reduce the impact on the individual and those around them
	Relaxation techniques shared with individual
Isolation of trigger factors	
Avoidance of trigger factors can lead to ritualistic behaviour. Bargaining against breathlessness, e.g. if I count to 5 then move I won't be as breathless, if I don't get dressed I won't get tired or breathless	Enable the individual to replace maladaptive behaviour with positive behaviour patterns
	Grade programme introducing variety of activities to increase wellbeing and ability to cope with varying levels of breathlessness and fatigue
Avoidance of all possible factors can lead to social isolation	Maintenance of good posture to eliminate unnecessary breathlessness
Reduced capacity for fulfilling occupations	Maintenance of environmental factors, e.g. good ventilation, temperature control
Questioning of own mortality	
Loss of reassurance that the body is working efficiently	Enabling grief process and adaptation to the diagnosis
Disease cannot be cured	Enable the individual to seek meaning in life through participation in occupational activities
Helplessness – loss of control	Changes in health have an effect on the individual's ability to maintain their control
Hopelessness – loss of choice	
Uselessness – loss of option	Redefinition of roles can enable the individual to lead a fulfilling life

Palliation

Although modern medical management can slow the progression of disease, it cannot prevent the eventual deterioration. It can be difficult to predict prognosis because progression is not consistent. During the terminal phase, it is essential to adopt open communication with individuals and carers to ascertain their expectations and fears for the future. Wherever possible, the preferred place of death should be discussed to facilitate a dignified and peaceful departure.

If the preferred place of death is at home, support should be given to the carer, family and friends as well as to the individual. When considering terminal care the following aspects should be addressed:

- The environment – the home environment will need to be adapted to facilitate care of the dying. Hoists, hospital beds, pressure-relieving equipment and specialist seating may be needed for individuals with major mobility problems. A balance between safe care techniques and intrusive medicalisation at home should be achieved to promote the wellbeing of the individual and carers.
- Practical care – should the individual become dependent upon assistance for personal care, it is important to maintain dignity. Continuity of care is essential for the individual and the carer during an emotional and private situation. Involvement of carers, as appropriate, can lessen distress.
- Psychological care – an important part of palliation is recognising the grieving process

that the individual and the family may be experiencing for the loss of a future life, loss of choice, loss of hope and loss of function. The occupational therapist should address these aspects within intervention, include the individual in planning care and environmental adaptations and, where possible, encourage the individual to partake in some aspects of normal activities, including leisure pursuits. Therapeutic activities can also be utilised to enable individuals to express their reaction to the disease in a non-threatening manner.

CONCLUSION

Chronic respiratory disease and heart failure represent a growing challenge for occupational therapy. The increased demand for services tailored to meet the needs of this group of people and their carers has led to changes in current practice which offer a new way forward. The management of the conditions and the problems they present depends upon good multidisciplinary working, with occupational therapists contributing to the coordination of care. Prophylactic intervention can alter the severity of the impact of the disease on an individual's ability to undertake occupational performance tasks. Through addressing the quality of each individual's life, there is potential to enable people to gain some satisfaction and fulfilment from continued occupational performance.

REFERENCES

Angle DP, Baum GL 1977 Psychological aspects of chronic obstructive pulmonary disease. Medical Clinics of North America 61:749–758

Bois RM 1992 Management of fibrosing alveolitis. British Journal of Hospital Medicine 47:680–683

Calverley PMA, Sondi S 1998 The burden of obstructive lung disease in the UK – COPD and asthma. Thorax 53(suppl 4):A83

Department of Health 2000 National service framework: coronary heart disease. HMSO, London

Gibbs L, Addington-Hall J, Simon J, Gibbs R 1998 Dying from heart failure: lessons from palliative care: many patients would benefit from palliative care at the end of their lives. British Medical Journal 371(7164):961–962

Goldstein RS, Gort EH, Stubbing D, Avendano MA, Guyatt GH 1994 Randomised control trial of respiratory rehabilitation. Lancet 344:1394–1397

Griffiths TL, Burr ML, Campbell IA et al 2000 Results at 1 year of outpatient multidisciplinary pulmonary rehabilitation: a randomised trial. Lancet 355:362–368

Hoffman L, Berg J, Rogers R 1989 Living with COPD. Postgraduate Medicine 86(6):153–166

Hough A 1997 Physiotherapy in respiratory care, 2nd edn. Chapman and Hall, London

Katz AM 2000 Heart failure. Lippincott Williams and Wilkins, Philadelphia

Kavanagh P 1998 Take heart! A proven step by step programme to improve your heart's health. Key Porter Books, Toronto

Lareau SC, Wilhite C, Specht NL et al 1999 Effects of pulmonary rehabilitation on activities, dyspnoea and fatigue. American Journal of Respiratory Critical Care Medicine 159(3):A763

McMurray J, Cleland J 2000 Heart failure in clinical practice. Martin Dunitz, London

McSweeney AJ, Grant I, Heaton RK et al 1982 Life quality of patients with chronic obstructive pulmonary disease. Archives of Internal Medicine 142:473–478

Murray J, Hart W, Rhodes G 1993 An evaluation of the cost of heart failure to the National Health Service in the UK. British Journal of Medical Economics 6:91–98

Office of National Statistics 2000 Death registrations 1999: cause England and Wales. Health Statistics Quarterly. Summer 2000

Rich 2000 In: McMurray J, Cleland J (eds) Heart failure in clinical practice. Martin Dunitz, London

Stewart S, Blue L 2001 Improving outcomes in chronic heart failure: a practical guide to specialist nurse intervention. BMJ Books, London

Sullivan SD, Ramsey SD, Lee TA 2000 The economic burden of COPD. Chest 117(2):5S–9S

Timmis A, Nathan A, Sullivan I 1997 Essential cardiology. Blackwell Sciences, London

Zaret B, Meser M, Cohen L 1992 Yale University School of Medicine: Heart book. Hearst Books, New York

FURTHER READING

Bourke SJ, Brewis RAL 1998 Lecture notes on respiratory medicine, 5th edn. Blackwell Sciences, Oxford

British Thoracic Society 1997 Guidelines for the management of chronic obstructive pulmonary disease. Thorax 52: Suppl 5

Morgan M, Singh S 1997 Practical pulmonary rehabilitation. Chapman and Hall, London

26

Parkinson's disease

Alison Beattie   Jan Harrison

INTRODUCTION

Parkinsonism is a progressive neurological disorder of the central nervous system characterised by tremor, rigidity and bradykinesia (poverty of movement). It is caused by dysfunction of the basal ganglia. Several disorders may produce this syndrome (Box 26.1) but the cause of the most common form of parkinsonism – idiopathic Parkinson's disease (PD) – remains unknown, although over recent years research has focused on environmental factors and genetics. The condition is named after Dr James Parkinson

---

Box 26.1   Parkinsonism and Parkinson's disease

Parkinsonism

Idiopathic (Parkinson's disease)
Drug induced (e.g. phenothiazines)
MPTP toxicity
Post-encephalitic
Wilson's disease

Parkinsonism plus

Progressive supranuclear palsy (Steele–Richardson syndrome)
Multiple system atrophies
– Olivopontocerebellar atrophy
– Striatonigral degeneration
– Progressive autonomic failure (Shy–Drager syndrome)

Parkinsonian 'features' occur in
● Alzheimer's disease
● Head trauma (e.g. boxers)
● Multiple cerebral infarcts

---

who, in 1817, wrote 'An Essay on the Shaking Palsy' (Parkinson 1817).

As there is no specific test for PD, diagnosis is based on the person's description of their symptoms and difficulties, these often being insidious in onset. The condition is associated with degeneration of neurons within the substantia nigra of the basal ganglia. There is also loss of pimentation in the substantia nigra and to a lesser extent in other pigmented nuclei. These changes lead to a reduction of available dopamine. Normal function is dependent on a balance of two chemical neurotransmitters, dopamine and acetylcholine, which influence controlled movement. The basal ganglia, together with associated motor areas, facilitate performance of well-learned voluntary motor skills and movement sequences. Actions can thus occur simultaneously and often automatically, allowing conscious attention to be focused elsewhere. Loss of dopamine disrupts this flow of movement.

The prevalence of idiopathic PD in Europe is approximately one or two per thousand and it is thought that it affects about 110 000 people in the United Kingdom, the majority of whom are elderly. The mean age of onset is 60 and thus it is one of the most common neurological conditions affecting older people (Fig. 26.1). Multiple pathology, for example, osteoarthritis, poor vision and hearing difficulties, is common in this age group and this adds to their problems. However, one in 20 diagnosed with PD are under the age of 40 and the needs of this group are usually quite different from elderly sufferers.

The treatment of PD was revolutionised in the 1970s by the introduction of L-dopa (levodopa) but several other drugs are also used. Drug therapy is the most important form of treatment for the condition and careful and regular monitoring is required. However, all of the drugs cause side-effects. Prior to the introduction of L-dopa, operative procedures were the main treatment and there has been a revival of surgical techniques, for example, thalamotomy, pallidotomy, brain implants using fetal brain tissue and thalamic stimulation.

PHYSICAL ASPECTS

The symptoms of PD result in the stooped posture, generalised slowness, mask-like facial expression, drooling of saliva and festination (shuffling gait) that are characteristic of this condition (Fig. 26.2).

One of the first noticeable problems for the person is tremor, which is most often experienced in the hands and arms and is referred to as 'pill rolling'. As the condition progresses, tremor may extend to other parts of the body, including the tongue and jaw. It is characteristically present at rest and has a rate of approximately four to six cycles per second. Tremor often reduces with activity although anxiety and fatigue exacerbate the problem.

Rigidity is caused by increased tone in the muscle groups of the affected areas and occurs throughout the range of movement. It is described as 'lead pipe rigidity' when sustained resistance is felt, for example, on passively moving a limb, and 'cog-wheel rigidity' when resistance is intermittent. The person may complain of stiffness, discomfort and even pain in the rigid muscles. There is often impaired spinal rotation and absence of natural arm swing.

Bradykinesia, or hypokinesia, refers to a slowness and poverty of voluntary movement. Basal ganglia dysfunction leads to difficulty in planning, preparing, initiating, sequencing and completing

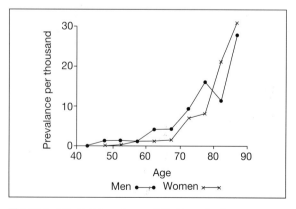

Fig. 26.1 Age and prevalence of Parkinson's disease (reproduced from Mutch et al 1986 Parkinson's disease: disability, review and management. British Medical Journal 293:675–677, with kind permission of the BMJ Publishing Group).

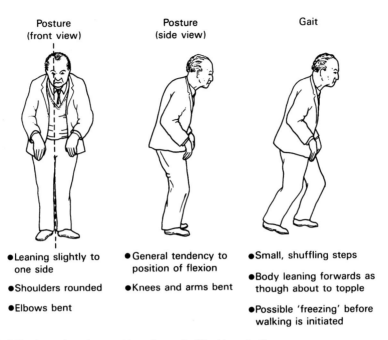

Posture (front view)	Posture (side view)	Gait
●Leaning slightly to one side	●General tendency to position of flexion	●Small, shuffling steps
●Shoulders rounded	●Knees and arms bent	●Body leaning forwards as though about to topple
●Elbows bent		●Possible 'freezing' before walking is initiated

Fig. 26.2 The characteristic stooped posture and hurrying gait of Parkinson's disease.

movements. These elements can be apparent in actions such as starting to walk, standing up from a chair or delay in responding to a request.

Another common symptom, known as 'freezing', occurs when the person suddenly stops and feels as if his feet are stuck to the ground. Postural instability is a further difficulty experienced by many and an impairment of righting reflexes causes problems in maintaining posture and frequently leads to falls. As the condition progresses the person may experience times when he can go from being quite active ('on') to becoming immobile ('off') in a short space of time – the 'on/off' phenomenon.

Other symptoms include impaired speech, which affects about half of all people with PD and is generally associated with the severity of the person's disability. The voice often becomes soft and lacks volume, there is lack of vocal variation and expression and speech can be hoarse and hesitant. Sometimes the person speaks too quickly or the voice fades. Dysphagia (difficulty in swallowing) leads to problems with eating and choking can sometimes be experienced. This is compounded by the physical difficulties of cutting up food and those that arise from tremor.

Muscular rigidity affects the process of lifting food to the mouth and can also result in 'trismus', which is difficulty in opening the mouth. Autonomic symptoms can be experienced and these include constipation, bladder dysfunction, postural hypotension and impotence. Weight loss is very common in PD and is multifactorial in origin. This often results in people being investigated for other conditions, for example, cancer.

The physical problems of PD vary from one individual to another, with some complaining of unilateral symptoms and others of bilateral. One of the most difficult features is that the disabling effects fluctuate, sometimes dramatically. Some people function well in the mornings, others in the evenings and for others there is no set pattern. Low stamina and fatigue are common features and may markedly affect performance.

COGNITIVE ASPECTS

Apart from a global slowing of movement, bradyphrenia (slowness of thought) can cause slow processing of information, problems maintaining a train of thought, distraction and loss of concentration. There may also be difficulty responding to more than one stimulus or in switching from one idea to another, and this can result in a seeming rigidity or inflexibility of thought or action. Problem solving can be affected and some people may be unable to monitor their own performance.

Memory impairment can also be found either as a cognitive symptom (Dewick & Playfer 1990, Oyebode 1995) or associated with depression (Hantz et al 1994). People with PD have a higher risk of developing dementia than age-matched comparisons (Aarsland et al 1996, Gibb & Luthert 1994). However, there is debate as to the incidence of dementia and it is not an early feature of the condition.

PSYCHOLOGICAL ASPECTS

Depression is a common symptom and some theorists believe it is part of the condition and attributable to the altered neurotransmitter functioning. There is significant debate as to the incidence of depression, which may be overlooked because of the lack of facial expression. Various studies have been undertaken (Hantz et al 1994, Taylor & Saint-Cyr 1990) and, whilst most agree that those with PD exhibit a higher level of depressive symptoms, the reported frequency ranges from 4 to 90%. The degree of depression may be linked to increasing disability and people under the age of 50 are more at risk of developing this problem. The obvious effect of reduction in quality of life, concern over financial matters and a changed occupational role may be contributory factors. A study by Ehmann et al (1990) found that people with PD had reduced coping strategies that made them more vulnerable to depressive illness.

Anxiety is another common symptom (Starkstein et al 1993) and is greater in people with PD than in a general population sample. The person is often worried about the future and how they will cope with the condition in the long term. Other factors that cause stress are problems with bodily functions, lack of self-efficacy, difficulties with interpersonal relationships and communication problems. Studies have found that there is a clear link between physical and psychological factors: tremor and rigidity increase with anxiety and the resulting tension further exacerbates the symptoms.

IMPACT OF THE CONDITION

As with other complex neurological conditions, PD can have a devastating effect on the individual and also on their close friends and relatives, potentially impacting on every aspect of life (Ring 1993).

Important features of the condition underlie its presentation: PD is chronic and progressive. However, the rate of change is usually slow and so the person has time to adjust to changes. It is variable: symptoms can alter from hour to hour and day to day. Different environments and emotional states can affect the presentation. PD is deceptive: many people may still be very mentally alert but unable to show it. They may appear withdrawn or uncooperative. Fatigue may result in someone appearing less able than is the case. Equally, the person may seem to be coping but may in fact be experiencing great difficulty.

The condition invariably leads to significant problems with functional mobility (Table 26.1), occupational performance and social roles. The person is likely to have problems with mobility both indoors and outdoors and this affects a range of activities. Speech difficulties and the facial mask can lead to social isolation. The combination of communication problems, mobility difficulties, cognitive impairment and other symptoms such as dribbling, sexual problems and incontinence often cause a downward spiral of anxiety, embarrassment, reduced confidence and a consequent decreased level of activity.

Self-care activities including bed mobility, bathing, dressing, hygiene and feeding are usually affected, as are the person's work, domestic and leisure pursuits. Established routines may be disturbed by the fluctuation in the condition's daily pattern and be difficult to maintain. It is, however, important for the individual to remain as active as possible in daily life as there is a tendency to become more passive, for example, to increase activities such as reading and watching television (Manson & Caird 1985). The person's roles may

Table 26.1 Most common disabilities

Symptom	In Aberdeen		Population of 250 000	
	No (%) of patients positive	No (%) uncertain	No of positive	No positive + uncertain
Walking slowly	207 (78)	33 (13)	376	437
Slower dressing	207 (78)	22 (8)	376	416
Difficulty getting out of chair	185 (70)	19 (7)	336	371
Difficulty turning in bed	178 (67)	32 (12)	324	382
Shuffling	176 (66)	29 (11)	320	373
Stooping when walking or falling to one side when sitting	176 (66)	24 (9)	320	364
Speech difficulty	172 (65)	22 (8)	313	353
Difficulty starting movements	171 (65)	22 (8)	311	351
Handwriting change	171 (65)	48 (18)	311	398
Tremor in arm:				
Right	145 (55)	15 (6)	264	291
Left	143 (54)	14 (5)	260	286
Control symptoms:				
Pins and needles in hands or feet	24 (9)	71 (27)	44	173
Flashing lights before eyes	25 (9)	65 (25)	45	163
Itching	10 (4)	59 (22)	18	126

Source figures derived from W Mutch et al 1986 Parkinson's disease in a Scottish city. British Medical Journal 292:534–536 (with kind permission of the BMJ Publishing Group). (Reproduced from 'Meeting a need?' published by the Parkinson's Disease Society.)

change fundamentally with the loss of social identities such as parent, employee, friend. It may be necessary for role reversal within the family, which, unless handled sensitively, can cause distress.

The impact of the condition will therefore be different for each person. Those closest often need to become carers and as the condition progresses more demands are put on them. In addition to, and possibly in reaction to, the physical stress of caring, emotional responses such as resentment, depression, guilt and anger can also build up (O'Reilly et al 1996). Because of all the difficulties, the carer too may become socially isolated.

THE INTERVENTION TEAM

For many people, their first contact is with their local medical practitioner, who will either make the diagnosis of PD or refer them to a specialist, usually either a neurologist or a geriatrician. In the early stages, drug therapy is the most important form of treatment and the value of specialist PD clinics has become recognised. Some have Parkinson's nurse specialists and most have physiotherapists, occupational therapists and speech and language therapists. Early intervention and support from these professionals is advantageous and their advice and counselling can help the person to adjust in a more positive way to the knowledge that they have this long-term condition.

The nurse specialist (McMahon 1999) provides general advice, for example, about when to take medication, and liaises with other team members. The physiotherapist (Parkinson's Disease Society 1997) advises on the need to maintain normal movement patterns and on the importance of exercises aimed at improving posture, rotation and arm swing. The speech and language therapist (Parkinson's Disease Society 1998) encourages the person to maintain the quality, speed and volume of their speech, thus reducing the likelihood of social isolation, and often addresses feeding difficulties. Therapy should involve the whole family and include advice about management of the condition and adjustments that may have to be made.

Box 26.2 The Parkinson's Disease Society

Many people benefit from membership of the PD Society (PDS) from which an extensive range of publications (including a pack by and for occupational therapists), videos, a freephone helpline (0808 800 0303) and information about local branches can be obtained. The PDS has a very active support network called YAPPERS (Young Alert Parkinsonians Partners and Relatives) for the young onset group.

The idea of short intensive courses (sometimes called 'Pitstops': Parkinson's Intensive Therapy, Speech Therapy, Occupational Therapy and Physiotherapy) lasting from between 3 and 10 days has proved useful. Attendance once or twice a year is thought to be beneficial but should be part of a broader, individual plan. A person with PD benefits from treatment at home where activities can be practised in familiar surroundings, and possibly with carers.

British studies in the 1980s (Beattie & Caird 1980, Mutch et al 1986, Oxtoby 1982) revealed general inadequacy in the provision of services and specialised equipment and the fact that few people had been seen by therapists in spite of need. The UK Parkinson's Disease Society (PDS; Box 26.2) has identified a model of care and requirements at various stages of the condition (Fig. 26.3) and produced data about the recommended level of input by professionals at each stage (Table 26.2).

As the condition progresses, typically some 6 years after diagnosis, drugs become less effective and the involvement of an increasing number of professionals may be required. Essential to the effectiveness of the team is coordination and good communication and so a key worker, often a nurse, might be appointed. At this stage, advice from a dietician, social worker and continence adviser may be needed, and sometimes a chiropodist, psychologist and community psychiatric

---

Diagnosis

AIMS
Development of disease awareness
Reduction in symptoms and distress
Acceptance of diagnosis

Assessment
(Medical and nursing)
Accurate diagnosis
Evaluate disability
Assess support available
Estimate patient understanding

MANAGEMENT
Develop care plan
Consider multidisciplinary referral
 • Specialist nurse
 • Physiotherapy
 • Occupational therapist
 • Social worker
 • Dietician
Assistance and advice with
    medication (not always required)
Provide patient/carer education on
 • Employment
 • Driving
 • Finances

OUTCOMES
Effective symptom control
Reduced patient distress

Maintenance

AIMS
Morbidity relief
Maintenance of function and self care
Promotion of normal activities

Reassessment
Avoid unnecessary medical dependency
Reduce symptoms
Avoid side-effects
Alert for complications e.g. constipation,
    postural hypotension

MANAGEMENT
Review care plan
Provide patient/carer education
Assistance and advice with medication
    single or dual drug therapy
Consider multidisciplinary referral
 • Speech (and language) therapy
 • Physiotherapy
 • Occupational therapist
 • Social worker
 • Dietician
Assess carer needs
 • Benefits
 • Support

OUTCOMES
Symptom reduction
Treatment compliance
Maintenance and promotion of normal activities

Complex

AIMS
Morbidity relief
Maintenance of function and self-care
    despite advancing disease
Assistance and adaptation of environment
    to promote daily living activities

Reassessment
Because of increasing disability and
    complexity
Symptom control

MANAGEMENT
Increasingly complex drug management from
    disease process and medication side-effects
Advice on practical problems and prevention
    of complications* (see below)
Referral/liaison may be required
 • as in stage I +
 • Psychiatrist / CPN
 • Neurosurgery

    *Complications
 • Motor fluctuations, dyskinesia
 • Depression, anxiety
 • Self care, feeding, dysphagia
 • Mobility, falls
 • Confusion, hallucinations

OUTCOMES
Optimum symptom control
Minimisation of disability
Compliance

Palliative

AIMS
Relief of symptoms and distress in
    patients and carers, morbidity relief
Maintenance of dignity, and remaining
    function despite advancing disease
Avoidance of treatment related problems

Reassessment
Symptom control

MANAGEMENT
Advice on administration of medication
Progressive dopaminergic drug withdrawal
 • Analgesia
 • Sedation
Counselling – psychology/psychiatry
Prevention and treatment of complications
 • Urinary incontinence
 • Pressure sores
 • Motor fluctuations

OUTCOMES
Absence of distress
Maintenance of dignity
Symptoms controlled

Fig. 26.3 Model of care and requirements at different stages of Parkinson's disease (reproduced from 'Moving and shaping – the future' with kind permission of the Parkinson's Disease Society).

Table 26.2 Patients' annual contacts with professionals (for a population of 250 000)

Years after diagnosis of PD	Contacts		Hours		
	GP	Consultant	Physio-therapist	Occupational therapist	Speech and language therapist
1	160	100	0	0	0
2–5	640	240	160	160	80
6–9	960	480	960	480	480
10–12	1440	480	1440	1440	960
Total	3200	1300	2560	2080	1520
WTE equivalent		Over 1	2	2	1–2

Reproduced from 'Meeting a need?' with kind permission of the Parkinson's Disease Society.
WTE, whole time equivalent.

nurse may also be required. Sometimes several professionals are involved with the same problem but they each contribute their own expertise; for example, difficulties with eating may require the input of the dietician, physiotherapist, speech and language therapist and also the occupational therapist. Collaboration rather than duplication is the key to success.

Ideally, assessment and intervention should be provided in, or local to, the individual's home. Hospital admission may be necessary, however, for regulation of medication. Such stays rarely offer the opportunity for effective intervention by therapists as the person is usually discharged as soon as the problems with the drug regimen are resolved. Difficulties with mobility or the need for specialist equipment, however, may come to light during admission and result in referral to the appropriate community services.

THEORETICAL FRAMEWORK

There has been too little research on occupational therapy and PD to provide firm evidence that can guide practice. However, the ideas underpinning models, theories and frames of reference presented and brought together over recent years can inform the therapeutic process and help encapsulate all the necessary aspects of a successful intervention. A stance that emphasises 'client centredness', that is, a full appreciation of an individual, his wishes, priorities and environment, is essential.

The concepts of human occupation and occupational performance, as proposed by Kielhofner (1995), Reed and Sanderson (1992) and Fisher (1999), amongst others, integrate all aspects of occupational therapy in PD. They focus on the impact of the condition on the person's ability to undertake the activities they want or need to do, that is, the occupational performance, rather than the mind/brain/body systems themselves. These client-centred models capture the complex interaction between the person, their culture and environment, the activity undertaken and the functional performance, and highlight the need for the therapist to understand all these elements to be able to assist the person effectively. The therapist can assist the individual to maintain or improve the ability to perform the activities and roles that they feel are essential to optimise functioning and contribute to a meaningful life.

The person

By the time referral is made to occupational therapy the individual will probably have started to demonstrate definite, typical signs and symptoms of PD and the physical manifestation of problems (the mind/brain/body performance subsystem) is likely to be quite obvious. Any underlying cognitive or psychological changes may not be as clearly defined. Both habits and roles can be disrupted early in the development of the condition. Volition is what guides and motivates a person and determines the meaningfulness of an activity. To an individual it can feel as though their whole choice of activity or locus of control lies with the PD rather than with themselves. It can affect their short- or long-term occupational decisions and commitments, sense of effectiveness and ability to enjoy activity.

The culture and environment

This includes the physical, social and cultural environments in which a person exists and with which they interact. Cultural and spiritual beliefs and customs are very important, all-pervading influences on the way a person does the things they do and the way they respond to events. Their culture will influence the way they choose and perform activities that are important to them and will influence how they cope with the condition. In terms of social environment, they may gradually lose touch with their social circle and markedly reduce social contact. The physical environment also often provides significant barriers. However, Kielhofner (1995) discusses how environments can both 'afford' opportunities for occupational behaviour or 'press' for particular types of behaviour. For the person with PD, the physical environment can 'afford' stimulus and tangible cues for action as well as providing barriers. A stimulating environment or keen therapists and relatives can 'press' for an expectation of maximal performance and achievement, whilst a dull living area in a residential home or an isolated life at home with little choice or challenge can produce the lowest level of occupational performance.

Activity/task

The activities an individual actually chooses to carry out in everyday life will vary from person to person, depending on factors such as culture, mentioned above. There needs to be a process between the person and the therapist to identify the activities that can be developed, limited, adapted, discarded, or carried out by others.

Performance

Occupational performance is the interaction between the person, the environment and the activity, relevant to his culture and roles. It is the way that he does something, and includes his level of ability, competence and satisfaction with the task, and is the main focus for occupational therapy.

THE ROLE OF THE OCCUPATIONAL THERAPIST

The therapist's role is to:

- assess the person in their preferred environment
- analyse the occupational performance
- clarify which skills are affected or intact
- analyse the sequence of activity
- establish the balance of daily routine
- assess the environment for barriers or opportunities
- consider any wishes a carer may have.

The therapist can then assist by:

- establishing priorities
- improving skills
- providing the resources for practising skills
- helping the person to organise and balance daily activity
- providing advice, information and education
- advising about specialist equipment
- advising on changes to the environment.

The therapist should ensure that the focus of her work is the impact of the condition on daily life, she should not be trying to treat the PD itself, and that the relevance and meaning of all input is obvious to the person and determined by them.

Occupational therapy outcomes, as outlined by Reed and Sanderson (1992; see also Chapter 3), should include:

- the achievement of optimum functioning within the person's own environment
- successful adaptation and adjustment to the circumstances
- an increased sense of accomplishment, satisfaction and control
- an increased sense of dignity and self-worth, through the knowledge that ability, not disability, is important to the quality of life.

INTERVENTIONS

THEORY

In terms of frames of reference, the most useful are probably those that encompass compensation and learning concepts (see Chapter 3). Whilst the therapist needs to ensure age-appropriate intervention, a strictly developmental approach with its emphasis on stage-on-stage development of skills is not relevant in this progressive condition. Likewise, a biomechanical approach is probably also an inappropriate frame of reference, although a certain amount of intervention to regain or maintain fitness, strength, range of movement and physical tolerance can be helpful. The maintenance of wellbeing and the prevention of unnecessary deterioration are important aspects for all members of the health team to emphasise but are not the primary focus for occupational therapy.

An educative approach, however, can be helpful. The person with PD goes through a process of dramatic change in their body and lifestyle. Therapists should provide education, advice and information about the effect of the condition on everyday life and also about sources of help. Although there is little specific research demonstrating that this input is effective, it is generally accepted that improved knowledge and education enhances the person's understanding and ability to adapt (Montgomery et al 1994).

The therapist may be able to provide a learning process (also known as a rehabilitative, remediation or restorative approach) to improve, restore or redevelop skilled and effective functional performance. This is an area that has been neglected in the past but work using cognitive strategies is beginning to show some promise in improving functional ability and is an area where further studies are required (Morris et al 1997). Evidence of sensory processing deficits in PD has been highlighted and therefore a sensory integrative approach has been mooted as a way forward, although no studies have been undertaken. The use of conductive education in PD has been known for some time and is occasionally employed by therapists. It uses rhythmical intention, verbalisation and goal-directed actions in a group setting to achieve a functional outcome and many people with PD find it helpful (Brown 1996).

In conjunction with a learning approach, or if skills cannot be relearned, the therapist can assist with the more traditional approach of compensatory or alternative strategies, adaptations, modifications or specialised equipment to attempt to overcome the loss of function. Again, there is no published research demonstrating the effectiveness of a compensatory or adaptive approach in PD, although the level of disability and dependency incurred would indicate a real need for it.

DATA GATHERING

The therapist needs to have an appreciation of the person, his environments, his activities (in self care, homecare, work and leisure) and his occupational performance in those activities. She should review information available from existing documentation, for example, case records and interviews of the individual and others, and from informal and formal observation of performance. The person may not be able to give visual or verbal feedback or use body language to express how he is feeling.

A range of assessments, particularly those of the Model of Human Occupation (Kielhofner 1995), can be used to gather specific and more structured information of concern to the therapist; it is not necessary to rely solely on informal data collection. The structured process of the Canadian Occupational Performance Measure (COPM; Law et al 1994) can help to establish which activities are the most important or of most concern to the individual. The therapist then needs to observe these activities to identify the problems. The Assessment of Motor and Process Skills (AMPS; Fisher 1999) and the Assessment of Communication and Interaction Skills (ACIS; Keilhofner 1995) can provide structured testing to identify specific problems with skills in performance and the way that the condition impacts on activity or communication. The

AMPS in particular can provide information about whether a person can still organise themselves logically, attend to the task, initiate actions, complete a task, solve problems and remember what they are doing. These skills are important with respect to relearning, as discussed previously. If further information on impairments, such as level of cognition or hand function, is required and this has not been supplied by performance testing, then it may be necessary to obtain it at this stage.

Some of the better-known assessments developed by other disciplines specifically for use in PD, such as the Hoehn and Yahr (1967) and the United PD Rating Scale (Lang & Fahn 1989) could be considered, although they each mix concepts of impairment and disability.

The therapist needs to know the pattern of the individual's daily activity and broader life plans. The use of a 24-hour activity sheet, checklist or diary is helpful in identifying difficult periods during the day. However, she also needs to have a sense of the individual's and family's hopes or fears for the future in the light of the diagnosis.

Initial assessments should act as baseline measures for later re-evaluation to demonstrate whether change has occurred. Many checklist-type assessments cannot be used in this way and are too insensitive to change. Corbett (1997) compared the AMPS, Hoehn and Yahr, UPDRS and Functional Independence Measure (FIM) and demonstrated that the AMPS (Fig. 26.4 and Boxes 26.3 and 26.4) was most sensitive to identifying change in PD. If formal tests have not been used, the therapist can still write a clear summary of performance in the relevant activities and this can provide a baseline for future evaluation and be used to set goals.

IDENTIFYING THE PROBLEM/PRIORITISING

Drawing on all available information (i.e. assessment results, knowledge of principles and intervention, experience and specific evidence) the therapist, the individual and relevant others as necessary can discuss how to proceed and how to prioritise the areas for intervention.

Box 26.3   Assessment of Motor and Process Skills (AMPS)

The AMPS was carried out with J. (see Box 26.4). The AMPS is a standardised observational assessment that measures a person's overall ability to perform everyday activities whilst providing information about which underlying skills are affected. The person chooses two or three familiar, relevant tasks to do. The occupational therapist assesses the quality of the performance by rating 16 motor skills (observable actions to move oneself or objects) and 20 process skills (observable actions to logically and effectively carry out an activity). J.'s graphic report results (see Fig. 26.4) demonstrate that he has enough difficulty with motor skills to affect his ability to be independent in everyday life. J. was found to be well below the cut-off point on the motor scale. Most people above this point have no difficulty with everyday tasks. The assessment also indicates that J. has limitations with some process skills and, at this level, he is unlikely to be able to manage alone in the community. J.'s AMPS results allow a more precise identification of his specific difficulties and level of ability, can guide therapy with him and give a baseline against which his abilities can be measured after intervention, drug treatment or over time.

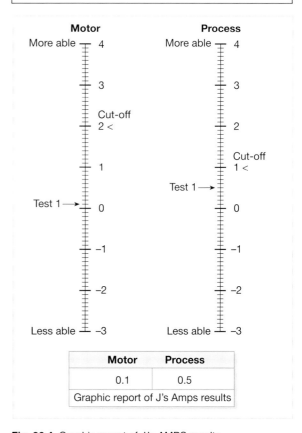

	Motor	Process
	0.1	0.5

Graphic report of J's Amps results

Fig. 26.4 Graphic report of J.'s AMPS results.

Box 26.4 Case study: J's own story

J. was born in London in 1945. He was diagnosed with idiopathic Parkinson's disease in 1979.

'After a travelling life, I settled down to a staff job with a BBC orchestra, in Glasgow. Looking back, things began to go wrong at this time, from 1974. I got strange sprains in strange places. The music seemed to be getting faster ... The reality was that I was getting slower. The first specific symptoms [tremor in left hand and arm on exertion] appeared after an operation to remove a ganglion. Following diagnosis my then neurologist took very early retirement. (He insisted the two events were not connected.) Later, I was helped considerably by a persistent occupational therapist who visited my home and rejected my protests that no help was needed. She arranged a wheelchair, devices to aid turning and getting in and out of bed, an intercom system, grabrails in strategic places, a shower room, a chair, trolleys and even a zimmer! The flat was transformed from an obstacle course. Referral was through a vigilant occupational therapist at Southern General Hospital, Glasgow. After a week of drug trials (I used to volunteer for everything!) she also made me aware of possible benefit payments, which I had not previously considered. For treatment I have been lucky: with my wise neurologist in London, a caring PD nurse specialist, my GP ... other Parkinson people are not so fortunate. There is also much support available through YAPP&Rs (Young Alert Parkinson Partners and Relatives) and the Parkinson's Disease Society HQ, branches and support groups. Most of all, I am blessed with a loving partner. Treatment-wise, I take an assorted cocktail of anti-Parkinson medication, adapted as new drugs become available. I have turned down the possibility of surgery on several occasions. Generally I look to the future with hope ...'

One option for intervention might be to choose the area that appears to have the easiest or quickest solution, particularly if time constraints are operating, for example, helping the person apply for benefits when finances are pressing and causing worry; or supplying a sloping cushion when standing up is problematic. However, although provision of equipment may seem the easiest solution to problems this is not always the case, and many items provided free are never used.

Another way of prioritising is to identify the most basic or underlying problem that impacts on many other areas, for example, difficulty in eating well due to tremor and loss of small muscle move-

ment may lead to loss of weight, increased fatigue, have an effect on drugs, cause decreased mobility and result in increased worry for the carer. In this case all attention would be directed to facilitating eating.

A different method of prioritising might be to choose the activity that is most important, annoying or worrying for the person, or alternatively to choose the activities that are most important or time consuming for the carer. Poor eating ability can again be the example for these guidelines – it can be embarrassing and frustrating for the person and take inordinate amounts of the carer's time. The important point is that the decision about which areas are dealt with is a collaborative process facilitated by the therapist.

INTERVENTION ACTIVITY

Intervention should occur only as a comprehensive plan that takes account of the person and their priorities, the person's family and other important relationships, variations in the manifestation of the condition, the effect of medication, the effect of environment and culture and the long-term nature of the disease. Interventions that work during the day might not work at night and those that work when the person is 'on' are unlikely to work when they are 'off', and so several options may be required. The therapist therefore needs to be very flexible and creative in her input. The priorities for a 40-year-old working woman with a family, newly diagnosed with PD, are likely to be very different from those of an 82-year-old man with long-standing PD and arthritis who is showing some signs of mental health problems.

A person with PD cannot be rushed and more time than normal is needed to elicit information, discuss, experiment and practise. To improve performance in activities, the individual will need to practise those activities, taking time because rushing usually only increases anxiety and tremor and ultimately the activity takes longer and causes more distress. For the older person with long-established habits and routines, much more time may be required to enable adaption to suggestions or change. The rate of progression of the condition can usually support the development of a therapeutic relationship, longer-term plans and the possibility for adjustment to occur. However, the earlier intervention can start, the better, and regular follow-up is essential.

Compromise is likely to be necessary to ensure the best solution and to achieve agreed goals. However, much is trial and error and what appears to be a good solution one day may not work the next. Goals may need to be broken down and set for specific parts of the day or particular places. It is important that both the therapist and the family recognise that the outcome may not be one that achieves 100% success every time for every activity. Sometimes, a small improvement in performance can be enough to be satisfying.

Traditionally, advice and lifestyle planning are given emphasis in intervention. This may include time management, prioritising and achieving balance in activity. People with PD usually have to think about which activities they wish to concentrate on because the whole normal daily routine may be disrupted. They need to work around the 'good' and 'bad' times and learn how to save their energy for the activities of their choice. Learning how to relinquish some activities, such as work, and possibly take on others, such as leisure, may need sensitive support. Alternatively, changes to the routine can happen over a long time and people may get into imbalanced patterns. For example, undue dependency on a spouse may have occurred, or the morning routine may have started to take up hours of time, or a person may have withdrawn into watching television all day. The therapist may be able to help people review the daily routine and suggest ways to organise time and restore balance. It is also important to assist with strategies for particular times when it is likely that the person will need to alter their daily routine, for example, at family occasions or admission to hospital.

Keeping healthy

It is important to advise on keeping fit, both mentally and physically. The person with PD in particular benefits from gentle fitness classes, yoga and relaxation classes. Encouragement to take a daily walk and do some stretching exercises to music or a video will prove useful. Eating well helps the correct absorption of drugs, alleviates problems of bowel management and maintains health. Psychological research is now demonstrating that 'use it or lose it' is as sound for mental processes as for physical and if the individual has limited opportunities for mental stimulation then some way of increasing these should be sought. Ideally, the solution could be found by improving social contact at the same time. If maintaining previous hobbies, interests and social interaction proves too difficult, the therapist should be as concerned with addressing this as with aspects of the home environment because it may be of great importance to the person. To overcome social embarrassment caused by immobility, festination, tremor and poor communication it may be necessary to learn strategies for coping in public places.

Skills acquisition and learning

More information is appearing about how cognitive functioning affects performance in PD: activities and skills that were previously carried out automatically may become increasingly difficult (Morris & Iansek 1997). However, people with PD can be rigid in their thought processes and slow to generalise learning. Cognitive strategies can help improve skills and prepare for an activity. Box 26.5 illustrates a checklist that the individual could use before beginning. These triggers or cues can also be used during activity if a person starts to slow down or stop, for example, during writing or if they freeze.

Carers should be involved as much as possible and it may be helpful to organise the environment so that performance is maximised. For example, a carer can be asked to lay out clothes so that the person has only to concentrate on dressing, or the chest of drawers containing clothes can be repositioned to ease access. People with PD often enjoy learning in groups and can benefit from the social contact provided (Gauthier et al 1987), although it must be ensured that anything learnt in groups can be applied elsewhere.

Box 26.5 Checklist

The person should:
- stop what they are doing and bring their full attention to the task
- ensure that only one activity or task at a time is attempted, or only one component if a complete task is too much
- try to relax, breathe deeply, concentrate, stretch if necessary
- organise and plan what needs to be done
- think or talk through the actions rather than just launch into them
- use written instructions or cue cards if necessary
- use visual, verbal and auditory cues, such as patterns on wallpaper, counting or music to reinforce actions
- visualise the action, this can sometimes give enough stimulation
- do the action and check it afterwards
- learn new things or complete familiar tasks in short sequences.

It may be helpful to:
- use practice and repetition to learn new activities
- rehearse the daily routine, making a day plan or timetable
- use appropriate memory strategies if memory is a problem
- reinforce strategies as much as possible in different locations
- check the relationship between performance and medication times
- attempt demanding tasks at times of optimal performance.

Compensatory strategies

The therapist might also need to consider compensatory strategies. One of these could be to try to perform activities in different ways, for example, if getting up from the bottom of the bath is a problem and neither verbal intention nor practice helps, then the person may need to try turning over onto their knees before trying to stand. If improvement is not achieved it might be at this point that the therapist needs to consider suggesting the use of equipment. Daily living aids should be seen as an adjunct to intervention, not an end in themselves. Their use should be negotiated with the person and family because the idea of special aids and adaptations needs sensitive introduction. If a piece of equipment is recommended it is essential that the person has an opportunity to practise using it with the therapist present and that its need is re-evaluated regularly. Objects in the home that can be awkward to other people with disabilities may not be so to people with PD, for example, a heavy pan can be easier to manage than a light one when there is tremor.

Functional mobility

To help the individual improve their functional mobility, all the cognitive and compensatory strategies suggested in the previous sections need to be used. If walking becomes too fast the person should be advised to stop, prepare himself and then start again. It is very important that carers realise that helping the person to adopt cues and strategies can be more useful than pulling on their arm. Counting, singing, chanting, putting the heel down first, focusing on points across a room, visualising lines on the floor, concentrating on arm swing and placing specific cues in places that are awkward to negotiate can all help. Sticks need to be of the correct height and rollators may be more useful than a frame that has to be lifted. Some obstacles, such as rugs and furniture, are a hindrance, whereas others are a positive help because they act as cues. Grabrails may be helpful if positioned appropriately.

Taking several steps in a circle is often safer than trying to turn on the spot and using supports that are stable and directly next to the person is essential to prevent overbalancing. If freezing occurs it may be possible to start moving again by using the same strategies as for initiating walking. Some people may try rocking their head or rotating their body to start them off. Keeping calm is essential and being distracted can help. Stairs do not often pose a problem, although some people become stuck at particular points. Strategies such as counting the steps when going up the stairs can help maintain momentum. Charting the individual's movements over time around the house may help to identify particular problem areas.

Good postural support and comfort are important when sitting and the individual's chair must facilitate his sitting to standing movement by being stable, having seat and armrests at the optimal height and possibly by having a forward-sloping seat. Some people may wish to use a riser chair but the balance mechanism needs to be adjusted carefully to prevent sudden propulsion. The person must ensure that they are balanced and standing upright before starting to walk. The concept of planning movement and applying strategies is often necessary for the sitting to standing action and for bed mobility. For the latter, it is helpful to have a firm mattress and it may be advantageous to place a silky sheet under the hips to aid sliding, and/or wear bedsocks for grip. A rail by the bed may be useful.

Specific goals and encouragement may be needed to maintain outdoor mobility. It is important that the full range of mobility allowances, benefits and local mobility schemes are made known. A wheelchair should not be the automatic solution to mobility problems because the emphasis should be on maintaining walking. However, many people find that the use of a lightweight or powered wheelchair for longer distances often becomes necessary. Good posture and comfort in the chair are important.

Assessment of driving ability and the possible need for car adaptations may be advisable. There is a legal responsibility to notify the authorities about the onset of certain medical conditions, including PD. However, many people with PD can continue to drive, although a car with automatic transmission and power steering might be easier to use.

Self care

It is very important to maintain self-esteem and dignity in PD and intervention can facilitate and maintain high standards of hygiene, particularly in oral, dental, hair, nail and skin care. Some small aids with long or large handles may help. If the person has lost confidence in using the bath, the therapist may be able to help by encouraging practice, change of technique and/or providing equipment. Showering, where possible, may be a preferred or safer option. Continence management must be thoroughly checked out with the medical practitioner. The therapist can assist by ensuring that the toilet is as accessible as possible.

Independence in dressing may be important to the person, or they may prefer to accept help, thus saving energy for other activities. Loose, stretchy and easy-to-manage clothes are the obvious first choice although some adaptations may need to be made, for example, wider openings, use of elastic or Velcro, larger buttons. Leather- or smooth-soled shoes may aid mobility if the person's feet tend to 'stick' to the floor and flat shoes may help if people feel they are falling forwards.

To improve communication, speech can be helped by ensuring that the person's posture is good and that they take time to express themselves. Relatives should be advised to exercise patience. Facial expression, which is often described as mask-like because of difficulties in frowning and smiling, can be improved by practising in front of a mirror. Writing, as with other activities, can be helped by applying strategies as described earlier before and during the action, and a thick-barrelled pen (roller balls require less pressure than ball points) may be useful. A word processor may overcome the problem.

Good posture is also important when eating, as is the need to take time. If chewing and swallowing are a problem, a change of diet to semi-solids or food supplements may be required. Sipping a drink along with a meal may assist swallowing and the provision of specialist equipment, such as a non-slip mat, a lipped plate or two-handled cup, can be helpful. Referral to a dietician or speech and language therapist may be necessary.

Home environment

Occupational therapists recognise that assessment of the individual's home needs to be approached with sensitivity, particularly when he is undergoing the major personal changes that the condition itself can create. It is best practice to try and ensure, however, that he is assessed in his own environment wherever possible.

In terms of risk management and safety, it is tempting to suggest the removal of obstacles. However, some objects can be used as visual cues to initiate or facilitate movement. A personal alarm can be worn as a bracelet or necklace and intercom alarms can be helpful for more dependent people. Environmental control systems can be useful to access switches and are usually fitted with alarms.

The therapist can offer advice about home adaptations, if required and if the person is ready to accept the changes and upheaval involved. For the more dependent person, ramps, door widening, bathroom or toilet alterations and stair or through-floor lifts may need to be considered. The therapist can advise on access to grants or funding for such work from statutory services. Rearrangement in the kitchen to make access easier may be advisable and some small household aids, such as plugs with large handles, may enable a higher level of independence.

Work

Many people are diagnosed with PD when still at work, running a household or involved in community activities. It is vital that they are encouraged and supported to continue with these for as long as possible. These activities will need to be viewed as an integral part of the person's life and discussed in terms of priority. It may be preferable to the individual to have help each morning for personal care so that energy can be saved for work with all the self-esteem, financial contribution and social interaction that employment provides. The therapist can explore labour-saving devices and techniques, changes to the work environment or organisation, transport arrangements to and from work, or discuss alternatives if the original work cannot be continued. She can advise on employment organisations that may assist. The worker or the homemaker may wish to consider prioritising tasks or sharing domestic tasks with others.

Leisure

As with work, it may be that maintaining leisure pursuits at the expense of mundane tasks is more beneficial to the person for the social contact and sense of achievement they can bring (Box 26.6). A major aspect of living with PD is that people become socially isolated and it is essential that the

---

Box 26.6 Case study: Mrs S.

Mrs S. is 75 years old and lives alone. Her problems began over 6 years ago when she noticed that her writing was becoming smaller and her grip weaker. She later developed a tremor and went to her GP, who diagnosed Parkinson's disease. Medication was prescribed and this helped significantly but she later began to experience problems with walking: she had difficulty initiating the movement, then took small steps and could not stop when she wanted to. She was also having problems getting in and out of the bath and doing up small fastenings. Her GP referred her to the community occupational therapist, who discussed all Mrs S.'s problems with her. Mrs S. complained about being worse in the mornings and that housework was becoming increasingly difficult and tiring.

The occupational therapist reassured Mrs S. that many people with Parkinson's disease share her problems. Mrs S. outlined her weekly routine and together they prioritised the activities she most enjoyed. A decision was made to employ a home help for heavy housework and shopping. Mrs S. was then able to conserve her energy for light housework and attending social activities in the afternoons. The occupational therapist also advised Mrs S. about walking: Mrs S. ensured that her posture was good, prepared herself to walk, tried to imagine stepping over a line when starting and sang a rhythmical tune to herself whilst she stepped out. The occupational therapist provided some equipment for the kitchen and bathroom. On follow-up, Mrs S. reported a significant improvement in mobility and ability to cope.

---

therapist considers ways to encourage confidence to continue engaging in leisure activities and the meaningful use of leisure time. Difficulties in transport and access can often be the main barrier to continuing social and leisure pursuits and this should be addressed with help from the therapist. Keep Fit programmes, little and often, can be helpful, as can relaxation, yoga or Tai'chi. Alternative sedentary hobbies may be necessary if adaptations to current ones cannot be made. People with PD positively benefit from mental stimulation and should be encouraged to participate in activities such as quizzes and games if possible.

CONCLUSION

Playfer (1990) states that involvement with those with PD is 'both a rewarding and an exasperating experience'. There are few other neurological disorders that respond so positively to medication. In recent years there has also been an increase in research into surgical techniques, as well as cognitive and psychological approaches, presenting a more optimistic outlook for future management.

Occupational therapists are concerned with the impact of the condition on daily life tasks and their expertise enables them to offer individuals and their families opportunities to live as positively as possible with the challenges PD can present.

ACKNOWLEDGEMENTS

Our sincere thanks go to The Parkinson's Disease Society for information and support and to Ana Aragon (senior occupational therapist, Bath & West Community NHS Trust) for information on cognitive strategies. Also, thanks to those with PD, and in particular, to J. for all his help and cooperation.

REFERENCES

Aarsland D et al 1996 Frequency of dementia in Parkinson's disease. Archives of Neurology 53:538–542

Beattie A, Caird F 1980 The occupational therapist and the patient with Parkinson's disease. British Medical Journal 280:1354–1355

Brown M 1996 Parkinson's and conductive education, PDS Information Sheet. Parkinson's Disease Society, c/o National Institute of Conductive Education, Birmingham

Corbett PJ 1997 Functional assessment in Parkinson's disease: comparison of four instruments to determine functional change, pre- and post apomorphine intervention. Master's thesis, the College of Occupational Therapists, London

Dewick H, Playfer JR 1990 Cognitive impairment in Parkinson's disease. Care of the Elderly 2(7):260–262

Ehmann TS, Beninger RJ, Gawel MJ, Riopelle RJ 1990 Coping, social support and depressive symptoms in Parkinson's disease. Journal of Geriatric Psychiatry and Neurology 3(2):85–90

Fisher AG 1999 Assessment of motor and process skills, 3rd edn. Three Star Press, CO

Gauthier L, Dalziel S, Gauthier S 1987 The benefits of group occupational therapy for patients with Parkinson's disease. American Journal of Occupational Therapy 41(6):360–365

Gibb WRG, Luthert PJ 1994 Dementia in Parkinson's disease and lewy body disease. In: Burns A, Levy R (eds) Dementia. Chapman & Hall, London, pp 719–737

Gisenberg MG, Grzessiak RC 1987 The Functional Independence Measure, a new tool for rehabilitation. Advances in Clinical Rehabilitation. Springer-Verlag, 1:6–18

Hantz P, Caradoc-Davies G, Caradoc-Davies T, Weatherall M, Dixon G 1994 Depression in Parkinson's disease. American Journal of Psychiatry 151(7):1010–1014

Hoehn MM, Yahr MD 1967 Parkinsonism: onset, progression and mortality. Neurology 17:427–442

Kielhofner G 1995 A model of human occupation: theory and application, 2nd edn. Williams & Wilkins, Baltimore, MD

Lang AET, Fahn S 1989 Assessment of Parkinson's disease. In: Quantification of Neurological Deficit. Butterworths, Stoneham, MA 02180, ch 21, pp 285–309

Law M, Baptiste S, Carswell A, McColl M, Polatajko H, Pollock N 1994 Canadian Occupational Performance Measure, 2nd edn. Canadian Association of Occupational Therapists Publications, Toronto, Ottawa

McMahon DG 1999 Parkinson's disease nurse specialist – an important role in disease management. Journal of Neurology (Suppl 3): S21–25

Manson L, Caird F 1985 Survey of the hobbies and transport of patients with Parkinson's disease. The British Journal of Occupational Therapy 48(7):199–200

Montgomery S et al 1994 Patient education and health promotion can be effective in Parkinson's disease: a randomised trial. American Journal of Medicine 97(5):429–435

Morris ME, Kirkwood B, Iansek R 1997 Moving ahead with Parkinson's disease. Victoria Printing, Blackburn

Mutch WJ, Dingwall-Fordyce I, Downie AW, Paterson JG, Roy SK 1986 Parkinson's disease in a Scottish city. British Medical Journal 292 (6519):534–536

O'Reilly F, Finnan F, Allwright S, Davey Smith G, Ben Shlomo Y 1996 The effects of caring for a spouse with Parkinson's disease on social, psychological and physical wellbeing. British Journal of General Practice 46:507–512

Oxtoby M 1982 Parkinson's disease patients and their social needs. Parkinson's Disease Society, London

Oyebode JR 1995 Cognitive and emotional aspects of Parkinson's disease. Health Psychology Update 22:14–17

Parkinson J 1817 An essay on the shaking palsy. Sherwood, Neely and Jones, London

Parkinson's Disease Society 1997 Parkinson's and the physiotherapist. Parkinson's Disease Society, London

Parkinson's Disease Society 1998 Parkinson's and the speech and language therapist. Parkinson's Disease Society, London

Playfer JR 1990 Parkinson's disease – the future prospects. Care of the Elderly 2(7):263–285

Reed K, Sanderson S 1992 Concepts of occupational therapy, 3rd edn. Williams & Wilkins, Baltimore, MD

Ring 1993 Psychological and social problems of Parkinson's disease. British Journal of Hospital Medicine 49(2):111

Starkstein SE et al 1993 Anxiety and depression in Parkinson's disease. Behavioural Neurology 6(3)

Taylor AE, Saint Cyr JA 1990 Depression in Parkinson's disease: reconciling physiological and psychological perspectives. Journal of Neurological Psychiatry 2(1):92–98

FURTHER READING

Andersen S 1996 The new role of the patient. The Parkinson (March). Available from the Parkinson's Disease Society, London

Bagley S, Kelly B, Tunnicliffe N, Turnbull G, Walker J 1996 The effect of visual cues on the gait of independently mobile Parkinson's disease patients. Physiotherapy 77:415–420

Buytenhuijs EL, Berger HJC, Vban Spaendonck KMP, Horstink MWI, Borm GF, Cools AR 1994 Memory and learning strategies in patients with Parkinson's disease. Neuropsychologia 32(3):335–342

Caird F (ed) 1991 Rehabilitation in Parkinson's disease. Churchill Livingstone, Edinburgh

Chesson R, Cockhead D, Maehle V 1995 Availability of therapy services to people with Parkinson's disease living in the community. Robert Gordon University, Aberdeen

Chrischilles EA, Rubenstein LM, Voelker MD, Wallace RB, Rodnitzky RL 1998 The health burdens of Parkinson's disease. Movement Disorders 13(3):406–413

European Parkinson's Disease Association. An insight into quality of life with Parkinson's disease: the global Parkinson's disease survey. Available from the European Parkinson's Disease Association, c/o Parkinson's Disease Society, London

Franklyn S, Perry A, Beattie A 1983 Living with Parkinson's disease. Parkinson's Disease Society, London (booklet and audio tape)

Freeman JS, Cody FWJ, Schady W 1996 The influence of external timing cues upon the rhythm of voluntary movements in Parkinson's disease. Journal of Neurology, Neurosurgery and Psychiatry 56:1078–1084

Mendelsohn GA, Dakof GA, Shaff M et al 1995 Personality change in Parkinson's disease and ageing. Journal of Personality 63(2):233–257

Miller E, Berrios G, Politynska BE 1996 Caring for someone with Parkinson's disease: factors that contribute to distress. International Journal of Geriatric Psychiatry 11:263–268

Oliveira RM, Gurd JM, Nixon P, Marshall JC, Passingham RSE 1997 Micrographia in Parkinson's disease: the effects of providing external cues. Journal of Neurology, Neurosurgery and Psychiatry 63:429–433

Oxtoby M, Williams A 2001 Parkinson's at your fingertips. Information pack available from the Parkinson's Disease Society, London. Class Publishing, London.

Parkinson's Disease Society 1992 Caring for people with Parkinson's 1995 DLF (1992) Advice notes for people who have Parkinson's disease. PDS/DLF Information Resource Paper ISD8. Parkinson's Disease Society, London

Parkinson's Disease Society 1994 Meeting a need? Parkinson's Disease Society, London

Parkinson's disease – physiotherapy evaluation Project UK. Correspondence to Professor R Plant, Institute of Rehabilitation, Hunters Moor Regional Rehabilitation Centre, Hunters Road, Newcastle Upon Tyne NE2 4NR

Pentland B et al 1987 The effects of reduced expression in Parkinson's disease on impression formation by health professionals. Clinical Rehabilitation 1:307–313

Percival R, Hobson P (eds) Parkinson's disease: studies in psychological and social care. The British Psychological Society, Leicester

Scott S, Caird FI, Williams BO 1983 Speech therapy for Parkinson's disease. Journal of Neurology, Neurosurgery and Psychiatry 46:140–144

Thomas S, Mac Mahon D, Henry S Moving and shaping – the future. Parkinson's Disease Society, London

Wermuth P et al 1995 Sexual problems in young patients with Parkinson's disease. Acta Neurologica Scandinavica 91(6):53–55

USEFUL CONTACTS

Parkinson's Disease Society, 215 Vauxhall Bridge Road, London SWIV 1EJ. Tel: 020 7931 8080 Fax: 020 7233 9908. Freephone 0808 800 0303. E-mail: www.parkinsons.org.uk

Disability Information Trust, Mary Marlborough Centre, Nuffield Orthopaedic Centre, Headington, Oxford OX3 7LD. Tel: 01865 227592

Institute of Complementary Medicines, PO Box 194, London SE16 7QZ. Tel: 020 7237 5165

27

Osteoarthritis

Paula Jeffreson   Alison Hammond

INTRODUCTION

Osteoarthritis (OA) is associated with increasing age but it is not an inevitable consequence of ageing. It is often considered of little importance and just part of 'getting old' but it is a major contributor to disability and dependence amongst older people, especially women (Hughes & Dunlop 1995). It is the most common form of arthritis and causes significant problems; one-quarter of elderly people with OA have ADL difficulties (Yelin & Katz 1990) and significant disability is found in walking, reaching, stooping and physical function needing endurance and strength (Verbrugge et al 1991). With an ageing population, the impact of OA on individuals, society and healthcare provision is increasing.

OA is a chronic joint disease caused by a disturbance in the normal balance of degradation and repair in the articular cartilage and subchondral bone. Peak onset is between 50 to 60 years of age and some 12% of people over 65 years have symptomatic OA. It can occur at any age in either sex and any joint can be affected, although it commonly affects the weight-bearing joints. Age and weight are the strongest determinants of OA, with prevalence rates for all joints rising with increasing age (Creamer & Hochberg 1997). Women tend to have more severe disease affecting multiple joints, particularly the knees and hands; OA in the hips is three times more common in men. Other joints commonly affected include the spine, shoulders, the carpometacarpal (CMC) joint of the thumb and the distal interphalangeal (DIP) joints of the fingers, ankles and toes. About 30% of adults have some degree of OA of the hand and it is the most common cause of hand pain in older adults (Chaisson & McAlindon 1997).

OA is multifactorial in origin and not simply a result of 'wear and tear' as is commonly thought. Pathological changes are reparative as well as destructive, with bone growth at joint margins as well as loss of cartilage and subchondral bone near the centre. It may not be a single disorder but a group of overlapping yet distinct diseases with risk factors, pathophysiology, clinical features and outcome varying according to the joints affected (Creamer & Hochberg 1997).

Both systemic and local biomechanical factors influence the development of OA (Dieppe 1994) (Fig. 27.1). Systemic factors (e.g. inherited susceptibility to OA, postmenopausal hormone deficiency, nutritional factors) can alter the structural make-up of articular cartilage and bone, making them more vulnerable to daily injuries and less capable of repair (Felson & Zhang 1998). Once these make a joint vulnerable, local biomechanical factors contribute to increasing joint breakdown. Abnormal stresses through joints alter biomechanical loading, thus damaging cartilage and bone. Such factors include injury, repetitive stress, joint deformity, obesity and muscle weakness.

OA could, in theory, be prevented. Greater body mass increases the risk of knee OA so reducing body weight directly reduces risk (Felson et al 1997). As abnormal joint loading increases risk, using ergonomic measures and joint protection can also reduce risk. Jobs involving kneeling, squatting and stair climbing are associated with higher rates of knee OA, whilst jobs requiring heavy lifting (such as farming) are associated with higher rates of hip OA (Creamer & Hochberg 1997). There is a clear link between repetitive joint use and hand OA. OA of the DIP joints is more common in people using repetitive finger movements and pincer grips to carry out their work than in the general population or those whose jobs required power grips (Hadler et al 1978).

PROBLEMS ASSOCIATED WITH OA

Pain, particularly on motion and after use, is a primary concern and is usually relieved by rest. Stiffness (the 'gel' phenomenon) is common after periods of inactivity and morning stiffness in affected joints can last up to 30 minutes. Muscle strength and joint movement deteriorate slowly, with progressive functional loss. These symp-

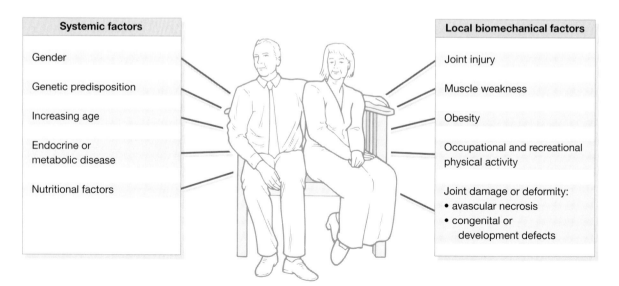

Fig. 27.1 Causes of osteoarthritis, including risk factors that predispose a person to the disease.

toms are caused by cartilage wear, particle debris in the joint and boney growths on the joint margins (called osteophytes), which interfere with the mechanical working of joints. Secondary inflammation and effusion may also add to pain and functional loss. Chronic pain can lead to muscle inhibition, atrophy and further muscle weakness, often occurring unequally round the joint. This further contributes to joint instability and deformity in the longer term. Symptoms do not necessarily correlate with the degree of damage to a joint. Further medical information is explained in Dieppe (1994) and Chadwick (1999).

THE IMPACT OF OA

OA symptoms exacerbate and remit but are steadily more progressive. Whilst not life threatening, quality of life deteriorates over time. Impact depends on the type and number of joints involved, the disease severity and on the individual's personality, work and lifestyle. If still working, increased sick leave, difficulty in job performance and consequent early retirement can have long-term economic consequences affecting pension income. Activities planned for retirement may become difficult or impossible. Declining mobility, chronic pain and progressive difficulties in ADL affect social life, reducing enjoyment and meaning and potentially leading to social isolation.

Ongoing losses may have a damaging effect psychologically and chronic pain can lead to growing irritability and depression. The whole family may be affected by this because it can be frustrating, distressing and lead to feelings of being powerless to help. The cycle of depression caused by inactivity, weakness and pain narrowing a person's life experiences and pleasures is summarised in Figure 27.2.

Older people with OA who perceive themselves as having more severe symptoms and serious OA use more passive coping methods (e.g. wish-fulfilling thoughts, depending on others, restricting function because of pain) and fewer active coping strategies (e.g. exercise, pain distraction, keeping physically and socially

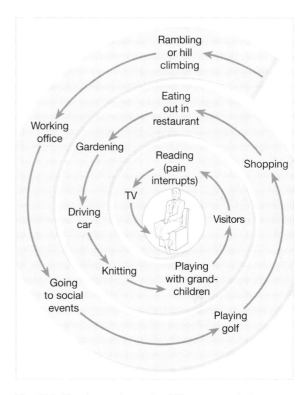

Fig. 27.2 The decreasing cycle of life events and pleasures.

active) than those who perceive themselves as better (Hampson et al 1996). Accepting the situation and resigning oneself to fate are common reactions amongst elderly women with OA (Downe-Wamboldt 1991). Those who cope with pain by restricting physical activity and resting are significantly more likely to have longer-term restrictions in mobility and function (Jensen et al 1991). People with OA are less physically fit than people of similar age who lead an inactive lifestyle. Thus the combination of poorer symptom appraisal, decreasing activity and decreasing mood promotes physical deconditioning, further decreasing activity and worsening mood and pain in a deteriorating spiral.

The relationship between beliefs about disease severity, coping strategies and mood has implications for therapy. Those who use more active coping strategies are less likely to be depressed longer term (Hampson et al 1996). Enhancing people's ability to self-manage their disease and use more active coping strategies can reduce pain, enhance mood and slow the progress of functional disability longer term, thus reducing costs to both families and society, as well as enhancing quality of life.

The majority of people do self-manage and compensate for increasing functional problems by finding alternative methods of task performance if pain, muscle weakness or loss of joint range of movement restricts an activity. Coping strategies such as distraction (taking a bath or shower, reading, exercising) and taking painkillers are commonly used to manage pain successfully. As a result, many people seek medical and therapy help if or when problems and pain become severe later in life. As OA occurs commonly in older people, they may by this stage have other physical impairments and medical conditions (such as heart disease or chronic obstructive airways disease), and the combined impact of these can be severe.

MANAGEMENT OF OA

OA is a degenerative condition and although recent research has improved the understanding of the disease process, there is currently no way of stopping its progression. Surgical techniques can make a dramatic impact by eliminating pain and restoring function. Nevertheless, there are increasing demands on healthcare professionals to find ways of helping people manage this disease (Hampson et al 1993), with a growing emphasis on self-management strategies (Hughes & Dunlop 1995). Active self-management can slow progress. Thus, earlier community-based intervention aimed at keeping people active and positive in outlook could do much to reduce functional loss and later stage medical, surgical and rehabilitation costs.

The aims of management for OA are:

- education about the disease, its treatment and self-management techniques
- relief of symptoms (pain and stiffness)
- maintaining optimal joint function and reducing disability

- modifying the environment to suit a person's needs
- maintaining and improving psychological status
- reduction of progression (stabilisation of damaged joints and/or prevention of OA appearing in new sites (Klippel & Dieppe 1997).

There is considerable variation in disease severity and many people never have treatment. OA can be undetected for years until symptoms are triggered by an acute inflammatory episode, severe cartilage loss or mechanical failure. Because of its chronic, degenerative nature, most treatment of OA takes place in the community. Admissions to hospital for rehabilitation are continuing to decline and improvements in surgical techniques are contributing to shorter lengths of stay in hospital following surgery.

A common approach to the management of OA is the pyramid approach shown in Figure 27.3.

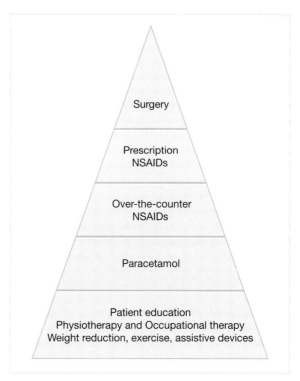

Fig. 27.3 The pyramid approach to the management of osteoarthritis (reproduced from Creamer & Hochberg 1997 Osteoarthritis. The Lancet 350 (9076):503–508 © by The Lancet Ltd, with kind permission).

Management starts at the base of the pyramid and treatment strategies are added from the next layer, and then the next, and so on, during the course of managing an individual's OA.

Drug treatment of OA needs to be suitable for the long-term treatment of older people with comorbidities and will be prescribed by the GP or rheumatology consultant (for people with more severe disease requiring outpatient management). Analgesic and non-steroidal anti-inflammatory drugs (NSAIDs) are widely used to treat pain and stiffness and are administered by one of three routes: oral, intra-articular and topical (rub-on creams). These do not alter the outcome of OA and NSAIDs are potentially toxic, with gastrointestinal side-effects (ulcers and haemorrhage) being common. Non-drug-related interventions (the base tier of Fig. 27.3) are best used first (Dieppe 1994). Current research is focused on the development of disease-modifying drugs.

THE INTERVENTION TEAM

Figure 27.4 depicts the members of the wider intervention team.

The orthopaedic surgeon will be involved with those individuals with more severe disease, who can be treated by:

- tidal lavage with saline introduced into the joint arthroscopically. This removes debris and inflammatory mediators
- osteotomy, that is, removing a wedge-shaped piece of bone to alter the biomechanical loading through a joint; this is useful in younger people
- partial or total arthroplasty, replacing bone ends with metal and plastic or silastic implants. This has been responsible for a dramatic improvement in the quality of life of many with OA.

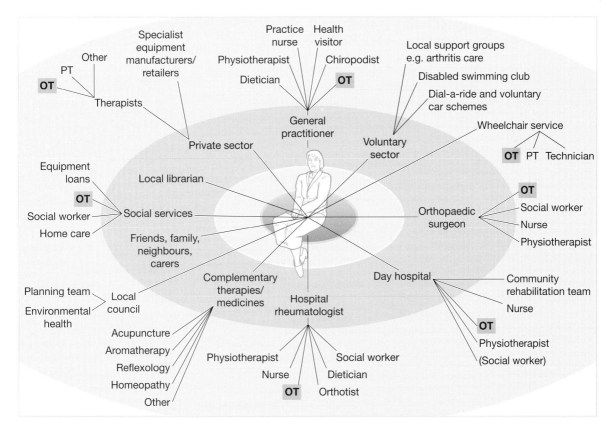

Fig. 27.4 The wider treatment team.

Community practice, hospital and clinic nurses help to monitor the health of an individual, provide information about OA and give advice concerning drug therapy, pain management and other treatments. As they come to know individuals and their families over a lengthening period of time, they are in a position to monitor the social and psychological wellbeing of a person and can refer them to other agencies as the need arises (Hill 1998).

The importance of exercise is well established and a systematic review of clinical trials has concluded exercise can improve pain and disability in OA in the hip and knee (van Baar et al 1999). The physiotherapist plays an important role in patient education, teaching correct exercise techniques to improve muscle strength and joint motion and developing individualised home exercise programmes. Hydrotherapy can be beneficial in the acute stages and is a good stepping stone to getting people involved in using their local swimming pool. Physiotherapy can relieve pain and stiffness through, for example, ice therapy, transcutaneous electrical nerve stimulation (TENS) and acupuncture, provision of walking aids, and support to improve joint stability, for example, patella taping or other forms of orthoses. Postural and gait re-education are important to assist in reducing abnormal loading on lower limb joints (Chadwick 1999).

Other team members play an important role. The orthotist may provide a variety of orthoses to support joints, reducing pain and joint stress and assisting function. Some people with cervical or spinal OA may be helped by a collar or corset.

Advice regarding footwear from podiatrists can be helpful, as are shoe insoles to alter the mechanical loading of damaged joints, support foot arches and take pressure off painful areas. Many people with OA of the spine, hips or knees find shock-absorbing insoles and good arch supports benefical in reducing activity-related pain (Dieppe 1995).

The dietician can provide benefical advice and support weight loss programmes if obesity is a primary cause of OA.

The social worker can provide help through:

- financial advice concerning benefits and grants

- information on how to access homecare or home meals provision
- coordination of community services to support a person when discharged from hospital
- liaison with employers
- provision of specialist counselling where appropriate.

Effective liaison is essential between the person with OA and the team members, and across different teams because comorbidity can mean that other specialists are involved.

People often seek help from complementary medicines such as acupuncture, aromatherapy, reflexology or from following special diets. Although evidence as to their efficacy remains scarce, many find them helpful in relieving symptoms.

The voluntary sector has a growing amount of support to offer. The Arthritis Research Campaign (ARC) and Arthritis Care publish information booklets about osteoarthritis, its management and practical self-help ideas. Arthritis Care runs a community-based educational, self-help programme called Challenging Arthritis, to inform and train people to manage their arthritis more effectively. Volunteers, with arthritis, are trained to deliver and facilitate the programme and it now runs throughout the United Kingdom. People with arthritis derive substantial and prolonged benefits in terms of perceived ability to manage arthritis, reduction in pain and improved psychological wellbeing from this programme (Barlow et al 1998).

THEORETICAL FOUNDATIONS FOR INTERVENTION

Dieppe (1994) describes three stages of prevention in the management of OA: primary, secondary and tertiary. Primary prevention seeks to reduce the risk factors that predispose a person to OA. Secondary prevention is the ability to detect OA early, monitor its progression easily and accurately, and have a targeted way of controlling the disease processes. Although primary and secondary prevention of OA are on the increase, most people have reached the tertiary stage, and have well-established OA with chronic pain and significant functional disability, before they are referred to a rheumatologist. It is at this stage that the occupational therapist usually becomes involved. The growth of primary care occupational therapy will increase GP access to occupational therapy services. Thus, in the future, occupational therapists are more likely to be involved at an earlier stage providing team care educating people to both self-manage OA and reduce predisposing risk factors. Mann et al (1999) identified that, with progressive age, elderly people with arthritis have an increasing need for assistive devices and home modifications but that few people had received such services from an occupational therapist.

The occupational therapist's main role at this tertiary stage is to work with the individual and others involved in their care to:

- regain function
- manage pain
- reduce stress to damaged joints
- develop positive coping strategies to enable the individual to live a more independent, fulfilling and pleasurable life.

In common with the treatment of other chronic disabling conditions, humanistic, person-centred models of practice guide therapists in their approach to people with OA (see Chapter 3). A holistic approach enables the therapist to gain an understanding of the psychological and social impact of the disease on an individual's life and she can use this knowledge with the individual to plan and prioritise appropriate treatment. To retain quality of life, the individual with widespread, severe OA must learn coping strategies to manage chronic pain and an unstoppable decline in physical health and function. The individual will be better able to do this with a belief that she or he can positively influence pain and impairment through active participation in treatment and maintenance of a healthy lifestyle. The occupational therapist can help facilitate this internal locus of control. The person-centred approach will ensure that treatment priorities are tailored

to meet those of the individual. For example, a person with spinal OA who is unable to dress himself may prefer to have help from his wife than struggle painfully with specialist dressing equipment and manage independently. Energy can then be used for more meaningful activities. Much of the discussion of the theoretical foundations for intervention in RA (Chapter 23) are relevant in OA.

OA affects the whole family and a social approach to the treatment of an individual involving the family, when appropriate, in education sessions and treatment decisions will help to strengthen and build the support network necessary for the individual to manage in the community. Although the importance of a holistic approach (Hagedorn 1997), seems clear for occupational therapists, it is becoming difficult to maintain in an increasingly reductionist work environment. Although occupational therapists have been treating people with OA for many years and are well-recognised members of the treatment team, there has been little evidence published to support what we do and there is an urgent need for evaluative research.

As people with OA are not usually referred for occupational therapy until they are experiencing significant functional difficulty, occupational therapists use a number of frames of reference to guide practice. Which predominates is often influenced by their work setting. For example, an occupational therapist working for a Social Services department often focuses on a compensatory/rehabilitative approach, while a therapist working on an orthopaedic ward with postsurgical patients may use a predominantly biomechanical approach. A therapist working in a day hospital, in primary care or another community rehabilitation setting may be engaged in a more health promotion role and use a primarily learning/cognitive approach. A variety of frames of reference can be used to help a person meet their individual needs and goals (Table 27.1).

Therapy is provided in a variety of settings and there is a trend towards community provision because of shorter hospital admissions. An interdisciplinary initiative to devolve hospital care to

Table 27.1 Frames of reference

	Frame of reference		
	Biomechanical	Compensatory	Learning
Approach	Biomechanical	Rehabilitative	Cognitive/behavioural
Techniques	Exercises and adapted activities to improve muscle strength and joint range of movement, transfer practice (toilet chair, bath, bed, car, etc.), orthoses	Person-centred programme, adapted tools and equipment, alternative techniques, environmental modifications, support from carers	Advice and education, developing coping strategies, problem solving, goal setting

the community, at the Fife Rheumatic Diseases Unit, found that 91% of patients surveyed preferred home-based treatment by therapists (Wilson & Cummings 1997). A research project into community occupational therapy rehabilitation provision in Kensington, Chelsea and Westminster found that the role of the occupational therapist within acute services is increasingly limited to that of discharge facilitation. The study recommended that most discharge facilitation, for example of people following joint replacements, could be undertaken by skilled technical, assistant and support staff, thus releasing qualified staff to undertake community rehabilitation (Hill et al 1998). Whatever the location, the essential components of therapy are similar.

ASSESSMENT

This will depend on the type and complexity of problems a person with OA is experiencing, and the presence of comorbidities. If, for example, they have difficulties getting in and out of the bath and up and down stairs because of OA in one knee, the assessment will be less complex than for a person with severe, generalised OA who has multiple problems managing at home. Assessment for the former may be a 'one-off', especially if they are expected to recover function with awaited surgery. The latter, however, will require ongoing assessment as their impairment progresses. For this latter group of people, the HAQ (Health Assessment Questionnaire; Kirwan & Reeback 1986) or the AIMS (Arthritis Impact Measurement Scale; Hill et al 1990) can be useful in identifying major problems and monitoring function over time.

Functional assessments

Generalised occupational therapy assessments such as the Canadian Occupational Performance Measure (COPM), the Functional Independence Measure (FIM) and the Occupational Performance History Interview (OPHI2) (see Chapter 6) are valuable, not only to identify need and prioritise treatment, but also as outcome measures. Some occupational therapists are required to use locally developed forms for data gathering and to record their assessments based on national guidelines, for example, in multidisciplinary collaborative care plans, care pathways or social services needs assessment. These should be done in conjunction with published, reliable and auditable assessments.

Home assessment

Stairs, bath, chair, toilet and bed transfers can be problematic when a person's lower limb joints or spine are affected. A home assessment enables the therapist to see what techniques, equipment and adaptations the individual currently uses at home and how problems are being managed. It may also provide the opportunity to discuss with family, friends and relatives the effects of these problems. This can help the therapist be more sensitive to the individual's culture, beliefs and wishes. The local environment and facilities can also be identified. As many people with OA are elderly and have comorbidities, the therapist must identify safety issues in the home, such as loose carpets or rugs (particularly near the top of stairs), steps and slippery or uneven floor surfaces in and around the house.

The assessment methods described in Chapter 23 can be used for upper limb, work, leisure and ADL assessment.

Work assessment

Hip, knee and CMC joint OA may be common reasons for work problems. The occupational therapy assessment will focus on how a person's disability impacts on:

- how the person gets to and from work
- what they are required to do
- the tools and equipment they have to do the job
- the work environment
- the person's motivation to perform the job
- the support they have from their employer, family or other carers
- the financial considerations that influence their decisions about work.

The Model of Human Occupation (MOHO) provides two assessment tools: the Worker Role Assessment and the Work Environment Assessment.

TREATMENT

As OA is chronic and degenerative in nature, an individual may return for treatment many times over the years. Each episode of care may focus on different aspects of their health and wellbeing. As with assessment, the amount and complexity of intervention will depend on how extensively OA has affected a person's lifestyle and whether there are comorbidities.

Psychosocial aspects

The individual may be experiencing a lot of pain, have a poor body image and been forced to give up many activities they found important or pleasurable. The therapist needs to show understanding and honesty and give information to help the person develop positive coping strategies. Gaining a good rapport and including family or other carers will help build long-term relationships. A comparative study of methods of teaching coping strategies to people with knee OA found that those attending education groups with their spouses showed greater improvement in psychological disability, pain behaviour, coping attempts, self-efficacy and marital adjustment than those attending without spouses (Keefe et al 1996). The therapist should avoid fostering dependency and encourage self-management. Attempts should be made to widen an individual's interests and social contact by working with them towards individually planned goals, for example, to participate in activities to help combat depression. Anxiety and depression have been shown to be powerful predictors of not maintaining important health behaviours, such as low impact exercise. Thus assessment of the person's mood and interventions to improve this may be important before providing other therapy interventions.

Education, self-management and facilitating self-efficacy

Understanding the cycle of negative attitudes, pain, passive coping methods, depression, reduced activity and physical deconditioning helps in motivating people to perceive and understand the importance of home-based self-management. Active self-management includes:

- low impact exercise (e.g. walking, swimming)
- range of motion exercises for specific joints
- applying heat or cold to painful joints
- relaxation
- joint protection
- massaging painful joints
- a balance of rest, exercise and meaningful activities compatible with level of disability
- the use of cognitive coping methods such as distraction, imagery and self-statements
- appropriate use of painkillers (Hampson et al 1993).

These methods are well described in Lorig and Fries (2000). The occupational therapist working collaboratively with the rheumatology team can do much to enable people to self-manage, through either individual or group education programmes. As in RA, using an educational, self-efficacy enhancing, behavioural instruction and goal-setting approach is more efficacious in enhancing adherence and reducing pain and disability than information provision alone. The degree of pain relief resulting from such an approach has been found to be 20–30% of that gained from NSAID treatment (Superio-Cabuslay et al 1996). This latter finding means that, longer term, NSAID use could be reduced through active self-management with subsequent benefits to the person in reduced side-effects and prescription costs, and benefits to the healthcare system in reduced drug costs, especially as OA is such a common condition. This is an underprovided area for people with OA.

Joint protection and energy conservation

The advice described in Chapter 23 is applicable for people with OA. If the person has localised OA, this advice will be tailored to the problems associated with the specific joint involved. See also Cordery and Rocchi (1998).

ADL training and assistive devices

Typical problems experienced by people with spinal or lower limb OA are walking, especially over rough ground, and transfers such as getting on and off chairs, toilet or bed, in and out of the bath, car and public transport, and up and down stairs and steps. Sitting, walking and standing to work can be very painful and maintaining one position for too long can cause stiffness. Bending to pick things up, or manage personal care and dressing is often difficult. OA in the neck or upper limb joints also causes problems with personal care, as well as with reaching and carrying. Hand involvement affects dexterity and grip, particularly if caused by painful CMC joints.

Ability, work tolerance and pain can be improved by the following:

- alternative techniques, such as altering the working position to use a better ergonomic posture and changing positions regularly
- joint protection advice, such as sitting to iron or weed the garden
- assistive devices, such as a walking stick, long-handled reacher or stairlift.

It is important to note that what helps one person might not help another and what works in a simulated situation in the occupational therapy department might not work in the person's own home.

George and Kerr (1988) found that in order for assistive devices to be most effective, the person should be properly assessed by an occupational therapist and given instructions on how to use the device. Gitlan and Levine (1992) emphasised the importance of home-based demonstrations by therapists. There is still relatively little scientific study of their prescription, provision and use (Rogers & Holm 1992). In a study of assistive devices used by elderly Americans, Mann et al (1995) found a high number and rate of use (about ten per person), an expressed need for additional devices and a high rate of satisfaction. There is increased use of assistive devices with age and most used are found effective (Sonn et al 1996). Hygiene (bath and toilet aids) and mobility devices are the most common. Their use can be an emotive issue, however, and the therapist should be sensitive to the wishes, beliefs and cultural background of the individual. A raised toilet seat may be a god-send to one person and unacceptable to another because it draws attention to their disability or because using it means 'giving in' to arthritis.

Having identified the source of the problem through activity analysis, methods or equipment that may offer a solution need to be tested and the following considered (Box 27.1).

Box 27.1 Considerations when prescribing equipment (Jefferson 1997)

- Does the identified equipment help to facilitate the task?
- Will it continue to do so in the person's home environment?
- Is the person able to operate the device independently or do they need help?
- Is the person able to install and/or use it safely? (the prescriber has responsibilities under the Consumer Protection Act 1987).
- Is the device available for the person to loan or will they have to buy it?

There are often long waiting times associated with the loan of social services equipment. An audit of waiting times for assistive devices (Wilson et al 1999) identified these were significantly reduced when small items were supplied by a hospital department.

There are many assistive devices designed to help people with arthritis (Fig. 27.5). Companies specialising in equipment produce catalogues and most occupational therapy service areas have a selection for demonstration and loan. The Disability Information Trust produces a series of

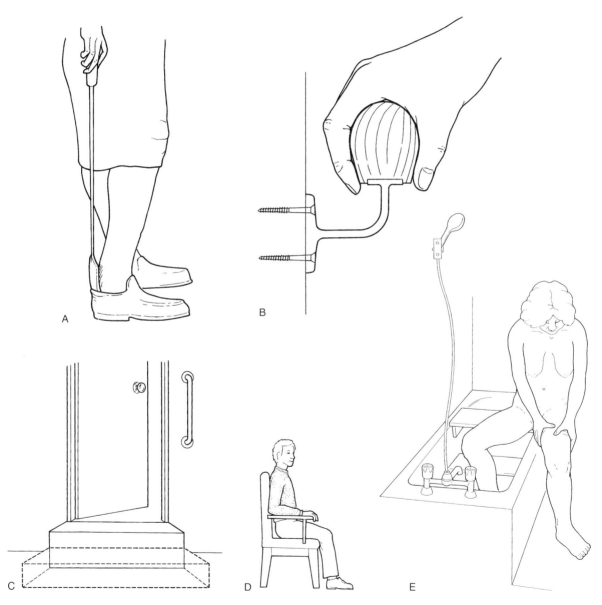

Fig. 27.5 (A) Long-handled shoe-horn to help avoid excess flexing of hip, (B) mop-stick rail, (C) half-step and grabrail at entrance, (D) chairs should be firm and high enough for easy rising, (E) typical use of bath board, (F) typical arrangement of bath equipment (cut-away bath panel for illustrative purposes only), (G) toilet with combined raise and frame, (H) use of perching stool for kitchen tasks, (I) trolley for carrying items.

Fig. 27.5 (F–I) *see overleaf*

F

G

H

I

Fig. 27.5 *continued*

books including 'Arthritis, an equipment guide' and the Disabled Living Foundation (DLF) Hamilton Index is a directory of product information on equipment for independent living.

The Medical Devices Agency at the Department of Health produces regular disability equipment assessment reports, which are widely distributed to Health and Social Services departments.

Mobility

Mobility can be greatly improved by a walking aid, supportive footwear or use of splints, for example, a knee brace. Assessment and provision of walking aids is usually carried out by the physiotherapist but in some areas the occupational therapist is also involved. The therapist should always reinforce instructions concerning safe use and maintenance of equipment. Care should be taken when walking outside on rough or slippery ground or on a slope. Ferrules on the bottom of sticks should be changed regularly and the brakes and tyre pressures on wheelchairs checked as a routine during treatment sessions.

Wheelchairs, if required, can be self- or attendant-propelled or powered. Scooters are useful if a person does not drive or wishes to shop independently. A person may be eligible for one of these from the wheelchair service or can purchase one from an independent company. Some wheelchair services operate voucher schemes that assist towards costs (See Chapter 7).

During a home visit, the therapist assesses the use of walking aids, wheelchairs, grab rails and the need for adaptations such as a half-step, rail or ramp to aid access into the house. When stair climbing is a problem, an alternative method of stepping may be suggested, for example, going sideways with two hands on the banister rail or fitting an extra rail. Installing a stairlift or through-floor lift can maintain a person's independent access to the first floor of their home. Kelsall (1996) found that stairlifts are usually preferred to moving to a bungalow. If it is not possible to install a lift, or if there are long delays in doing so and the bedroom and only toilet are upstairs, a commode downstairs can be used during the day, minimising painful stair climbing. If a person becomes unable to manage the stairs at all, the bed can be brought downstairs.

A trolley, as an indoor walking aid, has the additional advantage of enabling objects to be moved from room to room. A perching stool indoors or a 'shop-a-seat' walking aid outdoors enable activities to be carried out where standing tolerance is limited.

Many people with OA, especially of the spine, find driving difficult or painful. An automatic car with power steering may be all that is required to aid comfort and independence. Extra mirrors or a 'panoramic' mirror widen the field of vision and assist the driver with restricted mobility. Altering the position and angle of the seat can assist transfers. Supportive seat padding or a moulded seat shell aids comfort while sitting, especially on longer journeys.

Seating

Sitting to relax

OA of the spine and lower limb joints commonly causes discomfort while sitting and difficulty rising. A seating assessment is one of the most common referrals to a community occupational therapist. Factors influencing sitting comfort in an easy chair relate to: seat height, angle, construction and upholstery; the shape and tilt of the back rest; and the design of the armrests (Ellis 1988). Sweeney and Clark (1992) identified requirements depend on the disability. They recommended guidelines for selecting easy chairs for people with arthritis and low back pain. These include:

- careful measurement of a person to ensure correct seat height, depth, width and tilt
- the importance of a full-length back rest with adequately shaped padding to support the spine and head
- armrests should be at the correct height and partially padded for elbow comfort, with large rounded wooden handgrips to provide leverage for the person when rising from the chair.

Many people with difficulty rising from their existing armchair raise the seat by piling on cushions. This is not recommended because it reduces the length of the back rest and leaves the person with little arm support. Chair raisers should be fitted under the chair legs or castors to raise the seat height only.

Sitting to work

While comfort and ease in rising is important, the main consideration is positioning the person for the task. An adjustable-height perching stool may be ideal for kitchen, workshop or gardening tasks and there is a wide variety of adaptable office chairs available. People can try them out at specialist shops, disability equipment centres and some Occupational Therapy departments.

Portable seating

Specialist cushions, lumbar rolls and moulded seat inserts enable people to sit comfortably wherever they are.

Bathing

This can be a hazardous activity for those with poor mobility, reach or grip strength and getting into or out of the bath is a common site for falls. Ease and safety can be enhanced by correctly fitted bath aids such as a bath board and seat and a non-slip mat. There is a range of bath aids for a variety of bath types and the therapist should carefully assess their compatibility while considering the needs and wishes of the user. Powered bath seats will lower and raise a person into and out of the bath. Most have a back support for extra safety, although some people with good sitting balance prefer the backless variety, which allows them to recline in the bath. For someone with an over-bath shower, a slatted bath board can be used to sit upon as a safer alternative to standing. A grabrail by a bath or shower cubicle can assist transfers. For sitting whilst showering in a cubicle, a wall-mounted seat can be fitted or a free standing seat used, providing the shower base is strong enough. There is a wide range of level access showers on the market.

Personal care and domestic tasks

Common problems include:

- difficulty bending to wash, dress and pick things up
- difficulty reaching to dress, get things out of cupboards and operate environmental and electrical appliances
- reduced grip strength causing difficulties in brushing teeth, using toiletries, cutting food and carrying heavy objects in the hand.

After assessing the exact nature and cause of the problem and respecting the needs and wishes of the individual, the therapist will demonstrate alternative ways of carrying out the activity and select appropriate equipment for the person to try (see Chapter 7).

Home adaptations

The most common home adaptations among people with OA are:

- building a half step to reduce overall step height into the property
- building a ramp for wheelchair access into a property
- installing a shower
- installing a stairlift or through-floor lift
- raising or lowering work surfaces, for example, in the kitchen.

The assessment and application for home adaptations is almost always carried out by a social services occupational therapist, who will have expert knowledge about national legislation, local eligibility criteria and resources. Adaptations may be carried out via the Social Services department, the district council Housing department, the Environmental Health department or a combination of these. In many cases, the person will have to contribute towards the cost of the work to adapt their home. The social services occupational therapist will assist them in applying for a grant, such as the Disabled Facilities Grant or the Home Repair Assistance (leaflets available from the Department of the Environment) if they are eligible. The Home Repair Assistance is designed for small-scale works, such as a wheelchair ramp or grabrails; the Disabled Facilities Grant covers a range of work needed to help a disabled person live more independently in their home.

Work

Causal factors in OA are often linked to occupation and OA accounts for a high financial cost in terms of work hours lost. The therapist can offer similar treatment to that used with problems experienced in other activities in a person's life.

Advice includes modifying work activities to promote better:

- posture
- ergonomic function
- manual handling techniques.

Modifying work activities should also aim to reduce pain, fatigue and stress on affected joints. The therapist can give advice about the adaptation of existing equipment or the introduction of specialist equipment and can liaise with the Disability Employment Advisor (DEA) to assist the individual to gain financial assistance or training.

Leisure and hobbies

In a study of elderly persons with arthritis, Mann et al (1995) found the activity missed most was crafts. Yet these have been de-emphasised in occupational therapy education and clinical practice as the focus on ADL has increased. Using the same techniques as with other activities, the therapist should assist the individual to overcome barriers to leisure activities and crafts and to explore new interests. A knowledge of local leisure or sporting groups, clubs and voluntary driver schemes can be helpful in finding a way for someone with restricted mobility to regain access to society.

OA hands

The CMC joint is the most commonly involved and is most frequent in middle-aged women. Nagging pain during and after working with the affected hand occurs (Buurke et al 1999). The thumb is responsible for almost half of hand function and OA of the CMC significantly reduces grip strength and can also slow hand function and dexterity. Repetitive pinch, strong grip, twisting and applying force with the heel of the hand aggravate pain (Melvin 1989) and thus joint protection advice should focus on modifying these actions. Assistive devices such as jar openers, electric can openers and electric scissors all reduce the need for strong pinch and grip, as do enlarged and padded handles. Heat (e.g.

immersing in hot water or heat packs) can provide symptomatic relief.

Thumb CMC splints aim to immobilise or stabilise the CMC joint and so reduce or eliminate pain at the CMC during thumb loading activities but there is no scientific evidence available to demonstrate if this is true (Buurke et al 1999). A crossover trial of thumb CMC splints evaluated three commercial models: a thin, semirigid plastic thumbpost design; a firm, elastic thumbpost design incorporating a semirigid steel support on the dorsal side of the thumb; an elastic splint extending below the wrist, with a thumb support strap. All were similar in the degree of pinch strength reduction and pain relief obtained. The latter design was the most popular, being most comfortable, flexible and interfering least with palmar grip. Whilst less supportive, if such a splint is worn more often and provides a light pressure reminding the wearer to use their thumb more sparingly, it may be more effective long-term than a more rigid splint (Buurke et al 1999).

Rehabilitation for joint replacement surgery

Joint replacement surgery has made a huge impact on the lives of people with OA. Many joints are replaced routinely, most commonly the hip joint, with good long-term results in pain relief and improved function. It is the most common of the OA surgical procedures seen by the occupational therapist.

The aims of occupational therapy for people undergoing joint replacement surgery are to:

- promote a better understanding of the planned surgery, the expected benefits and postoperative precautions
- prepare for discharge in advance of surgery so that actual or potential problems can be identified and remedial action planned
- provide a link between hospital and home by liaising with carers and support services where this is indicated
- promote a return to function through a planned programme of simulated activities that reflect the person's lifestyle

- provide splints, if required, to support the surgery
- identify and provide equipment required to facilitate safe discharge and independence in ADL
- follow-up after discharge from the ward as required, for example, to exercise affected limb and to adjust splints
- monitor the functional effects of surgery.

Preoperative assessment and education

The effectiveness of presurgical education, training and counselling has been well reported. Butler et al (1996) identified that people who received a booklet from the hospital, explaining in advance the surgical procedure and postoperative rehabilitation programme, were less anxious on admission and discharge, had practised their exercises more frequently and required less occupational therapy than those who had not received the booklet.

As hospitals reduce pre- and postsurgical length of stay, there is less time available for patient education and rehabilitation. Beginning intervention before surgery (at the preoperative clinic visit as part of an interdisciplinary team programme) means the therapist can significantly increase time available to complete treatment. As well as preparing the person for surgery and discussing any worries they or their relatives may have, potential or actual problems can be identified, equipment needs assessed and community teams contacted. Those having lower limb joint surgery should be asked to measure their chair, toilet and bed heights at home so that the therapist can have this information when practising transfers with the person after surgery and ensure appropriate equipment is in place on discharge.

Preoperative functional assessment scores can be gathered to assist surgical and rehabilitation audit, for example, of mobility and ADL ability, grip strength, hand function and joint range of movement. Measurements can then be repeated at a given time postoperatively and results compared. If splints are required, their use and maintenance can be discussed, exercises practised and

questions the person may have about rehabilitation discussed.

Many hospitals have developed excellent interdisciplinary preoperative education programmes for people due to have joint replacement surgery. People are seen individually, with a relative or carer, and in groups. Teaching materials include booklets, slides and videos, which people can borrow. Most teams have devised their own in-house booklets (Box 27.2) and supplement these with published booklets, such as the patient information series published by the Arthritis Research Campaign (ARC) and Arthritis Care.

Postoperative rehabilitation

The rate at which rehabilitation proceeds will vary according to the individual and the therapist should be sensitive to their wishes, needs and abilities while encouraging effort and motivation to achieve maximum performance. It may be appropriate to involve a relative or carer from

---

Box 27.2 Suggested contents for patient booklets regarding joint replacement surgery

- Problems experienced by people for whom surgery is indicated.
- Benefits of surgery.
- Information about the new joint, including pictures. It may be useful to show how a joint is affected by OA.
- What to expect during hospital admission.
- Precautions following joint replacement.
- Pre- and postoperative exercise routines, including diagrams and an indication of the length of time rehabilitation can take.
- Activities of daily living, including diagrams of how to perform activities such as walking, stair climbing, transfers, meal preparation, childcare, personal care and sexual intercourse.
- Pictures of commonly used specialist equipment.
- Preparation needed for discharge with consideration of the home/work environment and any help needed.
- Follow-up appointment and home exercise programmes.
- When a person can expect to resume 'normal' activities.
- Common questions people ask and their answers.
- Sources of further information and help in the community.
- Invitation to the reader to send feedback to the hospital team on aspects of their care and suggestions for improvements.

the beginning of rehabilitation, especially if they will be required to carry out a task for the person, assist in transfers or help them with their home treatment programme.

Many hospitals have adopted an approach known as Care Pathways, an interdisciplinary programme with collaborative record keeping. A care pathway for a named surgery – total hip replacement, for example – specifies treatments that occur at given times, ensuring comprehensive, integrated and standardised quality rehabilitation. Variances in the pathway are recorded if an individual encounters difficulties.

In the initial postoperative session, the therapist discusses the surgery and may show the person an X-ray of their new joint to aid their understanding of the treatment rationale. The timetable of rehabilitation activities will be discussed, along with any concerns regarding their home circumstances. Instructions for the adoption of precautions will be reinforced by demonstrations and supervised practice of the desired behaviours with clear feedback to ensure correct techniques.

To reduce the risk of dislocation in the first 6 to 12 weeks after surgery, while the supporting ligaments and muscles recover, the hip should not be:

- flexed beyond 90° (avoid low seat heights and reaching for low objects)
- adducted (avoid crossing legs and use pillows between the legs when lying on one side and on the back)
- internally rotated (avoid twisting on one leg when standing). (Martin et al 1999)

With improved prosthetic design and surgical technique there is a growing debate among surgeons as to whether these precautions are still necessary. However, in the absence of robust research evidence to indicate a change in practice, the established precautions should still be taught.

For total shoulder replacement, for the first 4–6 weeks the individual should avoid:

- weight bearing through the operated arm
- resistive exercise
- extension and external rotation if subscapularis has been divided.

The arm is supported in a sling and not used for ADL in the first few days. Once range of movement and strengthening exercises are established, the arm can be used during light, bilateral tasks (Thornhill et al 1999).

For lower limb surgery, when the individual is able to start weight bearing the therapist should encourage correct gait and posture, in line with advice given by the physiotherapist. Advice about the safe use of walking aids during ADL, such as elbow crutches, sticks or walking frame, should be given and techniques practised. ADL training will include the adoption of precautionary behaviours during transfers, dressing, self care, kitchen and garden activities to avoid putting the new joint at risk. The therapist may discuss aspects of personal relationships, such as comfortable positions for sexual intercourse that will not affect the new joint.

Those who have had upper limb surgery may need a light-weight cup or long-handled cutlery. To extend their reach, a dish mop and a long narrow strip of towel with loop handles will help washing, while a dressing stick will assist in getting shirts on and off the shoulders. The operated arm should be dressed first and undressed last. A bottom-wiping gadget may be required if the unoperated arm is also severely affected by OA.

For lower limb surgery, the person should initially sit to wash and dress, put the operated limb in the garment first and pull up pants and trousers as far as possible before standing. Equipment to extend reach to aid dressing and washing include a long-handled sponge and toe wipe, long-handled shoe horn, helping hand, sock or tights aid. Bath or shower aids can be used to prevent excessive hip or knee flexion or straining a shoulder or elbow joint. An individual's bed, toilet and chair should be measured to ensure they can sit and rise without straining the new joint. Toilet raises come in various heights, with or without a frame. Chair- and bed-raiser units can usually be fitted to existing furniture. Equipment should be securely fitted and instructions given for safe use and maintenance.

All transfers and essential activities, using assistive equipment if required, should be assessed and practised under supervision to enable the individual to gain confidence and independence. In the kitchen, long-handled equipment can be used to reduce bending or stretching, a trolley can help in moving items around and a perching stool will ease standing to do tasks. In an audit of the provision and use of equipment following total hip replacement in Scotland, Davidson (1999) noted that most people found certain items, such as a raised toilet seat, long-handled shoe horn and helping hand, very useful in the first 6 to 12 weeks postsurgery. As this equipment in most cases is only required for short-term use, many hospitals hold a stock of equipment for loan.

With accurate knowledge of an individual's home situation and adequate simulated practice of essential ADL in hospital, a home visit should not be required for safe discharge home. However, if the therapist is not satisfied that the person will be able to cope safely, a home visit should be carried out and essential daily tasks practised there. It may be appropriate to arrange for carers or the community occupational therapist to be present if the person will require their services once they return home. Equipment can be fitted and positions for rails assessed if required. If the therapist is still not satisfied that the person will manage, an extended rehabilitation period or, following liaison with hospital and community teams, homecare services can be organised. Some people may need to be seen for follow-up treatment, for example, to strengthen muscles, improve range of movement or adjust splints.

CONCLUSION

Although OA is a chronic, degenerative condition that cannot, as yet, be cured, much can be done to reduce its destructive effects on a person's lifestyle. With the understanding of an individual's unique situation and an up-to-date knowledge of current practice and specialist equipment, the occupational therapist can help a person to develop coping strategies for pain relief and functional independence (Boxes 27.3 and 27.4).

The occupational therapist typically becomes involved in a person's care when he is already experiencing difficulties with ADL and intervention may sometimes be required for many years. As the causative factors become better understood, intervention may occur earlier, in the form of preventive health education and advice about suitable working positions and joint care. As hospital stays shorten, rehabilitation will become increasingly community based.

Box 27.3   Case study

Susan Campbell, a 30-year-old mother of a preschool child and secretary for a law firm, was referred from the rheumatology clinic with OA of both CMC joints. She complained of severe pain in the base of both thumbs and difficulties with both home and work tasks.

On examination, grip strength was reduced and a hand test showed slowed dexterity and all hand movements reduced by pain. Acute pain was reported on activity, with difficulty managing tasks requiring pinch, span or power grips, such as fastening clothes, opening jars, changing nappies, lifting heavy files at work and writing. Treatment aims were to reduce pain, improve function, improve understanding of the condition and facilitate altering behaviour to adopt joint protection methods for the CMC joints.

Ms Campbell was given information about the condition (verbal and written); trained in use of joint protection methods to reduce thumb stress; advised to pace work activities, to change hand activities regularly and take regular rests during word processing; recommended to purchase, following practice, appropriate kitchen gadgets (e.g. electric can opener); provided with equipment to enlarge grips and aid writing; taught a home exercise programme to maintain range of movement in the thumb CMCs and rest of the hand; and provided with bilateral thumbpost splints to reduce pain and provide support during function. At her 1-month review, Ms Campbell found the splints comfortable and providing pain relief and had increased her ability to perform ADL. Joint protection and energy conservation information was reinforced.

Box 27.4 Case study

Mr Owens, a sheep farmer who lives with his wife and son, was 67 when OA in both hips became severe, causing considerable pain and limiting mobility. His GP referred him to the orthopaedic surgeon and physiotherapist at the hospital for treatment and surgical assessment, and to the social services occupational therapist for a home assessment.

At the home visit, the primary problems identified were: rising from the sofa, bed, bath and toilet; difficulty with stairs, walking around the farm and prolonged standing; depressing the clutch to change gear when driving and getting in and out of his car. He had anxiety about declining function, continuing farming, financial responsibilities and reduced social activities. Treatment included: raising seating surfaces to aid transfers, provision of toilet and bath aids, provision of an extra stair rail, providing a perch stool for household activities and recommending a walking aid with integral seat support for use around the farm, providing advice about car adaptations and alternative models, joint protection and

energy conservation advice to reduce loading on the hips, recommending shock-absorbing insoles, reinforcing advice from the phsyiotherapist on exercise regimens and advising about appropriate benefits. The likely outcomes of hip replacement surgery were discussed with Mr Owens and his family to help relieve anxieties.

Later, when listed for hip replacements, the hospital occupational therapist met Mr Owens at the preoperative education programme, provided verbal and written information about surgery, postoperative rehabilitation and precautions and demonstrated and practised transfers, positioning and relevant ADL. Following his right total hip replacement, instruction on precautions was reinforced and transfers and relevant ADL were practised. Equipment for reach and to avoid bending was loaned.

A few months later Mr Owens had his left hip replaced. With pain eliminated and function restored, he was able to discard most of his equipment and resume many of his farming tasks.

REFERENCES

Barlow JH, Turner AP, Wright CC 1998 Long term outcomes of an arthritis self-management programme. British Journal of Rheumatology 37:1315–1319

Butler GS et al 1996 Pre-hospital education: effectiveness with total hip replacement surgery patients. Patient Education and Counselling 29:189–197

Buurke JH, Grady JH, de Vries J, Baten CTM 1999 Usability of thenar eminence orthoses: report of a comparative study. Clinical Rehabilitation 13:288–294

Chadwick A 1999 Osteoarthritis. In: David C, Lloyd J (eds) Rheumatological physiotherapy. Mosby, St Louis, MO, ch 9, pp 83–96

Chaisson C, McAlindon TE 1997 Osteoarthritis of the hand: clinical features and management. Journal of Musculoskeletal Management 14(5):66–68, 71–74, 77

Cordery J, Rocchi M 1998 Joint protection and fatigue management. In: Melvin J, Gall V (eds) Rheumatologic rehabilitation series. American Occupational Therapy Association, Bethesda, MD, vol 1: assessment and management, ch 12, pp 279–322

Creamer P, Hochberg MC 1997 Osteoarthritis. The Lancet 350(9076):503–508

Davidson T 1999 Total hip replacement: an audit of the provision and use of equipment. British Journal of Occupational Therapy 62(6):283–287

Dieppe PA 1994 Osteoarthritis. In: Klippel JH, Dieppe PA (eds) Rheumatology. Mosby, St Louis, MO, ch 7.1, pp 1–6

Dieppe P 1995 Therapeutics: towards effective therapy for OA. Primary, secondary and tertiary prevention. Rheumatology in Europe 24(3):118–120

Disability Information Trust 1997 Arthritis: an equipment guide, 2nd edn. Disability Information Trust, Oxford

Downe-Wamboldt B 1991 Coping and life satisfaction in elderly women with osteoarthritis. Journal of Advanced Nursing 16:1328–1335

Ellis M 1998 Choosing easy chairs for the disabled. British Medical Journal 296:701

Felson DT, Chaisson EE 1997 Understanding the relationship between body weight and osteoarthritis. Baillière's Clinical Rheumatology 11(4):671–681

Felson DT, Zhang Y 1998 An update on the epidemiology of knee and hip osteoarthritis with a view to prevention. Arthritis and Rheumatism 41(8):1343–1355

Felson DT, Zhang Y, Hannan MT et al 1997 Risk factors for incident radiographic OA in the elderly. Arthritis and Rheumatism 40(4):728–733

George J, Kerr AAJ 1988 Equipment for bathing. British Medical Journal (Clinical Research Addition) 296(6627):982–983

Gitlan LN, Levine RE 1992 Prescribing adaptive devices to the elderly: principles for treatment in the home. International Journal of Technology and Ageing 5(1):107–120

Hadler NM, Gillings DB, Levitin PM 1978 Hand structure and function in an industrial setting. Arthritis and Rheumatism 21(2):210–220

Hagedorn R 1997 Foundations for practice in occupational therapy, 2nd edn. Churchill Livingstone, Edinburgh

Hampson SE, Glasgow RE, Zeiss AM et al 1993 Self-management of ostearthritis. Arthritis Care and Research 6(1):17–22

Hampson SE, Glasgow RE, Zeiss AM 1996 Coping with osteoarthritis by older adults. Arthritis Care and Research 9(2):133–141

Hill J (ed) 1998 Rheumatology nursing. A creative approach. Churchill Livingstone, Edinburgh

Hill J, Bird HA, Lawton CA, Wright V 1990 The Arthritis Impact Measurement Scales: an anglicized version to assess the outcome of British patients with rheumatoid arthritis. British Journal of Rheumatology 29:193–196

Hill, Hauxwell, Furner 1998 The Victoria project. Community occupational therapy rehabilitation service. Research findings and recommendations. Riverside Community Health Care NHS Trust, Westminster, London

Hughes SL, Dunlop D 1995 The prevalence and impact of arthritis in older persons. Arthritis Care and Research 8(4):257–264

Jeffreson P 1997 Arthritis: using assistive devices to promote independence. British Journal of Therapy and Rehabilitation 4(1):528–534

Jensen MP, Turner JA, Romano JM 1991 Self-efficacy and outcome expectancies: relationship to chronic pain strategies and adjustment. Pain 44:263–269

Keefe FJ, Caldwell DS, Baucom D et al 1996 Spouse-assisted coping skills training in the management of osteoarthritic knee pain. Arthritis Care and Research 9(4):279–291

Kelsall A 1996 Stair lifts and through floor lifts. British Journal of Therapy and Rehabilitation 3:532–536

Kirwan JR, Reeback JS 1986 Stanford Health Assessment Questionnaire modified to assess disability in British patients with rheumatoid arthritis. British Journal of Rheumatology 25:206–209

Klippel JH, Dieppe PA (eds) 1997 Rheumatology, 2nd edn. Mosby, St Louis

Lorig K, Fries J 2000 The arthritis helpbook: a tested self-management programme for coping with arthritis, 5th edn. Perseus Books: Cambridge, MA

Mann W, Hurren D, Tomita M 1995 Assistive devices used by home based elderly with arthritis. American Journal of Occupational Therapy 49(8):810–820

Mann WC, Tomita M, Hurren D, Charvat B 1999 Changes in health, functional and psychosocial status and coping strategies of home-based older persons with arthritis over three years. Occupational Therapy Journal of Research 19(2):126–146

Martin SD, Zavadek K, Noaker J, Jacobs MA, Poss R 1999 Hip surgery and rehabilitation. In: Melvin J, Gall V (eds) Rheumatologic rehabilitation series. American Occupational Therapy Association, Bethesda, MD, vol 5: surgical rehabilitation, ch 5, pp 81–113

Melvin J 1989 Osteoarthritis. In: Rheumatic disease in the adult and child: occupational therapy and rehabilitation, 3rd edn. FA Davis, Philadelphia, PA

Rogers JC, Holm MB 1992 Assistive technology device use in patients with rheumatic disease: a literature review. American Journal of Occupational Therapy 46(2):120–127

Sonn U et al 1996 The use and effectiveness of assistive devices in an elderly urban population. Ageing, Clinical and Experimental Research 8(3):176–183

Superio-Cabuslay E, Ward MM, Lorig K 1996 Patient education interventions in osteoarthritis and rheumatoid arthritis: a meta-analytic comparison with non-steroidal antiinflammatory drug treatment. Arthritis Care and Research 9(4):292–301

Sweeney GM, Clark AK 1992 Easy chairs for people with arthritis and low back pain: results from an evaluation. British Journal of Occupational Therapy 55:69–72

Thornhill TS, Gall V, Vermette S, Griffin F 1999 Shoulder surgery and rehabilitation. Melvin J, Gall V (eds) Rheumatologic rehabilitation series. American Occupational Therapy Association, Bethesda, MD, vol 5: surgical rehabilitation, ch 3, pp 37–66

van Baar ME, Assenfeldt WJJ, Dekker J, Oostendoorp RA, Biljsma JW 1999 Effectiveness of exercise therapy in patients with osteoarthritis of the hip or knee. Arthritis and Rheumatism 42(7):1361–1369

Verbrugge LM, Lepkowski JM, Konkol LL 1991 Levels of disability among US adults with arthritis. Journal of Gerontology 46(2):S71–83

Wilson J, Cummings Y 1997 The Fife Rheumatic Diseases Unit – pioneering community rheumatology. Journal of the National Association of Rheumatology Occupational Therapy 11(1):16–17

Wilson J, McCracken E, Cummings Y 1999 Assistive devices: an audit of waiting times. British Journal of Occupational Therapy 62(6):269–271

Yelin E, Katz PP 1990 Transitions in health status among community dwelling elderly people with arthritis: a national, longitudinal study. Arthritis and Rheumatism 30(8):1205–1215

FURTHER READING

Banstead Mobility Centre 1998 Driving with arthritis. Banstead Mobility Centre, Carshalton, Surrey

Melvin J, Gall V 1998 Rheumatologic rehabilitation series. American Occupational Therapy Association, Bethesda, MD, vol 1: assessment and management

Melvin J, Gall V 1999 Rheumatologic rehabilitation series. American Occupational Therapy Association, Bethesda, MD, vol 5: surgical rehabilitation

Stein CM, Griffen MR, Brandt KD 1996 Osteoarthritis. In: Wegener ST, Belsa BL, Gall EP (eds) Clinical care of the rheumatic diseases. American College of Rheumatology, Atlanta, GA, ch 30

USEFUL CONTACTS

Arthritis Care
18 Stephenson Way, London NW1 2HD

Arthritis Research Campaign
Copeman House, St Mary's Gate, Chesterfield, Derbyshire S41 7TD

Banstead Mobility Centre
Damson Way, Fountain Drive, Carshalton, Surrey SM5 4NR

Disability Information Trust
Mary Marlborough Lodge, Nuffield Orthopaedic Centre, Oxford OX3 7LD

Glossary

Ability The measure of the level of competence with which a skill is performed.

Activity Being active in mind and/or body. Doing something, usually for a particular purpose.

Activity analysis Breaking down an activity into sequences of component tasks and identifying the skills required to perform these.

Adaptation The ability of an individual to adjust occupational performance in order to successfully master change.

Adaptive skills Those skills required, and acquired, to undertake adaptation.

Aim The direction of an action or actions.

Approach Ways and means of putting theory into practice.

Autonomy The ability to govern one's own actions.

Dysfunction Interruption in the ability to perform.

Frame of reference A system of theories serving to orientate or give particular meaning to a set of circumstances, which provides a coherent, conceptual basis for therapeutic intervention.

Function An action performed to fulfil an allocated task.

Goal The desired outcome or specific result.

Health A dynamic, functional state which enables the individual to undertake his normal occupational performance satisfactorily. 'The state of complete physical, mental and social wellbeing and not merely the absence of disease or infirmity.' (World Health Organization 1983)

Holism A perspective that considers all aspects of a person's circumstances simultaneously.

Models A simplified representation of the structure and content of a phenomenon or system that describes or explains the complex relationships between concepts within the system, and integrates elements of theory and practice.

Motivation An inner force that directs the will and causes the individual to act in a particular way.

Objective Definable actions undertaken to achieve a specific result.

Occupation That which defines and organises a sphere of action over a period of time and is perceived by the individual as part of his personal and social identity.

Occupational performance Actions executed, usually within patterns and habits, which form the normal and expected content of a person's existence and are aimed at meeting that individual's needs.

Occupational therapy The assessment and treatment of people using purposeful activity to prevent disability and develop independent function (Committee of Occupational Therapy for the European Communities 1990).

Occupational therapy process A series of ordered thoughts and actions undertaken in order to successfully complete occupational therapy intervention.

Philosophy Underlying beliefs and knowledge. The theory from which knowledge arises.

Potential One's innate aptitude, which is capable of development.

Process A sequence of actions ordered for a particular purpose to achieve a defined result.

Productivity The outcome of labour.

Reductionism A perspective that considers that the whole can be best understood by the study of individual parts.

Role The image and expectations a person holds about the positions he occupies in a variety of social contexts.

Skill A performance component that evolves with practice.

Task The constituent parts of an activity.

Wellbeing A sense of physical and mental comfort.

Work Any activity, physical or mental, undertaken to achieve a desired outcome.

Index